HIV/AIDS in the Post-HAART Era

MANIFESTATIONS, TREATMENT, AND EPIDEMIOLOGY

HIV/AIDS in the Post-HAART Era

MANIFESTATIONS, TREATMENT, AND EPIDEMIOLOGY

John C. Hall, MD
Department of Medical Dermatology
University of Missouri—Kansas City
Department of Dermatology, St. Luke's Hospital
Dermatology Staff, Kansas City Free Health Clinic
Kansas City, Missouri

Brian J. Hall, MD
Department of Pathology
University of Utah School of Medicine
Salt Lake City, Utah

Clay J. Cockerell, MD
Director, Division of Dermatopathology
University of Texas Southwestern Medical Center
Medical Director, Cockerell & Associates
Dermpath Diagnostics
Dermatopathology Laboratories
Dallas, Texas

2011
PEOPLE'S MEDICAL PUBLISHING HOUSE–USA
SHELTON, CONNECTICUT

People's Medical Publishing House-USA
2 Enterprise Drive, Suite 509
Shelton, CT 06484
Tel: 203-402-0646
Fax: 203-402-0854
E-mail: info@pmph-usa.com

PMPH-USA

11 12 13 14/PMPH/9 8 7 6 5 4 3 2 1

Printed in China by People's Medical Publishing House
Production/Book design: GYAT; Copy editor/indexer: Joanne M. Still; Staff Editor: Linda Mehta; Cover designer: Mary McKeon

Library of Congress Cataloging-in-Publication Data

HIV/AIDS in the post-HAART era : manifestations, treatment, and epidemiology / [edited by] John C. Hall, Brian J. Hall, Clay J. Cockerell.
  p. ; cm.
  ISBN-13: 978-1-60795-105-6 (alk. paper)
  ISBN-10: 1-60795-105-3 (alk. paper)
  1. AIDS (Disease) 2. HIV infections. I. Hall, John C., 1947– II. Hall, Brian J. (Brian John), 1981– III. Cockerell, Clay J.
  [DNLM: 1. Acquired Immunodeficiency Syndrome. 2. HIV Infections. WC 503]
  RA606.6H5834 2011
  616.97′92--dc22
                                        2011009217

Sales and Distribution

Canada
McGraw-Hill Ryerson Education
Customer Care
300 Water St
Whitby, Ontario L1N 9B6
Canada
Tel: 1-800-565-5758
Fax: 1-800-463-5885
www.mcgrawhill.ca

Foreign Rights
John Scott & Company
International Publisher's Agency
P.O. Box 878
Kimberton, PA 19442
USA
Tel: 610-827-1640
Fax: 610-827-1671

Japan
United Publishers Services Limited
1-32-5 Higashi-Shinagawa
Shinagawa-ku, Tokyo 140-0002
Japan
Tel: 03-5479-7251
Fax: 03-5479-7307
Email: kakimoto@ups.co.jp

United Kingdom, Europe, Middle East, Africa
McGraw Hill Education
Shoppenhangers Road
Maidenhead
Berkshire, SL6 2QL
England
Tel: 44-0-1628-502500
Fax: 44-0-1628-635895
www.mcgraw-hill.co.uk

Singapore, Thailand, Philippines, Indonesia, Vietnam, Pacific Rim, Korea
McGraw-Hill Education
60 Tuas Basin Link
Singapore 638775
Tel: 65-6863-1580
Fax: 65-6862-3354
www.mcgraw-hill.com.sg

Australia, New Zealand, Papua New Guinea, Fiji, Tonga, Solomon Islands, Cook Islands
Woodslane Pty Limited
Unit 7/5 Vuko Place
Warriewood NSW 2102
Australia
Tel: 61-2-9970-5111
Fax: 61-2-9970-5002
www.woodslane.com.au

Brazil
SuperPedido Tecmedd
Beatriz Alves, Foreign Trade Department
R. Sansao Alves dos Santos, 102 | 7th floor
Brooklin Novo
Sao Paolo 04571-090
Brazil
Tel: 55-16-3512-5539
www.superpedidotecmedd.com.br

India, Bangladesh, Pakistan, Sri Lanka, Malaysia
CBS Publishers
4819/X1 Prahlad Street 24
Ansari Road, Darya Ganj,
  New Delhi-110002
India
Tel: 91-11-23266861/67
Fax: 91-11-23266818
Email: cbspubs@vsnl.com

People's Republic of China
People's Medical Publishing House
International Trade Department
No. 19, Pan Jia Yuan Nan Li
Chaoyang District
Beijing 100021
P.R. China
Tel: 8610-67653342
Fax: 8610-67691034
www.pmph.com/en/

CONTENTS

CONTRIBUTORS*

Quarraisha Abdool Karim, MS, PhD [5]
Centre for the AIDS Programme of Research in
    South Africa
University of KwaZulu-Natal
Durban, South Africa
and Department of Epidemiology
Mailman School of Public Health
Columbia University, New York

Philip Alcabes, PhD [43]
Professor, School of Public Health
Hunter College
New York, New York

Andrew F. Angelino, MD [16]
Associate Professor of Psychiatry and Behavioral
    Sciences
Johns Hopkins University School of Medicine
Baltimore, Maryland

S. Anuradha, MD [21]
Professor of Medicine
Department of Medicine
Maulana Azad Medical College
Lok Nayak Hospital
New Delhi, India

Kamyar Arasteh, PhD [32]
Beth Israel Medical Center
New York, New York 10038

Share DeCoix Bane, PhD, MSW [31]
State Gerontologist
Missouri State Agricultural Extension Service
University of Missouri-Kansas City
Kansas City, Missouri

Giuseppe Barbaro, MD [11]
Cardiology Unit
Department of Medical Pathophysiology
University "La Sapienza"
Rome, Italy

Pablo Barreiro, MD, PhD [9]
Infectious Diseases Department
Hospital Carlos III
Madrid, Spain

José A. Bauermeister, MPH, PhD [29]
Assistant Professor, Department of Health Behavior
    and Health Education
The University of Michigan School of Public Health
Ann Arbor, Michigan

Ronald Bayer, PhD [1]
Professor, Center for the History and Ethics of
    Public Health
Department of Sociomedical Sciences
Columbia University Mailman School of
    Public Health
New York, New York

Preena Bhalla, MD [21]
Director Professor & Head
Department of Microbiology
Maulana Azad Medical College and
    Lok Nayak Hospital
New Delhi, India

Jyotirmay Biswas, MD [14]
Director and Head
Department of Uveitis and Ocular Pathology
Medical and Vision Research Foundations
Sankara Nethralaya
Chennai, India

Ruth M. Bland, MD [25]
Division of Developmental Medicine
University of Glasgow
United Kingdom
and Africa Centre for Health and Population Studies
University of KwaZulu-Natal
Somkhele,South Africa

Mark Bower, PhD, FRCP, FRCPath[24]
Consultant Medical Oncologist
Chelsea & Westminster Hospital
London, United Kingdom

Erin Boyce, MSW [31]
Research Assistant
School of Social Work
University of Denver
Denver, Colorado

Ivo Brito [3]
Sociologist
Chief of Prevention
Brazilian National AIDS Program,
    Ministry of Health
Brazilia, Brazil

Darigg C. Brown, PhD, MPH [28]
ORISE HIV Prevention in Communities of Color
    Post-Doctoral Research Fellow
Prevention Research Branch
Division of HIV/AIDS Prevention
National Center for HIV/AIDS, Viral Hepatitis, STD
    and TB Prevention
Centers for Disease Control and Prevention
Atlanta, Georgia

Pedro Cahn, MD, PhD [38], [42]
Chief, Division of Infectious Diseases
Hospital Juan A. Fernández
Buenos Aires, Argentina
and President, Fundación Huesped, Buenos Aires
Professor on Infectious Diseases, Buenos Aires
    University Medical School *and*
Past-President, International AIDS Society
Buenos Aires, Argentina

Pedro Chequer, MD, MPH [3]
UNAIDS Country Coordinator
Brazilia, Brazil

Contributors are listed in bold alphabetcally by last name. Bold bracketed numbers represent a contributor's chapter and the editors are distinguished by [Editor].

Lisa A. Clough, MD [4]
Assistant Professor of Medicine
Division of Infectious Diseases
University of Kansas Medical Center
Kansas City, Kansas

Clay J. Cockerell, MD [Editor], [8]
Professor, Department of Dermatopathology
University of Texas Southwestern Medical Center
and Medical Director, Cockerell & Associates
Dermpath Diagnostics
Dermatopathology Laboratory
Dallas, Texas

Debananda Das, PhD [40]
Staff Scientist, Experimental Retrovirology Section
HIV and AIDS Malignancy Branch
National Cancer Institute
Bethesda, Maryland

Jack A. DeHovitz, MD, MPH [36]
Professor, Department of Medicine
SUNY Downstate Medical Center
Brooklyn, New York

Don C. Des Jarlais, PhD [32]
Director of Research
Beth Israel Medical Center
New York, New York

Agatha N. Eke, PhD [28]
Behavioral Scientist, Prevention Research Branch
Division of HIV/AIDS Prevention
National Center for HIV/AIDS, Viral Hepatitis, STD
    and TB Prevention
Centers for Disease Control and Prevention
Atlanta, Georgia

Jean-Louis Excler, MD [37]
International AIDS Vaccine Initiative New York
New York, New York

Jason Faulhaber, MD [20]
Clinical Instructor, Department of Medicine
Harvard Medical School
Fenway Community Health
Boston, Massachusetts

Charles Feldman, MD, PhD [17]
Division of Pulmonology
Department of Internal Medicine
Charlotte Maxeke Johannesburg Academic Hospital
    and Faculty of Health Sciences
University of the Witwatersrand
Johannesburg, South Africa

Robert C. Gallo, MD [2]
Co-Director, Division of Basic Science and Vaccine
    Research
Director, Institute of Human Virology
Professor of Microbiology and Immunology
Professor of Medicine, School of Medicine
University of Maryland School of Medicine
Baltimore, Maryland

Massimo Ghidinelli, MD [37]
Regional Advisor, HIV/AIDS and STI
Department of Combatting Communicable Diseases
World Health Organization
Regional Office for the Western Pacific
Manila, The Philippines

Brian J. Hall, MD [Editor]
Department of Pathology
University of Utah School of Medicine
Salt Lake City, Utah

John C. Hall, MD [Editor]
Department of Medical Dermatology
University of Missouri—Kansas City
Department of Dermatology, St. Luke's Hospital
Dermatology Staff, Kansas City Free Health Clinic
Kansas City, Missouri

Jeffrey H. Herbst, PhD [29]
Lead Behavioral Scientist
Prevention Research Branch, Division of HIV/AIDS
    Prevention
National Center for HIV/AIDS, Viral Hepatitis, STD
    and TB Prevention
Centers for Disease Control and Prevention
Atlanta, Georgia

Darrel Higa, PhD, MSW [30]
ORISE Postdoctoral Fellow
Division of HIV/AIDS Prevention
Centers for Disease Control and Prevention
Atlanta, Georgia

Mark Hull, MD [12]
Division of HIV/AIDS
Department of Medicine
St. Paul's Hospital Providence Health Care and
    University of British Columbia

Rachel Jewkes, MBBS, MSc, MFPHM, MD [33]
Professor
Director, Gender & Health Research Unit
Medical Research Council
Pretoria, South Africa

Lars O. Kallings, MD PhD [39]
Professor Emeritus of Clinical Microbiology
Swedish Institute for Infectious Disease Control
Stockholm, Sweden
Former Special Envoy of the UN Secretary General
    for HIV/AIDS in Eastern Europe and Central Asia

Andrew Kambugu, MB, ChB, MMed [35]
Department of Medicine and Infectious Diseases
    Institute
School of Medicine, College of Health Sciences
Makerere University
Kampala, Uganda

Elly Katabira, FRCP(UK) [35]
Department of Medicine and Infectious Diseases
    Institute
School of Medicine, College of Health Sciences
Makerere Medical School
Kampala, Uganda

Ravinder Kaur, MD [21]
Professor, Department of Microbiology
Maulana Azad Medical College and
    Lok Nayak Hospital
New Delhi, India

Ayesha B. M. Kharsany, MSc, PhD [5]
Centre for the AIDS Programme of Research in
    South Africa
University of KwaZulu-Natal
Durban, South Africa

Donald Philip Kotler, MD [15]
Division of Gastroenterology & Liver Diseases
Professor, Department of Medicine
St. Luke's–Roosevelt Hospital Center
Columbia University College of Physicians and
    Surgeons
New York, New York

Pablo Labarga, MD, PhD [9]
Infectious Diseases Department
Hospital Carlos III
Madrid, Spain

Joep M. A. Lange, MD, PhD [35]
Department of Global Health
Academic Medical Center
University of Amsterdam
Amsterdam Institute for Global Health and
    Development
The Netherlands

Dmitry Lioznov, MD, PhD [36]
Chair, Department of Infectious Diseases and
    Epidemiology
Pavlov State Medical University
St. Petersburg, Russia

Ying-Ru Lo, MD [37]
Coordinator Prevention in the Health Sector
Department of HIV/AIDS
World Health Organization
Geneva, Switzerland

Eve Lofthus, BS [27]
Department of Oral Biology
School of Dentistry
University of Missouri-Kansas City
Kansas City, Missouri

Mona R. Loutfy, MD, FRCPC, MPH [26]
Division of Infectious Diseases
Department of Medicine
University of Toronto
Toronto, Ontario, Canada
and Department of Medicine
Women's College Hospital
Toronto, Ontario, Canada

Carole P. McArthur, MD, PhD [22], [27]
Professor, Department of Oral Biology
University of Missouri-School of Dentistry
and Department of Pathology
Truman Medical Center
University of Missouri-School of Medicine
Kansas City, Missouri

Donna Hubbard McCree, PhD, MPH, RPh [28]
Associate Director for Health Equity
Division of HIV/AIDS Prevention
National Center for HIV/AIDS, Viral Hepatitis, STD
    and TB Prevention,
Centers for Disease Control and Prevention
Atlanta, Georgia

Kenji Maeda, MD, PhD [40]
Research Fellow, Experimental Retrovirology
    Section, HIV and AIDS Malignancy Branch
National Cancer Institute
Bethesda, Maryland

Paul Man [12]
Division of Respiratory Medicine
Department of Medicine
St. Paul's Hospital Providence Health Care and
    University of British Columbia

Gordon Mansergh, PhD, MA, MEd [30]
Senior Behavioral Scientist
Division of HIV/AIDS Prevention
Centers for Disease Control and Prevention
Atlanta, Georgia

Luz Martin-Carbonero, MD, PhD [9]
Infectious Diseases Department
Hospital Carlos III
Madrid, Spain

Jose Medrano, MD [9]
Infectious Diseases Department
Hospital Carlos III
Madrid, Spain

Roberto Mejia, DDS, PhD [29]
Public Health Analyst and Contractor for
Prevention Research Branch, Division of HIV/AIDS
    Prevention
National Center for HIV/AIDS, Viral Hepatitis, STD
    and TB Prevention
Centers for Disease Control and Prevention
Atlanta, Georgia

Natalia Mendoza, MD [19]
Clinical Research Associate
Center for Clinical Studies
Houston, Texas

Fernando L. Merino, MD [4]
Assistant Professor of Medicine
Division of Infectious Diseases
University of Kansas Medical Center
Kansas City, Kansas

Hiroaki Mitsuya, MD, PhD [40]
Chief and Principal Investigator
Experimental Retrovirology Section
HIV and AIDS Malignancy Branch
National Cancer Institute
Bethesda, Maryland
and Professor and Chairman, Department of
    Hematology and Infectious Diseases
Kumamoto University School of Medicine
Japan

Julio S. G. Montaner, MD [12]
Division of HIV/AIDS
Department of Medicine, St Paul's Hospital
  Providence Health Care and
  University of British Columbia

L. Katie Morrison, MD [19]
Clinical Research Fellow
Center for Clinical Studies
Houston, Texas

David M. Murdoch, MD, MPH [17]
Assistant Professor of Medicine
Division of Pulmonary, Allergy &
  Critical Care Medicine
Duke University Medical Center
Durham, North Carolina

Jai P. Narain, MD, MPH [37]
Director, Department of Communicable Diseases
World Health Organization
Regional Office for South-East Asia
New Delhi, India

Mark Nelson, MD [18]
Department of GU/HIV Medicine
Chelsea and Westminster Hospital
London, United Kingdom

Marie-Louise Newell, MB, MSc, PhD [25]
Professor of Health and Population Studies
Africa Centre for Health and Population Studies
University of KwaZulu-Natal
Somkhele,South Africa
and MRC Centre of Epidemiology for Child Health
UCL Institute of Child Health
London, United Kingdom

Thi Thanh Thuy Nguyen, MD, MSc [37]
Medical Officer HIV/AIDS and STI
Department of Combatting Communicable Diseases
World Health Organization
Regional Office for the Western Pacific
Manila, The Philippines

Jürgen Noeske, PhD, MD[22]
German International Cooperation (GIZ)
Yaounde, Cameroon

Gerald M. Oppenheimer, PhD, MPH [1]
Broeklundian Professor of Public Health
Department of Health & Nutrition Sciences and
  Department of History
Brooklyn College and the Graduate Center
City University of New York
Brooklyn, New York
and Center for the History and Ethics of Public
  Health
Department of Sociomedical Sciences
Columbia University Mailman School of Public
  Health
New York, New York

Nicole Parrish, PhD [22]
Johns Hopkins University
Baltimore, Maryland

Peter Phillips, MD [12]
Division of Infectious Diseases
Department of Medicine
St Paul's Hospital Providence Health Care and
  University of British Columbia

Cristina Pimenta, PhD [3]
Executive Director, Brazilian Interdisciplinary AIDS
  Association
Professor, Department of Nursing
University Veiga de Almeida
Rio de Janeiro, Brazil

Walkyria Pereira Pinto, PhD [23]
Professor, Infectious Diseases Division
São Paulo University School of Medicine
São Paulo, Brazil

Richard W. Price, MD [13]
Professor Neurology, UCSF
Director, SFGH/UCSF HIV Neurology Research
  Program
Neurology Service
San Francisco General Hospital (SFGH)
San Francisco, California

John B. Pryor, PhD [34]
Distinguished Professor
Department of Psychology
Illinois State University
Normal, Illinois

Eloise Rathbone-McCuan, PhD [27], [31]
Professor, School of Social Work
University of Missouri-Kansas City
Kansas City, Missouri

Glenn D. Reeder, PhD [34]
Distinguished Professor (Emeritus)
Department of Psychology
Illinois State University
Normal, Illinois

Marvin Reitz, PhD [6]
Professor
Basic Science Division and Vaccine Research
Institute of Human Virology
University of Maryland School of Medicine
Baltimore, Maryland 21201

Pablo Rivas, MD [9]
Infectious Diseases Department
Hospital Carlos III
Madrid, Spain

Kristi Ruutel, MD, PhD [36]
Department of Infectious Diseases and
  Drug Abuse Prevention
National Institute for Health Development
Tallinn, Estonia

Andrew Scourfield, MD, MBBS [18]
Department of GU/HIV Medicine
Chelsea & Westminster Hospital
London, United Kingdom

Salaam Semaan, MPH, DrPH [32]
Deputy Associate Director for Science
Centers for Disease Control and Prevention
National Center for HIV/AIDS, Viral Hepatitis,
    STD, and TB Prevention
Atlanta, Georgia

Don Sin, MD [12]
Division of Respiratory Medicine
Department of Medicine
St Paul's Hospital Providence Health Care and
    University of British Columbia

Rohit Singhania, MBBS, SM [15]
Fellow
Division of Gastroenterology & Liver Disease
Department of Medicine
St. Luke's–Roosevelt Hospital Center
Columbia University College of
    Physicians and Surgeons
New York, New York

Vincent Soriano, MD, PhD [9]
Assistant Professor
University Complutense and Chief
Infectious Diseases
Hospital Carlos III
Madrid, Spain

Padmini Srikantiah, MD, MPH [37]
Assistant Professor, HIV/AIDS Division
San Francisco General Hospital
University of California
San Francisco, California

JoAna M. Stallworth, PhD, MPH [29]
Behavioral Scientist
Capacity Building Branch, Division of HIV/AIDS
    Prevention
National Center for HIV/AIDS, Viral Hepatitis, STD
    and TB Prevention
Centers for Disease Control and Prevention
Atlanta, Georgia

Carol W. Stanford, MD, FACP [41]
Associate Professor of Medicine
Department of Medicine
Division of Internal Medicine, Geriatrics, and
    Hospital Medicine
Truman Medical Center—Hospital Hill
University of Missouri-Kansas City School of
    Medicine
Kansas City, Missouri

James F. Stanford, MD, FACP [41]
Associate Professor of Medicine
Co-Director, HIV Research and Education
Department of Medicine, Division of Infectious
    Diseases
Director, Infection Prevention and Hospital
    Epidemiology
University of Missouri-Kansas City School of
    Medicine
Truman Medical Center—Hospital Hill
Kansas City, Missouri

**Justin Stebbing, MA, FRCP, FRCPath,
    PhD [24]**
Professor of Cancer Medicine and Medical
    Oncology
Imperial College Healthcare NHS Trust
Charing Cross Hospital
London, United Kingdom

S. Sudharshan, MD [14]
Consultant, Department of Uveitis
Medical and Vision Research Foundations
Sankara Nethralaya
Chennai, India

Omar Sued, MD, PhD [38]
Pan-American Health Organization
Buenos Aires, Argentina

Joseph S. Susa, DO [8]
Clinical Assistant Professor
Department of Dermatology
University of Texas Southwestern Medical Center
Dallas, Texas

Yi-Wei Tang, MD, PhD [7]
Professor of Pathology and Medicine
Director, Molecular Infectious Diseases Laboratory
Vanderbilt University Medical Center
Nashville, Tennessee

Claire Thorne, PhD [25]
MRC Centre of Epidemiology for Child Health
Institute of Child Health
University College London
London, United Kingdom

Glenn Treisman, MD, PhD [16]
Professor of Psychiatry and Behavioral Sciences and
    Internal Medicine
Director, AIDS Psychiatry Service
Co-Director, Pain Treatment Program
John Hopkins University School of Medicine
Baltimore, Maryland

Stephen K. Tyring, MD, PhD, MBA [19]
Director, Center for Clinical Studies
Department of Dermatology
University of Texas Health Science Center at
    Houston
Houston, Texas

Anneli Uuskula, MD, MSc, PhD [36]
Head, Department of Public Health
University of Tartu
Tartu, Estonia

Willem Daniel Francois Venter, MD [17]
Reproductive Health & HIV Research Unit,
    University of the Witwatersrand
Johannesburg, South Africa

Antonia M. Villarruel, PhD, FAAN [29]
Associate Dean for Research and Global Affairs
Professor & Nola J. Pender Collegiate Chair
University of Michigan School of Nursing
Ann Arbor, Michigan

Eugenia Vispo, MD [9]
Infectious Diseases Department
Hospital Carlos III
Madrid, Spain

Marco Antonio de Ávila Vitória, MD [23]
Department of HIV/AIDS
World Health Organization
Geneva, Switzerland

Sharon L. Walmsley, MD, FRCPC, MSc [26]
Division of Infectious Diseases
Department of Medicine
University of Toronto
Toronto, Ontario, Canada
and Division of Infectious Diseases
Department of Medicine
University Health Network
Toronto, Ontario, Canada

Laura Waters, MRCP [18]
Locum Consultant GU/HIV Medicine
Brighton and Sussex University Hospitals NHS Trust
Brighton, United Kingdom

C. Mel Wilcox, MD, MSPH [10]
Center for AIDS Research
University of Alabama at Birmingham
Division of Gastroenterology & Hepatology
Birmingham, Alabama

C. Beau Willison, MD [19]
Clinical Research Fellow
Center for Clinical Studies
Webster, Texas

FOREWORD

In the last few years we have gained confidence that
as individuals and all together we are not condemned passively
to allow the disease AIDS or the fears and forces which it can unleash
to dominate us. Against AIDS we will prevail together,
for we will refuse to be split, or to cast into the shadows
those persons, groups and nations that are affected.

—DR. JONATHAN MANN, 1989

For many of us, the HIV epidemic defines our lives in medicine. In 1981 when my UCLA colleagues and I reported five cases of *Pneumocystis pneumonia*, by no stretch of the imagination could anyone have foreseen the scope and impact of this event. We were unknowingly on the cusp of a scourge that over 30 years would claim 30 million lives and leave another 33 million infected, one that would profoundly affect the future of a continent and command the attention of world leaders.

In 2011 many of the events that happened over three decades feel as though they happened yesterday. I remember those first patients reported in *MMWR* in stark detail, more vividly than patients I saw just yesterday. I remember their faces, their life stories, the worry on the faces of their partners and parents, and their courage and forbearance as it dawned on them that we had no idea what their illness was or how to treat it. A highlights reel of significant events in the history of HIV/AIDS would take volumes, but from the clinical perspective the following loom large: the identification of the CD-4 deficiency, the discovery of HIV-1, the HIV-1 antibody test, AZT as a proof of principle that treatment was within the realm of possibility, viral load suppression as a benchmark for staging and treatment efficacy, and of course the advent of protease inhibitor-based HAART at the pivotal 1996 Vancouver International AIDS Conference.

Thirty years into HIV/AIDS, the progress in understanding the pathophysiology of a newly identified virus, and in treating an infection whose main target is the immune system itself has exceeded expectations. This progress was the result of firm resolve on the part of many as well as a measure of good luck. The gains we have seen in a comparatively short time stemmed from an urgent international research effort in the public sector and in industry, an effort that was fortunate in having access to concurrently emerging technologies in molecular biology and drug development. With control of viral replication now routinely achievable, the thrust of treatment research remarkably is now directed toward eradicating HIV from those already infected. These gains represent the life's work of clinicians and scientists in numerous disciplines, many of who authored chapters in this volume.

In 2011 the diagnosis of HIV is no longer regarded as a death sentence in the developed countries while in the developing world lack of access to life-prolonging HIV antivirals and to even the most basic health care remains not only tragic, but a moral eyesore. Decades from now the HIV epidemic may be looked back on as a tipping point in the West's awareness of the degree of poverty and preventable illness that is now the norm in sub-Saharan Africa and other regions. While necessary, widespread access to HIV treatment is not enough. HIV/AIDS necessitates an exceptional response at the highest levels, a response that includes debt cancellation, economic development, education, fair trade policies, and control of malaria and TB. Thirty years after the first reports, HIV in 2011 has unfortunately become endemic. A vaccine has been elusive, treatments are imperfect, and even after three decades intense social stigma and lack of basic human rights continue to hinder progress in prevention.

Many of us look back on our involvement in the HIV epidemic as the touchstone of our careers in medicine. While we have indeed come a long way in a brief time, HIV will unfortunately be even more prevalent in 2031 at the fiftieth anniversary of the epidemic. Looking ahead, barring unforeseen breakthroughs, the conquest of this latest plague of humanity will occupy the careers of generations of future physicians and researchers. The hopes of many millions for lives free from HIV depend on them.

—MICHAEL GOTTLIEB, MD
Los Angeles, California

PREFACE

Reading *"And the Band Played On"* defined for me what happened thirty years ago. Reading it a second time in preparing this book, much of the book remains pertinent today. More than a disease, AIDS focused the end of one century and the beginning of another through a lens of human endeavor in science and social change. It was remarkable in its consuming discussion of who we are in the world.

No single institution or scientist can hope to grasp the full scope of the plague upon us, so this book will use the world's experts in its attempt to unravel the mystery presented to us by AIDS. We seek not only definition, but also humankind's response to AIDS.

This humble tome reaches first into the history of the pandemic and then to a comprehensive discussion of the science, which are two inseparable topics. Transmission is broached early to emphasize its importance, its close association with historical fact, and its central role in the ultimate defeat of the virus.

The disease chapters incorporate the virology, laboratory diagnosis, the special role of Kaposi's sarcoma, and then a detailed analysis of how the various body systems are affected. The devastating consequences of the disease in the developing world are followed by malignancies in HIV and the too often ignored mental health consequences of the disease. The more recent discoveries of the metabolic consequences of the disease and the inflammatory reconstitution immune syndrome are next. This section concludes with the horrific medical and social science effects on the world's newly orphaned children.

The treatment section depicts attempts at controlling the virus itself and the opportunistic infections that the virus allows to run rampant in the immune system left, at times, hopelessly vulnerable.

The final division of the book is about the future directions in dealing with AIDS. It reviews the current state of prognosis, research, and where we currently stand and where we might be headed in our ongoing struggle with the HIV virus.

This book is a scientific treatise and social history of, arguably, the most significant event of the last thirty years. Not infrequently, it is hypothesized that what happens to our lives comes from forces beyond our control and our comprehension. This book defies this notion, as do all scientific ventures. It says that we can play a role in bettering the lives of others and ourselves through discovery and action. Let no future generation say we ever gave up, that we ever forgot those who succumbed or those who still suffer. May the next three decades bring us to the salvations of cure and prevention. Let us take the science we have gained and the social justice we have found and lift them up as monuments for our heroes. Here is a treatise that declares the human condition as one of science, struggle, perseverance, and hope.

—JOHN C. HALL, MD

INTRODUCTION

JOHN C. HALL AND BRIAN J. HALL

Each time history repeats itself, the price goes up.

—AUTHOR UNKNOWN

Tonight at a meeting of physicians from around the world, I mentioned to the doctor sitting next to me my enthusiasm over the completion of this book. His comment was that it's an old story, and why should a book be written about the acquired immunodeficiency syndrome (AIDS). He supplied the reason this book has been assembled with his question.

This is not the time in history to pretend AIDS has vanished. It's not an old story now, and it never will be old.

According to UNAIDS in a report dated December 2009, the total number of people infected with AIDS in Eastern Europe was 1.5 million, up 66% from 2001.[1] Even more disturbing is the fact that HIV infections in American youth is on the rise especially in minority youth.[2] In England and Wales, the prevalence of HIV infections in 15- to 44-year-olds has increased from 32,400 in 2001 to 54,500 in 2008,[3] equivalent to a rise in infection rate from 1.5 to 2.4 per 1,000 persons. In the Yunnan Province of China, HIV prevalence rates among injecting drug users (IDUs) has surpassed 40%.[4] Also, HIV prevalence rates among patients older than 50 is on the rise in the U.S., the United Kingdom, and around the world. The 50 and older age group now has a higher prevalence than the 15- to 24-year-old age group in South Africa. It is estimated that in the next 5–7 years, over 50% of the HIV-positive patients will be in the 50+ age group; and the number of new diagnoses in patients 50 and older in the United Kingdom rose from 299 in 2000 to 719 in 2007.[5] In another study involving 34 states in the U.S., the estimated number of new diagnoses of HIV increased 15% from 2004 to 2007.[6] Another recent report indicated that at least 3% of residents living in Washington, DC have HIV or AIDS, and almost 1 in 10 residents in the DC area aged 40–49 are infected with the virus.[7]

These are sobering statistics. To state that HIV/AIDS is an old story is false, and to pretend that the epidemic is going away would be an unwise assumption. The HIV/AIDS epidemic is still alive and is continuing to evolve. To take a stance of complacency and treat the epidemic as an "old story" at this point in time would be an international tragedy. Now is the time to re-educate clinicians, researchers, and patients to the trends, manifestations, and treatments of this disease. We hope to have accomplished this feat with the help of all of our colleagues and co-authors in the pages that follow.

Doctors Oppenheimer and Bayer are two of the true chronicle writers of the AIDS epidemic. They have authored an entire book on the subject, *AIDS Doctors: Voices from the Epidemic: An Oral History*, which is highly recommended to anyone interested in reading more about the history of HIV/AIDS. Their wordsmithing is unparalleled; they tell us the history and the history tells why this is the time to stay the course.

Doctor Robert Gallo is one of the greatest scientists of the last century, and his incredible research and perseverance has saved countless lives. He and Luc Montagnier were both credited with discovering the HIV virus and his legacy in the world of virology may never be matched. Dr. Gallo is credited with pioneering studies that led to the discovery of the first human RNA ret rovirus, human T-cell leukemia virus (HTLV-1), and its association with leukemia and lymphoma. The virus was originally isolated in his lab. Dr. Gallo is also the only recipient of two Lasker awards, which is one of the most respected science prizes in the world.

Doctors Pimenta, Brito, and Chequer enlighten the world on prevention. Dr. Chequer was co-Founder and Director of Brazil's National AIDS Programme and was one of the principal architects of Brazil's model response to HIV.

Doctors Clough and Merino discuss in detail the transmission of AIDS. Their expert discussion gives us a realistic look on how to break the disease's apparently inexorable spread throughout the world's population. Dr. Clough and Merino are both infectious disease experts with a clinical focus on HIV/AIDS from the University of Kansas.

Doctors Karim and Kharsany tell us information only found through the careful study of epidemiology. The constantly changing shifts in the epidemic from continents and countries tell us much about the disease. Dr. Karim has over two decades of HIV prevention research experience, and she has served as the first National Director of the South African National HIV/AIDS and STD Program. She and her husband recently completed a two and a half year research study showing that a new vaginal gel microbicide containing tenofovir was up to 54% effective in preventing HIV over a one-year period.[8]

Doctor Marvin Reitz shows his expertise as a premier virologist by providing invaluable information on the most adaptable organism to ever cause human disease. He also is studying how expression of chemokine genes is regulated to help understand how host defenses can deal with HIV-1 more effectively.

Doctor Tang takes on an almost impossible task of testing for a virus that defies testing. The ever-moving viral target has made the laboratory of the virus become a science of its own. His contribution, giving us the details of this topic, is encyclopedic and remarkable. Dr. Tang serves as Director of the Molecular and Infectious Disease Laboratory at Vanderbilt University and is an expert in 16S rRNA gene sequencing and PCR-based amplification techniques.

Doctor Cockerell has long led the dermatology community during the AIDS epidemic. Dr. Cockerell, along with Dr. Friedman-Kien, co-authored the *Color Atlas of AIDS*, and Dr. Cockerell also recently published another book, *Cutaneous Manifestations of HIV Disease*. He and Dr. Susa have done a great job covering the medical specialty that has long been a harbinger of the disease.

The AIDS virus has made some strange bedfellows among other infectious diseases. Hepatitis C is one of these diseases. Dr. Soriano et al. have brought to light how important this association is and why it cannot be ignored. Dr. Soriano is an infectious disease expert and hepatologist at Hospital Carlos III in Madrid, Spain and has been a lead author on guidelines for treatment of HCV/HIV co-infection.

Doctor Wilcox is an eminent clinician of gastrointestinal diseases and AIDS. He has authored over 200 peer-reviewed publications and book chapters and has authored his own book, *Atlas of Clinical Gastrointestinal Endoscopy.* He continues his extensive publication collection on this critical organ system in AIDS.

Cardiovascular disease has become more important as parts of the AIDS population have become victims of chronic, incurable illness. Dr. Barbaro puts this relatively new part of the epidemic in the forefront. He also has edited an entire book on the subject, *Cardiovascular Disease in AIDS.*

Doctor Julio Montaner is the current president of the International AIDS Society and has published extensively with regard to respiratory complications of AIDS and antiretroviral therapy for HIV infection. He also pioneered the use of adjunctive corticosteroids for AIDS-related *Pneumocystis carinii* pneumonia. The chapter on pulmonary diseases written in collaboration with colleagues helps make this project worthwhile.

Doctor Richard Price has authored numerous articles on the AIDS/dementia complex and HIV-1 CNS infections and injury. We are honored to have him as an author in this book, and he does a brilliant job of describing how HIV affects the nervous system.

Often overlooked in HIV disease but extraordinarily important early in the epidemic (and even more so now) is eye disease. No one could bring us more up to date on this topic than Drs. Sudharshan and Biswas have done. Dr. Biswas has published 240 articles in peer-reviewed journals and 34 chapters in books. He was one of the first to describe ocular lesions in AIDS patients in India.

AIDS and nutrition is very timely as survival has increased the importance of good nutrition. We are indebted to Drs. Kotler and Singhania for discussing nutrition and AIDS. Dr. Kotler is Vice President of the AIDS Community Research Initiative of America (ACRIA) and a well-respected world expert on metabolic complications of HIV/AIDS.

The psychiatric care of these patients is expertly discussed by Drs. Treisman and Angelino. Dr. Treisman has published numerous articles and authored a book on the subject, *The Psychiatry of AIDS: A Guide to Diagnosis and Treatment.* The stigma from society, the stamina needed for medicines and procedures, and the overall burden of disease cannot be ignored if we truly attempt to make AIDS patients whole.

The immune reconstitution inflammatory syndrome (IRIS) has become a disease within a disease. Drs. Murdock, Venter, and Feldman put their stamp on this book by expertly discussing a syndrome that we must constantly be watching for in order to care properly for our patients. Dr. Feldman is from the University of the Witwatersrand in Johannesburg South Africa, is an eminent pulmonologist, and has edited his own book, *Tropical and Parasitic Infections in the Intensive Care Unit.* Both he and Dr. Murdoch have previously collaborated on research into the role of IRIS in pulmonary tuberculosis.

Doctors Waters, Scourfield, and Nelson discuss what most likely is the most complex infection ever discovered. No organism has shown such adaptability to therapy. This chapter has taken a herculean task and brought in to the most complete resolution possible. Dr. Nelson is Service Director for the HIV Directorate, as well as Deputy Director of Research at Chelsea and Westminister Hospital in London, which is the largest HIV-treatment center in northern Europe

Doctor Tyring is the true giant of viral illnesses. He, along with his colleagues, have given us a true vision of the best viral facilitator in history, which is the HIV virus. In addition to his over 600 published articles, Dr. Tyring has written seven books of his own, including *Mucocutaneous Manifestations of Viral Diseases* and *Sexually Transmitted Infections and Sexually Transmitted Diseases.*

Doctor Faulhaber delineates in detail that the AIDS virus may be the best bacterial infection facilitator in medical history. Dr. Faulhaber is a clinical instructor at Harvard Medical School and an expert infectious disease clinician with a special interest in HIV treatment and resistance.

Fungal infections also have a friend in the HIV virus and have been with us since the AIDS epidemic began. No one could do a better job of this than Drs. Bhalla and Kaur. Dr. Bhalla has published innumerable articles on opportunistic infections and HIV.

Tuberculosis and AIDS have become the great synergistic twins, especially on the African subcontinent. Two chapters are devoted to what may be the most important development in the AIDS epidemic in this century. Dr. McArthur et al. and Pinto and Vitória speak from experience as well as from the scientific literature. Dr. McArthur is a PhD immunologist who has established an AIDS outpost in Cameroon, Africa, where 14 years of testing for TB drugs has been carried out. She is a tenured professor at the University of Missouri, Kansas City and Truman Medical Center. Dr. Pinto is an infectious disease specialist who has published widely on AIDS and infectious diseases and is largely responsible for making the STD/AIDS Reference and Training Center in Sao Paulo a great AIDS resource for all of South America. Dr. Vitória is a Medical Officer in the Department of HIV/AIDS at the WHO in Geneva and has done extensive work and research in HIV/AIDS.

The AIDS virus can not only coax other infections to appear, but also malignancies. As the epidemic deepens and the life expectancy of infected persons increases, this will only continue to grow in importance. Drs. Bower and Stebbing expose the malignancy and AIDS virus relationship with great expertise. Justin Stebbing is a Consultant Medical Oncologist and Professor of Cancer and Oncology at the Imperial College Healthcare NHS Trust. He has published over 300 peer-reviewed papers, and also chairs the World Vaccine Congress. Both Dr. Bower and Stebbing have published extensively on AIDS-related cancers.

Doctor Bland et al. will not let us forget why we fight AIDS. We fight for the young. Ruth Bland is a senior research fellow in the Division of Developmental Medicine at the University of Glascow. She is the Clinical Research Lead of the Wellcome Trust-funded Africa Centre for Health and Population Studies, University of KwaZulu-Natal, South Africa. Marie-Louise Newell has been Medical Coordinator for the European Collaborator Study on HIV infection in pregnant women and their children and the European Pediatric Hepatitis C Virus Network. She currently leads the Africa Centre for Health and Population Studies and is widely published on issues facing children and women.

Women are most apt to suffer from sexual contact, yet in many countries they get the least help to stem the suffering. Drs. Walmsley and Loutfy will not let us forget the loneliest victims of the most unforgiving infection. Sharon Walmsley is Assistant Director, Immuodeficiency Clinic Toronto Hospital and a member of the Steering Committee and co-chairman of the clinical development core of the Canadian HIV Trials Network, as well as a member of the scientific review committee of the Canadian Association for HIV Research. She is also on the governing council of the International AIDS Society. Mona Loutfy heads the women and HIV research program and Women's College Research Institute at Women's College Hospital in Toronto. She studies and has published on AIDS treatment in women and HIV post-exposure prophylaxis among other HIV topics.

Sex workers are an integral piece in the puzzle of AIDS transmission and Drs. Eloise Rathbone-McCuan, Lofthus, and McArthur explain what can be and has been done about it.

"African Americans and HIV" is a chapter worthy of a separate work on its own. Dr. Brown et al. elucidate an often forgotten subplot of AIDS in the United States. Darigg Brown is in the Prevention Research Branch of the Centers for the Disease Control in Atlanta and works on

AIDS transmission in African Americans. Agatha Eke is a behavioral scientist at the Centers for Disease Control and Prevention in the Division of HIV/AIDS Prevention. Dr. McCree is an expert on HIV in African Americans. Her work at the CDC has focused on testing strategies for African American women and behavioral interventions for heterosexually active African American men. She also co-edited an entire book entitled: *African Americans and HIV/AIDS: Understanding and Addressing the Epidemic.*

Hispanic/Latin communities are not left out of the AIDS epidemic and have their own story to tell. Dr. Herbst et al. tell us about this part of the epidemic. Roberto Mejia is head of the Division of HIV/AIDS Prevention at the Centers for Disease Control and Prevention. Dr. Jeffrey Herbst is also a part of the Division of HIV/AIDS Prevention of the CDC and recently completed a systematic review of HIV behavioral interventions targeting sexual risk reduction among Hispanics in the United States.

Lesbian, Gay, Bisexual, and Transgender communities have born the brunt of the epidemic, not only in numbers but also in experiencing social injustices. Drs. Mansergh and Higa tell the heartbreaking story. Darrel Higa is at the Center for Disease Control and Prevention currently working in the Prevention Research Branch and focusing on men who have sex with men. Dr. Mansergh is a behavioral scientist at the CDC and is also part of the Division of HIV/AIDS Prevention. He has published extensively on HIV infection and MSM.

AIDS and aging must now be faced by all who are affected by the epidemic. We must become more aware of this ever-enlarging group of victims. Dr. Rathbone-McCuan et al. tell us what challenges are occurring in this newest epidemiologic group. Dr. Rathbone-McCuan has published multiple articles and books on the elderly and aging, including *North American Elders: United States and Canadian Perspectives (Contributions to the Study of Aging)* and *Self-Neglecting Elders: A Clinical Dilemma.*

From the beginning of the AIDS epidemic, intravenous drug abuse has been a major route of transmission. Dr. Des Jarlais et al. detail the continuing association between abuse of drugs and abuse by the virus. Don Des Jarlais is Director of Research with the Baron Edmond de Rothschild Chemical Dependency Institute at Beth Israel Medical Center in Boston and is a world leader and expert in research on the epidemiology of HIV transmission among injection drug users. He has also recently been appointed to the Scientific Advisory Board for The U.S. President's Emergency Plan for AIDS Relief (PEPFAR).

The rights of women have been linked to the AIDS epidemic from the beginning, and violence has been an unfortunate result of many attempts to maintain those rights. Dr. Rachel Jewkes has published over 150 articles on gender-based health and violence. She is Director of the Gender and Health Research Council of South Africa.

Prejudice against any minority seems universal. In AIDS it is immeasurably cruel and remarkably incomprehensible since we are all potential victims. Professors Glenn Reeder and John Pryor help us understand HIV-related stigmas. They have both published extensively on prejudice and stereotyping as well as HIV-related stigma. Both are also professors of psychology at Illinois State University.

Africa has become the epic battleground for the AIDS epidemic, and Dr. Lange and his colleagues add this essential piece to the book. Andrew Kambugu directs an HIV training program for physicians in Sub-Saharan Africa. Joep Lange is Senior Scientific Advisor to the International Antiviral Therapy Evaluation Centre. He is former president of the International AIDS Society and also the founding editor of the journal *Antiviral Therapy.* Among many other AIDS-related organizations, he is a founding member of the PharmAccess Foundation, which aims to improve access to AIDS therapy. Elly Katabira has been President of the International AIDS

Society Governing Council. He has been a World AIDS Foundation International Scholar and has worked extensively in the care and support for people living with AIDS

Doctor Lioznov gives a fresh look at a unique part of the AIDS epidemic. Eastern Europe and Central Asia have their own story to tell about AIDS, which encompasses different forms of the virus, disease manifestations, and social milieu wherever it strikes. Anneli Uuskula is the recipient of grants from the National Institutes of Health to study AIDS prevention and is widely published on AIDS. Dr. Jack A. DeHovitz has published articles on AIDS and is Director of The HIV Center for Women and Children, SUNY Downstate Medical Center. He is principal investigator for numerous AIDS-centered research projects. Dr. Ruutel is from Estonia and is the coordinator of the National HIV/AIDS Prevention Strategy, is a member of the National HIV/AIDS Commission, and was Estonia's representative to the Northern Dimension Partnership Group on HIV/AIDS. Dr. Lioznov has published extensively on various aspects of the AIDS epidemic and is a collaborator in PANCEA, an NIH-funded research project designed to provide information to help increase the efficiency of HIV prevention programs.

Asia and the Pacific have produced their own experts on the AIDS epidemic. Dr. Lo et al. are among those experts and contribute greatly to the text. Dr. Narin is Director of Communicable Diseases for the World Health Organization and is the author of *AIDS in Asia, The Challenge Ahead*. He has published extensively. Dr. Lo is coordinator of the Health Sector Unit of WHO's HIV/AIDS Department. She has published numerous publications and book chapters. Dr. Ghidinelli is WHO Regional Advisor in HIV/AIDS and Sexually Transmitted Infections for the Western Division. He is an advocate for condom use and his work on AIDS is widely respected internationally. Dr. Srikantia served in the Epidemic Intelligence Service for the CDC and is a fellow in infectious diseases at the University of California, San Francisco. Dr. Exceler is Medical Director of the International AIDS Vaccine Initiative.

Latin America and the Caribbean are at the crossroads of many cultures, and Drs. Cahn and Sued reveal how the AIDS epidemic has affected this part of the world. Dr. Cahn is a past President of the International AIDS Society, has published over 80 AIDS-related articles, and has worked tirelessly in missions around the world for AIDS organizations.

As with all parts of life, the future belongs to the young. Dr. Kallings allows us a glimpse into where this demographic group stands in the AIDS epidemic. Lars Kallings has served as the United Nations Secretary General's Special Envoy on HIV/AIDS in Eastern Europe and was Founding President of the International AIDS Society. He has served as Chairman of the Global Commission on AIDS, advisor to WHO, and Senior Advisor to the Global Programme on AIDS on Scientific and Policy Affairs.

New AIDS treatments bring us to the frontiers of modern genetics, immunology, and virology. Drs. Maeda, Das, and Mitsuya bring us to the leading edge of AIDS science. Dr. Mitsuya is chief of the Experimental Virology Section of the National Cancer Institute. He has done epochal studies on AIDS drug discovery, implementation, and resistance, which have benefitted all who seek to purge the virus from mankind. Dr. Mitsuya's research in 1985 led to the discovery of the anti-HIV drugs azidothymidine (AZT), dideoxyinosine (ddI), and dideoxycytidine (ddC). He was awarded the first NIH World AIDS Day Award for his work in developing drugs for AIDS. Dr. Maeda is a Research Fellow at the Center for Cancer Research and the National Cancer Institute and has published extensively on AIDS medications.

The holy grail of AIDS prevention is a vaccine. Drs. James and Carol Stanford tell where we have been and where we are going in this venture to save countless lives. Dr. James Stanford is Co-Director of the University of Missouri—Kansas City Center for AIDS Research and Education and has participated in AIDS vaccine research. Carol Stanford is Advisor to the

American Medical Women's Association and directs the Dermatology Clinic at Truman Medical Center.

Doctor Cahn tells us what the future may and may not hold. This chapter was written in the hope that the road ahead will be a bright one.

Doctor Alcabes tells what this epidemic of epic proportions can or cannot teach us about the next potential infectious disease calamity. Philip Alcabes is an infectious disease epidemiologist who has extensively written about AIDS epidemiology and has consulted on AIDS prevention projects in Latin America, Eastern Europe, and the Soviet Union.

The incredible ensemble of chapters produced by our internationally renowned, expert authors will never be repeated. That is part of the joy of bringing together researchers, epidemiologists, and clinicians of this caliber to create a book such as this. We owe so much to all of our authors and co-authors who have helped make this book what it is. To all of them we will be forever thankful.

A final word in this introduction is to thank one of the most important names in discovering and describing the epidemic. Doctor Michael Gottlieb honors us all with his foreword to the book. He co-authored the first report on the AIDS epidemic in 1981 and is a Trustee of the Global AIDS Interfaith Alliance, which performs AIDS relief in Africa. He still practices full time as an AIDS-treating physician in Los Angeles, California.

References

1. Cohen J. Late for the epidemic: HIV/AIDS in Eastern Europe. Science. 2010 Jul 9;329(5988):160, 162–164.

2. Lehmann C, D'Angelo LJ. Human immunodeficiency virus infection in adolescents. Adolesc Med State Art Rev. 2010 Aug;21(2):364–387, xi. Review.

3. Presanis AM, Gill ON, Chadborn TR, Hill C, Hope V, Logan L, Rice BD, Delpech VC, Ades AE, De Angelis D. Insights into the rise in HIV infections, 2001 to 2008: a Bayesian synthesis of prevalence evidence. AIDS. 2010 Nov 27;24(18):2849–2858.

4. Jia M, Luo H, Ma Y, Wang N, Smith K, Mei J, Lu R, Lu J, Fu L, Zhang Q, Wu Z, Lu L. The HIV epidemic in Yunnan Province, China, 1989–2007. J Acquir Immune Defic Syndr. 2010 Feb;53 Suppl 1:S34–40.

5. Arie S. HIV infection is rising among over 50s across the world, figures show. BMJ. 2010 Jul 27;341:c4064. doi: 10.1136/bmj.c4064.

6. Centers for Disease Control and Prevention (2009), HIV/AIDS Surveillance Report 2007, (Vol. 19).

7. Vargas JA, Fears D. "At Least 3 Percent of D.C. Residents Have HIV or AIDS, City Study Finds; Rate Up 22% From 2006." Washington Post 15 March 2009: A01. Print.

8. Abdool Karim Q, Abdool Karim SS, Frohlich JA, Grobler AC, Baxter C, Mansoor LE, Kharsany AB, Sibeko S, Mlisana KP, Omar Z, Gengiah TN, Maarschalk S, Arulappan N, Mlotshwa M, Morris L, Taylor D; CAPRISA 004 Trial Group. Effectiveness and safety of tenofovir gel, an antiretroviral microbicide, for the prevention of HIV infection in women. Science 2010 Sep 3,329(3996):1168–1174. Epub 2010 Jul 19.

ABBREVIATIONS AND ACRONYMS

In the vast body of literature pertaining to HIV/AIDS, a profusion of acronyms and abbreviations are commonly used. The following list is provided as a quick reference. Abbreviations for anti-HIV drugs are in bold.

AARP—American Association of Retired Persons
ABC—abacavir
ABV—doxorubicin, bleomycin, and vincristine (chemotherapy regimen)
ACRIA—AIDS Community Research Initiative of America
ACT-UP—AIDS Coalition to Unleash Power
Ad5—adenovirus type 5
ADA—Americans With Disabilities Act
ADC—AIDS dementia complex
ADCC—antibody-dependent cellular cytotoxicity
ADLs—activities of daily living
ADV—adefovir
AFASS—acceptable, feasible, affordable, sustainable, and safe (breastfeeding alternatives)
AGEP—acute generalized eruptive pustulosis
AIDS—acquired immunodeficiency syndrome
AIM—acute infectious mononucleosis
AIN—anal intraepithelial neoplasia
ALCL—anaplastic large cell lymphoma
ALT—alanine aminotransferase
ALVAC—canarypoxvirus
ANI—asymptomatic neurocognitive impairment
APP—amyloid precursor protein
APV—amprenavir
AR—actinic reticuloid
ARDS—adult respiratory distress syndrome
ARN—acute retinal necrosis
ARR—acquired rifampin resistance
ARRM—AIDS risk reduction model
ARS—acute retroviral syndrome
ART—antiretroviral therapy
ARV—antiretroviral (drug/medication)
ATL—adult T cell leukemia/lymphoma
ATLL—adult T cell leukemia/lymphoma
ATT—anti-tuberculous therapy
AUC—area under the curve
AZT—zidovudine (originally, azidothymidine)
AZT-MP—zidovudine monophosphate
AZT-TP—zidovudine triphosphate
AZV—atazanavir

BA—bacillary angiomatosis
BAL—bronchoalveolar lavage
BCA—bichloroacetic acid
BCC—basal cell carcinoma

BCG—Bacille Calmette-Guérin
BHITS—Breastfeeding and HIV International Transmission Study Group
BHIVA—British HIV Association
BLV—bovine leukemia virus
BMD—bone mineral density
BNAb—broadly neutralizing antibody
BSL—biosafety level

CAD—chronic actinic dermatitis
CA-MRSA—community-acquired methicillin-resistant *Staphylococcus aureus*
CARE Act—Ryan White Comprehensive AIDS Resource Emergency Act of 1990
CAREC—Caribbean Epidemiological Center
cART—combination antiretroviral therapy
CD4BS—CD4+ cell binding site
CDD—catalytic core domain
CDC—U.S. Centers for Disease Control and Prevention
CDC/CAR—U.S. Centers for Disease Control and Prevention Central Asia Region
CDE—cyclophosphamide, doxorubicin, etoposide (chemotherapy regimen)
CHOP—cyclophosphamide, hydroxydaunorubicin (doxorubicin), Oncovin (vincristine), and prednisone/prednisolone chemotherapy regimen
CIE—counter immunoelectrophoresis
CIN—cervical intraepithelial neoplasia
CLI—community-level intervention
CM—cryptococcal meningitis
C_{max}—maximum concentration
CM-IRIS—cryptococcal meningitis IRIS
CMV—cytomegalovirus
CNS—central nervous system
CONASIDA—National AIDS Commission
COPD—chronic obstructive pulmonary disease
CPE—cerebrospinal fluid penetration efficacy
CPT—cotrimaoxazole preventive therapy
CRABP-1—cytoplasmic retinoic-acid binding protein-1
CRFs—circulating recombinant forms
CRP—C-reactive protein
CS—cesarean section
CSF—cerebrospinal fluid
CSW—commercial sex worker

CT—computed tomography
CTD—carboxy-terminal domain
CTL—cytotoxic T lymphocyte
CVD—cardiovascular disease

DAIDS—Division of Acquired Immunodeficiency Syndrome (of the U.S. National Institutes of Health, National Institute of Allergy and Infectious Diseases)
DAPY—diarylpyrimidine
DATA—diaryltriazine
DBS—dried blood spots
DEBI—diffusion of effective behavioral interventions
ddC—zalcitabine
ddI—didanosine
DFA—direct fluorescent antibody
d4T—stavudine
DHHS—U.S. Department of Health and Human Services
DIH—drug-induced hepatitis
DLBCL—diffuse large B cell lymphoma
DLBL—diffuse large B cell lymphoma
DLV—delavirdine
DMPA—depot medroxyprogesterone acetate
DNA—deoxyribonucleic acid
dNMP—deoxyribonucleoside monophosphate
dNTP—deoxyribonucleoside triphosphate
DOT—directly observed treatment
DOTS—directly observed treatment, short course
DRESS—drug rash with eosinophilia and systemic symptoms
DRTB—drug-resistant tuberculosis
DRV—darunavir
DSM—*Diagnostic and Statistical Manual of Mental Disorders*
DSPN—HIV-related distal sensory polyneuropathy
DST—drug susceptibility testing
DTH—delayed-type hypersensitivity
dTTP—deoxythymidine triphosphate

EACS—European AIDS Clinical Society
EBV—Epstein-Bar virus
ECM—extracellular matrix
ECT—electroconvulsive therapy
EFV—efavirenz
eGFR—estimated glomerular filtration rate
EI—entry inhibitor
ELISA—enzyme-linked immunosorbent assay
ENF—enfuvirtide
EPF—eosinophilic pustular folliculitis
EPOCH—etoposide, prednisolone, Oncovin (vincristine), cyclophosphamide, doxorubicin (chemotherapy regimen)

EPS—extrapyramidal symptom(s)
ETR—etravirin
ETV—entecavir
EVG—elvitegravir
EWIs—early warning indicators

FDA—U.S. Food and Drug Administration
FDG-PET—F-fluorodeoxyglucose positron emission tomography
FeLV—feline leukemia virus
FIND—Foundation for Innovative New Diagnostics
5-FU—5-fluorouracil
FM—fluorescence microscopy
FPV—fosamprenavir
FRET—fluorescence resonance energy transfer
FTA-ABS—fluorescent treponemal antibody absorbed (test)
FTC—emtricitabine

GA—granuloma annulare
GaLV—gibbon ape leukemia virus
G-CSF—granulocyte colony stimulating factor
GFATM—Global Fund to Fight AIDS and Malaria
GI—gastrointestinal
GI—granuloma inguinale
GLBT—gay, lesbian, bisexual, and transgender
GLI—Global Laboratory Initiative
GLI—group-level intervention
GM-CSF—granulocyte/macrophage colony-stimulating factor
GMS—Grocott's methenamine silver (stain)
GPA—World Health Organization Global Programme on AIDS
GPCR—G protein-coupled, seven-transmembrane segment receptor
GXM—glucuronoxylomannan

H&E—hematoxylin and eosin (stain)
HAD—HIV-associated dementia
HAM—HTLV-1-associated myelopathy
HAM/TSP—HTLV-1-associated myelopathy/tropical spastic paraparesis
HAND—HIV-associated neurocognitive disorder
HBM—health belief model
HBV—hepatitis B virus
HCA-MRSA—healthcare-acquired methicillin-resistant *Staphylococcus aureus*
HCV—hepatitis C virus
HDL—high-density lipoprotein
HEPS—heavily exposed, persistently seronegative (individuals)
HER—HIV Epidemiologic Research study

HGSIL—high-grade squamous intraepithelial lesion
HHV-8—human herpesvirus-8
HIV—human immunodeficiency virus
HIV-DR—drug-resistant HIV
HIVE—HIV encephalitis
HPV—human papillomavirus
HRC—Harm Reduction Coalition
HR2—heptad repeat 2 (amino acid sequence)
HSCT—hematopoietic stem cell transplantation (bone marrow transplantation)
HSV—herpes simplex virus
HSV-1—herpes simplex virus type 1
HSV-2—herpes simplex virus type 2
HTLV—human T-cell leukemia virus
HTLV-1—human T cell leukemia virus type 1
HTVN—U.S. HIV Vaccine Trials Network
HZO—herpes zoster ophthalmicus

IAS—International AIDS Society
ICF—intensified case finding
ICP—intracranial pressure
ID—infective dermatitis
IDU—injecting-drug user
IDF—indinavir
IFN—interferon
IL—interleukin
ILI—individual-level intervention
IMB—information-motivational-behavioral (skills model)
IMT—intima-media thickness
INH—isoniazid
IPD—invasive pneumococcal disease
IPI—international prognostic index
IPT—isoniazid preventive therapy
IRIS—immune reconstitution inflammatory syndrome
IRU—immune recovery uveitis
IRV—immune recovery vitritis
ISTI—integrase strand transfer inhibitor
ITT—intent-to-treat
ITU—imidoylthiourea
IUATLD—International Union Against Tuberculosis and Lung Disease
IUD—intrauterine device

JCV—JC virus

KCS—keratoconjunctivitis sicca
KOH—potassium hydroxide
KS—Kaposi's sarcoma
KSHV—Kaposi's sarcoma-associated herpesvirus

LAC—Latin America and the Caribbean

LCB—lactophenol cotton blue mount
LCMV—lymphocytic choriomeningitis virus
LDH—lactate dehydrogenase
LdT—telbivudine
LED—light-emitting diode
LEE—liver enzyme elevation
LEEP—loop electrosurgical excision procedure
LGBT—lesbian, gay, bisexual, and transgendered persons
LGSIL—low-grade squamous intraepithelial lesion
LGV—lymphogranuloma venereum
LIP—lymphocytic interstitial pneumonitis
LLETZ—large loop excision of transitional zone
LRP—lipoprotein-receptor–related protein
LS—lipodystrophy syndrome
LTR—large terminal repeat (sequences)
LV—lupus vulgaris
LyP—lymphomatoid papulosis

MAC—*Mycobacterium avium* complex
MACS—Multicenter AIDS Cohort study
MAI—*Mycobacterium avium-intracellulare*
MARPs—most-at-risk populations
MC—molluscum contagiosum
MDR—multidrug-resistant
MDR-TB—multidrug-resistant tuberculosis
MF—mycosis fungoides
MGIT—Mycobacterium Growth Indicator Tube
MHA-TP—microhemagglutination assay for antibody to *Treponema pallidum*
MI—myocardial infarction
MIC—minimum inhibitory concentration
MMWR—*Morbidity and Mortality Weekly Report*
MND—minor neurocognitive disorder
MODS—microscopic observational drug susceptibility
MRI—magnetic resonance imaging
mRNA—messenger ribonucleic acid
MRSA—methicillin-resistant *Staphylococcus aureus*
MSM—*Médecins Sans Frontieres* (Doctors Without Borders)
MSM—men who have sex with men
MSMW—men who have sex with men and women
MTCT—mother-to-child transmission (of infection)

NAAT—nucleic acid amplification test
Nabs—neutralizing antibodies
NADR/ATOM—National AIDS Demonstration Research/AIDS Targeted Model
NAHOF—New York Association of HIV Over Fifty
NAM—nucleoside analog mutation

NDWG—New Diagnostic Working Group (of Stop TB Partnership)
NFV—nelfinavir
NGO—nongovernmental organization
NHL—non-Hodgkin's lymphoma
NIAID—National Institute of Allergy and Infectious Diseases
NIH—National Institutes of Health
NIMH—National Institute of Mental Health
NK—natural killer (cell)
NNIBP—non-nucleoside inhibitor binding pocket
NNPI—nonpeptidic protease inhibitor
NNRTI—non-nucleoside reverse transcriptase inhibitor
NRTI—nucleoside reverse transcriptase inhibitor
NRTI-TP—nucleoside reverse transcriptase inhibitor triphosphate
NSAID—nonsteroidal anti-inflammatory drug
NSP—needle and syringe (exchange) program
NTM—nontuberculous mycobacteria
NTP—national tuberculosis program
NVP—nevirapine

OARAC—Office of AIDS Research Advisory Council
OB—optimized background (treatment regimen)
OHL—oral hairy leukoplakia
OI—opportunistic infection
OST—opioid substitution therapy

PAH—pulmonary arterial hypertension
PAHO—Pan American Health Organization
PaO_2—partial pressure of oxygen (in arterial blood)
PAS—periodic acid Schiff (stain)
PBMC—peripheral blood mononuclear cell
PBP—penicillin-binding protein
PCL—primary central nervous system lymphoma
PCNSL—primary central nervous system lymphoma
PCP—*Pneumocystis carinii* pneumonia
PCR—polymerase chain reaction
PCT—porphyria cutanea tarda
PD—photosensitive dermatitis
PEG—percutaneous endoscopic gastrostomy
PEL—primary effusion lymphoma
PEP—postexposure prophylaxis
PIC—preintegration complex
PITC—provider-initiated (HIV) testing and counseling
PJP—*Pneumocystis jirovecii* pneumonia
PLR—persistent light reaction
PLWHA—persons living with HIV/AIDS

PML—progressive multifocal leukoencephalopathy
PMTCT—prevention of mother-to-child transmission (of HIV)
PORN—progressive outer retinal necrosis
PPD—purified protein derivative (antigen)
PrEP—pre-exposure prophylaxis
PTSD—post-traumatic stress disorder
PY—patient years

QD—once daily
QOL—quality of life

RAL—raltegravir
RAM—resistance-associated mutation
REAL—Revised European-American Lymphoma (classification system)
rhGH—recombinant human growth hormone
RIA—radioimmunoassay
RNA—ribonucleic acid
RPHRN—rapidly progressive herpetic retinal necrosis
RR—relative risk
RTF—Retooling Task Force (of Stop TB Partnership)
RTI—reverse transcriptase inhibitor

SAGE—Services & Advocacy for GLBT (Gay, Lesbian, Bisexual, and Transgendered) Elders (previously, Senior Action in a Gay Environment)
SAPIT—Starting Antiretroviral Therapy at Three Points in Tuberculosis study
SCC—squamous cell carcinoma
SD—seborrheic dermatitis
SEPs—syringe exchange programs
SHIV—chimeric HIV/SIV infection model
SI—syncytium inducing (regarding HIV isolates)
SIL—squamous intraepithelial inflammatory lesion
SIRS—systemic inflammatory response
SIV—simian immunodeficiency virus
SIVcpz—simian immunodeficiency virus, chimpanzee species
SIVgor—simian immunodeficiency virus, gorilla species
SIVmac—simian immunodeficiency virus infection, rhesus macaques
SIVsm—simian immunodeficiency virus infection, sooty mangabeys
SJS—Stevens-Johnson syndrome
SLE—systemic lupus erythematosus
SLPI—secretory leukocyte protease inhibitor
SMART—Strategies for Management of Antiretroviral Therapy study

SQV—saquinavir
SREBP—sterol regulatory element-binding protein
SSRI—selective serotonin reuptake inhibitor
SSTIs—skin and soft tissue infections
STD—sexually transmitted disease
STI—sexually transmitted infection
STLV—simian T cell leukemia virus
SW—sex worker

TAG—Treatment Action Group
TAMPEP—European Network for HIV/STI
    Prevention and Health Promotion Among
    Migrant Sex Workers
TAM—thymidine analog mutation
TAR—Tat activation region
TB—tuberculosis
TB-IRIS—*Mycobacterium tuberculosis* IRIS
TBP—TATAA binding protein
TCA—trichloroacetic acid
TDF—tenofovir
TDM—therapeutic drug monitoring
TDR—UNICEF/UNDP/World Bank/WHO Special
    Program for Research and Training in
    Tropical Diseases
Th1—T helper cell type 1
Th2—T helper cell type 2
THF—tetrahydrofuranyl
3TC—lamivudine
TIBO—tetrahydroimidazobenzodiazepinone
TMP-SMX—trimethoprim-sulfamethoxazole
TNF—tumor necrosis factor
TNFR—tumor necrosis factor receptor
TPN—total parenteral nutrition

TPPA—*Treponema pallidum* particle agglutination
    (test)
TPR—tipranavir
Tregs—T regulatory cells
TRIM—tripartite motif
TSP—tropical spastic paraparesis
TST—tuberculin skin test
^{201}Th-SPECT—thallium single-photon emission
    computed tomography

ULN—upper limits of normal
UNGASS   United Nations General Special
    Session
UNICEF—United Nations Children's Fund
UNODC—United Nations Office on Drugs and
    Crime
USAID—United States Agency for International
    Development
UV—ultraviolet

VDRL—Venereal Disease Research Laboratory
    (test)
VDRL/RPR—VDRL rapid plasma reagin
VISP—vaccine-induced seropositivity
VLDL—very-low-density lipoprotein
VRC—Vaccine Research Center
VZIG—varicella-zoster immune globulin
VZV—varicella zoster virus

WHO—World Health Organization
WIHS—Women's Interagency HIV Study

XDR-TB—extensively drug-resistant tuberculosis

Part I

HISTORY

Chapter **1** AN EPIDEMIC OF UNKNOWN PROPORTION: THE FIRST DECADE OF HIV/AIDS

GERALD M. OPPENHEIMER AND RONALD BAYER

The hottest places in hell are reserved for those,
who in a time of great moral crisis,
maintain their neutrality.

—Dante (1265–1327)

Introduction

June 5, 1981 marks the official point zero of the human immunodeficiency virus (HIV) epidemic. On that date, the U.S. Centers for Disease Control and Prevention (CDC) published what has become a landmark communication in its *Morbidity and Mortality Weekly Report (MMWR).*[1] Written by Michael Gottlieb, a young infectious disease doctor, and colleagues, it alerted the public health community that between October 1980 and May 1981 five young and previously healthy homosexual men had been treated in Los Angeles hospitals for biopsy-confirmed *Pneumocystis carinii* pneumonia (PCP). From this information, the CDC suggested a possible link between PCP and homosexual sex or "lifestyle." As if to reinforce that point, Gottlieb's paper was closely followed by another from New York City and San Francisco; it reported that in the 30 months preceding July 1981, Kaposi's sarcoma (KS) had been diagnosed in 26 gay males 26 to 51 years of age.[2] KS was known as a rare cancer that occurred primarily in elderly males and in immunosuppressed organ recipients. Its appearance in a relatively large number of young men was startling, as was that of PCP in individuals without a clinically based cause for immunodeficiency. As they read of the reports, doctors on both coasts recognized similar patients who had passed through their emergency rooms and services since the late 1970s. Others remembered young patients who had died of infections that were difficult to diagnose and devastating in their course.[3]

Over the next 18 months, the news of the burgeoning epidemic became darker, heralded by the headlines of the *MMWR.* On July 9, 1982, the CDC announced that Kaposi's sarcoma and opportunistic infections had been diagnosed in Haitians.[4] A week later the *MMWR* reported PCP in hemophiliacs.[5] On December 10, it alerted its readers to the possible transmission of the new disease, now called acquired immune deficiency syndrome (AIDS), through blood transfusions.[6] On December 17, 1982 and January 7, 1983, respectively, the agency reported unexplained immunodeficiency in infants and in female sex partners of men with AIDS.[7,8] What emerged was a profile of the epidemic as the burgeoning of a new, sexually transmitted and blood-borne disease. In 1982, the extent to which AIDS had spread was unknown. That would remain so until the responsible viral agent would be discovered and characterized and a blood test developed and used in sero-surveys.

But the landmark reports in the *MMWR* tell only part of the story, the seemingly ineluctable evolution of the outbreak. They do not characterize how physicians and nurses responded to their patients, how they understood the epidemiologic significance of their clinical experiences, or the extent to which growing fears about possible infection from AIDS generated resistance in them selves or their colleagues. Looking back, some who treated patients recalled that "the anxiety of those early years was palpable."[9] Nonetheless, in the first years, even that minority of doctors who would commit themselves to AIDS work had no reason to believe that the grim clinical picture would produce a grave social burden. As the epidemic took off, there was a reluctance on the part of many to acknowledge its potential proportions. Donna Mildvan, an infectious disease doctor in New York who had seen some of the earliest cases of AIDS, recalled years later that "everyone was resistant in stages."[10]

For example, as gay doctors hypothesized that the epidemic was sexually transmitted, some sought to warn their communities. By 1983, San Francisco's Bay Area Physicians for Human Rights issued guidelines on sexual risk reduction. In New York City, Dr. Dan William, a gay public health official, tried to do the same before it was too late. Recalling the initial years of the Third Reich, he observed, "[AIDS is] really not unique. I mean it's our own holocaust.... And [in] every holocaust there were warnings. There was Crystal Night in Germany."[11]

But for many gay men, a lifestyle involving the experience of multiple sexual encounters was part of a precious and newly won freedom. To be told this freedom was implicated in a life-threatening disease was especially disturbing, even oppressive. To counsel restraint was tantamount to a rejection of their liberation; their initial response to those, like William, who offered such advice was often dismissive. It took time for the message to sink in that sex with many partners was significantly related to the etiology of KS and PCP and should be curtailed. Such admonitions, expressed in the gay press and, to a more limited degree, in the medical journals, were increasingly buttressed by clinical and epidemiologic studies.

Explaining a Disease of Unknown Origin

That research began in mid-1981, when the CDC initiated a special task force charged with surveillance on KS and opportunistic infections. Its purpose was to confirm that the observed disorder was new and that all new cases were verified.[12] To determine if KS had occurred before 1980 in young individuals, the task force queried epidemiologists at state and local tumor registries. Because the CDC was the sole supplier of pentamidine, a drug used to treat PCP, its own files could reveal whether the infection had been seen previously in adults without an underlying illness. By August, 1981, the CDC requested of all state health departments that they report all suspected cases of KS.

What was the etiology of this new disorder? What relationship did it bear to sex? What caused immunosuppression in previously healthy young gay men? As a start, the CDC performed a brief survey in San Francisco, New York, and Atlanta of 420 men attending clinics for sexually transmitted diseases (STDs).[13] The 35 cases of KS or PCP culled from this unrepresentative sample were interviewed in depth with the hope of developing scientific leads. Researchers found that these men, all homosexuals, had had many sexual partners the previous year and had frequently used recreational drugs like marijuana, cocaine, and amyl or butyl nitrite. The rate of nitrite use was closely associated with number of partners, suggesting a relationship between the two. It was possible that nitrite use was simply a confounding factor, appearing to be linked to PCP and KS because it was part of the men's sexual activity (a median number of 87 partners in the past year). But that 86% of the gay and bisexual men in the CDC's survey had used amyl nitrite in the previous 5 years, compared to only 15% of heterosexual males, was a striking finding, and amyl nitrite became one of the first hypothetical determinants to be investigated. Amyl nitrite seemed worth examining, particularly as it appeared to be a component of the "gay lifestyle" hypothesis that was riveting the epidemiologic researchers at the time. From 1981 until the middle of the decade, researchers pursued the association, positing that amyl nitrite might predispose homosexual men to immune deficiency.[14]

An alternative hypothesis, also investigated by the CDC, was the possibility that the new syndrome was caused by cytomegalovirus (CMV), a microbe suspected of both being sexually transmitted and a cause of KS. A small clinical study published in 1981 by Michael Gottlieb and colleagues found a high rate of CMV in homosexual men with KS or PCP; the latter group also suffered from a low count of T4 lymphocytes (also known as T4 helper cells). Although it was possible that CMV infection might result from T4-cell deficiency and the reactivation of a dormant infection, the authors of this study preferred to suspect the virus, based on earlier research that found much higher rates of CMV infection in gay men compared to heterosexual men.[15]

A third hypothesis focused on multiple factors which, in concert, overloaded the immune system and led to its dysfunction. An editorial in the *New England Journal of Medicine* posited that the joint effects of persistent, sexually transmitted viral infection (possibly CMV) and a recreational drug like amyl nitrite precipitated immunosuppression in genetically predisposed males.[16] In the *Journal of the American Medical Association*, Dr. Joseph Sonnabend, who treated many of the early AIDS cases in Greenwich Village, proposed a model in which repeated sexual contact with many partners exposed a subgroup of homosexual men to CMV and allogeneic sperm, over time leading to a damaged and suppressed immune system.[17] In his article, as in the gay press, Sonnabend indicted the "unprecedented level of promiscuity" over the last decade in urban enclaves like the Village.[18] However, he could not explain why the same disease should be seen in Haitians and hemophiliacs. Instead, he looked to possible alternative factors, suggesting a list of variables that, ironically, presaged the arguments of future HIV denialists like Peter Duesberg—namely, malnutrition, recreational drugs, and acute viral infections.

The early focus on gay men and their "lifestyle" made it difficult to recognize that AIDS was also occurring in other groups. Here, too, people were resistant in stages. Among public health officials, there was a reservoir of resistance to the idea that AIDS could be heterosexually transmitted—in particular, that women could infect men. The notion that the agent, whatever it was, could be transmitted from mother to child, either in utero or during birth, produced more than the normal level of scientific skepticism from both professional colleagues and the public health community, even in light of clinical and epidemiologic studies. When in 1982 James Oleske, a pediatrician based in Newark, New Jersey, submitted a manuscript describing AIDS in the babies he treated, reviewers of the journal rejected his diagnosis. "There was such distaste for this disease," he recalled. "How could this sort of filthy disease occur in children?"[19]

As epidemiologic evidence accumulated, the lifestyle hypothesis—despite its initial appeal—became increasingly untenable. The occurrence of PCP in hemophiliacs who had no other underlying disease but were dependent on factor VIII therapy, raised the possibility that blood was a vehicle for some transmissible agent. That theory was strengthened by a CDC report of the appearance of immunodeficiency and opportunistic infection in a 20-month-old child who had previously received multiple transfusions from a donor later found to have AIDS.[14]

On March 4, 1983, a few months before Oleske's article was finally published in *JAMA*, a Public Health Service (PHS) interagency report in the *MMWR* formalized a major shift in the conceptualization of the epidemic.[20] The weight of the evidence, including cases of immunodeficiency and opportunistic infections in the female sex partners of bisexuals and intravenous drug-using men, and of their children, pointed to the existence of a transmissible infectious agent. Although the microbe was unknown, it appeared from the case distribution to be analogous to hepatitis B, a virus transmitted sexually, parenterally, and through blood and blood products. In this reconfiguration of the known variables, lifestyle did not drop out, but instead became an indirect cause of AIDS.

Although identification of the virus was still months away (see Chapter 2 by Robert Gallo), the hepatitis B model suggested a direction for public health intervention. The PHS recommended that actions known to limit the spread of the hepatitis B virus be applied to the new epidemic. In particular, the PHS strongly advised against sexual contact with persons suspected of having AIDS. In addition, it requested of groups at higher risk of the disease that they not donate blood or plasma, and encouraged doctors to recommend autologous transfusions to their patients. Finally, the PHS called for the development of blood-screening procedures.[14]

In the same *MMWR*, the CDC made reference to "high-risk groups" whose members carried a greater probability of infection and of causing infection, carrying a microbe that could be transmitted through the vehicle of bodily fluids. Although the CDC stressed that "each group contains many persons who probably have little risk of acquiring AIDS," in reality, no such distinction could be drawn. In the absence of a screening or diagnostic test, risk group designation was, in effect, synonymous with carrier status for its members.

One of the results of creating "high risk groups" was to reinforce the linkage between AIDS and socially "marginal" members of society. Conceptually, although each group represented a threat to the rest of the community, public health strictures were to contain the contamination. The hope was that the epidemic could be cordoned at the borders, among a residue who were "different" from the majority. A risk group designation, however inadvertently, created a source of blame and a target for discrimination.

Working in the Dark

The first decade of the AIDS epidemic was characterized by one contemporary physician as "medieval."[21] How far the disease would spread, no one knew. Public interest oscillated between indifference and panic. Fear of infection by risk groups produced widespread discrimination in the workplace, at schools, and in medical facilities. For American medicine, the outbreak represented a startling reversal. After decades of medical advances, doctors were now confronted with a disease that seemed to parry their interventions. Of course, they had managed debilitating chronic diseases and other incurable conditions, but what rendered AIDS so different was that it was an infectious threat, something that physicians in the U.S. had come to think of as chiefly an affliction of the less developed world. In addition, it primarily struck down the young, inverting the "natural order" of things in advanced industrial countries. As in war, the old were burying their children.

The advent of the AIDS epidemic forced doctors in those countries to face the most basic questions. If I cannot cure my patients, what can I do? What is my role as a doctor? And what is my duty to patients who pose a threat to my own life? As doctors sought answers to these questions, they had to reflect on professional experience before antibiotics, when healers routinely fell victim to contagion. And they had to do so surrounded by a degree of suffering for which few among them had been prepared. In describing his patients in the first years of the epidemic, for example, one physician noted, "we didn't have anything to offer them. [They] died, and the deaths they died, I recall, were very terrible deaths; they were deformed and disfigured and wasted away, Kaposi's sarcoma lesions all over their bodies."[22]

To therapeutic limits and fear of infection, another burden was added to those who committed themselves to caring for patients with AIDS. They often experienced institutional, professional, and social hostility. Although some doctors received support from their institutions and colleagues, this was frequently not the case. In many hospitals across the country, both public and private, the story was one of professional isolation or rejection. In the epidemic's first years, administrators and other shapers of policy acted to distance their facilities from the epidemic, to limit related research or to reduce patient admissions, believing that the stigma of AIDS or the fear it engendered might tarnish their institutions. They worried that the new disease would repel new house officers or private donors. AIDS also represented a threat to established research commitments and allocation of resources. Further, those who cared for such patients might encounter the antipathy of colleagues as well. Such responses often affected their ability to provide care to their patients. Specialists rejected their referrals, trying to hold AIDS as arm's length out of homophobia, antipathy for the disease, or fear of infection. The stigma suffered by their patients became a burden with which those who treated AIDS too had to contend.

Some AIDS doctors tried to change the behavior of other clinicians by providing a model of care. One pediatrician, for example, observing that nurses and residents were avoiding HIV-infected infants and children, tried to normalize the disease: "Without saying anything else, I would examine all these babies without wearing gowns, gloves. Only for drawing blood, then I would insist that we have to wear gloves. Teach and talk about the disease as something natural, something common."[23]

Although this pediatrician, Hermann Mendez, was empathic, understanding the fears of others, there were times that those who treated AIDS were appalled by those who failed to meet their professional obligations, rejecting infected patients or referring them to the minority who committed themselves to treating patients with AIDS.

Faced with institutional and professional antipathy and profound therapeutic limitations, physicians in the earliest years of the epidemic reached out to others like themselves for social and clinical support. As clinicians, they were anxious for any intelligence on new diagnostic tests, advice on managing their patients, and any sign of effective treatment. Although articles began to appear in medical journals by the end of 1981, AIDS doctors depended heavily on local linkages, both formal and informal, to obtain the most current information.

In New York City, the Department of Health held meetings at which physicians presented their cases. These "inner city rounds" provided doctors with the opportunity to exchange information on diagnosis, treatment, and care. At the University of California in San Francisco, the Kaposi's sarcoma clinic under Marcus Conant played a similar role, bringing in physicians from multiple specialties to examine patients and conduct grand rounds. More often, physicians depended less on such organized efforts than on informal networks. At times, these served as the context for the earliest clinical studies on the transmission and treatment of HIV infection.[24]

Confronted by disorders of unknown origin, AIDS doctors began to search for interventions against the cascade of diseases they encountered. They turned to whatever experience they could cull and tried what seemed likely to work. Wafaa El-Sadr, now engaged in organizing AIDS programs in sub-Saharan Africa, was a physician at the Veterans Hospital in New York when she first encountered AIDS. She recalled, "It was really scary. We had no clue what we were doing, and in retrospect we made a lot of mistakes…. We didn't anticipate things. We were just reacting."[25]

Some of the earliest treatments were radical, guided mainly by hope. Oncologists adopted aggressive treatments, perceiving AIDS as an aggressive disease. At a number of academic medical centers, doctors attempted to reconstitute their patients' immune systems using bone marrow transplants, with fatal results. The same was true of chemotherapy. But treatment was already available for a number of the opportunistic infections, including toxoplasmosis, bacterial meningitis, and cryptococcal meningitis; these were unusual only in that they ran a more aggressive course. A drug for the treatment of PCP, pentamidine, existed before the epidemic, but it was so rarely needed that the CDC maintained a limited supply that it sent to doctors as required. In fact, as we noted above, the sudden upsurge in calls for pentamidine in 1981 had served to alert the CDC that something strange and unexpected was afoot. Another therapy against PCP, Bactrim, had also become available in the 1970s. Physicians had learned to use it prophylactically in cancer and organ transplant patients whose weakened immune systems put them at a high risk of *Pneumocystis* infection. Ironically, doctors were slow to apply the same lessons to patients with AIDS. The relatively few who did found their position buttressed when, in 1988, *JAMA* published the results of a clinical trial headed by Margaret Fischl, director of the AIDS Clinical Research Unit in Miami's Jackson Memorial Hospital.[26]

Although most of the pharmaceuticals used initially were already part of doctors' armamentarium, physicians were forced by their patients' plight to find new medications. Gancyclovir was still an experimental drug when it became the first agent found effective against CMV. So too was acyclovir, which proved successful in the treatment of herpes lesions. Fred Siegel, at Mount Sinai in New York City, who desperately requested acyclovir from Burroughs Wellcome & Company on a compassionate use basis, spoke of its therapeutic power in wonder. "One of the most dramatic things I've ever seen in medicine was the resolution of this tremendous herpes ulcer in five days with acyclovir. My father used to tell me about the day he first used penicillin on a woman with post-abortion infection of the uterus who was dying…[She] was cured. It was the biggest miracle he had ever seen. So here I was reliving this with acyclovir."[27]

Learning to manage infections spurred by a disease that had first seemed outside their control proved to have a powerful psychological effect on doctors treating patients with AIDS. It was possible to do something; suffering could be mitigated and survival time extended. But, as physicians realized, an effective intervention would only be found once the underlying cause of AIDS was identified. Or so they hoped. With the isolation of HIV in 1983, many became naively optimistic that they could learn to target the virus.

From Subjects to Participants: Reframing Biomedical Research

The unique constellation of forces unleashed by AIDS—sociopolitical as well as clinical—had a profound impact on the conduct of research designed to address the scientific challenges posed by the epidemic. In the mid-1970s, the National Commission for the Protection of Human Subjects of Biomedical and Behavioral Research issued its Belmont Report which codified a set of ethical principles that ought to inform the work of researchers. Those norms provided the foundations for regulations subsequently enacted by the Department of Health and Human Services and the Food and Drug Administration. At the core of those guidelines was the radical distinction between research designed to produce socially necessary, generalizable knowledge and therapy designed to benefit individuals. Against the former, individuals—but especially those who were socially vulnerable—needed protection against conscription.

During the 1980s, AIDS forced a reconsideration of this formulation. The role of the randomized clinical trial, the importance of placebo controls, the centrality of academic research institutions, the dominance of scientists over subjects, the sharp distinction between research and therapy, and the protectionist ethos of the Belmont Report were all brought into question.

Although scholars concerned with the methodologic demands of sound research and ethicists committed to the protection of research subjects played a crucial role in the ensuing discussions, both as defenders of the received wisdom and as critics, the debate was driven by the articulate demands of those most threatened by AIDS. Most prominent were groups such as the People with AIDS Coalition and the AIDS Coalition to Unleash Power (ACT-UP), organizations made up primarily of white, gay men. But advocates of women's, children's, and prisoners' rights also made their voices heard. What was so stunning—disconcerting to some and exciting to others—was the rhythm of challenge and response. Rather than the careful exchange of academic arguments, there was the mobilization of disruptive and effective political protest.

The threat of death hovered over the process. As Carol Levine noted in her 1988 essay "Has AIDS Changed the Ethics of Human Subjects Research?": "the shortage of proven therapeutic alternatives for AIDS and the belief that trials are, in and of themselves, beneficial have led to the claim that people have a *right to be* research subjects. This is the exact opposite of the tradition starting with Nuremberg—that people have a *right not to be* research subjects."[28] That striking reversal resulted in a rejection of the model of research conducted at remote academic centers, with restrictive (protective) standards of access and strict adherence to the "gold standard" of the randomized clinical trial. Blurring the distinction between research and treatment—"A Drug Trial is Health Care Too"—those insistent on radical reform sought to open wide the points of entry to new "therapeutic" agents both within and outside of clinical trials; they demanded that the paternalistic, ethical warrant for the protection of the vulnerable from research be replaced by an ethical regime informed by respect for the autonomous choice of potential subjects who could weigh for themselves the possible risks and benefits of new treatments for HIV infection. Moreover, the revisionists demanded a basic reconceptualization of the relationship between researchers and subjects. In place of protocols imposed from above, they proposed a more egalitarian and democratic model in which negotiation would replace scientific authority.

Contemporary competing analyses of the unfolding events reveal how the debate had touched on profound moral and scientific matters. Martin Delaney, an activist-founder of Project Inform in San Francisco, for example, stated that "regulatory practices contribute to the failure of science, demean the public good, and tread heavily on our civil liberties.... Science and patient alike would be better served by a system that permits life-threatened patients some form of access to the most promising experimental therapies, peacefully coexisting alongside a program of unencumbered clinical research."[29]

Those who were less sanguine spoke in a very different voice. Legal scholar George Annas warned that the blurring of the distinction between research and treatment could only harm the desperate. "It is not compassionate to hold out false hope to terminally ill patients so that they spend their last dollars on unproven 'remedies' that they might live longer."[30] Jerome Groopman of New England Deaconess Hospital in Boston went further. He saw the contemporary liberalization as a threat to the research enterprise itself: "If the philosophy is that anyone can decide at any point what drugs he or she wants to take, then you will not be able to do a clinical trial."[31] A stringent and provocative analysis of this critical moment in the history of AIDS has been provided by Steven Epstein in his volume *Impure Science*.[32]

The Search for Antiviral Therapy

It is in this context that the history of efforts to identify an antiviral agent must be understood. Among the first drugs tested against HIV using human subjects was suramin, an antiparasitic medication used in the treatment of African sleeping sickness. It appeared to be promising, inhibiting viral replication in vitro. In New York, Los Angeles, and San Francisco, hubs of the epidemic, oncologists and infectious disease doctors like Donna Mildvan, Alexandra Levine, Don Abrams, and Paul Volberding enrolled their patients in clinical trials. They saw their work as the beginning of antiretroviral therapy, a positive moment in the epidemic. Unfortunately, suramin proved toxic. Although physicians learned a great deal about HIV infection by following their patients, the trial was a failure, causing the deaths of study participants. For those treating AIDS, suramin marked the beginning of a series of roller coaster rides of initially high expectations followed by crushing disappointments.

Although the 1985 suramin trial was short-lived, the search for an effective antiretroviral agent intensified and crystallized in the late 1980s in clinical research involving AZT, which appeared to inhibit HIV reproduction in vitro. The saga of that drug—the hopes it initially inspired and the disappointment and anger it ultimately precipitated—provides an insight into the desperation that surrounded the treatment of AIDS during the epidemic's first decade.

Beginning in February 1986, 282 individuals with AIDS or serious symptoms associated with HIV infection were enrolled in a randomized, double-blind controlled trial under the auspices of the National Institute of Allergy and Infectious Disease. Six months later it was halted by its data monitoring board on the ethical grounds that those on AZT were clearly benefitting compared to subjects receiving a placebo. Nineteen of the latter died out of 137 participants, compared to one of the 145 on the new drug. What was so striking was that many of those on AZT underwent a stunning revitalization, gaining weight and energy; opportunistic infections began to clear away as patients' T-cell counts rose.

After half a decade or more of seeing young patients sicken and die, the prospect of an effective drug was overwhelming for many who treated AIDS. There was palpable excitement, as doctors could now order a medication that seemed to allow them to manage both the disease and the opportunistic infections associated with it. But some physicians remained skeptics: the results were too good, the trial was too small and of short duration. Not all patients were helped and too many suffered toxic side affects: significant anemia, nausea, and myositis. The skeptics' hesitation and criticism, unfortunately, proved prescient. By 1988, it had become clear that the positive effects of AZT were short-lived, with patients whose conditions had improved returning to a downward, fatal course as viral resistance increased. For doctors and patients who had become enthusiasts, the limitations of AZT were devastating.[32]

Although some physicians reversed course and discounted the drug entirely, research continued on its power to slow AIDS progression. In 1989, another clinical trial—this to determine the effect of AZT on asymptomatic HIV-infected patients—was halted early; again a data monitoring board found there was sufficient positive evidence to make the trial's continuation ethically unsupportable.[33] Oncologist Paul Volberding, director of the AIDS clinic at San Francisco General Hospital and the study's principal investigator, saw the trial as a turning point in the history of the epidemic. "Community organizations used it as a reason to encourage people to be tested [for HIV]: *'Be here for the cure.'* It brought lots of people into medical care for the first time."[34] A concurrent editorial in the *New England Journal of Medicine* by Gerald Friedland, a pioneer in describing and treating AIDS in IV drug users, was entitled "Early Treatment for HIV: The Time

Has Come."[35] Treatment enthusiasm had returned. Eight years into the epidemic, those who treated AIDS patients and pursued therapeutic research desperately needed some success.

That enthusiasm was challenged in 1993, when the Concorde trial, a European study that mirrored Volberding's, reported its results. Unlike its American counterpart, the Concorde trial had continued to run its full course of 3 years. Its findings contradicted those of the earlier trial and stood as a sharp rebuke to those who had claimed that life could be prolonged if AZT treatment was started early in asymptomatic patients.[36] In the years between 1989 and 1993, many who treated AIDS had begun to view AZT as a drug of limited utility, given viral resistance. Concorde seemed to confirm their worst fears. Others, in examining the study, found it methodologically flawed. But as a consequence of its negative results, it was no longer clear when to initiate AZT therapy or whether to use it at all.

To forestall further confusion, the Public Health Service issued guidelines balancing advice that avoided unreasonable expectations and therapeutic nihilism. But for many, the time was one of exasperation or worse. Two months after the initial report of the Concorde trial in *Lancet*, the IXth International Conference on AIDS convened in Berlin. The results hung like a pall over the meeting. That malaise continued for clinicians who now felt they had lost their therapeutic thread.

As doctors came to a realistic assessment of the place of AZT in the treatment of HIV infection and as patients contemplated the failure of the drug to measure up to its initial promise, a process of disenchantment set in that would, on occasion, take on a kind of fury. What at first had symbolized to many the success of science came to represent to some its utter failure. And those who might have derived some limited benefit from AZT were too discouraged to consider its utility.

The controversy swirling around AZT only darkened as the drug became the object of increasing political animosity. Its reception among some African Americans was affected by deep suspicions that AIDS had been created to kill them and the perception that this new therapy was designed to further harm them. Among the mainly white activists in ACT-UP, there were those who felt that already meager scientific resources had been squandered in fruitless endeavors. AZT, they charged, was a toxic medication that only led to further suffering. Using demonstrations, street theater, and the media, they expressed their outrage against the torpid response of government and industry to developing effective drugs.[32] For this, they also held the clinical trialists to blame, hurling their rage at the most prominent among them, like Margaret Fischl in Miami and Martin Hirsch of the Harvard Medical School, and publicly attacking them when they spoke.

Drugs, Doctors, and Patients: The Burden of Ignorance

As the search for effective drugs to arrest the fatal epidemic appeared to stall, a large number of patients began to insist that their relationship with physicians had to be transformed, becoming one of collaboration and equality. Such patients were mainly educated, middle-class individuals who came to their doctors well armed with information culled from networks and organizations to which they belonged. Patients wanted to question their providers, challenge their proposed therapeutic plans, and introduce novel treatments outside the boundaries of conventional medicine. They pressed for changes that went far beyond the transformations that the critics of medical paternalism had demanded in the years prior to AIDS. To a surprising degree, their doctors were receptive. Recognizing their own limited capacity to successfully treat HIV infection, physicians seemed ready to share their authority, at least for this disease. As one contemporary AIDS clinician recalled, "we began to use words we wouldn't otherwise use with patients with other diseases, things like, 'You know, this has to be a partnership.'"[37] Where doctors faced clinical limitations on what they had to offer, sharing the burden of uncertainty made caring for AIDS patients more tolerable.

But collaboration under such circumstances could produce a tension between the demands of patients and physicians trained in the canons of scientific medicine. This was especially true when the requests involved drugs whose efficacy was in doubt. African American patients who rejected AZT at times sought Kemron, a drug marketed with great fanfare by the Kenyan government as capable of eliminating the symptoms of AIDS and perhaps the virus as well. From the onset, the claims made for Kemron—a low dose of alpha interferon—were met with skepticism on the part of most scientists and doctors, perhaps adding to its luster among those who mistrusted mainstream biomedicine. Its lack of effectiveness for those infected with HIV was finally demonstrated in 1993 through a clinical trial conducted in Africa by Ugandan scientists. The World Health Organization, which sponsored the study, announced its results at the same Berlin International AIDS Conference that had showcased the negative findings of the Concorde trial.

More dangerous, because of its toxicity, was another drug, compound Q. In 1989, the *Proceedings the National of Academy of Sciences* reported that laboratory studies of this derivative made from the Chinese cucumber appeared to kill HIV-infected cells. As patients began to import the drug from China, an activist group in San Francisco, Project Inform, inaugurated an underground clinical trial in New York, Los Angeles, San Francisco, and Fort Lauderdale, Florida. Approved neither by the Food and Drug Administration nor an institutional review board—both vital given compound Q's potential toxic effects—the study sparked a bitter dispute among AIDS activists, researchers, and physicians, some of whom served as study coordinators. Treatment enthusiasts provided compound Q on an experimental basis; other physicians reacted with fierce resistance, opposing the use of compound Q as heroic medicine at its worst, leading to toxicity and death.

Nevertheless, to be effective clinicians, doctors often felt compelled to hold their tongue as patients tried new agents. This allowed physicians to at least gain their patients' trust and to be apprised of what drugs, herbs, and potions they were consuming. As a contemporary AIDS doctor explained, "If I did not give my blessing to patients using these drugs, they would simply go elsewhere. I attempted to integrate the use of ribavirin and isoprinosine into whatever other therapies we had."[38]

Patients' turning toward untested agents—to isoprinosine and ribavirin, among others—underscored the desperation and confusion that marked the end of the epidemic's first decade. For physicians, this was a grim and frustrating period, an ordeal without an apparent end, and a time marked by the deaths of so many patients in their private practices and hospital wards.

Bearing the Weight of Death and Dying

No training was sufficient to prepare physicians for the number of deaths they encountered in this new epidemic, for the suffering of the dying, and for the youth of the patients they ministered to. The mortality statistics for an infectious disease in a developed country were staggering. In 1981, 120 AIDS fatalities were recorded, probably an undercount. Five years later, accrued deaths had risen to 12,000. By 1990, that number stood at 100,000, almost a third in that year alone. AIDS became the leading cause of death in men aged 24 to 44 in 1992, the fourth leading cause in young women. But for young black women, it was the leading cause of death in 10 American cities that year.[39,40] In the antibacterial era, numbers like these were staggering, beyond the experience of anyone who had not practiced in third world countries. The infectious diseases they used as possible models of AIDS, like hepatitis B, at first led doctors to hope for a limited case fatality rate. This proved to be another form of denial. By 1987, they understood, given the epidemiologic data and their own experiences, that AIDS was almost universally fatal. One AIDS doctor recalled that when he encountered a new patient, still strapping and attractive, his response was, "I'm looking at a healthy dead person; it's just a matter of time."[41] Revealing a positive HIV test to a patient became a trial for many doctors. Having been taught little in medical school to prepare them, a remarkable number of physicians first learned through AIDS how to inform patients they suffered from a fatal disease.

Since death was almost always inevitable, physicians sought to demonstrate their professional mastery by organizing their patients' dying and death. What that meant varied: controlling pain, helping a patient come to terms with the stigma of AIDS and the trial of dying, reconnecting patients and families, and helping all—including the doctors themselves—to recognize when further interventions would be futile. Reconnecting with centuries past, doctors spoke of orchestrating a "good death," one in which their patients died with some dignity, despite the ravages of the disease. For many physicians, this was demanding and new. Summing up, one AIDS doctor observed, "It will sound macabre, but I realized I was a travel agent for death, and that my role was to make the process as drawn out, as comfortable, and as full of interesting things as it was possible to do. I couldn't prevent the ultimate outcome, but I could manage it."[42]

In addition to that technical prowess that allowed them to care for the dying and those around them, doctors had to learn something else not commonly taught in medical school. They would discover that these deaths of young patients would challenge their own sense of well-being. During the bleakest years of the epidemic, when therapeutic options were frustratingly few, clinical distance would fail them; they could not shield themselves from the sadness that developed in the course of their work. "You have a lot of ghosts in you," one early AIDS doctor noted.[43]

As patients approached death, doctors had to make personal and strategic decisions about how close they would become to patients, some of whom they had accompanied from initial diagnosis through multiple acute illnesses. Unable to forestall death, they had also to come to grips with their own sense of competence and failure. Although they usually recognized that nothing could be done to prevent a final, fatal outcome, the socialization of doctors often contributed to a lingering attachment to the curative role. As one contemporary physician recalled, "I think we all have these feelings that if I had only done this, if only I had done that, maybe he wouldn't have died." [44]

For physicians to continue their work, they had to shield themselves, recognizing the need to maintain sufficient distance to avoid burnout. In turns, they became stoical or moderated their expectations. "If you think you can save the world, don't go into AIDS care," one doctor observed.[45] But at times, coping mechanisms failed under the onslaught of intense clinical involvement, followed by a patient's death. Doctors and nurses became depleted or chronically depressed and had to leave AIDS work, at least temporarily. Others buffered their involvement by assuming collateral responsibilities that took them away from constant patient care. For example, they became administrators, managing AIDS services, or became absorbed in research, focusing on clinical trials and teaching.

But such absences came at a price, particularly for very sick patients felt abandoned at a time of great vulnerability. Worse still was when doctors themselves died. By 1990, when the medical newsletter *Medical World News* published an account of doctors who had died of AIDS, the CDC had estimated that 350 physicians had been struck down by the epidemic.[46] Many of them, virtually all of whom were gay, treated patients with HIV infection.

Public Health and "HIV Exceptionalism"

Just as AIDS had deeply affected clinical medicine and biomedical research in the first decade, it also compelled a reconsideration of how public health officials could best meet the challenge of limiting the spread of HIV. As had been true of the shape of the controversies about care and research, it was the sociopolitical context of HIV that both defined the contours of debate and the resolutions that merged. Once again, AIDS required a rethinking of fundamental principles and norms that had informed practice over prior decades.

Did the history of responses to lethal infectious diseases provide lessons about how best to contain the spread of HIV infection? Should the policies developed to control STDs or other communicable conditions be applied to AIDS? If AIDS were not to be so treated, what would justify such differential policies?

To understand the importance of these questions, it is necessary to recall that conventional approaches to public health threats were typically codified in the latter part of the 19th or the early part of the 20th century. Even when public health laws were revised in subsequent decades, they tended to reflect the imprint of their genesis. They provided a warrant for mandating compulsory examination and screening, breaching the confidentiality of the clinical relationship by reporting to public health registries the names of those with diagnoses of "dangerous diseases," imposing treatment, and—in the most extreme cases—confining persons through the power of quarantine.[47]

As the century progressed, the most coercive elements of this tradition were rarely brought to bear because of changing patterns of morbidity and mortality and the development of effective clinical alternatives. Nevertheless, it was the specter of these elements that most concerned proponents of civil liberties and advocates of gay rights as they considered the potential direction of public health policy in the presence of AIDS.[18] Would there be widespread compulsory testing? Would the names of the infected be recorded in central registries? Would such registries be used to restrict those with HIV infection? Would the power of quarantine be used, if not against all infected persons, then at least against those whose behavior could result in the further transmission of infection?

Although there were public health traditionalists who pressed to have AIDS and HIV infection brought under the broad statutory provisions established to control the spread of STDs and other communicable diseases, they were in the distinct minority. Ultimately, it was those who called for "HIV exceptionalism" who came to dominate public discourse, at least in the first decade of the epidemic.[48] It was then that an alliance of gay leaders, civil libertarians, physicians, and public health officials began to shape a policy for dealing with AIDS that reflected the exceptionalist perspective. Only as that decade began to draw to a close could one detect the signs that exceptionalism was being subject to important challenges. Those challenges would only intensify with the end of the era of radical therapeutic limits.

Exemplifying this perspective and its trajectory over time was the question of HIV testing. The HIV-antibody test, first made widely available in 1985, was the subject of great controversy from the outset. Out of often stormy debates emerged a broad consensus that, except in a few, well defined circumstances, people should be tested only with their informed, voluntary, and specific consent. Mandatory testing, so much a feature of the public health response to epidemic disease in the past—and even routine testing with presumed consent—were deemed counterproductive and violative of the ethical principle of autonomy and of basic norms of civil liberties. However, when the clinical importance of identifying those with asymptomatic HIV infection became clear in the late 1980s, the political context of the debate over testing underwent a fundamental change.

Gay organizations began to urge homosexual and bisexual men to have their antibody status determined under confidential or anonymous conditions; others sought to loosen the strictures on testing. Physicians pressed for AIDS to be returned to the medical mainstream and for the HIV-antibody test to be treated like other blood tests—that is, given with the presumed consent of the patient. Thus, for example, four clinical societies in New York State—including the New York Medical Society—sued, (unsuccessfully it must be noted) the commissioner of health in 1989 to compel him to define AIDS and HIV infection as sexually transmitted and communicable diseases.[49] Among the goals of the suit was the liberalization of the stringent consent requirements for HIV testing. In 1990, the House of Delegates of the American Medical Association called for HIV infection to be classified as an STD. Although the delegates chose not to act on a resolution that would have permitted testing without consent, their decision on classification had clear implications for a more routine approach to HIV screening, one in which the standard of specific informed consent would no longer prevail.[50]

The movement toward routine or mandatory testing was especially marked in the case of pregnant women and newborns. Pregnant women were already tested in this way for syphilis and hepatitis B. The screening of newborns for phenylketonuria and other congenital conditions was standard. The publication in the *Morbidity and Mortality Weekly Report* on March 15, 1991 of recommendations for the prophylaxis of *Pneumocystis carinii* pneumonia in newborns would affect the discussion of the importance of identifying infants born to mothers with HIV infection.[51]

Like the debates over HIV testing, the contention over whether HIV infection should be subject to mandatory public health reporting focused on the traditions of disease control and fundamental questions of privacy and liberty. Clinical AIDS had been a reportable condition in every state since 1983. But since the inception of HIV testing, there had been a sharp debate about whether the names of all infected persons should be reported to confidential registries of public health departments. Gay groups and their allies adamantly opposed HIV reporting as a matter of principle. Many public health officials opposed such a move because of its potential effect on the willingness of people to seek HIV testing and counseling voluntarily.

By 1991 only a few states, typically those with relatively few AIDS cases, had required such reporting. But divisions had begun to appear in the alliance against the reporting of names in states where the prevalence of HIV infection was high and where gay communities were well organized. In New York State, the same four medical societies that had proposed a change in testing policy demanded that HIV infection be made a reportable condition. In 1989, Stephen Joseph, then commissioner of health in New York City, stated that the prospects of early clinical intervention warranted "a shift toward a disease-control approach to HIV infection along the lines of classic tuberculosis practices," including the "reporting of seropositives."[52] Although political factors thwarted the commissioner, it is clear that his call represented part of a national trend.

At the end of November 1990, the Centers for Disease Control declared its support for HIV reporting. In a carefully crafted editorial note in the *Morbidity and Mortality Weekly Report,* the agency stated that by using measures to maintain confidentiality, the implementation of a standardized system for HIV reporting to state health departments could enhance the ability of local, state, and national agencies to project the levels of required resources "[and aid] in the establishment of a framework for providing partner notification and treatment services…"[53]

Most important in the move toward the reporting of names was the belief on the part of public health officials that effective programs of partner notification required the reporting of the names of persons with HIV infection as well as the names of those with a diagnosis of AIDS. Despite the long-established role of health departments in the control of venereal diseases, notification of the sexual and needle-sharing partners of patients with HIV infection or AIDS had been the exception rather than the rule. Opponents of such notification or contact tracing denounced it as a coercive measure, even though it had always depended on cooperation with the index patient and protection of that patient's anonymity.

The early opposition to partner notification by gay and civil-liberties groups began to yield as a better understanding of the practice developed. From 1988 on, the CDC made the existence of partner-notification programs in states a condition for the granting of funds from its HIV-prevention program. Such programs were also endorsed by the Institute of Medicine, the National Academy of Sciences, the Presidential Commission on the HIV Epidemic, the American Bar Association, and the American Medical Association.

More controversial still was the debate over the "duty to warn." Many of the early strict-confidentiality statutes relating to HIV infection and AIDS appeared to prevent physicians from acting when confronted with infected patients who indicated that they would neither inform their partners nor alter their sexual practices. By the end of the 1980s, however, it was possible to witness change. Both the American Medical Association and the Association of State and Territorial Health Officials endorsed legislative provisions that would have permitted disclosure to people placed at risk by the HIV infection of a partner. By 1990, only two states had imposed on physicians a legal duty to warn spouses that they were at risk for HIV infection. Approximately a dozen states had passed legislation granting physicians a "privilege to warn or inform" sexual and needle-sharing partners, thus freeing clinicians from liability whether or not they issued such warnings. In a remarkable acknowledgment of the extreme sensitivity of the issues involved, some of the legislation stipulated that the warnings could not involve revealing the identity of the source of the threat to the person being informed.

Finally, public health officials were confronted with the question of whether the power of quarantine had any role to play in inhibiting the transmission of HIV. On epidemiologic, pragmatic, and ethical grounds, there had been virtually no support for the use of such public health authority with all HIV-infected persons. There had however, been periodic discussion of whether the tradition of restricting liberty in the name of the public health should be invoked when a person's behavior posed a risk for HIV transmission. Such proposals typically came from those identified with a politically conservative posture. Although bitter opposition greeted all attempts to bring such behavior within the scope of existing quarantine statutes, more than a dozen states did so from 1987 through 1990. Noteworthy, when such measures had been enacted, they had generally provided an occasion to revise state disease-control laws to reflect contemporary constitutional standards of due process.

More common, though still relatively rare, was the use of the criminal law under such circumstances. From 1987 through 1989, 20 states enacted statutes permitting the prosecution of persons whose behavior posed a risk of HIV transmission, a move broadly endorsed by the Presidential Commission on the HIV Epidemic.[54] The 1990 Ryan White Comprehensive AIDS Resources Emergency (CARE) Act required that all states receiving funds have the statutory capacity to prosecute those who engaged in behavior linked to the transmission of HIV infection to unknowing partners. Perhaps more crucial, aggressive local prosecutors had relied on the general criminal law to bring indictments against some people for HIV-related behavior. In the absence of statutes specifically defining such behavior as criminal in the vast majority of instances, such prosecutions resulted either in acquittal or in a decision to drop the case. Nevertheless, where there had been guilty verdicts, the penalties were at times unusually harsh.[55]

When the exceptionalist perspective first took hold in the early years of the epidemic, many of its proponents viewed it as providing the opportunity to address the traditional authoritarian dimensions of public health. They asserted that modern public health need not involve limitations on the rights of individuals. Indeed, they argued that a public health that respected rights world be both more effective and more ethical.[18] The most striking impacts of this outlook occurred in the epidemic's first years. But, by the late 1980s, the hold of this perspective had been subject to erosion as the era of therapeutic impotence yielded to an enhanced capacity to manage opportunistic infections, even if the picture surrounding antiretroviral therapy remained bleak.

In the mid-1990s, fundamental transformations occurred as therapeutic prospects like the use of AZT to dramatically reduce maternal-fetal transmission and the emergence of HAART radically transformed every dimension of the HIV epidemic. Under these altered circumstances, the exceptionalist perspective would be subject to further challenge. Nevertheless, even as critical elements of public health policy would assume more traditional dimensions, the legacy of exceptionalism would remain clear in the extent to which the claims of individual rights and the importance of consultations with stakeholders had become defining features of contemporary public health theory and practice.

The therapeutic advances of the mid-1990s brought to an end so much that came to define AIDS in its first years, at least in countries like the United States. A disease that seemed to reveal the limits of medicine would become a complex, sometimes difficult to manage chronic disease. And with that change the narratives of death and suffering that had defined AIDS would, in time, become something increasingly difficult to recall. But as the toll exacted by HIV in the advanced industrialized nations took on more "normal" dimensions, attention would shift to the extraordinary and stark picture of the epidemic's course elsewhere, especially in sub-Saharan Africa and parts of Asia. In these resource-poor areas, the therapeutic advances that had transformed HIV/AIDS in other parts of the world remained out of reach of all but a few, focusing global attention on issues of life and death arising from inequality and inequity. It was in these economically challenged countries that the next chapter in the history of AIDS would be written.

References

1. CDC. *Pneumocystis* pneumonia—Los Angeles. MMWR 1981;30:250–252.
2. CDC. Kaposi's sarcoma and *Pneumocystis* pneumonia among homosexual men—New York City and California. MMWR 1981;30:305–308.
3. Bayer R, Oppenheimer G. AIDS Doctors: Voices from the Epidemic. New York: Oxford University Press; 2000.
4. CDC. Opportunistic infections and Kaposi's sarcoma among Haitians in the United States. MMWR 1982;31:353–354.
5. CDC. *Pneumocystis carinii* pneumonia among persons with hemophilia A. MMWR 1982;32:365–367. MMWR 1982;365–367.
6. CDC. Possible transfusion-associated acquired immune deficiency syndrome (AIDS)—California. MMWR 1982;31:652–654.
7. CDC. Unexplained immunodeficiency and opportunistic infections in infants—New York, New Jersey, California. MMWR 1982;31:665–667.
8. CDC. Immunodeficiency among female sexual partners of males with acquired immune deficiency syndrome (AIDS)—New York. MMWR 1983;31:697–698.
9. Bayer R, Oppenheimer G. AIDS Doctors: Voices from the Epidemic. New York: Oxford University Press; 2000 (p. 22).

10. Bayer R, Oppenheimer G. AIDS Doctors: Voices from the Epidemic. New York: Oxford University Press; 2000 (p. 22).

11. Bayer R, Oppenheimer G. AIDS Doctors: Voices from the Epidemic. New York: Oxford University Press; 2000 (p. 23).

12. Centers for Disease Control Task force on Kaposi's Sarcoma and Opportunistic Infections. Epidemiologic aspects of the current outbreak of Kaposi's sarcoma and opportunistic infections. N Engl J Med 1982;306: 248–252.

13. Astor G. The Disease Detectives. New York: New American Library; 1983.

14. Oppenheimer GM. In the Eye of the Storm: The Epidemiological Construction of AIDS. In: Fee E, Fox DM, editors. AIDS: The Burdens of History. Berkeley, California: University of California Press; 1988. pp. 267–300.

15. Gottlieb MS, Schroff R, Schanker HM, et al. Pneumocystis carinii pneumonia and mucosal candidiasis in previously healthy homosexual men: evidence of a new acquired cellular immunodeficiency. N Engl J Med 1981;305:1425–1431,

16. Durack DT. Opportunistic infections and Kaposi's sarcoma in homosexual men. N Engl J Med 1981;305:1465–1467.

17. Sonnabend J, Witkin SS, Purtilo DT. Acquired immunodeficiency syndrome, opportunistic infections, and malignancies in male homosexuals: A hypothesis of etiologic factors in pathogenesis. JAMA 1983;249:23470–2374.

18. Bayer R. Private Acts, Social Consequences: AIDS and the Politics of Public Health. New York: The Free Press, 1989. pp. 24.

19. Bayer R, Oppenheimer G. AIDS Doctors: Voices from the Epidemic. New York: Oxford University Press; 2000. p.31.

20. CDC. Prevention of acquired immune deficiency syndrome (AIDS): Report of inter-agency recommendations. MMWR 1983;32:101–104.

21. Bayer R, Oppenheimer G. AIDS Doctors: Voices from the Epidemic. New York: Oxford University Press; 2000 (p. 63).

22. Bayer R, Oppenheimer G. AIDS Doctors: Voices from the Epidemic. New York: Oxford University Press; 2000 (p. 70).

23. Bayer R, Oppenheimer G. AIDS Doctors: Voices from the Epidemic. New York: Oxford University Press; 2000 (p. 106).

24. Bayer R, Oppenheimer G. AIDS Doctors: Voices from the Epidemic. New York: Oxford University Press; 2000 (pp. 110–111).

25. Bayer R, Oppenheimer G. AIDS Doctors: Voices from the Epidemic. New York: Oxford University Press; 2000 (p. 119).

26. Fischl M. Dickinson GM, LaVoie L. Trimethoprim-sulfamethoxazole prophylaxis for pneumocystis carinii pneumonia in AIDS. JAMA 1988;259:1185–1189.

27. Bayer R, Oppenheimer G. AIDS Doctors: Voices from the Epidemic. New York: Oxford University Press; 2000 (p. 124).

28. Levine C. Has AIDS changed the ethics of human subjects research? Law Med Health Care 1988;16:167–173.

29. Delaney M. The case for patient access to experimental therapy. J Infect Dis 1989;159:416–419.

30. Annas GJ. Faith (healing), hope and charity at the FDA: The politics of AIDS drug trials. Vill Law Rev 1989;34:771–797.

31. CDC. Parallel system defended. AIDS Weekly 1989;11: 3.

32. Epstein S. Impure Science: AIDS, Activism, and the Politics of Knowledge. Berkeley, California: University of California Press; 1996.

33. Volberding P, Lagakos SW, Koch MA, et al. Zidovudine in asymptomatic human immunodeficiency virus infection. N Engl J Med 1990;322:941–949.

34. Bayer R, Oppenheimer G. AIDS Doctors: Voices from the Epidemic. New York: Oxford University Press; 2000 (p. 137).

35. Friedman G. Early treatment for HIV: The time has come. N Engl J Med 1990;322:1000–1002.

36. Concorde Coordinating Committee. Concorde: MRC/ANS randomised double-blind controlled trial of immediate and deferred zidovudine in symptom-free HIV infection. Lancet1994;343:871–881.

37. Bayer R, Oppenheimer G. AIDS Doctors: Voices from the Epidemic. New York: Oxford University Press; 2000 (p. 157).

38. Bayer R, Oppenheimer G. AIDS Doctors: Voices from the Epidemic. New York: Oxford University Press; 2000 (p. 168).

39. CDC. Update: Mortality attributable to HIV infection/AIDS among persons aged 25–44 years—United States, 1990 and 1991. MMWR 1993;42:481–486.

40. CDC. Update: Mortality attributable to HIV infection/AIDS among persons aged 25–44 years—United States, 1994. MMWR 1996;45:121–125.

41. Bayer R, Oppenheimer G. AIDS Doctors: Voices from the Epidemic. New York: Oxford University Press; 2000 (p. 174).

42. Bayer R, Oppenheimer G. AIDS Doctors: Voices from the Epidemic. New York: Oxford University Press; 2000 (p. 171).

43. Bayer R, Oppenheimer G. AIDS Doctors. Voices from the Epidemic. New York: Oxford University Press; 2000 (p. 172).

44. Bayer R, Oppenheimer G. AIDS Doctors: Voices from the Epidemic. New York: Oxford University Press; 2000 (p. 185).

45. Bayer R, Oppenheimer G. AIDS Doctors: Voices from the Epidemic. New York: Oxford University Press; 2000 (p. 209).

46. Depleting the Front Lines: Medicine's Loss. Med World News. April 9, 1990; 24–29.

47. Fairchild AL, Bayer R, Colgrove J. Searching Eyes: Privacy, the State, and Disease Surveillance in America. Berkeley: University of California Press; 2007.

48. Bayer R. Public health policy and the AIDS epidemic: An end to AIDS exceptionalism? N Engl J Med 1991;324:1500–1504.

49. New York State Society of Surgeons et al. v. Axelrod, 1989.

50. Jones L. HIV infection labeled as STD; board to clarify testing policy. Amer Med News; 1990;3:28.

51. Working Group on PCP Prophylaxis in Children. Guidelines for prophylaxis against *Pneumocystis carinii* pneumonia for children infected with human immunodeficiency virus. MMWR 1991;40:1–13.

52. Joseph SC. Remarks at the Fifth International Conference on AIDS, Montreal, June 4–9, 1989.

53. CDC. Update: Public health surveillance for HIV infection—United States, 1989 and 1990. MMWR 1990;39:859–861.

54. Report of the Presidential Commission on the Human Immunodeficiency Virus Epidemic: submitted to the President of the United States. Washington, D.C.: Presidential Commission on the Human Immunodeficiency Virus Epidemic; 1988.

55. Gostin LO. The AIDS litigation project: A national review of court and human rights commission decisions, part 1: the social impact of AIDS. JAMA 1990; 263:1961–1970.

Chapter 2 A PERSONAL HISTORY OF THE DISCOVERY OF HIV

ROBERT C. GALLO

There are two ways to live: you can live as if nothing is a miracle;
you can live as if everything is a miracle.

—ALBERT EINSTEIN

Introduction

For years, retroviruses had been recognized as the primary cause of many kinds of leukemias and related hematopoietic tumors in a wide variety of animals, leading to the expectation that this would also be true for humans. In addition, retroviruses were known to cause non-neoplastic diseases, including anemia and immune suppression. Despite this, there was almost no evidence for the involvement of retroviruses in any human diseases or even for their presence. However, the development of sensitive, specific molecular techniques for detecting and identifying retroviruses and for the large-scale culturing of T lymphocytes throughout the 1970s culminated in the discovery of the first human retrovirus, HTLV-1, and its implication as the cause of adult T cell leukemia/lymphoma (ATL), a relatively rare and geographically localized leukemia prevalent in southern Japan, parts of the Caribbean, and Africa. HTLV-1 was also identified as the cause of tropical spastic paraparesis (TSP) (also known as HTLV-associated myelopathy), a demyelinating neuropathy resembling multiple sclerosis. Although no retroviruses have so far been demonstrated for other human leukemias or related diseases, many of the techniques that were developed to identify HTLV-1 were instrumental for the isolation of HIV-1, its identification as the causal agent of AIDS, the ability to grow HIV-1 in quantity, the consequent development of a blood test that has saved innumerable lives, and the development of effective antiretroviral drugs. The latter development has made HIV-1 infection a somewhat manageable chronic condition rather than an invariably lethal disease. An effective vaccine remains one of our most important needs, but has thus far proven elusive.

Background

The discovery of retroviruses occurred at the beginning of the twentieth century, when Ellerman and Bang recognized that cell-free filtrates contained an agent that could cause leukemia in chickens.[1] Shortly thereafter, Rous, using the same technique, showed the transmission of sarcomas to chickens.[2] Much later, similar findings were reported for mice, both for breast tumors by Bittner[3] and for leukemia by Gross.[4] The involvement of retroviruses in leukemia was soon extended to other mammals by Jarrett, who showed that feline leukemia was due to infection with a retrovirus.[5,6] Jarrett's work and subsequent work by Essex and Hardy[7] clearly show that this virus was naturally transmitted from cat to cat. This was important because it was the first example of transmissible leukemia in an outbred species. Kawakami and Theilen and colleagues then showed that some leukemia in primates, specifically in gibbon apes and new world monkeys, was due to retroviral infections.[8,9]

The findings that retroviruses caused leukemias and lymphomas in a variety of animals, including nonhuman primates, caused an expectation by many that leukemias would prove to be generally of retroviral etiology, which generated extensive efforts to identify retroviruses in human leukemias. The discovery of reverse transcriptase in 1970 was of incalculable importance, as it provided the first highly sensitive, relatively unambiguous, and generalized tool to detect and characterize retroviruses present at low levels, and it was the first demonstration of the reversal of what was considered to be the invariant flow of genetic information, from DNA to RNA to protein. As a result, these viruses were designated for the first time as retroviruses. Many laboratories, including my own, made extensive efforts to refine this tool in order to identify human retroviruses, especially in leukemias. Our approach was two-fold, and included refining the available techniques for the detection and characterization of reverse transcriptase as well as developing methods for culturing the types of cells relevant to leukemias.

It was important to concentrate on developing techniques sensitive and specific enough to discriminate between reverse transcriptase and cellular DNA polymerases, but sufficiently general and robust for detecting reverse transcriptase from a wide variety of retroviruses. Sensitivity was especially an issue because of the possibility that a human retrovirus might only replicate at low levels. Although this was thought unlikely because the known animal retroviruses were generally expressed at high levels, it turned out to be true for human T cell leukemia virus type 1 (HTLV-1). One of the early diagnostic characteristics of reverse transcriptase was the presence of RNAse-sensitive DNA synthesis in particulate fractions having the density of retroviral particles (1.16–1.18 g/mL) treated with nonionic detergent and supplied with labeled DNA precursors.[10] Although convenient, this kind of activity could often be due to RNA-primed but DNA-dependent DNA synthesis by mitochondrial DNA polymerase γ in membrane fragments having the same approximate density as retroviral particles.[11,12] More rigorous criteria were soon developed. These included a template preference by both purified and unpurified reverse transcriptase for synthetic polyribonucleotides over polydeoxyribonucleotides,[13,14] as well as the ability of the sufficiently purified polymerase to reverse transcribe natural RNA into DNA.[15,16]

The second approach, to try to reproducibly grow and obtain sufficient amounts of the relevant hematopoietic cell types, focused on using conditioned media as a source of cell growth factors. These efforts led to our identification of T cell growth factor, subsequently called interleukin 2 (IL-2). IL-2 was one of the first cytokine growth factors to be identified and characterized, and it allowed the growth of large quantities of T cells over an extended time period.[17,18] Both the discovery of IL-2 and the availability of accurate and sensitive reverse transcriptase assays proved critical to the discovery of HTLV-1, because it is a virus that is generally expressed only at low levels and is not easy to transmit and grow.

Prejudices Against the Existence of Human Retroviruses

Prior to the discovery of HTLV-1, there was a pervasive belief that human retroviruses did not exist. There were several reasons for this. For one thing, reports of human retroviruses in the past had often turned out to be contaminations with animal retroviruses. Retroviral cross-contamination occurs more readily than one might expect. Secondly, the known animal retroviruses tended to be abundantly expressed, and the reasoning by analogy was that this would be true for any human retroviruses, making them easy to detect if present. As we now know, that was not the case for the human T cell leukemia virus (HTLV), and is certainly not true for all of the currently recognized animal retroviruses. There was little evidence at the time for retroviruses as oncogenic agents in nonhuman primates except for gibbon ape leukemia virus (GaLV). Human serum is lytic for some retroviruses, engendering a belief that humans would be immune to retroviral infections. Many of the leading retrovirologists were therefore convinced human retroviruses did not exist. These prejudices are summarized in **Table 2–1**.

TABLE 2–1	**Why Prejudices Were So Strong Against the Possible Existence of Human Retroviruses**
	• Decades of repeated failed attempts.
	• High replication in animals (i.e., they should have been easy to find if they existed).
	• Little evidence in primates as disease-causing agents.
	• Human sera are lytic for many animal retroviruses; therefore, humans were protected.

Even more pervasive was the generalized belief that infectious diseases were a thing of the past, especially in the industrialized world. The idea that viruses could cause cancer in humans was also not widely espoused.

Why We Pursued Human Retroviruses

In spite of this, there were some encouraging factors that kept us focused on the hunt. One was the availability if IL-2, which allowed us to grow primary T cells in large quantity. Another was the availability of sensitive and specific reverse transcriptase assays. Bovine leukemia virus (BLV) had also been recently discovered. It caused leukemia in cattle and was transmitted from cow to cow, yet was hard to detect, difficult to grow, and not highly expressed. We were also encouraged by the demonstrations that GaLV strains caused various types of leukemia in primates. GaLV had been transmitted on one occasion from a pet gibbon to a pet wooly monkey, suggesting that cross-species transmission of viruses could occur. In fact, GaLV itself is thought to have originated by transmission from an Asian mouse species. These factors are summarized in **Table 2–2**.

Discovery of HTLV, the First Human Retrovirus

We were driven to look for retroviruses in human T cell malignancies by two considerations. First, we had isolated a strain of gibbon ape leukemia virus (GaLV$_H$) from a gibbon with a T cell leukemia.[19] One of the strains of GaLV reported by Kawakami was also from an animal with a T cell leukemia, albeit of a different type.[8] Second, the only growth factor readily available at that

TABLE 2-2	Encouraging Factors to Keep Searching for Human Retroviruses
	BLV story
	Il-2 discovery (allowed us to grow primary T cells)
	Reverse transcriptase (gave us sensitive assays)
	GaLV story (first time a retrovirus shown to cause a leukemia in primates in nature)
	GaLV interspecies transmissions (ape to a monkey—why not humans?)

time was IL-2, which would only support the growth of T cells. The availability of IL-2 made it possible to grow relatively large quantities of T cells from T cell malignancies. One of the types of hematopoietic diseases upon which we focused[20] was from patients diagnosed at the time as having the CD4+ T cell malignancies mycosis fungoides or Sézary syndrome. In retrospect, it is clear that some of these patients instead had adult T cell leukemia/lymphoma (ATL). Reverse transcriptase assays and electron microscopy (**Figure 2–1**) indicated the presence of a retrovirus in one such cell line, from a patient diagnosed with mycosis fungoides.[21] Shortly thereafter, we isolated a similar virus from primary cells obtained from a second patient, one diagnosed with Sézary syndrome.[22] The availability of HTLV-1 from large-scale cultures made it possible to generate nucleic acid and protein reagents for a detailed characterization of the virus and for various clinical studies, including a blood test for the serum antibodies to the virus that would indicate infection. By nucleic acid homology and protein serology, HTLV-1 was clearly distinct from all previously characterized animal retroviruses.[23,24] It was absent in most types of leukemia. It was, however, present in T cells but not B cells from ATL patients,[25] suggesting a causative role in the disease. Miyoshi confirmed the presence of a retrovirus in primary ATL T cells and in a cell line generated by cocultivation of ATL T cells with normal cord blood T cells.[26] Importantly, the infected cell line was of the opposite sex from the ATL donor. This demonstrated that this virus was both infectious and able to transform target T cells. This virus, originally called ATL for adult T cell leukemia virus, was later shown to be identical to HTLV-1, and the nomenclature was adjusted to HTLV accordingly.[27,28] Transformation of T cells further suggested that HTLV-1 was the cause of the disease. Much of this is dealt with in detail in reviews.[29,30]

The identification of HTLV-1 from patients with ATL, along with the demonstration in T cells of those patients and of the transforming ability of HTLV-1, was highly suggestive of a causative association. ATL was first recognized as a distinct entity by Takatsuki and colleagues, who characterized it is as representing a distinct subset of leukemias highly endemic to certain areas of southern Japan.[31,32] This work made it much easier to associate HTLV-1 with leukemia, since it is not prevalent in other types of leukemia and because ATL is a rare and unique leukemia. The development of the HTLV-1 blood test allowed us to make the association of HTLV-1 with ATL not only in Japan, but also in the Caribbean and other areas.[33–36] It also led to the realization that the virus causes a variety of other diseases as well, notably a multiple sclerosis-like disease called tropical spastic paraparesis (TSP), also known as HTLV-associated myelopathy.[37,38] HTLV-1 is transmitted most efficiently by breast feeding,[39,40] a finding which has led to significant reductions in mother-to-child transmission, an important route of infection with HTLV-1. Consequently, the incidence in Japan of both infection and ATL has declined precipitously.

The same techniques led to the isolation and characterization of the second human retrovirus, HTLV-2, from a T cell line derived from a patient with hairy cell leukemia.[41,42] HTLV-2 is

numerous isolates of HIV. Our papers resulting from this work described viral detections and some true isolates (in the sense of continuous culture and production of virus) from a total of 48 different patients.[55] We were able to produce six of these isolates in continuously growing T cell lines.[56] This was important because now, for the first time, sufficient virus could be produced for a detailed characterization and for the development of a practicable blood test for serum antibodies to HIV. This test, along with the isolates of the same virus from many AIDS patients, provided confidence that this virus (called HTLV-3 by us and LAV[Bru] by Montagnier's group) was indeed the cause of AIDS.[57]

A controversy occurred during this time period that stemmed from the unusually high similarities between Montagnier's LAV(Bru) and our HTLV-3B. It was recognized by then that each HIV 1 isolate differed significantly from all other isolates, LAV(Bru) and HTLV-IIIB were nearly identical, and both labs had exchanged cultures. This controversy was largely resolved when it was discovered that a contamination from a third culture had occurred in both labs. Both our lab[58] and, shortly thereafter, Montagnier's lab[59] sequenced early cultures of LAV(Bru) and, to our surprise, found it to be distinct from the published sequences of both LAV(Bru) and HTLV-3B. However, later cultures of LAV(Bru) were found to contain a different virus, one that was identical to both published sequences. This virus, LAV(Lai) originated from another patient in Montagnier's lab[59] and is an extremely aggressively growing virus. It was most likely present as a minor population in materials sent to us from Montagnier and one which contaminated several of our cultures, as it also did in Montagnier's lab. In some respects, this was a fortunate occurrence as it made available a virus that was easy to grow and it helped accelerate subsequent work such as the development of a blood test and proof that HIV was the cause of AIDS.

Proving HIV to be the cause of AIDS provided some special challenges. One was the long period between the initial infection and the onset of AIDS, which can be longer than fifteen years. A second difficulty was that AIDS results in numerous other infections, raising the question of which is the relevant infection. There were also concerns that rapid progress required rapid verification, and two factors complicated this goal. First, samples from AIDS patients were hard to obtain, and some institutions even forbade their entry because of fears of infection. Second, T-cell culture techniques, although practiced by immunology laboratories, were not widely used in virology laboratories. These factors made it difficult to rapidly and conclusively confirm HIV isolations. This made the blood test quite urgent for a number of reasons. First, it could prevent transmission of HIV by contaminated blood. Second, it would allow us to follow the epidemic from the earliest period of infection. Third, it would be required for showing HIV to be the cause of AIDS. The test that was developed for serum antibodies proved to be simple, inexpensive, safe, rapid, sensitive, and accurate, and consisted of an initial ELISA test followed by a confirmatory Western blot if the ELISA were positive. Although the HIV blood test was quickly adapted by large companies that could make the test available on an industrial scale, we probably could have done better. For example, we could have tested the products used by hemophiliacs in 1984 even without large scale production of the test.

To briefly revisit that period (1983–1986), I will mention some of the noteworthy advances here. These include discovering HIV;[54–56] providing convincing evidence that it was the cause of AIDS;[57,60,61] understanding the routes of transmission; completely sequencing the viral genome;[62–64] identifying and defining most genes and their protein products (although some of their functions were not understood);[65–67] identifying the main target cells (CD4+ T cells, macrophages, and brain microglial cells);[68,69] the generation and distribution of reagents to scientists all over the world; a realization of the genomic heterogeneity, including microvariation within a single patient;[70,71] development of the blood test, the first practical life-saving advance;[61,72] establishment of the SIV-monkey model;[73,74] initiating antiretroviral therapy;[75] and beginning to understand some of the pathogenic mechanisms.[76]

We were lucky in many respects that AIDS came when it did and not earlier. The replication cycle of animal retroviruses was largely elucidated in the 1970s, so we had a fundamental idea of the biology involved once HIV was shown to be the cause. Many of the basic tools of molecular biology were also in place by this time. These included monoclonal antibodies, the ability to grow human T cells with IL-2, and experience with other human retroviruses. However, we were also unlucky in some respects that AIDS came when it did, since people had become much less concerned about infectious diseases. Society appears to have a memory span no longer than one generation. Here are three examples: First, there was surprise and lack of preparation in 1918 for the great influenza epidemic, due to forgetting lessons of the late 19th century.[77] Second, there was also surprise and lack of preparation at the onset of the polio epidemic in the late 1940s and early 1950s.[78] Accounts of that period show that both medical science and society as a whole believed serious infectious diseases had been conquered. Third, the same attitude was again prevalent in the 1970s, as shown by closure of microbiology departments and threats of decreasing support to the U. S. Centers for Disease Control and Prevention (CDC).

The Future

Understanding the cause of the epidemic was not accomplished by a single group. Montagnier's group and my own identified the virus and showed it to be the etiologic agent. The CDC, however, was instrumental in identifying and tracking the epidemic, but did not—and cannot—have expertise with every category of microbe. They had no expertise in animal or human retroviruses. I became involved only after a lecture by the James Curran of the CDC calling for help from virologists. I believe that the government should provide base support for national virus centers, with expertise in all categories of viruses. These centers would be able to provide needed expertise to the CDC for etiologic agents, diagnostics, and perhaps therapy and prevention.

References

1. Ellerman V, Bang O. Experimentelle leukämie bei hühnern. Zentralbl Bakteriol Parasitenkd Infectionskr Hyg Abt Orig 1908;46:595.
2. Rous P. A transmissible avian neoplasm (Sarcoma of the common fowl). J Exp Med 1910;12:696.
3. Bittner JJ, Evans CA, Green RG. Survival of the mammary tumor milk agents of mice. Science 1945;101(2613):95–97.
4. Gross L. Neck tumors, or leukemia, developing in adult C3H mice following inoculation, in early infancy, with filtered (Berkefeld N), or centrifugated (144,000 X g), Ak-leukemic extracts. Cancer 1953;6(5):948–958.
5. Jarrett WF, Crawford EM, Martin WB, Davie F. A virus-like particle associated with leukemia (lymphosarcoma). Nature 1964;202:567–569.
6. Jarrett WF, Martin WB, Crighton GW, Dalton RG, Stewart MF. Transmission experiments with leukemia (lymphosarcoma). Nature 1964;202:566–567.
7. Hardy WD, Jr., Old LJ, Hess PW, Essex M, Cotter S. Horizontal transmission of feline leukaemia virus. Nature 1973;244(5414):266–269.
8. Kawakami TG, Huff SD, Buckley PM, Dungworth DL, Synder SP, Gilden RV. C-type virus associated with gibbon lymphosarcoma. Nat New Biol 1972;235(58):170–171.
9. Theilen GH, Gould D, Fowler M, Dungworth DL. C-type virus in tumor tissue of a woolly monkey (Lagothrix spp.) with fibrosarcoma. J Natl Cancer Inst 1971;47(4):881–889.
10. Schlom J, Spiegelman S. Simultaneous detection of reverse transcriptase and high molecular weight RNA unique to oncogenic RNA viruses. Science 1971;174(11):840–843.

11. Reitz MS, Smith RG, Roseberry EA, Gallo RC. DNA-directed and RNA-primed DNA synthesis in microsomal and mitochondrial fractions of normal human lymphocytes. Biochem Biophys Res Commun 1974;57(3):934–948.

12. Bobrow SN, Smith RG, Reitz MS, Gallo RC. Stimulated normal human lymphocytes contain a ribonuclease-sensitive DNA polymerase distinct from viral RNA-directed DNA polymerase. Proc Natl Acad Sci U S A 1972;69(11):3228–3232.

13. Robert MS, Smith RG, Gallo RC, Sarin PS, Abrell JW. Viral and cellular DNA polymerase: comparison of activities with synthetic and natural RNA templates. Science 1972;176(36):798–800.

14. Goodman NC, Spiegelman S. Distinguishing reverse transcriptase of an RNA tumor virus from other known DNA polymerases. Proc Natl Acad Sci U S A 1971;68(9):2203–2206.

15. Abrell JW, Gallo RC. Purification, characterization, and comparison of the DNA polymerases from two primate RNA tumor viruses. J Virol 1973;12(3):431–439.

16. Abrell JW, Reitz MS, Gallo RC. Transcription of 70S RNA by DNA polymerases from mammalian RNA viruses. J Virol 1975;16(6):1566–1574.

17. Morgan DA, Ruscetti FW, Gallo R. Selective in vitro growth of T lymphocytes from normal human bone marrows. Science 1976;193(4257):1007–1008.

18. Ruscetti FW, Morgan DA, Gallo RC. Functional and morphologic characterization of human T cells continuously grown in vitro. J Immunol 1977;119(1):131–138.

19. Gallo RC, Gallagher RE, Wong-Staal F, et al. Isolation and tissue distribution of type-C virus and viral components from a gibbon ape (Hylobates lar) with lymphocytic leukemia. Virology 1978;84(2):359–373.

20. Poiesz BJ, Ruscetti FW, Mier JW, Woods AM, Gallo RC. T-cell lines established from human T-lymphocytic neoplasias by direct response to T-cell growth factor. Proc Natl Acad Sci U S A 1980;77(11):6815–6819.

21. Poiesz BJ, Ruscetti FW, Gazdar AF, Bunn PA, Minna JD, Gallo RC. Detection and isolation of type C retrovirus particles from fresh and cultured lymphocytes of a patient with cutaneous T-cell lymphoma. Proc Natl Acad Sci U S A 1980;77(12):7415–7419.

22. Poiesz BJ, Ruscetti FW, Reitz MS, Kalyanaraman VS, Gallo RC. Isolation of a new type C retrovirus (HTLV) in primary uncultured cells of a patient with Sezary T-cell leukaemia. Nature 1981;294(5838):268–271.

23. Kalyanaraman VS, Sarngadharan MG, Poiesz B, Ruscetti FW, Gallo RC. Immunological properties of a type C retrovirus isolated from cultured human T-lymphoma cells and comparison to other mammalian retroviruses. J Virol 1981;38(3):906–915.

24. Reitz MS, Poiesz BJ, Ruscetti FW, Gallo RC. Characterization and distribution of nucleic acid sequences of a novel type C retrovirus isolated from neoplastic human T lymphocytes. Proc Natl Acad Sci U S A 1981;78(3):1887–1891.

25. Gallo RC, Mann D, Broder S, et al. Human T-cell leukemia-lymphoma virus (HTLV) is in T but not B lymphocytes from a patient with cutaneous T-cell lymphoma. Proc Natl Acad Sci U S A 1982;79(18):5680–5683.

26. Miyoshi I, Kubonishi I, Yoshimoto S, Shiraishi Y. A T-cell line derived from normal human cord leukocytes by co-culturing with human leukemic T-cells. Gann 1981;72(6):978–981.

27. Popovic M, Reitz MS, Jr., Sarngadharan MG, et al. The virus of Japanese adult T-cell leukaemia is a member of the human T-cell leukaemia virus group. Nature 1982;300(5887):63–66.

28. Gallo R, Wong-Staal F, Montagnier L, Haseltine WA, Yoshida M. HIV/HTLV gene nomenclature. Nature 1988;333(6173):504.

29. Blayney DW, Blattner WA, Jaffe ES, Gallo RC. Retroviruses in human leukemia. Hematol Oncol 1983;1(3):193–204.

30. Shaw GM, Broder S, Essex M, Gallo RC. Human T-cell leukemia virus: its discovery and role in leukemogenesis and immunosuppression. Adv Intern Med 1984;30:1–27.

31. Takatsuki K, Uchiyama T, Sagawa K, Yodoi J. [Surface markers of malignant lymphoid cells in the classification of lymphoproliferative disorders, with special reference to adult T-cell leukemia (author's transl)]. Rinsho Ketsueki 1976;17(4):416–421.

32. Uchiyama T, Yodoi J, Sagawa K, Takatsuki K, Uchino H. Adult T-cell leukemia: clinical and hematologic features of 16 cases. Blood 1977;50(3):481–492.

33. Kalyanaraman VS, Sarngadharan MG, Bunn PA, Minna JD, Gallo RC. Antibodies in human sera reactive against an internal structural protein of human T-cell lymphoma virus. Nature 1981;294(5838):271–273.

34. Robert-Guroff M, Ruscetti FW, Posner LE, Poiesz BJ, Gallo RC. Detection of the human T cell lymphoma virus p19 in cells of some patients with cutaneous T cell lymphoma and leukemia using a monoclonal antibody. J Exp Med 1981;154(6):1957–1964.

35. Blattner WA, Kalyanaraman VS, Robert-Guroff M, et al. The human type-C retrovirus, HTLV, in Blacks from the Caribbean region, and relationship to adult T-cell leukemia/lymphoma. Int J Cancer 1982;30(3):257–264.

36. Yoshida M, Miyoshi I, Hinuma Y. Isolation and characterization of retrovirus from cell lines of human adult T-cell leukemia and its implication in the disease. Proc Natl Acad Sci U S A 1982;79(6):2031–2035.

37. Osame M, Usuku K, Izumo S, et al. HTLV-I associated myelopathy, a new clinical entity. Lancet 1986;1(8488):1031–1032.

38. Gessain A, Barin F, Vernant JC, et al. Antibodies to human T-lymphotropic virus type-I in patients with tropical spastic paraparesis. Lancet 1985;2(8452):407–410.

39. Kinoshita K, Amagasaki T, Hino S, et al. Milk borne transmission of HTLV-I from carrier mothers to their children. Jpn J Cancer Res 1987;78(7):674–680

40. Ando Y, Nakano S, Saito K, et al. Transmission of adult T-cell leukemia retrovirus (HTLV-I) from mother to child: comparison of bottle- with breast-fed babies. Jpn J Cancer Res 1987;78(4):322–324.

41. Kalyanaraman VS, Sarngadharan MG, Robert-Guroff M, Miyoshi I, Golde D, Gallo RC. A new subtype of human T-cell leukemia virus (HTLV-II) associated with a T-cell variant of hairy cell leukemia. Science 1982;218(4572):571–573.

42. Reitz MS, Popovic M, Haynes BF, Clark SC, Gallo RC. Relatedness by nucleic acid hybridization of new isolates of human T-cell leukemia-lymphoma virus (HTLV) and demonstration of provirus in uncultured leukemic blood cells. Virology 1983;126(2):688–72.

43. Chen YM, Jang YJ, Kanki PJ, et al. Isolation and characterization of simian T-cell leukemia virus type II from New World monkeys. J Virol 1994;68(2):1149–1157.

44. Watanabe T, Seiki M, Tsujimoto H, Miyoshi I, Hayami M, Yoshida M. Sequence homology of the simian retrovirus genome with human T-cell leukemia virus type I. Virology 1985;144(1):59–65.

45. Guo HG, Wong-Staal F, Gallo RC. Novel viral sequences related to human T-cell leukemia virus in T cells of a seropositive baboon. Science 1984;223(4641):1195–1197.

46. Giri A, Markham P, Digilio L, Hurteau G, Gallo RC, Franchini G. Isolation of a novel simian T-cell lymphotropic virus from Pan paniscus that is distantly related to the human T-cell leukemia/lymphotropic virus types I and II. J Virol 1994;68(12):8392–8395.

47. Liu HF, Vandamme AM, Van BM, Desmyter J, Goubau P. New retroviruses in human and simian T-lymphotropic viruses. Lancet 1994;344(8917):265–266.

48. Calattini S, Chevalier SA, Duprez R, et al. Discovery of a new human T-cell lymphotropic virus (HTLV-3) in Central Africa. Retrovirology 2005;2:30.

49. Wolfe ND, Heneine W, Carr JK, et al. Emergence of unique primate T-lymphotropic viruses among central African bushmeat hunters. Proc Natl Acad Sci U S A 2005;102(22):7994–7999.

50. Wernicke D, Trainin Z, Ungar-Waron H, Essex M. Humoral immune response of asymptomatic cats naturally infected with feline leukemia virus. J Virol 1986;60(2):669–673.

51. Essex M, McLane MF, Lee TH, et al. Antibodies to cell membrane antigens associated with human T-cell leukemia virus in patients with AIDS. Science 1983;220(4599):859–862.

52. Gallo RC, Sarin PS, Gelmann EP, et al. Isolation of human T-cell leukemia virus in acquired immune deficiency syndrome (AIDS). Science 1983;220(4599):865–867.

53. Gelmann EP, Popovic M, Blayney D, et al. Proviral DNA of a retrovirus, human T-cell leukemia virus, in two patients with AIDS. Science 1983;220(4599):862–865.

54. Barre-Sinoussi F, Chermann JC, Rey F, et al. Isolation of a T-lymphotropic retrovirus from a patient at risk for acquired immune deficiency syndrome (AIDS). Science 1983;220(4599):868–871.

55. Gallo RC, Salahuddin SZ, Popovic M, et al. Frequent detection and isolation of cytopathic retroviruses (HTLV III) from patients with AIDS and at risk for AIDS. Science 1984;224:500–503.

56. Popovic M, Sarngadharan MG, Read E, Gallo RC. Detection, isolation, and continuous production of cytopathic retroviruses (HTLV-III) from patients with AIDS and pre-AIDS. Science 1984;224(4648):497–500.

57. Sarngadharan MG, Popovic M, Bruch L, Schupbach J, Gallo RC. Antibodies reactive with human T-lymphotropic retroviruses (HTLV-III) in the serum of patients with AIDS. Science 1984;224(4648):506–508.

58. Guo HG, Chermann JC, Waters D, et al. Sequence analysis of original HIV-1. Nature 1991;349(6312):745–746.

59. Wain-Hobson S, Vartanian JP, Henry M, et al. LAV revisited: origins of the early HIV-1 isolates from Institut Pasteur. Science 1991;252(5008):961–965.

60. Schupbach J, Sarngadharan MG, Gallo RC. Antigens on HTLV-infected cells recognized by leukemia and AIDS sera are related to HTLV viral glycoprotein. Science 1984;224(4649):607–610.

61. Safai B, Sarngadharan MG, Groopman JE, et al. Seroepidemiological studies of human T-lymphotropic retrovirus type III in acquired immunodeficiency syndrome. Lancet 1984;1(8392):1438–1440.

62. Wain-Hobson S, Sonigo P, Danos O, Cole S, Alizon M. Nucleotide sequence of the AIDS virus, LAV. Cell 1985;40(1):9–17.

63. Sanchez-Pescador R, Power MD, Barr PJ, et al. Nucleotide sequence and expression of an AIDS-associated retrovirus (ARV-2). Science 1985;227(4686):484–492.

64. Ratner L, Haseltine W, Patarca R, et al. Complete nucleotide sequence of the AIDS virus, HTLV-III. Nature 1985;313(6000):277–284.

65. Muesing MA, Smith DH, Cabradilla CD, Benton CV, Lasky LA, Capon DJ. Nucleic acid structure and expression of the human AIDS/lymphadenopathy retrovirus. Nature 1985;313(6002):450–458.

66. Arya SK, Guo C, Josephs SF, Wong-Staal F. Trans-activator gene of human T-lymphotropic virus type III (HTLV-III). Science 1985;229(4708):69–73.

67. Robey WG, Safai B, Oroszlan S, et al. Characterization of envelope and core structural gene products of HTLV-III with sera from AIDS patients. Science 1985;228(4699):593–595.

68. Shaw GM, Gonda MA, Flickinger GH, Hahn BH, Gallo RC, Wong-Staal F. Genomes of evolutionarily divergent members of the human T-cell leukemia virus family (HTLV-I and HTLV-II) are highly conserved, especially in pX. Proc Natl Acad Sci U S A 1984;81(14):4544–4548.

69. Harper ME, Marselle LM, Gallo RC, Wong-Staal F. Detection of lymphocytes expressing human T-lymphotropic virus type III in lymph nodes and peripheral blood from infected individuals by in situ hybridization. Proc Natl Acad Sci U S A 1986;83(3):772–776.

70. Saag MS, Hahn BH, Gibbons J, et al. Extensive variation of human immunodeficiency virus type-1 in vivo. Nature 1988;334(6181):440–444.

71. Hahn BH, Shaw GM, Taylor ME, et al. Genetic variation in HTLV-III/LAV over time in patients with AIDS or at risk for AIDS. Science 1986;232(4757):1548–1553.

72. Joyce C, Anderson I. US licenses blood test for AIDS. New Sci 1985;105(1446):3–4.

73. Chakrabarti L, Guyader M, Alizon M, et al. Sequence of simian immunodeficiency virus from macaque and its relationship to other human and simian retroviruses. Nature 1987;328(6130):543–547.

74. Chalifoux LV, Ringler DJ, King NW, et al. Lymphadenopathy in macaques experimentally infected with the simian immunodeficiency virus (SIV). Am J Pathol 1987;128(1):104–110.

75. Mitsuya H, Weinhold KJ, Furman PA, et al. 3'-Azido-3'-deoxythymidine (BW A509U): an antiviral agent that inhibits the infectivity and cytopathic effect of human T-lymphotropic virus type III/lymphadenopathy-associated virus in vitro. Proc Natl Acad Sci U S A 1985;82(20):7096–7100.

76. Lane HC, Fauci AS. Immunologic abnormalities in the acquired immunodeficiency syndrome. Annu Rev Immunol 1985;3:477–500.

77. Barry JM. The Great Influenza: The Epic Story of the Deadliest Plague in History. New York: Viking;2004.

78. Oshinsky DM. Polio: An American Story. New York: Oxford University Press; 2005.

Part II

PREVENTION

second characteristic is more important, since it perceives the problem of AIDS as related to sexuality not as a generic and abstract problem, but rather as "socially discriminated forms of sexuality," deviant forms incompatible with normal sexual behavior. This medical and social normalization arose as a counterpoint aimed at controlling "sexual deviants" and "social deviants" or drug users and, based on this, established prevention measures for risk groups.[8]

Despite there being sufficient evidence that the epidemic was not restricted solely and exclusively to groups considered to be risk groups, major disease control agencies in various countries continued to defend the argument that it was a very specific epidemic concentrated in those groups and that, therefore, a natural gap would prevent it from spreading to the general population. This normative and behavioral reference became incorporated into prevention practice approaches. A set of mechanisms seeking to investigate the sexual behavior of these groups was brought into operation with initial cohort studies and, consequently, prevention strategies were designed mostly seeking to intervene based on a normative perspective of sexuality.

It was on the basis of cognitive/rational approaches centered on the concept of risk groups that behavioral theories were incorporated into prevention initiatives. This focus influenced prevention practices for many years and became the theoretical reference for most national programs throughout the world. Thus, an arsenal of normative mechanisms was put into practice in the field of prevention, aimed at disciplining and regulating people's sexual practices.[9]

In the early 1990s it was recognized that information and education efforts to prevent and reduce the risk of infection should also be extended to young adults and adolescents, as well as to the general population, considering the extension of the epidemic in countries where traditionally homosexual practices were not recognized as existing or labeled as such, and to female non-drug users, and that secondary and tertiary prevention procedures should also be incorporated.[10]

At the time, socially constructed concepts of sexuality and vulnerability began to be developed by scholars and public health officials. It can been seen, however, that the prevention measures developed in the 1980s and 1990s were directed exclusively towards meeting the public health needs of HIV-negative people. At that time, care for people living with HIV/AIDS was primarily palliative care or of a social welfare nature.

Consequently, throughout the 1990s progress was observed in controlling the epidemic in various regions of the world such as in Thailand in Asia, Uganda in Africa, and Brazil in the Americas, with the continuous practice of safer sex activities, such as reduced number of sex partners, increased male condom use and the introduction of the female condom as an alternative (albeit with limited access), and syringe and needle exchanges for injecting drug users, as well as the incorporation of bio-safety standards to reduce occupational accidents in laboratory or healthcare settings as reported by UNAIDS and referred to by many authors.[11,12]

An annual report recently released by the Joint United Nations Programme on HIV/AIDS (UNAIDS) and the World Health Organization (WHO) highlights that HIV prevention programs are making a difference.[13] As expressed by the Executive Director of UNAIDS, Michel Sidibé: "The good news is that we have evidence that the declines we are seeing are due, at least in part, to HIV prevention. However, the findings also show that prevention programming is often off the mark and that if we do a better job of getting resources and programs to where they will make most impact, quicker progress can be made and more lives saved."

Nevertheless, at the beginning of the third decade of the epidemic, HIV infection continues to spread and to affect poorer population groups and previously unaffected groups, including the female population and younger people throughout the world. The UNAIDS 2009 report estimates that 33.4 million [31.1 million–35.8 million] people are living with HIV worldwide; 2.7 million [2.4 million–3.0 million] people were newly infected in 2008; and that 2 million

[1.7–2.4 million] people died of AIDS-related illness in 2008. The data brings us to the ultimate question: What have we done right in respect to prevention approaches and strategies and what can be done to accelerate progress in the control of the epidemic globally?

Prevention Strategies and Approaches

Cognitive-Behaviorist Theories in the Field of HIV Prevention

Prevention strategies disseminated by the public health normative agencies and incorporated by health services and nongovernmental organizations particularly in the 1980s and 1990s were fundamentally based on individual behavior change with regard to sexual practices or in relation to the sharing of syringes and needles among injecting drug users.

Many of the original works outlining the major theories that are the basis for current knowledge about behavioral change theories were published in the 1970s and 1980s. These include Icek Ajzen's[14,15] articles on theories of reasoned action and planned behavior, Albert Bandura's writings on social cognitive theory,[16] and James Prochaska and Carlo DiClemente's works on what they called the "transtheoretical model."[17] More recently, interest in behavioral change theories has arisen because of their application in the areas of health, education, and criminology, leading to further research backed by institutions like the National Institutes of Health (NIH) and the UK Prime Minister's Strategy Unit. With this renewed interest, however, there is also a shift towards research into understanding the maintenance of behavioral change in addition to broadening the research base for revising current theories that focus on initial change. Most of the models used for initial HIV prevention approaches were based on one or more of the following theoretical references: (a) health belief model (Janz and Becker, 1984; Rosenstock, Strecher and Becker, 1994—found in a 1996 AIDSCAP publication)[18]; (b) social cognitive learning theory (Bandura, 1989; Castiel, 1996)[18]; and (c) theory of reasoned action (Ajzen and Fishbein, 1975 & 1980)[18]; and (d) the AIDS risk reduction model (ARRM) (Catania, Kegeles, and Coates, 1990).[19]

The health belief model (HBM) assumes that people's attitudes and beliefs influence their health status, given that in everyday life they face situations that require decisions in the light of the threat or risk of contracting a disease and, consequently, their evaluation of the medical and social resources available to them, such as health services, correct information, and guidance and prevention commodities. That is to say, when an individual has been the subject of an action intended to change behavior, they feel capable of perceiving the benefits and the barriers with regard to their behavior.

The principal criticism of this model is that it focuses all its action on the individual, completely ignoring other factors that influence health-related behavior, such as socioeconomic factors, the social norms of the group to which a person belongs and, the social representations of ways of coping with illness and death. This model does not allow for the comprehension of the health-illness process as a socially experienced and shared condition and, therefore, is unable to situate itself within the context of the culture that involves a set of social experiences, repertoires, and dramas that have a great impact on the family structure, people's emotional relationships, and networks of social interaction.

Social cognitive learning theory is a learning theory based on the ideas that people learn by observing what others do ("modeling") and that human thought processes are central to understanding personality. While social cognitists agree that there is a fair amount of influence on development generated by learned behavior displayed in the environment in which one grows up, they believe that the individual person (and therefore cognition) is just as important in determining moral development.[16] People learn by observing others, with the environment, behavior, and cognition all as the chief factors in influencing development. These three factors are not static or independent; rather, they are all reciprocal. For example, each behavior witnessed can change a person's way of thinking (cognition). Similarly, the environment one is raised in may influence later behaviors.

This model prioritizes the stages of learning in adopting safer sex practices. According to Castiel, the learning stages include the following: (1) the moment when behavior change starts; (2) the measurement of the efforts made; and (3) the duration of efforts in the face of obstacles.[20] The author points out that one of the weakest points of this approach is the fact that it induces guilt and victimization in individuals or "cultural" groups who engage in high-risk practices. The sequence of the learning process is said to be directly related to the individual's possible cognitive capacity to judge what is right and what is wrong and, therefore, decide on the most appropriate behavior in the face of risky situations.

Social cognitive theory is applied today in many different arenas, such as mass media, public health, education, and marketing. A familiar example is the use of celebrities to endorse or promote products or behaviors such as condom use to certain segments of the population. By choosing the proper gender, age, and ethnicity, the use of social cognitive theory is said to help ensure the success of an AIDS campaign pitched to urban city youth by promoting identity with a recognizable peer, a greater sense of self-efficacy, and imitation of the actions presented in order to learn the proper prevention and actions for a more highly informed, AIDS-aware community.[21]

The theory of reasoned action (TRA) was proposed by Ajzen and Fishbein.[14,15] The components of TRA are three general constructs: behavioral intention (BI), attitude (A), and subjective norm (SN). TRA suggests that a person's behavioral intention depends on the person's attitude about the behavior and subjective norms. A person's voluntary behavior is said to be predicted by his/her attitude toward that behavior and how he/she thinks other people would view them if they performed the behavior. It is also based on the principle that behavior is defined by four components: action, objective, context, and time. It is a more comprehensive and complex theory than the previous ones, in that it posits the changing of a risk behavior is the result of individual *and* collective action. Action is not the product of particular behaviors between people, but rather human behavior that depends on the actions of others motivated by objectives and values, in addition to being determined historically.

The great limitation of this theory is that it supposes that all behaviors and attitudes in the face of a situation involving risk have intentionality, are rationally assimilated, and are marked by the values of the group to which the person belongs. A human action does indeed comprise these components, but the response on the subjective level can be very different and interspersed by pragmatic actions without the interference of rationally motivated behaviors.

One aspect of this theory should be highlighted, since it allows progress to be made in the relationship between epidemiology and the socio-cultural dimension in terms of HIV/AIDS prevention work. As the action is normative, it can be perceived by the individual or group, and this enables the individual or group to recognize that other people are changing their behavior and those with whom they interact most closely can provide support with the change. The normative force of the group acts on people, creating feelings of self-confidence and self-esteem. The problem resides, fundamentally, in failing to recognize that the normative structures also act against individuals. This can be seen in the countless situations in which the rights of people living with HIV and AIDS are violated, as a result of the widespread prejudice and the exclusion of the group when different opinions and views are raised against such structures.

The AIDS Risk Reduction Model (ARRM) was introduced in 1990 and provides a framework for explaining and predicting the behavior change efforts of individuals specifically in relationship to the sexual transmission of HIV/ AIDS. A three-stage model, the ARRM incorporates several variables from other behavior change theories, including the Health Belief Model, "efficacy" theory, emotional influences, and interpersonal processes. The stages, as well as the hypothesized factors that influence the successful completion of each stage (please see attached diagram), are as follows:[19]

Stage 1: Recognition and labeling of one's behavior as high risk;

Stage 2: Making a commitment to reduce high-risk sexual contacts and to increase low-risk activities;

Stage 3: Taking action. This stage is broken down into three phases: (1) information seeking; (2) obtaining remedies; (3) enacting solutions. Depending on the individual, phases may occur concurrently or phases may be skipped.

A general limitation of the ARRM model, as with others, is its focus on the individual. For instance, many women feel at risk for HIV, not due to their own behavior but because of the behaviors of their sexual partners, and report it as an issue outside of their control.[22] Thus, when applying behavioral models, there is a need to take into greater consideration the social-cultural issues that influence or limit an individual's behavior choices and ability to take action.

The behavioral models we have presented above are some of the models in practice (mostly in the 1980's and 90's) for those working with STD/HIV/AIDS prevention. These are theories used to seek responses in the practical field and to guide different strategies in order to move towards safer sexual practices among the most affected populations. Some of the early strategies adopted were: the peer education approach, communication campaigns, capacity building and training of outreach workers to operate in specific social networks (CSW and MSM), and training of community health workers among others. Nevertheless, few studies truly evaluate the impact of these strategies and practices on changing risk behaviors of persons and groups. Under a similar perspective, Martin Bloom[23] gives us a broad and practical view point of primary prevention practices based on cognitive learning theories that also considers the person's social context (environment) and life course events (time frame) as important elements necessary for interaction to take place and adequate functioning or elimination of the harmful environmental agent to occur. Bloom considered primary prevention to be those promotive actions that support a person in making environmental changes and strengthening resistance. Bloom's "configurational equation" for achievement of high-level potentials is summarized in the **Figure 3–1**.

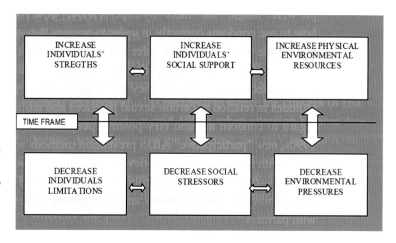

Figure 3–1. *Primary prevention practice—configuarational equation. Source: Bloom, M. 1996. Primary prevention practices. Thousand Oaks, CA: SAGE. Used with permission.*

social and economic conditions inherent to the lack of power, are the risk factors that most influence precarious health conditions.[39] This is also the process by which socially excluded or marginalized people mobilize themselves to gain control over their health and lives. The fight by groups against gender and racial oppression, economic exploitation, political repression, or foreign intervention helps to build the self-confidence needed for their actions.

An empowered or strengthened community uses its resources, the skills of its members and its organizations, to meet community or collective needs. Interventions using empowerment approaches need to consider concepts regarding practices and beliefs related to interpersonal, community, and organizational changes, while also focusing collective capacity building and community mobilization as being crucial for more dynamic and innovative efforts in response to the structural factors of the epidemic.

The teachings of Freire[37] related more to the tradition of popular education in Latin America. He considered that the "raised awareness" of a person or group is the result of a dialogue-based participation of an individual or community affected by a situation in common in the collective planning and implementation of a response to that problem or situation. Social change is said to take place through collective construction and the perception of the social, cultural, economic, and political strength that structures reality, and acts against the forces perceived to be oppressive.

Under the pedagogical formulations of Paulo Freire,[37] the educational process is described as libertarian and dialogic. It is a socio-political approach, intended to build a critical perception of the socio-cultural and political-economic forces that structure reality, motivating and facilitating action against oppressive forces. This view is in contrast to the model that sees education as an act of specialists offering information and knowledge to the "uneducated", without the construction of the critical perception of socio-cultural forces or the joint identification of the needs and vulnerabilities of the community or group, or the participatory planning of possible strategies and local responses.

The socio-political approach considers individuals as active agents in their communities and subcultures, capable of reaching an understanding of their symbolic universe through a process of sensitization and raising of awareness, thus being able to modify or recreate it, instead of passively accepting it. With regard to the socio-political view, Gayle Rubin,[40] when examining gender and race politics from a social construction point of view, also considers that when sexuality and sex are understood through social analysis and historical comprehension, a political and social view of sexuality becomes possible, whereby "sexual policy" is thought of in terms of population, communities, forms of migration, settlement, conflict, marginalization, inequality, and forms of oppression.

Further developments of Freire's reflections are presented by Paiva,[41] who opts for "libertarian education" as a means of encouraging collective organization and believes in the production of responses by those who are directly affected and living in the context of vulnerability. She observes that approaches to prevention and the promotion of safer sex, such as "lectures, leaflets and campaigns do not create 'sexual subjects', nor do they improve people's self-esteem so that they decide to avoid risk, and they do not impose safe practices as priorities put into everyday practice, rather than just the intention to do so. ..."[41]

Paiva emphasizes the need to politicize the psycho-educative spaces and proposes the notion of "psychosocial emancipation" as one of the references for enhancing the application of the notion of vulnerability. She states that: "in the psycho-educative spaces, the process has gained from slow learning and from the impact of safer sex workshops on a group or community or, more recently, the organization of interactive sessions of medication adherence groups in reference services or non-governmental organizations."[41] Nevertheless, the author observes that the sexuality dealt with in such contexts is "everyone's sexuality," as if everyone had the same sexual practices, "without considering their particular aspects in each sexual scene, in each socio-cultural context." Furthermore, as a consequence of the simplified view, "the target population is always considered to be HIV negative and to need to protect itself from potentially HIV positive people."[42]

Pedagogical approaches that attempt to encourage the capacity of being critical and thinking systematically, based on the individual's own positions in life, tend to be more consistent, long-lasting, and, therefore, more successful. Such approaches generally start from matters of everyday life and the concerns of groups and people, rather than the concerns of specialists, in contrast to the pedagogical approach that sees the minds of those who are being educated as "empty receptacles" waiting to be filled with the good and intelligent ideas of specialists in intervention and communication.

In summary, the adoption of preventive or protective measures is not restricted to individual decision, or to access to correct information about forms of transmission and protection. The understanding and incorporation of safer sex practices in relation to HIV/AIDS and sexual health are the result of a dynamic process, built based on social experiences or, using the terminology of Gagnon and Simon,[29] the result of social and cultural scenarios and interpersonal scripts or, putting it more simply, the vision of the world by the subjects in question.

Having moved from the concepts of risk and individual responsibility to the concept of vulnerability and, therefore, to the conceptualization of the social dimensions and dynamics of HIV infection, we can see that there has been a fundamental transformation, over the course of time, of the paradigms that have formed and guided the responses to the epidemic in the last decades. This transformation has taken place in relation to the notions of education about AIDS, moving from individualist information-driven models, to more multidimensional models of collective awareness raising and community mobilization, as potentially more effective strategies, which aims to produce more resistant and long-lasting responses.

Further developments of this reflection include Paulo Freire's notion of awareness raising as a constructive social process based on dialogue, that enables one to act with others to correct social injustices and inequalities as the essence of community "qualification" and mobilization as a strategy for fighting AIDS. The participatory working methodology, which sees a person as the "subject and protagonist" of their responses and which promotes the commitment of local networks, is capable of generating a sense of solidarity and fighting for a common objective and for citizenship.

We therefore reach the conclusion that, in order for us to advance and be more effective with prevention work, prevention models need to be built by integrating various levels of theoretical frameworks and concepts. It needs to work on the diverse dimensions of vulnerability (individual, social and programmatic), through proposals for structural and cultural interventions that take into consideration the subjects and their peers in their social and collective environment, but which also consider the subject on the individual level, with feelings and subjectivities, as the owner of his or her own personal history, and with unique interpersonal and sexual scripts and scenarios.

Community Participation and Solidarity

The discussion on how to reduce social exclusion and social inequalities as factors of vulnerability to HIV is present in current national and international debates in various areas, such as the transmission per unprotected sexual act.[75] A threshold below which HIV transmission does not occur has not been established. Women may intermittently shed HIV in breast milk, and HIV RNA has been detected in more than 80% of women when more than one breast milk sample was analyzed.[64] In a longitudinal study of serial samples of breast milk over a 2-year period of time, women who had higher detectable HIV levels and were consistent shedders of virus in their breast milk were more likely to transmit HIV to their infants.[47] Transmission of HIV infection through breast milk can occur at any time during lactation, but the highest risk seems to occur during the first few weeks of life. During this period, the milk is high in cellular content and appears to have higher viral loads than milk produced later in pregnancy.[40] Beyond the first month of breastfeeding, the rate of HIV transmission remains relatively stable.

A number of other risk factors have been associated with breastfeeding, including presence of overt or subclinical mastitis, breast abscess, maternal HIV seroconversion in the postpartum period, maternal systemic illness, nonexclusive breastfeeding, abrupt weaning, and oral thrush in infants younger than 6 months of age.[67,76–79]

The exact mechanism of breast milk transmission is not well defined. HIV could be directly introduced into the intestinal submucosa through defects in the epithelial cell layer of the intestinal mucosa or tight junctions between intestinal epithelial cells. Once HIV penetrates this epithelial layer, the virus has direct access to CD4 cells that reside in the Peyers patch of the intestinal submucosal layer. Alternatively, HIV could be actively transported through highly specialized cells in the intestinal mucosa to submucosal lymphocytes. Recent evidence supports the suggestion that HIV-specific immunity is critical to the prevention of neonatal HIV infection and likely involves innate, humoral, and cellular responses. Innate immune responses thought to be important to HIV vertical transmission include chemokine[80] and mucosal surface proteins.[80] Breast milk, cervicovaginal secretions, and placental tissue all contain detectable levels of chemokines, which may block or downregulate the HIV coreceptors CCR5 and CXCR4 and interfere with viral infection of host cells. The mucosal surface protein SLPI is found in breast milk, genital secretions, and saliva and has anti-HIV properties.[81] Higher levels of SLPI in vaginal secretions and infant saliva have been shown to correlate with lower levels of HIV transmission.[82] Each 100 ng/mL increase in salivary SLPI was associated with a 50% decreased risk in HIV transmission after 1 month.[82]

Humoral immune responses, mainly neutralizing antibodies, play an important role in preventing infant HIV infection. In a study comparing mothers who transmitted HIV with those who did not, in utero transmitters were much less likely to have neutralizing antibodies to their own HIV strain than those who did not transmit virus. Interestingly, infants were not inherently resistant to neutralizing antibody from other mothers, suggesting that viral selection as a result of antibody pressure may occur.[83] Infants have also been shown to generate their own neutralizing antibodies in response to challenge with HIV antigens.[84,85]

Cellular immune responses are also found to be important in maternal and infant response. Maternal cellular response includes CD8$^+$ cytotoxic lymphocyte (CTL) and CD4$^+$ T-helper responses. A similar selective pressure occurs as HIV-exposed infants often become infected with a viral strain that has escaped maternal CTL response.[40]

Transmission by Intravenous Drugs

Introduction of HIV into the injecting drug user (IDU) community likely occurred very early in the HIV epidemic. Serosurvey studies conducted on banked serum samples from IDUs entering treatment centers in New York revealed that 9% (1 of 11) of specimens collected in 1978 tested positive for HIV. Once introduced into this population, HIV appeared to spread quickly. By 1979, seroprevalence rose to 26%, increased further to 38% in 1980, and reached a plateau of 55%–60% by 1984.[86] A similar trend was described in Europe, with 51% of IDUs in Edinburgh, Scotland, and 62% of IDUs in Milan, Italy, showing evidence of HIV infection by the mid-1980s.[87–89] In Asia, HIV spread at an even more alarming rate among IDUs. In Bangkok, Thailand, seroprevalence among IDUs was estimated at 1% in 1987, 15% by March of 1988, and 43% by December of that same year.[90]

Recent evidence suggests that HIV transmission through injection drugs continues to increase globally.[86,87] Injecting drug use accounts for 10% of HIV transmissions globally and up to 30% of new HIV infections each year outside of Sub-Saharan Africa. An increasing number of IDUs have been reported from countries with previously low rates of injecting drug use. Recent reports suggest that 42% of IDUs in Ukraine and 38% of IDUs in Russia are infected with HIV.[86] China, which has the largest population of IDUs in the world, is also at risk for a transition to a generalized HIV epidemic. Although HIV prevalence among IDUs in China is reported to be 12%, there are localized areas—such as Dehong Prefecture, in Yunnan Province— where HIV prevalence is estimated to be 54%, and IDUs make up the majority of persons living with HIV.[86]

Transmission of HIV among IDUs occurs primarily through contamination of injection equipment, which is reused by an uninfected IDU. Behaviors that increase the magnitude and frequency of exposure increase the risk for infection. Among IVDs in the U.S., race, ethnicity, low income, male gender, and a diagnosis of antisocial personality have all been associated with a higher prevalence of infection. African Americans and Hispanics have significantly higher seroprevalence than white, non-Hispanics. Gender risk appears to differ on the basis of geographic variation. In New York, seroprevalence has been reported to be 13% higher in male than female IVDs, whereas in San Francisco, no significant gender difference has been noted. Antisocial personality has been associated with more frequent needle sharing, sharing with a greater number of partners, and greater concomitant use of alcohol and cocaine.

Sharing needles, syringes, and other equipment is a major risk factor for HIV transmission and is largely driven by legal and economic necessity. HIV seroprevalence correlates with reported frequency of needle sharing.[89,91] In Edinburgh, seroprevalence was 30% among users who denied sharing equipment, 56% among those who reported sharing sometimes, and 75% among those who reported that they consistently shared needles or equipment.[89] Sharing with multiple partners is also a risk. In a San Francisco study, HIV seroprevalence was 3% among IDUs who denied sharing, 9% in those who reported sharing with only one other person, and 15% among those reported to share with two or more people on a regular basis.[92] Risk of HIV transmission is also increased in IDUs who frequent "shooting galleries," where drug equipment is made available for rent or sharing, and the potential for exposure to dozens of users is great.[93]

Sexual transmission among IDUs is a major driving force of the HIV epidemic. For female IDUs, having a male sexual partner who is HIV-positive is an independent risk factor for acquiring HIV infection.[94] In Milan, an IDU with a seropositive partner is four times more likely to seroconvert, after controlling for syringe sharing and other risk factors.[95] High-risk sexual behavior is more common among IDUs, and often includes partners outside the IDU community. A study of IDUs in Russia reported that more than 80% of IDUs had sex without condoms and that 44% of IDUs had sex with a partner who did not inject drugs.[96] Frequent trading of sex for money or drugs is common and is an independent risk factor for acquiring HIV infection. In several Russian studies, more than 30% of IDUs have reported a history of sex work.[97] Homosexual and bisexual IDUs are at significantly increased risk for HIV infection, not only because of sexual transmission but also because of the exceedingly high prevalence of HIV in their needle-sharing group.

Significant effort has been spent on programs and measures to reduce the transmission of HIV through injecting drug use. Needle and syringe exchange programs, drug counseling and treatment, education regarding safe injection, and safer sexual practices and testing programs have been shown to reduce HIV transmission.[96]

Transmission by Blood, Blood Product, and Tissue Transplantation

HIV transmission through contaminated blood products is very efficient. More than 90% of recipients transfused with an HIV-seropositive blood component become infected.[98] Transmissions have been documented for red cells, whole blood, fresh-frozen plasma, platelets, and clotting factors.[99] Storage and processing may affect infectiousness of the product.[100] Risk for infection decreases as storage time increases. Unwashed HIV-contaminated red blood cells are 95% infectious if stored for fewer than 8 days. When stored for greater than 3 weeks, the unit is only 50% infectious.[98] Risk for transmission is also associated with donor's HIV RNA blood levels, but other donor factors have not been shown to affect transmission rates.[101] The probability of transfusion transmission also appears to be independent of the age and sex of the recipient, and reason for transfusion.[99]

Patients who acquire HIV infection from a contaminated blood product appear to have a similar rate of HIV disease progression when compared to those who acquire HIV through other modes.[102] In the U.S., 1-year overall mortality is similar among persons infected through blood transfusion versus other routes. However, one study conducted in Zaire, demonstrated that patients transfused with HIV-positive blood are 33% more likely to die within the year than are patients transfused with HIV-negative blood.[103] The explanation for this apparent geographic difference has not been determined.

The U.S. Centers for Disease Control and Prevention (CDC) estimates that, before the HIV testing of blood donations, 12,000 to 15,000 cases of transfusion-associated AIDS may have resulted.[104] Following the introduction of HIV-1 antibody testing in 1985 and the subsequent inclusion of HIV-2 antibody testing in 1986, a significant reduction in transmission risk was noted. The addition of P24 antigen testing, which was designed to identify cases of recently infected donors who had not developed antibody (window period), further reduced transmission risk. Estimates are broad, but suggest that, following the implementation of those screening methods, transmission risk in the U.S. ranged from 1/200,000 to 1/2,000,000 per unit transfused.[105,106] In 2002, the U.S. Food and Drug Administration (FDA) approved nucleic acid testing and further reduced the window period from 22 to 12 days.[107] More recent estimates suggest that risk for HIV transmission from a transfused unit of red cells is between 1/1.4 million and 1/1.8 million.[108,109] Further improvement in donor screening has also played a role in reducing HIV transmission. Eligibility screening questionnaires are routinely used to identify potential high-risk donors. However, the effectiveness of these questionnaires depends on accurate donor reporting and, unfortunately, a proportion of HIV-infected donors recognize their risk but fail to exclude themselves.[110]

Despite improved screening methods, transmission through contaminated blood products may still occur in resource-rich countries. Donations may be collected during acute HIV infection, a period in which our current screening methods fail. A limited number of chronic carriers may not develop HIV antibody and may, therefore, escape screening, and some HIV serotypes do not react to form a positive antibody test. Although unusual, technical or clerical errors may still occur.

Unfortunately, transmission of HIV through contaminated blood products continues to occur throughout many resource limited countries. Despite a much larger donation pool, only 43% of the 191 World Health Organization (WHO) states test blood for HIV, hepatitis C, and hepatitis B. At least 80,000 to 160,000 infections are thought to occur annually throughout the world as a result of transfusion-transmitted HIV. This represents 2%-4% of all cases of HIV transmission worldwide.[108,111] Impediments to safe blood transfusions in these regions include inadequate funding for measures such as HIV testing, blood donor screening, education, and counseling. Furthermore, in order to have an effective prevention screening program, it is necessary to have effective quality assessment programs, standardized test manufacturing practices, and ongoing staff training.

HIV transmission from plasma-derived products is unusual but can occur when inadequate processing is performed. Albumin and plasma are extracted with cold ethanol and then pasteurized. They do not transmit HIV when processed adequately. Immune globulin products are treated with a lower concentration of cold ethanol and cannot be pasteurized without loss of activity. However, there have not been any documented cases of HIV disease in recipients of these products. There have been reports of recipients of hepatitis B immunoglobulin becoming transiently HIV antibody positive by passive acquisition of antibodies from the product, but there has not been evidence of transmitted infections.[112,113]

HIV has been transmitted through transplantation of the kidney, liver, heart, pancreas, bone, and skin. There have not been reported cases of transmission from non-blood–containing organs or low vascular tissue such as cornea, fresh-frozen bone without marrow, lyophilized tendon, or irradiated dura mater.[114] These observations are supported by seroconversions among 48 transplant recipients who received an organ or tissue donation from a single HIV-seronegative donor without known HIV risk factors. Among the 48 recipients, 41 were tested and seven were found to be HIV positive. Four of the seven received infected organ transplants, the remaining three received fresh-frozen bone. Of the remaining 34 noninfected recipients, 25 received ethanol-treated bone, corneas, soft tissue, or dura mater.[115]

Special Populations

It is important to recognize that unique groups which share common characteristics and are at increased risk of acquiring and transmitting HIV infection exist. Identifying these groups and improving our understanding of these unique characteristics provides the opportunity for implementing interventions and altering HIV transmission cycles.

Acute HIV

Acute HIV infection has been recently recognized as a period of special importance in the dynamics of HIV transmission. Individuals with acute infection have high viral loads and lack protective antibodies. They are considered more infectious and, therefore, contribute to a higher percentage of new infections.[116] Individuals with acute infection are often unaware of their HIV seropositive status. Estimates of the total burden of HIV in the population rely on sophisticated mathematical models derived from epidemiologic data, as well as observed and projected incidence and prevalence rates. Based on these models, it is believed that 25% of those infected with HIV in the U.S. are unaware of their seropositive status. They represent a substantial risk group for HIV transmission, with estimates suggesting that they account for 54% of new HIV infections.[11] Early identification of HIV-infected individuals is considered a critical step in the global approach to limiting HIV transmission as well.[117] As a result, new recommendations for HIV testing of adults were recently updated.[118] Perhaps the most worrisome of these recent data is the observation that rates of new infection exceed rates of persons initiating HIV therapy. According to UNAIDS published data, for every two persons who start ART, five become newly infected. On the basis of these mathematical models, some authors advocate two new strategies, known as "test and treat" and "pre-exposure prophylaxis," in order to decrease rates of HIV transmission.[33] The "test and treat" approach emphasizes increased testing and earlier initiation of treatment; the "pre-exposure" method emphasizes implementing measures such as safe drug injection, condom use, and male circumcision. Both strategies recognize that uncontrolled HIV is a major driving force in an ongoing epidemic and strive to decrease exposure of HIV among uninfected persons. More research is needed in order to validate these strategies in both resource-rich and -limited countries.

Drug and Alcohol Dependence

Drug and alcohol users are a population at significant risk for acquiring and transmitting HIV infection. Marginalization, imprisonment, poor access to health care, stigmatization, and limited access to drug treatment programs represent some of the main challenges.[86,119] Active substance abuse is also associated with higher rates of comorbid medical conditions, including pyogenic bacterial infections, STDs, tuberculosis, hepatitis, and cancer. The rates of hepatitis B and hepatitis C coinfection can be as high as 86% among drug users living in urban areas, and the prevalence increases with the number of years of injection drug use.[120]

As a result of these complex medical conditions and limited access to health care, HIV-infected substance abusers are less likely to remain adherent to HIV medications and are more likely to develop HIV-resistant isolates. In turn, this group is more likely to transmit resistant strains in the community and limit treatment options in the future.

Multiple studies among a variety of populations and geographic areas have shown that sex under the influence of drugs or alcohol is associated with high-risk sexual behavior. In a recent study of 505 heterosexual men in substance abuse treatment programs, 73% admitted to having sex under the influence in the prior 90 days, and almost 40% during their most recent sexual event. Sex under the influence at the most recent event was more likely to involve anal intercourse, sex with a casual partner, and less condom use.[121]

Psychiatric illness is also a major problem among individuals addicted to drugs and alcohol.[122] HIV-infected persons diagnosed with psychiatric conditions are a vulnerable population with regard to HIV transmission. The prevalence of HIV infection in people with severe mental illness is much higher than in the general population.[123] In fact, many metropolitan areas in the U.S. during the first 2 decades of the HIV epidemic experienced a marked increase in a population characterized by HIV infection, personality disorder, homelessness, and substance abuse. This combination of comorbid conditions presented a significant challenge to public health authorities and continues to present a significant burden to these communities. As a whole, this group engages in high-risk behaviors that significantly contribute to the ongoing transmission of HIV. In a study of 101 persons with bipolar disorder and substance use, 75% of the population was sexually active, 69% of those reported unprotected intercourse, 39% reported multiple partners, 24% reported sex with prostitutes, and 10% reported commercial sex practices.[124]

Homeless persons infected with HIV are typically disenfranchised from access to health care, and only a minority of them benefit regularly from HIV care provided by outreach programs such as community health van initiatives. Homeless persons are also more likely than individuals in the general population to engage in high-risk behaviors. A recent study of 8,075 HIV-infected persons compared drug, alcohol, and sexual HIV transmission risk behaviors between homeless and housed persons living with HIV. Homeless respondents were more likely to abuse alcohol and drugs and engage in injection drug use. Sexually active homeless persons had more sex partners, and engaged more in sex exchange for money or drugs, as well as in unprotected vaginal or anal sex with an unknown serostatus partner. Housing remained a significant predictor of the number of sex partners, commercial sex, unprotected sex with a partner of unknown status, and drug and alcohol use variables.[125]

Comprehensive care of the HIV-infected drug and alcohol users must include routine preventive care, improved education for reducing high-risk behavior, and comprehensive mental health as well as substance abuse counseling and treatment programs.

Prisons

An estimated 2 million people are incarcerated in the U.S. on any given day. Recent increases in inmate populations have largely been driven by legislative changes directed toward controlling drug trafficking and use. These changes have led to an increased number of prisoners with active substance abuse and the behavioral problems that inherently accompany this condition. In turn, increased rates of commercial sex work, STDs including HIV, and mental illness are observed in inmates compared to the general population.[126]

Transmission of infectious diseases—in particular, HIV—among prisoners has always been difficult to assess. No reliable data are available for evaluation. Up to two-thirds of HIV-infected inmates are diagnosed and initiate HIV treatment for the first time during their incarceration.[127,128] Studies have shown that HIV-infected individuals who are unaware of their diagnosis are more likely to engage in high-risk sexual behavior and more likely to transmit virus. Thus, within the prison system, the cycle of infection and reinfection often continues to go unchecked in a highly susceptible population. Given the high rates of intermittent medication adherence, the risk of transmitting resistant virus is particularly high in this confined population.

Although these trends provide a significant challenge to the elimination of HIV transmission within correctional facilities, they also create a new environment for broader implementation of prevention and treatment programs. In order to be effective, such programs must include not only HIV care, but also mental health and substance abuse counseling. Not all correctional facilities in the U.S. offer comprehensive HIV programs at present. Programs have been implemented in states such as Connecticut, New York, and Massachusetts. Data published by these programs, as well as official reports from the Bureau of Justice Statistics,[129] have shown remarkable improvement in outcomes and a decrease in HIV-associated mortality of more than 75% in state prisons. A recent financial analysis of HIV health care for inmates found that comprehensive HIV care for prisoners is more cost effective than inadequate treatment.[130]

Recent data show that reincarceration is associated with worse HIV clinical outcomes.[126] The explanation for this phenomenon is likely multifactorial, but may be associated with relapse in substance abuse, disconnection with health care, and subsequent discontinuation of therapy following prison release. Relapse of behaviors that increase risk of transmission should be considered a missed opportunity, particularly in those with good virologic control while incarcerated. These missed opportunities have significant consequences, as such behaviors are likely to increase the risk for transmitting resistant virus. Careful discharge planning that stresses continuity of medical care in the community has been postulated as a key factor in achieving good clinical outcomes after prison release. The potential benefit of decreasing HIV transmission in the community by ex-inmates who have successful, long-term suppression of HIV viremia while incarcerated deserves further analysis.

Commercial Sex Workers

Commercial sex workers constitute a very heterogeneous social group, with wide variation in social acceptance among different countries. However, despite the variety of social practices, a common characteristic among all commercial sex workers is their high risk for acquiring and transmitting HIV. In most instances, commercial sex workers are exposed to more than one risk factor for HIV transmission. They tend to live fractionated, marginal lives, engaging in behaviors that are high-risk. Multiple studies have shown substantially lower rates of condom use among commercial sex workers compared to the general population.[131] Unprotected sexual encounters leads to increased rates of other STDs, further increasing the risk for HIV acquisition and transmission.[19,23] Injection drug use is also common in sex workers in most of the world. Even those who do not voluntarily use drugs are likely to be exposed to or forced into drug use as part of the trade. Behavior-modifying drugs tend to decrease the overall adherence to safe-sex practices and increase HIV transmission risk. The combination of multiple risk factors for HIV transmission is not uncommon in certain social groups. A recent study in Mombasa, Kenya, showed that transactional sexual encounters between women and MSM sex workers are frequent, and both vaginal and anal sex are often performed unprotected.[132,133] Lack of awareness of HIV seropositivity in clients seeking sex from commercial sex workers is a significant problem. Similarly, commercial sex workers are often unaware of their HIV serostatus. A recent study from the Netherlands showed that only 19% of the 108 heterosexual attendees at a STD clinic found to be HIV-positive in an anonymous survey were aware of their HIV seropositive status.[134] Lack of awareness leads to a false sense of security, increased high-risk behavior, and increased risk for disease transmission.

Therefore, broad exposures to both sexually and parenterally transmitted infections are common among and are likely underappreciated by commercial sex workers. Despite a clear need for routine health care to prevent, diagnose, and treat HIV and its associated complications in many countries, access to care is very fragmented, if at all existent. To complicate matters, physical and sexual abuse, exploitation in the form of human trafficking, and financial instability add to the social stigma and further prevent access to regular health care. Even in countries where prostitution has been legalized, the social consideration of sex workers has not improved.[135] Unfortunately, despite this bleak picture, prostitution is often presented with a hint of tolerance in Western media and the performing arts, and even with a suggestion that it is a trendy, profitable activity. Although, the motivations to join activities related to sex trade vary, awareness of the associated health risks—in particular, the risk for HIV transmission—are not always appreciated. Open discussions of safe sex practices with clients are often missing, even though such communication is vitally important. Furthermore, because workers are often forced into unsafe and unwanted practices despite understanding of the risks, interventions to improve conditions and empower choice are also important.

Occupational Exposures

Health care workers, including laboratory workers, are at risk for acquiring HIV when in contact with infectious body fluids. The complete elucidation of infective body fluids was a necessary step to implement strategies to minimize HIV transmission by occupational exposure. Fluids considered a potential source of HIV infection include blood, semen, vaginal secretions, amniotic fluid, cerebrospinal fluid, and any body fluid contaminated with blood. Conversely, urine, saliva, feces, and sweat have not been convincingly linked to HIV transmission, irrespective of whether HIV can be isolated in any of those fluids.

Preventive strategies to avoid occupational transmission of HIV supported by the CDC include the routine use of barriers (gloves, masks, etc.), meticulous washing of skin exposed to potentially contaminated body fluids, and careful handling and disposing of sharp instruments during and after use.[132] As of December 2001, the CDC had received reports of 57 documented cases of HIV seroconversion in the healthcare setting in the U.S. An additional 138 infections were considered possibly the result of occupational transmission. Underreporting is likely, given the inherent difficulty in obtaining accurate epidemiologic data outside of hospital environments. For the same reasons, the number of cases associated with occupational transmission of HIV throughout the world is not known.

A variety of accidents involving HIV-contaminated body fluids can take place in direct patient care and laboratory settings. However, the most common mechanism of occupational transmission of HIV is, by far, a percutaneous exposure to infected blood caused by a hollow-bore device (needle, catheter, etc.)—commonly referred to as "sharps." The average risk for transmission of HIV is thought to be approximately 0.3% after a percutaneous exposure to HIV-infected blood, and less than 0.1% after a mucous membrane exposure.[136,137] Intact skin exposed to contaminated body fluids is not considered a signicant risk for HIV transmission. Factors that have been recognized to increase the risk for transmission include the presence of visible blood in the device, insertion of the device into a blood vessel, deep injury, and the death of the source patient within 2 months after exposure.[136] Cumulative risk for HIV infection from occupational exposure depends on three factors: the prevalence of HIV infection among patients, the risk for HIV transmission after a single exposure, and the nature and frequency of exposures.[138]

Despite all coordinated efforts to avoid exposure to contaminated body fluids, accidents that could potentially be linked to transmission of blood-borne pathogens are common, and the CDC estimates that over 380,000 sharps injuries occur in U.S. hospitals every year. Postexposure prophylaxis in the form of combination ART should be available in all healthcare settings for immediate administration to affected personnel. Guidelines for basic and expanded regimens of postexposure prophylaxis are routinely updated. Even in the best possible circumstances, the protection offered by preventive strategies that include rapid initiation of ART for postexposure prophylaxis is not complete. As many as 21 cases of HIV infection have been documented in healthcare workers treated with standard regimens of postexposure prophylaxis.

References

1. BoilyMC, et al. Heterosexual risk of HIV-1 infection per sexual act: systematic review and meta-analysis of observational studies. Lancet Infect Dis 2009;9(2):118–129.
2. Baggaley RF, White RG, Boily MC. HIV transmission risk through anal intercourse: systematic review, meta-analysis and implications for HIV prevention. Int J Epidemiol 2010;39(4):1048–1063.

3. Vittinghoff E, et al.Per-contact risk of human immunodeficiency virus transmission between male sexual partners. Am J Epidemiol 1999;150(3):306–311.

4. Jin F, et al. Per-contact probability of HIV transmission in homosexual men in Sydney in the era of HAART. AIDS2010;24(6):907–913.

5. Miller CJ, Shattock RJ. Target cells in vaginal HIV transmission. Microbes Infect 2003;5(1):59–67.

6. Coombs RW, Reichelderfer PS, Landay AL. Recent observations on HIV type-1 infection in the genital tract of men and women. AIDS 2003;17(4):455–480.

7. Moriyama A, et al. Secretory leukocyte protease inhibitor (SLPI) concentrations in cervical mucus of women with normal menstrual cycle. Mol Hum Reprod 1999;5(7):656–661.

8. Bomsel M. Transcytosis of infectious human immunodeficiency virus across a tight human epithelial cell line barrier. Nat Med 1997;3(1):42–47.

9. Wawer MJ, et al. Rates of HIV-1 transmission per coital act, by stage of HIV-1 infection, in Rakai, Uganda. J Infect Dis 2005;191(9):1403–1409.

10. Keele BF. Identifying and characterizing recently transmitted viruses. Curr Opin HIV AIDS 2010;5(4):327–334.

11. Marks G, Crepaz N, Janssen RS. Estimating sexual transmission of HIV from persons aware and unaware that they are infected with the virus in the USA. AIDS 2006;20(10):1447–1450.

12. Donoghoe MC, et al. Setting targets for universal access to HIV prevention, treatment and care for injecting drug users (IDUs): towards consensus and improved guidance. Int J Drug Policy 2008;19 Suppl 1:S5–S14.

13. Fideli US, et al. Virologic and immunologic determinants of heterosexual transmission of human immunodeficiency virus type 1 in Africa. AIDS Res Hum Retroviruses 2001;17(10):901–910.

14. Quinn TC, et al. Viral load and heterosexual transmission of human immunodeficiency virus type 1. Rakai Project Study Group. N Engl J Med 2000;342(13):921–929.

15. Chakraborty H, et al. Viral burden in genital secretions determines male-to-female sexual transmission of HIV-1: a probabilistic empiric model. AIDS 2001;15(5):621–627.

16. Donnell D, et al. Heterosexual HIV-1 transmission after initiation of antiretroviral therapy: a prospective cohort analysis. Lancet 2010;375(9731):2092–2098.

17. Wilson DP et al. Relation between HIV viral load and infectiousness: a model-based analysis. Lancet 2008;72(9635):314–320.

18. HPTN 052 trial at http:// www.hptn.org/research_studies/hptn052.asp.

19. Cameron DW, et al. Female to male transmission of human immunodeficiency virus type 1: risk factors for seroconversion in men. Lancet 1989;2(8660):403–407.

20. Dyer JR, et al. Association of CD4 cell depletion and elevated blood and seminal plasma human immunodeficiency virus type 1 (HIV-1) RNA concentrations with genital ulcer disease in HIV-1-infected men in Malawi. J Infect Dis 1998;177(1):224–227.

21. Ghys PD, et al. The associations between cervicovaginal HIV shedding, sexually transmitted diseases and immunosuppression in female sex workers in Abidjan, Cote d'Ivoire. AIDS 1997;11(12):F85–F93.

22. Telzak EE, et al. HIV-1 seroconversion in patients with and without genital ulcer disease. A prospective study. Ann Intern Med 1993;119(12):1181–1186.

23. Fleming DT, Wasserheit JN. From epidemiological synergy to public health policy and practice: the contribution of other sexually transmitted diseases to sexual transmission of HIV infection. Sex Transm Infect 1999;75(1):3–17.

24. Gray RH, et al. Probability of HIV-1 transmission per coital act in monogamous, heterosexual, HIV-1-discordant couples in Rakai, Uganda. Lancet 2001;357(9263):1149–1153.

25. Grosskurth H, et al. Control of sexually transmitted diseases for HIV-1 prevention: understanding the implications of the Mwanza and Rakai trials. Lancet 2000;355(9219):1981–1987.

26. Auvert B, et al. Randomized, controlled intervention trial of male circumcision for reduction of HIV infection risk: the ANRS 1265 Trial. PLoS Med 2005;2(11):e298.

27. Bailey RC, et al. Male circumcision for HIV prevention in young men in Kisumu, Kenya: a randomised controlled trial. Lancet 2007;369(9562):643–656.

28. Gray RH, et al. Male circumcision for HIV prevention in men in Rakai, Uganda: a randomised trial. Lancet 2007;369(9562):657–666.

29. Gust DA, et al. Circumcision status and HIV infection among MSM: reanalysis of a Phase III HIV vaccine clinical trial. AIDS 2010;24(8):1135–1143.

30. Brewer DD, Golden MR, Handsfield HH. Unsafe sexual behavior and correlates of risk in a probability sample of men who have sex with men in the era of highly active antiretroviral therapy. Sex Transm Dis 2006;33(4):250–255.

31. Hart GJ, Elford JJ. Sexual risk behaviour of men who have sex with men: emerging patterns and new challenges. Curr Opin Infect Dis 2010;23(1):39–44.

32. Sullivan, PS, et al. Estimating the proportion of HIV transmissions from main sex partners among men who have sex with men in five US cities. AIDS 2009;23(9):1153–1162.

33. Burns DN, Dieffenbach CW, Vermund SH. Rethinking prevention of HIV type 1 infection. Clin Infect Dis 2010;51(6):725–731.

34. Trends in HIV/AIDS diagnoses among men who have sex with men—33 states, 2001–2006. MMWR 2008; 57(25):681–686.

35. Smith DM, Richmandd, Little SJ, HIV superinfection. J Infect Dis 2005;192(3):438–444.

36. Little SJ, et al. Antiretroviral-drug resistance among patients recently infected with HIV. N Engl J Med 2002;347(6):385–394.

37. Feng TJ, et al. Prevalence of syphilis and human immunodeficiency virus infections among men who have sex with men in Shenzhen, China: 2005 to 2007. Sex Transm Dis 2008;35(12):1022–1024.

38. UNAIDS, 2009 AIDS epidemic update. UNAIDS/09.36E/JC1700E. Geneva, Joint United Nations Programme on HIV/AIDS AND World Health Organization. 2009.

39. Mofenson LM. Technical report: perinatal human immunodeficiency virus testing and prevention of transmission. Committee on Pediatric Aids. Pediatrics, 2000. 106(6):E88.

40. Lehman DA, Farquhar C. Biological mechanisms of vertical human immunodeficiency virus (HIV-1) transmission. Rev Med Virol 2007;17(6):381–403.

41. Lewis SH, et al. HIV-1 in trophoblastic and villous Hofbauer cells, and haematological precursors in eight-week fetuses. Lancet 1990;335(8689):565–568.

42. Dickover RE, et al. Identification of levels of maternal HIV-1 RNA associated with risk of perinatal transmission. Effect of maternal zidovudine treatment on viral load. JAMA 1996; 275(8):599–605.

43. Fawzi, W, et al. Predictors of intrauterine and intrapartum transmission of HIV-1 among Tanzanian women. AIDS 2001;15(9):1157–1165.

44. Garcia PM, et al. Maternal levels of plasma human immunodeficiency virus type 1 RNA and the risk of perinatal transmission. Women and Infants Transmission Study Group. N Engl J Med 1999;341(6):394–402.

45. Mock PA, et al. Maternal viral load and timing of mother-to-child HIV transmission, Bangkok, Thailand. Bangkok Collaborative Perinatal HIV Transmission Study Group. AIDS 1999;13(3):407–414.

46. Mofenson LM, et al. Risk factors for perinatal transmission of human immunodeficiency virus type 1 in women treated with zidovudine. Pediatric AIDS Clinical Trials Group Study 185 Team. N Engl J Med 1999;341(6):385–393.

47. Nduati R, et al. Effect of breastfeeding and formula feeding on transmission of HIV-1: a randomized clinical trial. JAMA 2000;283(9):1167–1174.

48. Sperling RS, et al. Maternal viral load, zidovudine treatment, and the risk of transmission of human immunodeficiency virus type 1 from mother to infant. Pediatric AIDS Clinical Trials Group Protocol 076 Study Group. N Engl J Med 1996;335(22):1621–1629.

49. Brahmbhatt H, et al. The effects of placental malaria on mother-to-child HIV transmission in Rakai, Uganda. AIDS 2003;17(17):2539–2541.

50. Brahmbhatt H, et al. Association of HIV and malaria with mother-to-child transmission, birth outcomes, and child mortality. J Acquir Immune Defic Syndr, 2008;47(4):472–476.

51. Ayisi, J.G, et al. Maternal malaria and perinatal HIV transmission, western Kenya. Emerg Infect Dis 2004;10(4):643–652.

52. Mwapasa V, et al. The effect of Plasmodium falciparum malaria on peripheral and placental HIV-1 RNA concentrations in pregnant Malawian women. AIDS 2004;18(7):1051–1059.

53. Tkachuk, AN, et al. Malaria enhances expression of CC chemokine receptor 5 on placental macrophages. J Infect Dis 2001;183(6):967–972.

54. Menendez C, et al. The impact of placental malaria on gestational age and birth weight. J Infect Dis 2000;181(5):1740–1745.

55. ter Kuile FO, et al. The burden of co-infection with human immunodeficiency virus type 1 and malaria in pregnant women in sub-saharan Africa. Am J Trop Med Hyg 2004;71(2 Suppl):41–54.

56. Taha TE, et al. A phase III clinical trial of antibiotics to reduce chorioamnionitis-related perinatal HIV-1 transmission. AID 2006;20(9):1313–1321.

57. Wawer MJ, et al. Control of sexually transmitted diseases for AIDS prevention in Uganda: a randomised community trial. Rakai Project Study Group. Lancet 1999;353(9152):525–535.

58. Bulterys M, et al. Sexual behavior and injection drug use during pregnancy and vertical transmission of HIV-1. J Acquir Immune Defic Syndr Hum Retrovirol 1997;15(1):76–82.

59. Burns DN, et al. Influence of other maternal variables on the relationship between maternal virus load and mother-to-infant transmission of human immunodeficiency virus type 1. J Infect Dis 1997;175(5):1206–1210.

60. Matheson PB, et al. Heterosexual behavior during pregnancy and perinatal transmission of HIV-1. New York City Perinatal HIV Transmission Collaborative Study Group. AIDS 1996;10(11):1249–1256.

61. Rodriguez EM, et al. Association of maternal drug use during pregnancy with maternal HIV culture positivity and perinatal HIV transmission. AIDS 1996;10(3):273–282.

62. Turner BJ, et al. Cigarette smoking and maternal-child HIV transmission. J Acquir Immune Defic Syndr Hum Retrovirol 1997;14(4):327–337.

63. Semba RD, et al. Maternal vitamin A deficiency and mother-to-child transmission of HIV-1. Lancet 1994;343(8913):1593–1597.

64. Gaillard P, et al. Vaginal lavage with chlorhexidine during labour to reduce mother-to-child HIV transmission: clinical trial in Mombasa, Kenya. AIDS 2001,15(3).389–396.

65. Neely MN, et al. Cervical shedding of HIV-1 RNA among women with low levels of viremia while receiving highly active antiretroviral therapy. J Acquir Immune Defic Syndr 2007;44(1):38–42.

66. Drake AL, et al. Herpes simplex virus type 2 and risk of intrapartum human immunodeficiency virus transmission. Obstet Gynecol 2007;109(2 Pt 1):403–409.

67. John GC, et al. Correlates of mother-to-child human immunodeficiency virus type 1 (HIV-1) transmission: association with maternal plasma HIV-1 RNA load, genital HIV-1 DNA shedding, and breast infections. J Infect Dis 2001;183(2):206–212.

68. Chen KT, et al. Genital herpes simplex virus infection and perinatal transmission of human immunodeficiency virus. Obstet Gynecol 2005;106(6):1341–1348.

69. McClelland RS, et al. Association between cervical shedding of herpes simplex virus and HIV-1. AIDS 2002;16(18):2425–2430.

70. Landesman SH, et al. Obstetrical factors and the transmission of human immunodeficiency virus type 1 from mother to child. The Women and Infants Transmission Study. N Engl J Med 1996;334(25):1617–1623.

71. The mode of delivery and the risk of vertical transmission of human immunodeficiency virus type 1—a meta-analysis of 15 prospective cohort studies. The International Perinatal HIV Group. N Engl J Med 1999;340(13):977–987.

72. Fowler MG. Newell ML. Breast-feeding and HIV-1 transmission in resource-limited settings. J Acquir Immune Defic Syndr 2002;30(2):230–239.

73. Coutsoudis A, et al. Late postnatal transmission of HIV-1 in breast-fed children: an individual patient data meta-analysis. J Infect Dis 2004;189(12):2154–2166.

74. Creek TL, et al. Hospitalization and mortality among primarily nonbreastfed children during a large outbreak of diarrhea and malnutrition in Botswana, 2006. J Acquir Immune Defic Syndr 2010;53(1):14–19.

75. Richardson BA, et al. Breast-milk infectivity in human immunodeficiency virus type 1-infected mothers. J Infect Dis 2003;187(5):736–740.

76. Dunn DT, et al. Risk of human immunodeficiency virus type 1 transmission through breastfeeding. Lancet 1992;340(8819):585–588.

77. Ekpini ER, et al. Late postnatal mother-to-child transmission of HIV-1 in Abidjan, Cote d'Ivoire. Lancet 1997;349(9058):1054–1059.

78. Embree JE, et al. Risk factors for postnatal mother-child transmission of HIV-1. AIDS 2000;14(16):2535–2541.

79. Semba RD, et al. Mastitis and immunological factors in breast milk of human immunodeficiency virus-infected women. J Hum Lact 1999;15(4):301–306.

80. Farquhar C, et al. CC and CXC chemokines in breastmilk are associated with mother-to-child HIV-1 transmission. Curr HIV Res 2005;3(4):361–369.

81. Pillay K, et al. Secretory leukocyte protease inhibitor in vaginal fluids and perinatal human immunodeficiency virus type 1 transmission. J Infect Dis 2001;183(4):653–656.

82. Farquhar C, et al. Salivary secretory leukocyte protease inhibitor is associated with reduced transmission of human immunodeficiency virus type 1 through breast milk. J Infect Dis 2002;186(8):1173–1176.

83. Dickover R, et al. Role of maternal autologous neutralizing antibody in selective perinatal transmission of human immunodeficiency virus type 1 escape variants. J Virol 2006;80(13):6525–6533.

84. Johnson DC, et al. Safety and immunogenicity of an HIV-1 recombinant canarypox vaccine in newborns and infants of HIV-1-infected women. J Infect Dis 2005;192(12):2129–2133.

85. McFarland EJ, et al. HIV-1 vaccine induced immune responses in newborns of HIV-1 infected mothers. AIDS 2006;20(11):1481–1489.

86. Mathers BM, et al. Global epidemiology of injecting drug use and HIV among people who inject drugs: a systematic review. Lancet 2008;372(9651):1733–1745.

87. Aceijas C, et al. Global overview of injecting drug use and HIV infection among injecting drug users. AIDS 2004;18(17):2295–2303.

88. Nicolosi A, Lazzarin A. HIV seroconversion rates in intravenous drug abusers from northern Italy. Lancet 1989;2(8657):269.

89. Robertson JR, et al. Epidemic of AIDS related virus (HTLV-III/LAV) infection among intravenous drug abusers. Br Med J (Clin Res Ed) 1986;292(6519):527–529.

90. Choopanya K, et al. Risk factors and HIV seropositivity among injecting drug users in Bangkok. AIDS 1991;5(12):1509–1513.

91. Sasse H, Salmaso S, Conti S, Risk behaviors for HIV-1 infection in Italian drug users: report from a multicenter study. First Drug User Multicenter Study Group. J Acquir Immune Defic Syndr 1989;2(5):486–496.

92. Chaisson RE, et al. Human immunodeficiency virus infection in heterosexual intravenous drug users in San Francisco. Am J Public Health 1987;77(2):169–172.

93. D'Aquila RT, et al. Race/ethnicity as a risk factor for HIV-1 infection among Connecticut intravenous drug users. J Acquir Immune Defic Syndr 1989;2(5):503–513.

94. Schoenbaum EE, et al. Risk factors for human immunodeficiency virus infection in intravenous drug users. N Engl J Med 1989;321(13):874–879.

95. Nicolosi A, et al. Parenteral and sexual transmission of human immunodeficiency virus in intravenous drug users: a study of seroconversion. The Northern Italian Seronegative Drug Addicts (NISDA) Study. Am J Epidemiol 1992;135(3):225–233.

96. Neaigus A, et al. Effects of outreach intervention on risk reduction among intravenous drug users. AIDS Educ Prev 1990;2(4):253–271.

97. Abdala N, et al. Sexually transmitted infections, sexual risk behaviors and the risk of heterosexual spread of HIV among and beyond IDUs in St. Petersburg, Russia. Eur Addict Res 2008;14(1):19–25.

98. Donegan E, et al. Transfusion transmission of retroviruses: human T-lymphotropic virus types I and II compared with human immunodeficiency virus type 1. Transfusion 1994;34(6):478–483.

99. Donegan E, et al. Infection with human immunodeficiency virus type 1 (HIV-1) among recipients of antibody-positive blood donations. Ann Intern Med 1990;113(10):733–739.

100. Donegan E, et al. Transmission of HIV-1 by component type and duration of shelf storage before transfusion. Transfusion 1990;30(9):851–852.

101. Busch MP, et al. Factors influencing human immunodeficiency virus type 1 transmission by blood transfusion. Transfusion Safety Study Group. J Infect Dis 1996;174(1):26–33.

102. Giesecke J, et al. Incidence of symptoms and AIDS in 146 Swedish haemophiliacs and blood transfusion recipients infected with human immunodeficiency virus. BMJ 1988;297(6641):99–102.

103. Colebunders R, et al. Seroconversion rate, mortality, and clinical manifestations associated with the receipt of a human immunodeficiency virus-infected blood transfusion in Kinshasa, Zaire. J Infect Dis 1991;164(3):450–456.

104. Kalbfleisch JD, Lawless JF, Estimating the incubation time distribution and expected number of cases of transfusion-associated acquired immune deficiency syndrome. Transfusion 1989;29(8):672–676.

105. Lackritz, E.M, et al. Estimated risk of transmission of the human immunodeficiency virus by screened blood in the United States. N Engl J Med 1995;333(26):1721–1725.

106. Schreiber GB, et al. The risk of transfusion-transmitted viral infections. The Retrovirus Epidemiology Donor Study. N Engl J Med 1996;334(26):1685–1690.

107. Dodd RY, Notari EPT, Stramer SL. Current prevalence and incidence of infectious disease markers and estimated window-period risk in the American Red Cross blood donor population. Transfusion 2002;42(8):975–979.

108. Goodnough LT, Shander A, Brecher ME. Transfusion medicine: looking to the future. Lancet 2003;361(9352):161–169.

109. Busch MP, Kleinman SH, Nemo GJ. Current and emerging infectious risks of blood transfusions. JAMA 2003;289(8):959–962.

110. Cleary PD, et al. Sociodemographic and behavioral characteristics of HIV antibody-positive blood donors. Am J Public Health 1988;78(8):953–957.

111. Bharucha ZS, Risk management strategies for HIV in blood transfusion in developing countries. Vox Sang 2002;83(Suppl 1):167–171.

112. Tedder RS, et al. Hepatitis B transmission from contaminated cryopreservation tank. Lancet 1995;346(8968):137–140.

113. Sugg U, et al. Safety of immunoglobulin preparations with respect to transmission of human immunodeficiency virus. Transfusion 1987;27(1):115.

114. Simonds RJ, HIV transmission by organ and tissue transplantation. AIDS 1993;7 (Suppl 2):S35–S38.

115. Simonds RJ, et al. Transmission of human immunodeficiency virus type 1 from a seronegative organ and tissue donor. N Engl J Med 1992;326(11):726–732.

116. D'Souza MP, et al. Acute HIV-1 infection: what's new? Where are we going? J Infect Dis 2010;202(Suppl 2):S267–S269.

117. Cohen MS, et al. The detection of acute HIV infection. J Infect Dis 2010;202(Suppl 2):S270–S277.

118. Branson BM, et al. Revised recommendations for HIV testing of adults, adolescents, and pregnant women in health-care settings. MMWR Recomm Rep 2006;55(RR-14):1–17; quiz CE1–4.

119. Vlahov D, Robertson AM, Strathdee SA. Prevention of HIV infection among injection drug users in resource-limited settings. Clin Infect Dis 2010;50(Suppl 3):S114–S121.

120. Amon JJ, et al. Prevalence of hepatitis C virus infection among injection drug users in the United States, 1994–2004. Clin Infect Dis 2008;46(12):1852–1858.

121. Calsyn DA, et al. Sex under the influence of drugs or alcohol: common for men in substance abuse treatment and associated with high-risk sexual behavior. Am J Addict 2010;19(2):119–127.

122. O'Connor PG, Selwyn PA, Schottenfeld RS. Medical care for injection-drug users with human immunodeficiency virus infection. N Engl J Med 1994;331(7):450–459.

123. Rosenberg SD, et al. Prevalence of HIV, hepatitis B, and hepatitis C in people with severe mental illness. Am J Public Health 2001;91(1):31–37.

124. Meade CS, et al. HIV risk behavior among patients with co-occurring bipolar and substance use disorders: associations with mania and drug abuse. Drug Alcohol Depend 2008;92(1–3):296–300.

125. Kidder DP, et al. Housing status and HIV risk behaviors among homeless and housed persons with HIV. J Acquir Immune Defic Syndr 2008;49(4):451–455.

126. Springer SA, et al. Effectiveness of antiretroviral therapy among HIV-infected prisoners: reincarceration and the lack of sustained benefit after release to the community. Clin Infect Dis 2004;38(12):1754–160.

127. Mostashari F, et al. Acceptance and adherence with antiretroviral therapy among HIV-infected women in a correctional facility. J Acquir Immune Defic Syndr Hum Retrovirol 1998;18(4):341–348.

128. Altice FL, Mostashari F, Friedland GH. Trust and the acceptance of and adherence to antiretroviral therapy. J Acquir Immune Defic Syndr 2001;28(1):47–58.

129. Maruschak L. HIV in prisons and jails, in U.D.o.J.B.o.J.S.O.o.J. Programs, Editor. 2001;NCJ publication: Washington, D.C.

130. Bozzette SA, et al. Expenditures for the care of HIV-infected patients in the era of highly active antiretroviral therapy. N Engl J Med 2001;344(11):817–823.

131. Vanwesenbeeck I. Another decade of social scientific work on sex work: a review of research 1990–2000. Annu Rev Sex Res 2001;12:242–289.

132. Smith A, M.A., Agwanda C, Kowuor D, vander Elst E, Davies A, Graham S, Jaffe H, Sanders E. Female clients and partners of MSM Sex Workers in Mombasa, Kenya in 17th Conference on Retrovirus and Opportunistic Infections. 2010; San Fransisco, Ca.

133. Gerberding JL. Occupational risks from exposure to HIV in the health care environment. J Am Podiatr Med Assoc 1988;78(3):143–146.

134. Van der Bij AK, et al. Low HIV-testing rates and awareness of HIV infection among high-risk heterosexual STI clinic attendees in The Netherlands. Eur J Public Health 2008;18(4):376–379.

135. Rekart ML, Sex-work harm reduction. Lancet 2005;366(9503):2123–2134.

136. Cardo DM, et al. A case-control study of HIV seroconversion in health care workers after percutaneous exposure. Centers for Disease Control and Prevention Needlestick Surveillance Group. N Engl J Med 1997;337(21):1485–1490.

137. Updated U.S. Public Health Service Guidelines for the Management of Occupational Exposures to HBV, HCV, and HIV and Recommendations for Postexposure Prophylaxis. MMWR Recomm Rep 2001;50(RR-11):1–52.

138. Bell DM. Occupational risk of human immunodeficiency virus infection in healthcare workers: an overview. Am J Med 1997;102(5B): 9–15.

139. Lattimore S, Thornton A, Delpech V, Elford J. Changing PAtterns of Sexual Risk Behavior Among London Gay Men: 1998–2008. Sex Transm Dis. 2010 Oct 1.

Chapter 5 EPIDEMIOLOGY OF HIV/AIDS

QUARRAISHA ABDOOL KARIM AND

AYESHA B.M. KHARSANY

Federal officials consider it an epidemic. Yet you rarely hear a thing about it. At first it only seemed to strike one segment of the population. Now Barry Peterson tells us this is no longer the case.

—DAN RATHER, CBS Nightly News, August 12, 1982

Introduction

The identification of several cases of *Pneumocystis carinii* among homosexual men across several cities in the United States in 1981 signaled what would soon become known as acquired immune deficiency syndrome (AIDS),[1,2] a more widespread and even more complex phenomenon than anticipated. Following the isolation of human immunodeficiency virus (HIV) in 1983, a causal relationship with AIDS was established.[3-5] Within three decades, the virus has spread across the globe, infecting more than 60 million people and resulting in about 25 million deaths.[6] These statistics mask the devastating impact of the HIV/AIDS pandemic on morbidity and premature mortality on families, communities, and societies, most notably in sub-Saharan Africa that continues to bear the brunt of the disease burden.

By the mid-1990s, the development and availability of life-prolonging combination antiretroviral (ARV) treatment, also known as highly active antiretroviral therapy (HAART), transformed what was an inevitably fatal disease to a chronic, manageable condition. Even more remarkable and unprecedented was that within a decade through global solidarity, political leadership and commitment ARV treatment became available in resource constrained settings. Notwithstanding this major advance,[7] the continued spread of HIV remains a challenge. While there are a growing number of countries demonstrating control and/or declines in the number of new HIV infections, advances in preventing sexual transmission of HIV remains daunting.

This chapter reviews the complex diversity of the evolving HIV pandemic and implications and challenges for HIV prevention.

Transmission of HIV

HIV continues to spread sexually, through unsafe injecting substance use practices, perinatally, through unsafe blood supplies, and nosocomially through poor practice of universal precautions in health care delivery.

Sexual transmission remains the major route of HIV transmission and accounts for about 80% of all HIV infections globally. Transmission through this route occurs through any unprotected penetrative sex act where one partner is infected with HIV (discordant sex acts). The risk of becoming infected depends on the likelihood that the sex partner is infected (a function of background prevalence in the population), number of sex partners and frequency of change, concurrent partnerships with a high frequency of unprotected sex acts, the type of sex act (receptive anal versus receptive vaginal), and the amount of virus (viral dose) present in the semen, vaginal, or cervical secretions of the infected partner. The viral dose is dependent on the stage of HIV infection with individuals who have recently been infected having the highest amount of virus, followed by those with a concomitant sexually transmitted disease (STD), followed by those with advancing HIV disease and a high concentration of HIV receptor cells at the site of infection, which increases the risk of acquiring and transmitting HIV.[8–16]

Injection drug use accounts for about 10% of all HIV infections globally. In countries such as those in Asia and Eastern Europe, it remains the dominant mode of transmission, accounting for about 80% of all HIV infections in these settings. Inadequate screening of blood and blood products and poor practice of universal precautions in health care settings accounts for about 4% of transmission. Perinatal transmission accounts for about 6% of all infections; transmission can occur during pregnancy, during labor and delivery, and postpartum through breast feeding. This is the one area where substantial progress has been made in terms of interventions to reduce transmission to the point where, in some industrialized country settings, transmission has been close to eliminated. In resource-constrained settings, it continues to be a challenge as uptake of prevention of mother to child transmission (PMTCT) services remains low to modest because of fear of violence, stigma, and discrimination or loss of security.[17–19]

Monitoring the HIV Pandemic

As HIV is linked in time, place, and population group, understanding where new HIV infections are occurring (incidence) and the total number of HIV infections (prevalence), where these infections are geographically, and how they are being acquired (modes of transmission) has been important for monitoring temporal trends of the evolving pandemic, guiding the targeting of prevention efforts, assessing the impact of interventions, and planning for health care delivery needs.[20] In many countries, the extent and magnitude of HIV infection remains uncertain as a result of weak disease surveillance systems and diagnostic capabilities.

In the first decade of the epidemic, reporting of AIDS cases was the mainstay of surveillance. By early 1997, over 1.7 million cases of AIDS had been reported to the World Health Organization (WHO) from 197 countries. Notwithstanding lack of uniformity in reporting, case definition and completeness of reporting these data provided a reasonable picture of the evolving epidemic. The development of HIV antibody tests and more widespread access to HIV testing in the late 1980s helped identify countries with emerging HIV epidemics, and gave us a better understanding of the modes of transmission and natural history of the infection.

Given the 5- to 7-year delay between infection with HIV and the development of AIDS, the limited utility of AIDS cases for planning purposes became apparent, and surveillance systems based on HIV infection started to emerge. In countries where heterosexual transmission is the dominant mode of transmission, anonymous testing of pregnant women became and remains the mainstay of HIV surveillance. Since the introduction of HIV antibody testing, routine screening of blood supplies has eliminated this mode of transmission in most countries. During much of the 1990s and early 2000s, HIV data from other sentinel groups provided supplemental data to assist with understanding the evolving epidemics.[21–25] An important adjunct to the sentinel surveillance has been the implementation of population-based surveys, especially in generalized epidemic settings. By 2001, more than 30 developing countries in the Caribbean, sub-Saharan Africa, and Asia had implemented nationally representative population-based household surveys with HIV testing, generating important data in men and women throughout the life cycle. These surveys have improved the reliability of national HIV estimates in countries with generalized epidemics.[26–29]

The World Health Organization/Joint United Nations Program on HIV/AIDS (WHO/UNAIDS) annually generates data on the status of the pandemic globally, regionally, and at a country level. These estimates are only as good as the data provided by member countries. The quality of these data is constantly reviewed and improved on by the WHO/UNAIDS Surveillance Reference Group.[30] The mathematical projections generated by this group provide additional insights into the evolving epidemics at a country level and globally[30] and monitoring the effectiveness of prevention and care efforts.[31]

The introduction of ARV treatment and resultant increased life expectancy of HIV-infected individuals has decreased the utility of HIV prevalence data for surveillance purposes.[32] The development of more sensitive laboratory measures for incident/new HIV infections and a deeper appreciation of monitoring behavioral patterns has lead to the development of third-generation surveillance systems.[33–36] At this point in the pandemic, the most sensitive way to monitor trends in the pandemic is to measure new HIV infections or incidence rates; however, major limitations include lack of availability of robust laboratory methods and costs of undertaking these tests.[36,37]

HIV Epidemic Typologies

From the first described AIDS cases among men who have sex with men and injecting drug users in North America, Europe, and Australia and heterosexually acquired infections in eastern and central Africa with a concomitant epidemic in infants born to HIV-infected mothers, the HIV pandemic has evolved to become a complex mosaic of epidemics across the world, differing in disease burden, modes of transmission, and intensity, with not a single country in the world spared.[38–40]

WHO/UNAIDS classifies the current epidemics into several typologies to capture dominant characteristics of the evolving epidemic at a country or regional level.[41]

Low-level epidemics describe settings where HIV infection has been present for many years, but has never spread to significant levels to the general population. This epidemic state suggests that sexual networks of risk are not diffuse and there are low levels of partner change or concurrent sexual relationships, or that the virus has been introduced only very recently. Generally, the HIV prevalence is between 1% and 5%. An example of this type of epidemic is that in Senegal in West Africa.

In contrast, *concentrated epidemics* typifies HIV spread within a defined subpopulation, such as men who have sex with men, injecting drug users, or sex workers and their clients. HIV remains at high levels in these subpopulations. This epidemic typology suggests active networks of risk within a defined subpopulation that does not bridge or cross into other populations. The disease burden and infection rates may vary substantially between countries. Within these concentrated epidemics, mode of transmission may change even as epidemics within subpopulations may continue. The epidemic in the United States typifies this epidemic classification.

In *generalized epidemics*, HIV is firmly established in the general population. Heterosexual transmission sustains this epidemic, and countries with generalized epidemics report an HIV prevalence of about 5% in pregnant women and more than 5% in adults, with a concomitant epidemic of perinatally acquired infections. Most countries in sub-Saharan Africa fit this profile.

A special and unique typology of generalized epidemics is *hyperendemic* epidemics. This typology is used to describe the epidemic in southern Africa where, despite HIV being rare prior to 1990, the prevalence is at an unprecedented high level—in excess of 15% in the general population—and new infection rates higher than 5% per year occur despite high and increasing morbidity and mortality rates. All sexually active persons have an elevated risk of acquiring HIV infection in these settings.

In countries with low level and concentrated epidemics, the central prevention focus is on populations at greatest risk. To reduce the likelihood that a low-level or concentrated epidemic will become generalized, prevention programs also focus on potential epidemiologic bridges, such as the sex partners of injecting drug users or men having sex with men. In generalized epidemics, in which infection extends beyond discrete populations at elevated risk, greater investment is required in broader, population-based interventions, such as mass media, school-based education, community mobilization, workplace interventions, and strategies to alter social norms. In contrast, hyperendemic settings require broad-based societal mobilization to address the sociocultural and economic practices that contribute to unsafe sexual behavior. This expanded focus should complement intensive knowledge on HIV transmission networks, behavior change, and biomedical and structural interventions with access to antiretroviral treatment to reduce the likelihood of HIV acquisition.[42-46]

A key lesson in terms of altering epidemic trajectories in this decade of the pandemic—both at a country level and globally—has been the importance of knowledge of the epidemic at a country level in terms of the virus, populations most affected, and modes of transmission to better inform and target interventions and customize combinations of interventions.

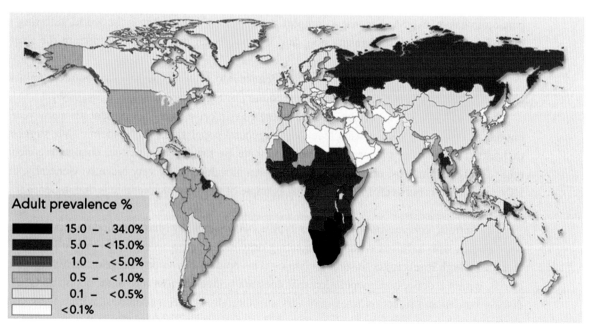

Figure 5–1. *Global view of HIV infection, 2007. Source: WHO/UNAIDS 2008 AIDS Epidemic Update Report.*

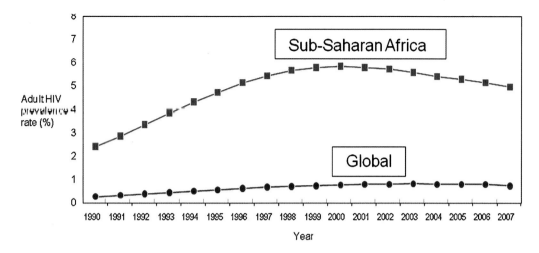

Figure 5–2. *Estimated adult HIV prevalence (%) globally and in sub-Saharan Africa, 1990–2007. Source: WHO/UNAIDS 2007 AIDS Epidemic Update Report.*

Global Epidemiology of HIV/AIDS

By the end of 2008, WHO/UNAIDS estimated that there were 33.4 million (31.1 million–35.8 million) people living with HIV globally (**Figure 5–1**), with 2.7 million (2.4 million–3.0 million)* new HIV infections and 2.0 million (1.7 million–2.4 million) deaths from AIDS.[47] Significantly—and in contrast to the first decade of the HIV pandemic—about 50% of all new HIV infections have occurred in women, and an estimated 45% of new HIV infections occurred in young people between 15 and 24 years of age.

Sub-Saharan Africa

Sub-Saharan Africa, despite being home to about 10% of the world's population, continues to bear a disproportionate burden of HIV infection (**Figure 5–2**). In 2008, an estimated 1.9 million (1.6 million–2.2 million) new infections occurred, accounting for 67% of the global HIV infections [22.4 million (20.8 million–24.1 million)] (**Figure 5–2**). Despite laudable efforts through the President's Emergency Plan for AIDS Relief (PEPFAR) and the Global Fund for TB, Malaria, and HIV,[48] about 75% [1.4 million (1.1 million–1.7 million)] of AIDS-related deaths occurred in this region.[47] Southern Africa continues to be the epicenter of the pandemic with about a third of all new HIV infections occurring here as well as about 32% of all AIDS deaths. Although there has been some decline in the number of new HIV infections, HIV incidence and AIDS mortality rates remain unacceptably high.

Within sub-Saharan Africa, there is considerable heterogeneity in the distribution of HIV infection, both in magnitude and breadth, and women bear a disproportionate burden of infections (**Figure 5–3**), with rates of HIV infection at least three times higher than those in men.[49–51] Infection in young women between 15 and 24 years of age serves as a proxy measure for HIV incidence rates,[51,52] and remains unacceptably high in southern Africa. The HIV epidemic in

---

*The ranges around the estimate define the boundaries within which the actual numbers lie, based on the best available information.[47]

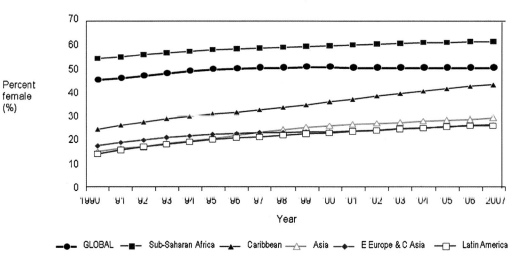

Figure 5–3. *Estimated adult female HIV prevalence (%) in sub-Saharan Africa in comparison to global estimates 1990–2007. Source: UNAIDS 2007 AIDS Epidemic Update Report.*

this region is a major obstacle to countries in achieving their Millennium Development Goals (MDG) in relation to life expectancy, infant mortality rates, and maternal deaths.[53,54]

The HIV prevalence in several countries such as Swaziland (25.9%), Botswana (25.0%), Lesotho (23.4%), South Africa (16.9%), Zambia (15.6%), and Zimbabwe (18.1%) exceeds 15% and in these settings is described as generalized hyperendemic-epidemics.[6,38,39,50,55,56] In countries such as Cameroon (5.5%), the Central African Republic (6.2%), Malawi (12.7%), Kenya (7.8%), Uganda (6.4%) and the United Republic of Tanzania (5.7%), the generalized epidemics continue, with HIV prevalence remaining above 5%. In West and Central Africa, data from population-based surveys showed HIV prevalence remains <5% among the adult general population (women and men) between 15 and 49 years of age. Countries such as Senegal (0.7%), Guinea (1.5%), and Benin (1.2%) continue to experience HIV prevalence of <2%.[6,56] An increasing number of countries are reporting declines in HIV infections, including the United Republic of Tanzania, Zambia, Zimbabwe, and Botswana.

A key lesson from the pandemic is that there is no room for complacency. In the early 1990s, HIV prevalence in Uganda was about 14% in adults and about 30% in pregnant women. With strong political leadership, commitment, and strong prevention campaigns, HIV prevalence declined to 5% by the end of 2001, and adult national HIV prevalence has stabilized at 5.4%.[57,58] However, there are signs of concern to be noted in the increasing rate of new infections in young women in rural Uganda.

Southern Africa remains the worst affected region, with South Africa having an estimated 5.7 million people living with HIV. In Swaziland, the adult HIV prevalence of 26% (from a national population-based survey) is the highest ever documented. In East Africa the HIV epidemic is considered to be comparatively smaller and prevalence has remained relatively low. Most of the comparatively smaller HIV epidemics in West Africa are stable or are declining. HIV prevalence among pregnant women in urban areas fell from 10% in 2001 to 6.9% in 2005. The largest epidemic in Nigeria, the continent's most populous country, appears to have stabilized at 3.1%, according to HIV infection trends among women attending antenatal clinics. Although HIV data from antenatal clinics suggest that most epidemics in sub-Saharan Africa appear to be stabilizing, the actual number of infected individuals continues to grow because of ongoing new infections and increasing access to antiretroviral therapy. However, there is no evidence yet of major changes in HIV-related behavior.[59–61]

The epidemic in these regions is largely driven by heterosexual intercourse between discordant couples (unprotected sex with a known HIV-positive partner). As epidemics have matured in generalized and hyperendemic epidemic settings, the exceptionally high background prevalence increases risk and HIV transmission unrelated to sex work, and is driven by complex combinations of sexual networks and structural, social, and political factors.[62] The significant contribution and role of early sexual debut, concurrent sexual partnerships, high prevalence of regular nonmarital partners among married individuals, often culturally acceptable multiple sexual partners, extensive labor migration, and high prevalence of intergenerational sexual partnerships play an important role in increasing risk of HIV infection and facilitating the spread of HIV. However, almost one-third to one-half of new infections occur in low-risk partnerships, among people in stable or serodiscordant monogamous relationships, in steady long-term heterosexual partnerships or in individuals with only one sex partner. A signal characteristic of heterosexual transmission infection in sub-Saharan Africa is the age and sex difference in HIV acquisition, with young women acquiring infection about 5 to 7 years earlier than men and women having about three-fold higher rates of infection than men.[63] Altering HIV infection rates in young women under 20 years of age is key to altering epidemic trajectories in these settings.

The region's epidemic is much more varied and diverse, with sex workers, men having sex with men, and injecting drug users, though less central, also contributing to the high rates of transmission. West Africa's epidemic is largely driven by female sex workers, with more than a third of sex workers surveyed being HIV-infected. HIV transmission in injecting drug users is important in epidemics in the East, southern Africa, and Mauritius, where more than half of the infections occur through contaminated injecting equipment. Due to political and social barriers, reliable data on men having sex with men are limited; however, recent studies suggest that in Zambia, Mombassa, and Dakar, 33%, 43% and 22% of men having sex with men, respectively, were HIV-infected; these data confirm the widespread existence of these groups across Africa having high rates of HIV infection.[64,65] Among heterosexual discordant couples, primary and late-stage HIV infection contribute significantly to transmission.[9, 66, 67]

Middle East and North Africa

Limited information is available on the spread of HIV in the Middle East and North Africa. In 2008, the total number of adults and children living with HIV was estimated to be 310,000 (250,000–380,000), including the 35,000 (24,000–46,000) people who were newly infected with the virus and 20,000 (15,000–25,000) AIDS-related deaths which occurred in the same year.[47] With the exception of the Sudan, the epidemics in this region are comparatively small and HIV prevalence has not exceeded 0.3%.[68] Unprotected paid sex and use of contaminated drug injecting equipment are the primary sources of HIV transmission. In Libyan Arab Jamahiriya, Tunisia, Algeria, Morocco, Syrian Arab Republic, and Iran, HIV infection is concentrated among subpopulations; and among injecting drug users, HIV prevalence ranges from 15% to 23%. Although socially stigmatized, sex between men plays a part in HIV transmission, and in Egypt and Sudan, HIV prevalence in these groups was 6.2% and 9%, respectively. Increasing numbers of women diagnosed with HIV through heterosexual transmission overlap with injecting drug use, sex work, and men having sex with men. Although varying combinations of risk factors are associated with HIV transmission, the epidemic in the Middle East and North Africa regions remains concentrated in key subpopulations.[69–72]

Eastern Europe and Central Asia

In Eastern Europe and Central Asia, the HIV/AIDS epidemic is rapidly expanding. In 2008, the estimated number of people living with HIV in Eastern Europe and Central Asia rose to 1.5 million (1.4 million–1.7 million), of which an estimated 110,000 (100,000–130,000) people became infected and some 87,000 (72,000–110,000) died of AIDS in the same year.[47] Almost 90% of those infected live in either the Russian Federation (69%) or Ukraine (29%), the worst affected regions where the epidemics continue to grow, with newly emerging epidemics in Tajikistan and Uzbekistan.

Multiple HIV epidemics in this region are concentrated largely among injecting drug users, sex workers, and their various sexual partners. The majority (62%) of new HIV infections are attributable to injecting drug use, but these new infections are geographically dispersed, with varying levels of HIV prevalence ranging from 3% to more than 50%. Less than 1% of new HIV infections are acquired through unprotected sex between men, and HIV prevalence remains relatively low, from 0.9% to 11%; however, this is probably an underestimate of the role of this mode of HIV transmission. The main driver of the epidemic in this region is the overlapping of injecting drug use and sex work, with more than one-third of female sex workers also being injecting drug users. Injecting drug users bridge from being bisexual to heterosexual; this contributes to the growing number of women infected. HIV prevalence among pregnant women who are injecting drug users exceeds 1%.[73–77]

Asia

In Asia, the HIV/AIDS epidemic appeared much later, around the mid 1980s, and by early 1990, Thailand and India accounted for the majority of infections. In Thailand, HIV prevalence among injecting drug users increased rapidly, from less than 1% in late 1987 to about 50% in 1990. A decline in new infections followed, with Thailand's exemplary success with its 100% condom promotion campaign among sex workers and clients. Similarly, in the Yunnan province in China, HIV infections were generally concentrated among injecting drug users and sex workers; by 1993, 10% to 30% of injecting drug users were found to be HIV-infected.

Asia, home to about 60% of the world's population, follows sub-Saharan Africa in terms of the number of people living with HIV. In 2008, an estimated 4.7 million (3.8 million–5.5 million) people were living with HIV, including 350,000 (270,000–410,000) who became newly infected; during that year, 330,000 (260,000–400,000) AIDS-related deaths occurred.[47] In Southeast Asia, where national HIV infection levels are highest, the epidemic trends are dissimilar. In India, between 2 and 3.1 million people are living with HIV, yet the HIV prevalence remains below 1%. Epidemics in Indonesia, Pakistan, and Vietnam are growing rapidly. In Vietnam, the estimated number of people living with HIV more than doubled between 2000 and 2005, and in heavily populated countries such as Bangladesh and China, the numbers of new HIV infections are increasing steadily.[47,68,78–90] Due to the vastness of the countries and populations, the national adult HIV prevalence in most of the Asian countries is likely to mask serious concentrated epidemics.

Asia's epidemic is most diverse and is driven by injecting drug use, men having sex with men and women, and sex work; the overlapping of these subpopulations helps contribute to the growing epidemic. In the northeastern part of India and in several large cities, more than half of the people living with HIV are injecting drug users and spread the virus through unprotected sex with regular partners and/or transactional sex.[91–95] In China and Vietnam, high proportions of women are injecting drug users and are also involved in paid sex work. Unprotected sex work—in brothels, street-based, or home-based—is the most important risk factor for the spread of HIV in several Asian countries. Declining HIV prevalence in Thailand, Cambodia, and Tamil Nadu followed successful condom promotion programs in all of these countries.[96–100]

Latin America

In Latin America, the number of new HIV infections in 2008 was an estimated 170,000 (150,000–200,000), bringing to 2 million (1.8 million–2.2 million) the total number of people living with HIV in this region. In the same year, 77,000 (66,000–89,000) people died of AIDS in Latin America.[47] The trends in the overall levels of HIV infections in Latin America have changed little in the past decade. The largest HIV epidemic is in Brazil, where about 730,000 people are living with HIV. Due to widespread access to antiretroviral treatment, the number of deaths has declined; however, the adult HIV prevalence is greater than 2%.[68] Transmission is mainly among men having sex with men, with a number of hidden epidemics uncovered recently. HIV infection is much lower among female sex workers, at around 3% to 10%; in contrast, men having sex with men have the highest rates of infection, often exceeding 10%. Drawing attention to the increasing role of heterosexual transmission in Latin America, HIV infection is increasing in women who are infected by male sexual partners who, in turn, have acquired HIV during unprotected sex with another man or through use of contaminated drug injecting equipment. Condom promotion efforts in recent years have resulted in declines in HIV prevalence.

Caribbean Countries

In the Caribbean, an estimated 240,000 (220,000–260,000) people were living with HIV in 2008, with the majority being concentrated in the Dominican Republic and Haiti. An estimated 20,000 (16,000–24 000) people were newly infected with HIV in this region, and some 12,000 (9,300–14,000) people died of AIDS.[47] HIV surveillance systems are still inadequate in several Caribbean countries, but available information indicates that most of the epidemics in the region appear to have stabilized or, in some urban areas, have declined. In the Dominican Republic, HIV prevalence declined from 1.0% in 2002 to an estimated 0.8% in 2007. Unprotected heterosexual intercourse, sex work, and sex between men significantly drive the epidemic in this region. With declining HIV prevalence among sex workers suggesting that sex workers are protecting themselves and their clients against HIV infection, men having sex with men account for more than 80% of all reported HIV cases in some areas.

North America, Western and Central Europe

In North America, Western and Central Europe the HIV epidemic has remained stable for several years. In 2008, an estimated 2.3 million (1.9 million–2.6 million) were living with HIV; 75,000 (49,000–97,000) new infections and 38,000 (27,000–61,000) deaths from AIDS occurred in the same year.[47] Access to life-prolonging antiretrovial treatment has led to an increase in the number of people living with HIV. In the United States, the HIV prevalence in the general population remains low, at 0.6%. Recent data suggest that new HIV epidemics are emerging among women and in minority ethnic groups. The main modes of HIV transmission is attributed to high-risk heterosexual intercourse, men having sex with men, and injecting drug use. A substantial proportion of newly diagnosed HIV infections and AIDS cases were attributable to high-risk heterosexual intercourse; many of these infections occurred in people born in countries with high HIV prevalence—mainly, the countries of sub-Saharan Africa and the Caribbean. Transmission by multiple uses of contaminated injecting equipment accounts for a lesser number of new HIV diagnoses, with declines in the number of new HIV diagnoses in this group.

Oceania

In Oceania, an estimated 59,000 (51,000–68,000) people were living with HIV in 2008, about 3,900 (2,900–5,100) of whom were newly infected; an estimated 2,000 (1,100–3,100) died from AIDS in the same year.[47] In Papua New Guinea, the epidemic has grown; this country is home to more than 70% of HIV infected people in the region, and the number of new HIV diagnoses more than doubled between 2002 and 2006. Unprotected paid sex is the main mode of HIV transmission. In the surrounding regions of Australia and New Zealand, HIV prevalence has remained below 1% and is concentrated among men having sex with men.

Demographic Impact of the HIV/AIDS Pandemic

In a matter of three decades, the HIV/AIDS pandemic has had a devastating impact on young men and women in the prime of their lives and continues to threaten economic and social development. In resource-constrained settings, gains in human development achieved over centuries have been reversed in a short space of time, setting households into deeper poverty. In the context of the current global economic crisis, many individuals and communities are being rendered even more vulnerable.[54,101–110] In these settings, the high burden of HIV, the continuing increase in the number of new infections, and antiretroviral treatment coverage levels remaining low to modest provide a glimpse of the devastation yet to come.

HIV/AIDS is the leading cause of death in sub-Saharan Africa. Worldwide, about 15 million [13–19 million] children have been orphaned to date; about 80% of these children live in sub-Saharan Africa.[111,112] In countries where governments have failed to implement national programs to effectively manage HIV/AIDS, AIDS-related morbidity and mortality, increases in the number of orphans, and declining life expectancy have caused profound changes in the population structure, with considerable alterations in the demographic profile.[68] Life expectancy in sub-Saharan African countries has generally been low compared to that in most developed countries, and the HIV epidemic has had a substantial impact on lowering life expectancy even more (**Figure 5–4**). Average life expectancy in sub-Saharan Africa is now 47 years; without AIDS, it could have been 62 years. In South Africa, total deaths (from all causes) increased by 87% between 1997 and 2005.[113] During this period, death rates more than tripled for women aged 20 to 39 years, and more than doubled for males aged 30 to 44 years, with at least 40% of deaths attributable to HIV. The impact of HIV in the province of KwaZulu-Natal, the epicenter of the pandemic, AIDS-related morbidity and premature mortality increased substantially,[101,105,114,115] and by 2004, life expectancy in the province had declined by about 10 years. Life expectancy is 53.8 years for women and 49.4 years for men.[102]

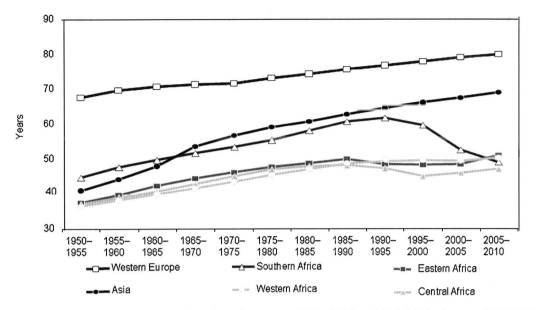

Figure 5-4. *Life expectancy at birth, selected regions, 1950–1955 to 2005–2010. Source: WHO/UNAIDS 2008 AIDS Epidemic Update Report.*

Epidemiology of HIV/AIDS in Children

Heterosexual intercourse remains the driving force in countries with generalized hyperendemic epidemics, and the high rate of sexual transmission has given rise to the world's largest population of children living with HIV. In 2008, an estimated 2.1 million (1.2 million–2.9 million) children under 15 years of age were living with HIV, 1.8 million (1.7 million–2.0 million) in sub-Saharan Africa. An estimated 280,000 (150,000–410,000) HIV-infected children younger than 15 years died of AIDS, more than 90% of them in sub-Saharan Africa.[68]

Drivers of the Pandemic

Insight on the variation in levels of risk in populations is central to the understanding of how HIV infection spreads. The speed of spread of HIV through a population depends on a combination of structural, social, and political factors that shape behavior, vulnerability, and risk. In regions of political turmoil and disturbance, disruption of family life, logistics, and access to health care are important factors driving the spread of HIV. Among the the structural drivers that increase vulnerability and contribute to HIV transmission are: indigenous sexual and ethnic practices, women's status in certain societies, social rejection of condoms in certain populations, restrictive national policies as barriers to the implementation of important interventions, limitations on access to interventions (for example, condoms for youth and sex workers and prevention benefits for marginalized populations), stigma, and discrimination.

In generalized hyperendemic epidemics, HIV infection extends beyond discrete populations of men having sex with men, injecting drug users, and sex workers, and background prevalence of HIV is the single biggest risk factor for HIV acquisition. The majority of HIV-infected individuals are unaware of their HIV status, and this remains a barrier for both treatment access and prevention. For many women, being married is the single biggest risk factor for HIV acquisition.

34. Zaba B, Slaymaker E, Urassa M, Boerma JT. The role of behavioral data in HIV surveillance. AIDS 2005;19 Suppl 2:S39–52.

35. World Health Organisation and Joint United Nations Programme on HIV/AIDS. Guidelines for Second Generation HIV Surveillance: The next decade. Working group on Global HIV/AIDS and STI Surveillance. WHO/CDC/EDC/2000.5 UNAIDS/00.03E 2000:orld

36. McDougal JS, Pilcher CD, Parekh BS, Gershy-Damet G, Branson BM, Marsh K, Wiktor SZ. Surveillance for HIV-1 incidence using tests for recent infection in resource-constrained countries. AIDS 2005;19 Suppl 2:S25–30.

37. Rehle T, Shisana O, Pillay V, Zuma K, Puren A, Parker W. National HIV incidence measures--new insights into the South African epidemic. S Afr Med J 2007;97:194–199.

38. Abdool Karim Q, Hassanally L. HIV Epidemic Types and Customized Prevention Responses. FOCUS, A Guide to AIDS Research and Counseling 2008;v23 n4 Fall:1–4.

39. Abdool Karim SS, Abdool Karim Q, Baxter C, Gouws E. Global Epidemiology of HIV-AIDS. Infectious Disease Clinics of North America 2007;21:1 17.

40. UNAIDS. Joint United Nations Programme on HIV/AIDS. Practical Guidelines for Intensifying HIV Prevention: Towards Universal Access. ISBN 978 92 9173 557 0 (NLM classification: WC 503.2) 2007.

41. Joint United Nations Programme on HIV/AIDS (UNAIDS) and World Health Organization (WHO). Practical Guidelines for Intensifying HIV Prevention: Towards Universal Access. ISBN 978 92 9173 557 0 (NLM classification: WC 503.2) 2007,Geneva.

42. Rothenberg R. HIV transmission networks. Current Opinion in HIV and AIDS 2009;4:260–265.

43. Coates T, Aggeton P, Gutzwiller F, Jarlais DD, Kihara M, Kippax S, et al. HIV prevention in developed countries. Lancet 1996;348:1143–1148.

44. Coates TJ, Richter L, Caceres C. Behavioural strategies to reduce HIV transmission: how to make them work better. Lancet 2008,;72:669–684.

45. Shelton JD. Why multiple sexual partners? Lancet 2009;374:367–369.

46. Padian NS, Buvé A, Balkus J, Serwadda D, Cates W Jr. Biomedical interventions to prevent HIV infection: evidence, challenges, and way forward. Lancet 2008;372:585–599.

47. Joint United Nations Programme on HIV/AIDS (UNAIDS) and World Health Organization (WHO). AIDS epidemic update, 2009. Accessed at, http://data.unaids.org/pub/Report/2009/2009_epidemic_update_en.pdf 2009,Geneva.

48. The Global Fund to Fight AIDS, Tuberculosis and Malaria. Accessed 25 November 2009 at, http://www.theglobalfund.org/en/about/.

49. Berkley S, Naamara W, Okware S, Downing R, Konde-Lule J, Wawer M, et al. AIDS and HIV infection in Uganda—are more women infected than men? AIDS 1990;4:1237–1242.

50. Abdool Karim Q, Abdool Karim SS. The evolving HIV epidemic in South Africa. International Journal of Epidemiology 2002;31:37–40.

51. Cowan F, Pettifor A. HIV in adolescents in sub-Saharan Africa. Curr Opin HIV AIDS 2009;4:288–293.

52. Ghys PD, Kufa E, George MV. Measuring trends in prevalence and incidence of HIV infection in countries with generalised epidemics. Sex Transm Infect 2006;82 Suppl 1:i52–56.

53. Millineum Development Goals. Accessed 25 November, 2009 at, http://www.un.org/millenniumgoals/aids.shtml.

54. Chopra M, Lawn JE, Sanders D, Barron P, Abdool Karim SS, Bradshaw D, et al. Achieving the health Millennium Development Goals for South Africa: challenges and priorities. Lancet 2009,374:1023–1031.

55. Kilmarx PH. Global epidemiology of HIV. Curr Opin HIV AIDS 2009;4:240–246.

56. World Health Organization. Regional Office for Africa. HIV/AIDS epidemiological surveillance report for the WHO African Region: 2007 update. 2008,ISBN 978 92 9023 105 9 (NLM classification: WC 503.4.HA1).

57. Stoneburner RL, Low-Beer D. Population-level HIV declines and behavioral risk avoidance in Uganda. Science 2004;304:714–718.

58. Green EC, Halperin DT, Nantulya V, Hogle JA. Uganda's HIV prevention success: the role of sexual behavior change and the national response. AIDS Behav 2006;10:335–346; discussion 347–350.

59. Shisana O, Rehle T, Simbayi LC, Zuma K, Jooste S, Pillay–van-Wyk V, et al. South African national HIV prevalence, incidence, behaviour and communication survey 2008: A turning tide among teenagers? Cape Town: HSRC Press. 2009.

60. Gouws E, Stanecki KA, Lyerla R, Ghys PD. The epidemiology of HIV infection among young people aged 15–24 years in southern Africa. AIDS 2008;22 Suppl 4:S5–16.

61. South African National Department of Health. Department of Health Summary Report : National HIV and Syphilis Antenatal seroprevalence Survey in South Africa (2007) 2008.

62. Gupta GR, Parkhurst JO, Ogden JA, Aggleton P, Mahal A. Structural approaches to HIV prevention. Lancet 2008;372:764–775.

63. Leclerc-Madlala S. Age-disparate and intergenerational sex in southern Africa: the dynamics of hypervulnerability. AIDS 2008;22 Suppl 4:S17–25.

64. Monasch R, Mahy M. Young people: the centre of the HIV epidemic. World Health Organ Tech Rep Ser 2006;938:15–41; discussion 317–341.

65. Smith AD, Tapsoba P, Peshu N, Sanders EJ, Jaffe HW. Men who have sex with men and HIV/AIDS in sub-Saharan Africa. www.thelancet.com Published online July 20, 2009,DOI:10.1016/S0140-6736(09)61118-1.

66. Guthrie BL, de Bruyn G, Farquhar C. HIV-1-discordant couples in sub-Saharan Africa: explanations and implications for high rates of discordancy. Curr HIV Res 2007;5:416–429.

67. Hollingsworth TD, Anderson RM, Fraser C. HIV-1 transmission, by stage of infection. J Infect Dis 2008;198:687–693.

68. UNAIDS/WHO. Report on the global HIV/AIDS epidemic 2008. "UNAIDS/08.25E / JC1510E". ISBN 978 92 9 173711 6 2008.

69. Ehrhardt AA, Sawires S, McGovern T, Peacock D, Weston M. Gender, empowerment, and health: what is it? How does it work? J Acquir Immune Defic Syndr 2009;51 Suppl 3:S96–S105.

70. Sawires S, Birnbaum N, Abu-Raddad L, Szekeres G, Gayle J. Twenty-five years of HIV: lessons for low prevalence scenarios. J Acquir Immune Defic Syndr 2009;51 Suppl 3:S75–82.

71. Shawky S, Soliman C, Sawires S. Gender and HIV in the Middle East and North Africa: lessons for low prevalence scenarios. J Acquir Immune Defic Syndr 2009;51 Suppl 3:S73–74.

72. Peacock D, Stemple L, Sawires S, Coates TJ. Men, HIV/AIDS, and human rights. J Acquir Immune Defic Syndr 2009;51 Suppl 3:S119–125.

73. Bozicevic I, Voncina L, Zigrovic L, Munz M, Lazarus JV. HIV epidemics among men who have sex with men in central and eastern Europe. Sex Transm Infect 2009;85:336–342.

74. Burruano L, Kruglov Y. HIV/AIDS epidemic in Eastern Europe: recent developments in the Russian Federation and Ukraine among women. Gend Med 2009;6:277–289.

75. Podlekareva D, Bannister W, Mocroft A, Abrosimova L, Karpov I, Lundgren JD, Kirk O. The EuroSIDA study: Regional differences in the HIV-1 epidemic and treatment response to antiretroviral therapy among HIV-infected patients across Europe—a review of published results. Cent Eur J Public Health 2008;16:99–105.

76. Wiessing L, van de Laar MJ, Donoghoe MC, Guarita B, Klempova D, Griffiths P. HIV among injecting drug users in Europe: increasing trends in the East. Euro Surveill 2008,13.

77. Williamson LM, Buston K, Sweeting H. Young women and limits to the normalisation of condom use: a qualitative study. AIDS Care 2009;21:561–566.

78. Wang L, Wang N, Wang L, Li D, Jia M, Gao X, et al. The 2007 Estimates for People at Risk for and Living With HIV in China: Progress and Challenges. J Acquir Immune Defic Syndr 2009;50:414–418.

79. Azim T, Khan SI, Haseen F, Huq NL, Henning L, Pervez MM, et al. HIV and AIDS in Bangladesh. J Health Popul Nutr 2008;26:311–324.

80. Azim T, Rahman M, Alam MS, Chowdhury IA, Khan R, Reza M, et al. Bangladesh moves from being a low-prevalence nation for HIV to one with a concentrated epidemic in injecting drug users. Int J STD AIDS 2008;19:327–331.

81. Islam MM, Conigrave KM. HIV and sexual risk behaviors among recognized high-risk groups in Bangladesh: need for a comprehensive prevention program. Int J Infect Dis 2008;12:363–370.

82. Mercer A, Khanam R, Gurley E, Azim T. Sexual risk behavior of married men and women in Bangladesh associated with husbands' work migration and living apart. Sex Transm Dis 2007;34:265–273.

83. Reddy A, Hoque MM, Kelly R. HIV transmission in Bangladesh: an analysis of IDU programme coverage. Int J Drug Policy 2008;19 Suppl 1:S37–46.

84. Sarkar K, Bal B, Mukherjee R, Chakraborty S, Saha S, Ghosh A, Parsons S. Sex-trafficking, violence, negotiating skill, and HIV infection in brothel-based sex workers of eastern India, adjoining Nepal, Bhutan, and Bangladesh. J Health Popul Nutr 2008;26:223–231.

85. Sharma M, Oppenheimer E, Saidel T, Loo V, Garg R. A situation update on HIV epidemics among people who inject drugs and national responses in South-East Asia Region. AIDS 2009;23:1405–1413.

86. Silverman JG, Decker MR, Kapur NA, Gupta J, Raj A. Violence against wives, sexual risk and sexually transmitted infection among Bangladeshi men. Sex Transm Infect 2007;83:211–215.

87. Hesketh T. HIV/AIDS in China: the numbers problem. Lancet 2007;369:621–623.

88. Wang H, Chen RY, Ding G, Ma Y, Ma J, Jiao JH, et al. Prevalence and predictors of HIV infection among female sex workers in Kaiyuan City, Yunnan Province, China. Int J Infect Dis 2009;13:162–169.

89. Wong FY, Huang ZJ, Wang W, He N, Marzzurco J, Frangos S, et al. STIs and HIV among men having sex with men in China: a ticking time bomb? AIDS Educ Prev 2009;21:430–446.

90. Yao Y, Wang N, Chu J, Ding G, Jin X, Sun Y, et al. Sexual behavior and risks for HIV infection and transmission among male injecting drug users in Yunnan, China. Int J Infect Dis 2009;13:154–161.

Chapter 6 VIROLOGY OF HIV

MARVIN S. REITZ

I've got something here that's bigger than Legionnaire's.
What's the shortest time between submission and publication?

—MICHAEL GOTTLIEB, MD, UCLA, April 4, 1981

Identification of a New Disease

Reports of what is now known as AIDS (acquired immunodeficiency syndrome) first appeared in the early 1980s.[1-5] AIDS was not immediately recognized as a single entity because the manifestations were quite diverse, ranging from various opportunistic infections, especially *Pneumocystis carinii* pneumonia (PCP) (a fungal infection common in humans but not generally pathogenic) and Kaposi's sarcoma (KS) (a previously rare and generally indolent skin lesion primarily seen in elderly men of Mediterranean extraction). Homosexuals were the first identified risk group. Other risk groups were soon identified, including Haitians, heroin users, and hemophiliacs. This, along with the identification of disease clusters, suggested that AIDS was infectious in origin. Many suggestions were made regarding a possible causative agent. In 1982, Gallo's lab and that of Essex suggested that the causative agent was an human T cell leukemia (HTLV)-related virus,[6-8] based on the facts that HTLV-I infects CD4+ T cells, the main cell population affected in AIDS, and that retroviruses such as feline leukemia virus (FeLV) cause immunodeficiency in addition to leukemia. Indeed, HTLV-I, the causative agent of adult T cell leukemia (ATL), itself causes a modest immune impairment that can be manifested even in the absence of ATL. The notion that AIDS was caused by a new retrovirus related to HTLV was obviously quite attractive.

HIV-1: Discovery and Identification as the Cause of AIDS

Montagier and his colleagues were the first to detect the retrovirus now known as human immunodeficiency virus type 1 (HIV-1) in 1983.[9] Shortly thereafter, the Gallo laboratory made a large number of detections and isolations of what proved to be the same virus. Several of these isolates were put into T cell lines for large-scale production.[10-13] The virus was soon shown to be novel and to not be closely related to HTLV-1. The availability of large quantities of viral proteins facilitated the development of a blood test for the presence of the antibodies to the virus. It was proven to be the cause of AIDS and was named HIV-1. The blood test also allowed most infected blood products to be identified, greatly reducing subsequent infections of hemophiliacs and transfusion recipients and saving countless thousands of lives.

HIV Origins

In addition to providing protein reagents, large-scale production of HIV-1 also made viral nucleic acid reagents available. This resulted in the discovery of HIV-2, a related but distinct virus, in western Africans.[14,15] At about the same time, related viruses, collectively called simian immunodeficiency viruses (SIVs), were discovered in several species of Old World monkeys, including African green monkeys.[16] Phylogenetic studies suggest that HIV-2 originated recently by zoonotic transmission from monkeys to humans,[17,18] and that such transmission most likely occurred through infection of hunters and butchers involved in the bush meat trade.

More recently, it has been suggested that the chimpanzee *Pan troglodytes* ssp. *troglodytes* is the source of HIV-1,[19,20] and that chimpanzees may themselves have been infected by cross-species transmission, perhaps upon multiple occasions. In fact, the chimpanzee virus (SIV_{cpz}) appears to be a result of recombination between different SIVs.[21] Transmission of SIV_{cpz} to humans seems to have occurred at least three times, and a transmission in southeastern Cameroon likely accounts for group M, the prevalent HIV-1 group. Similar zoonotic transmissions have probably occurred on many other occasions. If this is so, the resultant viruses have not been detected or been disseminated in human populations, and the three successful zoonoses (groups M, N and O) are the only ones that appear to have survived. One wonders to what extent future transmissions of this sort are likely to occur.

It has been recently suggested that following transmission to humans, HIV-1 was introduced into Haiti from Africa, and that it then entered the U.S. in the 1960s.[22] It then would have spread and given rise to clade B HIV-1(M), the predominant clade of HIV-1 in the U.S, Europe, and other locations. Clade B is but one of nine clades within the HIV-1(M) group, and there are many interclade recombinants that are in active circulation. Africa contains the widest variety of clades and inter-clade recombinants, consistent with the origin of HIV-1 in Africa, although clade C is the most common form of HIV-1 in both Africa and India.

A recent report has suggested that the distant evolutionary origin of HIV is represented by an endogenous lentivirus of European rabbits. This virus, called RELIK, is estimated to have entered the rabbit genome seven million years ago and could represent the ancestral form of all lentiviruses.[23]

HIV Virology

HIV-1 is a lentivirus, a group that also includes bovine and feline immunodeficiency viruses, equine infectious anemia virus, Maedi-visna virus, and caprine arthritis-encephalomyelitis virus. However, HIV-1 also bears some interesting similarities to HTLV. One is its preference for CD4+ T cells in the host. Both are also genetically complex retroviruses. Unlike the simple retroviruses such as murine leukemia virus, which have only *gag*, *pol*, and *env* genes and a single spliced mRNA, HIV and HTLV have additional genes and mRNAs that result from a complex pattern of multiple RNA splicing, as summarized in **Figure 6–1**. Both viruses have genes which are necessary for viral replication that are functionally similar. One gene product (Tax/Tat) upregulates viral RNA synthesis many-fold and the other (Rex/Rev) regulates viral RNA splicing patterns.

Unlike HTLV, however, HIV-1 is highly competent for infection of its target cells, which can include primary CD4+ T cells, CD4+ T cell lines, and macrophage-monocytes. The cell surface protein CD4 was identified as a host cell receptor for HIV-1,[24,25] partially explaining the viral host cell range. Howevder, this did not completely explain the host cell range. HIV-1 isolates fall broadly into two cell tropism groups.[26,27] One group had been referred to as T cell line-tropic or syncytium inducing (SI). These were viruses that could infect both primary T cells and T cell lines, but were poorly infectious for macrophages. They also form multicellular syncytia following infection. The other group were called macrophage-tropic or non-syncytium–inducing (NSI). They infect both macrophages and primary T cells, but do not generally infect T cell lines very well and do not form large syncytia.

The basis for this dichotomy was revealed following the identification of three β-chemokines, MIP-1α, MIP-1β, and RANTES, as naturally produced factors that blocked infection by NSI HIV-1.[28] Shortly thereafter, Berger's lab realized that SI isolates use a chemokine receptor (now called CXCR4) as an obligate second receptor.[29] CXCR4 does not recognize MIP-1α, MIP-1β, or RANTES, and these chemokines do not inhibit infection with SI viruses. It was then recorded by multiple groups that NSI isolates depended upon a different chemokine receptor, CCR5, for which all three chemokines are ligands.[30–35] The molecular basis for the tropism differences of the two HIV-1 groups was now clear. As a result, NSI and SI isolates are now designated as R5 and X4 isolates, respectively. The first binding event upon encountering the cell surface is to CD4. This triggers a conformational change in gp120, the viral surface envelope protein, which unmasks the binding site for the chemokine receptor. Once the gp120 binds to the chemokine receptor, a second conformational change occurs which exposes the fusion domain of gp41, the viral transmembrane envelope protein. Fusion then leads to cell entry, as summarized in **Figure 6–2**.

When HIV is transmitted between individuals, it is almost always exclusively the R5 virus. Some individuals have a deletion mutation of CCR5. This mutation, CCR5Δ32, results in a lack of CCR5 expression, and people who are homozygous for CCR5Δ32 are highly resistant to infection as a result.[36–39] There are no obvious deleterious effects of the CCR5Δ32 mutation, which suggested that targeting CCR5 could be a viable therapeutic or preventative option. In fact, small molecules that target CCR5 have been developed and have begun to enter clinical use.

After the virus fuses with the cell membrane and enters the cell, a preintegration complex (PIC) is released into the cytoplasm and reverse transcription occurs. During reverse transcription, the PIC is transported to the nucleus. Upon completion of reverse transcription, viral DNA is integrated into the host cell genome. Unlike simple retroviruses, the HIV-1 PIC can actively enter the nucleus of a nondividing cell.[40–43] This is due, at least in part, to nuclear targeting signals on the Vpr, integrase, and matrix (p17) proteins contained in the PIC,[41–44] as shown schematically in **Figure 6–3**.

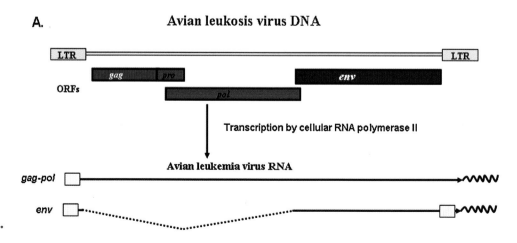

Figure 6–1A.

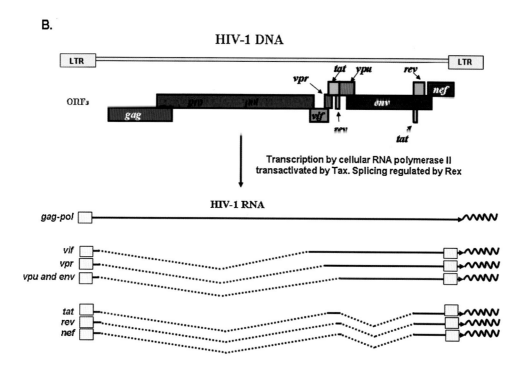

Figure 6–1B.

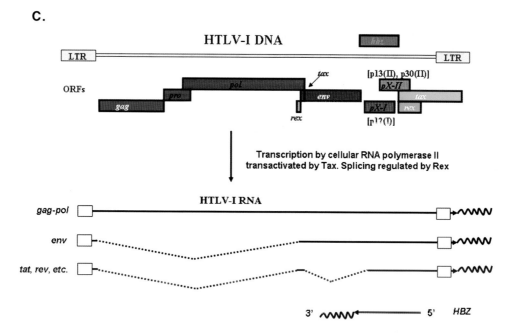

Figure 6–1C.

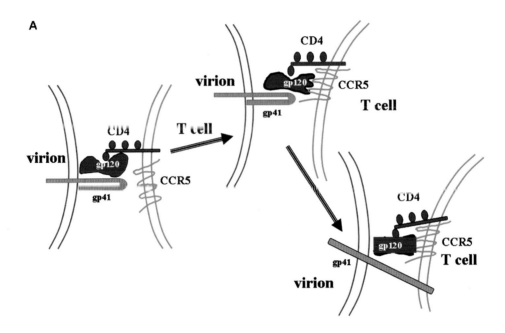

Figure 6–2A.

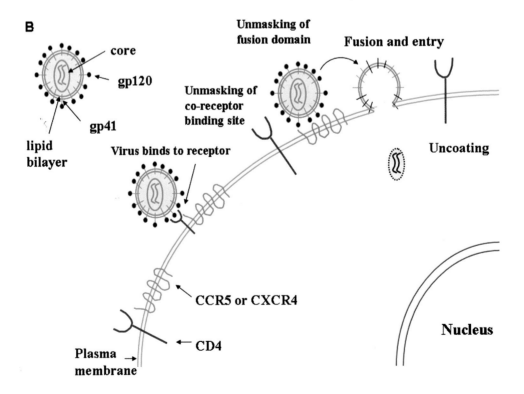

Figure 6–2B.

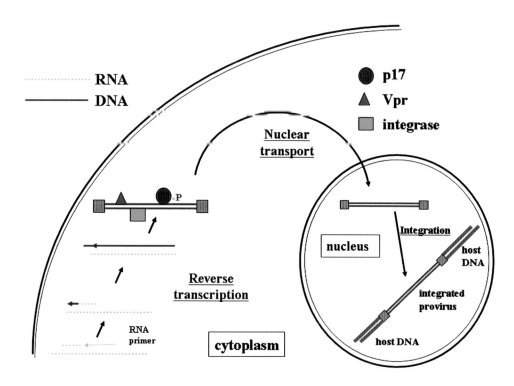

Figure 6-3.

The Viral Genome

The HIV genome, shown schematically in **Figure 6-1**, is about 9,750 nucleotides long.[45-48] As mentioned earlier, the HIV genome bears little sequence identity with HTLV, but functionally it bears a strong resemblance, encoding numerous accessory proteins and having a complex RNA splicing pattern, shown schematically in **Figures 6-1** and **6-4**. Like other retroviruses, a viral promoter/enhancer for cellular RNA polymerase and a polyadenylation/transcription stop signal are contained in the large terminal repeat (LTR) sequences. In addition, the LTRs contain a Tat activation region (TAR), which is a binding site for the HIV transcriptional transactivator, Tat.[49-52] Tat is functionally analogous to the HTLV-I Tax protein. Full-length viral RNA is also the mRNA for the Gag gene products, translated as a polypeptide precursor and processed by the viral protease into the myristoylated p17 matrix protein, the p24 capsid protein, the p7 nucleocapsid protein, and a p6 protein.[53,54] A translational frameshift permits translation of the Pol protein as a Gag-Pol precursor polypeptide,[55,56] which is processed by the viral protease into the p32integrase, the p66/51 reverse transcriptase/RNase H, and the p10 protease.[57] The highly glycosylated envelope protein is translated from a singly spliced mRNA.[58-60] After cleavage of the signal peptide, the gp120 surface protein and transmembrane gp41 protein are generated by cleavage by furin, a cellular protease.[61] The gp41 remains associated with the gp120, and the two proteins are present on the surface of the virus particles as a trimer. Vpu is cotranslated from the singly spliced Env transcript.[60]

The primary function of Vif is to block the antiviral activity of the cellular protein APOBEC-3G.[119,120] APOBEC-3G is one of a family of cytidine deaminases that are involved in RNA editing and hypermutation of cellular genes. In the absence of Vif, APOBEC-3G edits viral RNA and causes multiple G to A mutations that hypermutate the viral genome.[121] Vif blocks APOBEC-3G incorporation into virus particles. The role of APOBEC-3G in antiviral responses is discussed further below.

HIV-Host Cell Interactions

Because viruses are by their nature quite limited in genetic capacity, they typically rely on many cellular factors, some of which are described above, to facilitate viral replication. Conversely, infected cells have a wide variety of antiviral responses. Thus, viral-host cell interactions are important because they determine the efficiencies of both viral infections and antiviral responses. These interactions potentially provide opportunities for rational design of antiviral therapies. Recently, in a large study using individual siRNA knockdown expression of all known human genes, more than 250 cellular genes appeared to be important for support of viral replication.[122] It may be possible to target some of these interactions for antiviral therapy, although clearly specificity will be critical to avoid the possibility of targeting important cell-cell protein interactions and generating untoward side effects. One virus-cell interaction that has been targeted is that of the Env protein with the CCR5 coreceptor, and drugs that target this interaction have recently entered clinical practice, as discussed below.

Many virus-host interactions are antiviral. Two obvious and broad examples are humoral and cellular adaptive immune responses. Neutralizing antibodies primarily target the surface Env protein, gp120, although a few such antibodies are directed against the ectodomain of the transmembrane Env protein, gp41. Antibodies against other viral proteins may mediate antibody-directed cellular cytotoxicity (ADCC), but their significance is not entirely clear. However, targeting gp120 with neutralizing antibodies presents difficulties. The gp120 is extremely variable, particularly within the five hypervariable regions, and single point mutations in the gp120 (or even the gp41) can abrogate neutralization, even by broadly neutralizing natural antibodies.[123–126]

The carbohydrate residues and hypervariable regions are on the surface of virion-associated gp120 trimers and tend to occlude the more conserved regions that comprise the CD4 and CCR5 binding sites. These sites might be transiently exposed during infection, allowing access to appropriate neutralizing antibodies. Indeed, following CD4 binding, the CCR5 binding site of the envelope is exposed.[127–131] This site may be a conformationally restrained site because of the necessity to maintain its function and efforts are being made to generate antibodies against it. These efforts include the use as antigens of gp120-CD4 chimeric proteins which are joined by a peptide tether. Interestingly, this approach has generated antibodies that show a rather broad neutralization profile.[132,133]

An example of cellular immunity is CTL recognition of viral proteins expressed by infected cells. CTL epitopes exist on most HIV proteins, and since these proteins are generally more conserved than is gp120, many vaccine approaches have depended upon eliciting CTL responses to them. One disadvantage to this approach is that it depends on cells being already infected.[134] A recent large vaccine trial based upon this approach failed.[135] However, another recent vaccine trial that combined this approach with the generation of neutralizing antibodies has shown a transient weak (but significant) protective effect,[136] suggesting that a combined vaccine approach may be required.

A third type of host antiviral interaction, represented by innate immunity, has been receiving increased interest. Innate immunity involves a wide variety of mechanisms, including natural killer cell activity, the actions of chemokines and cytokines and their receptors, inflammatory responses, and various intracellular activities. Recent discoveries have increased our appreciation of innate immunity. In the case of HIV-1, the first report of this type of activity, as mentioned above, identified the cellular CCR5 ligands MIP-1α, MIP-1β, and RANTES as potent antiviral factors that blocked the interaction of gp120 with its CCR5 coreceptor.[28] Interestingly, a number of reports have shown a correlation of expression levels of these chemokines with greater resistance to infection in HIV-exposed people, as well as with a slower progression to AIDS in infected people.[137–141] As a caveat, higher levels of chemokine expression may simply be a marker for better preservation of immune competence. A more recent report has shown that β defensins may also provide significant anti-HIV activity,[142] although the mechanism differs. Antiviral activity appears to depend upon binding to CCR6 followed by induction of APOBEC-3G (see below).

APOBEC-3G and related family members have recently been found to mediate intracellular antiviral activity, which is counteracted by the HIV-1 Vif protein. The APOBEC family may represent an ancient host defense mechanism against retroviruses; APOBEC-3G inhibits replication of retroviruses in general. It is normally incorporated into virions, where it binds to viral RNA. It becomes activated when the virion enters a target cell and initiates reverse transcription.[143–145] Resting CD4 T cells contain an active low molecular weight form of APOBRC.[146] T cell activation results in the formation of an inactive high molecular weight form. Vif prevents APOBEC incorporation into virions by depleting cytoplasmic APOBEC. This occurs by a dual mechanism that includes both inhibiting translation of APOBEC mRNA and facilitating degradation of the protein by the 26S proteasome.[145] A recent report suggests that the antiviral activity of APOBEC does not seem to depend upon its cytidine deaminase activity.[146]

Another recently described intracellular antiviral activity is mediated by members of the tripartite motif (TRIM) family.[147] The tripartite motif contains a RING domain at its N-terminus, a B box-2 domain, and a coiled-coil domain.[148] The TRIM family, as with the APOBEC family, appears to represent another ancient antiretroviral innate host defense. TRIM5α, the best studied of the group, may be a functional homolog of the Fv1 restriction element, which regulates the susceptibility of murine cells of different genetic backgrounds to infection with B-tropic versus N-tropic murine leukemia viruses (MuLV), and was identified forty years ago.[149] The capsid protein is the target of both factors, and the restriction of N-tropic MuLV infection by both proteins depends upon recognition of residue 110 of the MuLV capsid protein.[150] HIV-1 has evolved a partial resistance to human TRIM5α,[151] which may help to explain its successful transmission from chimpanzees to humans. In contrast, macaque TRIM5α strongly restricts HIV-1.[147,150] TRIM5α binds to viral capsid hexamers[152] and it inhibits replication at the post-entry level. The mechanism is not entirely clear, however, and there may be several mechanisms. One likely mechanism is to accelerate uncoating of the viral capsid, resulting in a nonfunctional PIC.[152,153] The antiviral activity of TRIM5α is increased by its trimerization.[154]

A third recently described mechanism of intracellular antiviral activity is mediated by CD317, also known as tetherin.[155] Tetherin causes the retention of fully formed virions on the surface of infected cells. This interaction is species specific. Vpu from murine cells is not active against HIV.[156] The viral Vpu protein overcomes this antiviral activity by down-regulating surface levels of tetherin by accelerating its degradation by the 20S proteasome.[156] This function appears to be assumed by Nef in some SIV strains.[157,158]

HIV Pathogenesis

Many mechanisms have been proposed for HIV pathogenesis, and they include both direct and indirect mechanisms. Proposed direct mechanisms are those that kill infected cells, and they include syncytium formation, apoptosis, cell cycle arrest, and other mechanisms. At times, the prevalent view has been that most of the pathogenesis is due to direct cell killing. However, although this clearly occurs, infected cells are generally only a small minority of the total CD4+ T cell population, and so direct killing does not seem to account for the large-scale collapse of the immune system that occurs during infection. Direct killing also fails to explain pathologies that are common in HIV-infected people that involve cells not infected with HIV, including HIV-associated neuropathy and nephropathy. Recently it was reported that HIV-1 and SIV infections quickly result in the rapid infection and killing of large numbers of CD4+ T cells in the gastrointestinal tract.[159,160] Although this could be an example of direct cell killing, progression to AIDS is generally slow. To explain the slow course, it has been proposed that gastrointestinal integrity is compromised due to the rapid depletion of gut-associated lymphoid tissue, and that this leads to leakage of bacteria from the gut and chronic immune activation.[161] This model of AIDS progression thus includes elements of direct and indirect mechanisms, but to date it has not been widely accepted.

To kill uninfected cells, it is necessary to invoke indirect mechanisms. One way this might occur is through chronic antigenic stimulation by HIV proteins, eventually resulting in clonal depletion and immune exhaustion. Another possibility is that uninfected cells could be adversely affected by circulating proteins. These could be virus-encoded proteins such as gp120 or Tat, or cellular proteins such as cytokines released from infected cells. As a possible example of the latter, interleukin-10 (IL-10), which is elevated in AIDS patients, is involved in facilitating functional immune exhaustion, resulting in chronic lymphocytic choriomeningitis virus (LCMV) infections in mice.[162] Blockade of the IL-10 receptor in infected mice prevents both chronic LCMV infection and immune exhaustion.[162] Cellular and viral proteins might act in concert. As another possible example, excess production of interferon by T cells from AIDS patients, in combination with extracellular Tat, leads to reduced expression of antiviral chemokines and the generation of suppressor T cells.[163] The auxiliary proteins of HIV, discussed above, can modify cellular signal transduction pathways, leading to induction of expression of cytokines or other soluble cell proteins. It is probable that HIV pathogenesis is the result of multiple factors.

Prospects for Future HIV Therapies

Retroviral infection, because viral DNA is integrated into host cell DNA, lasts for the life of the cell. This means that once an infection is established, it is impossible for all practical purposes to clear the body of every infected cell. This is particularly true when long-lived cells are latently infected, as has been demonstrated for HIV.[164] Since infection by a retrovirus is essentially lifelong, eradication of HIV from populations will depend upon widespread prevention of infection, and this will likely depend upon the development of a protective vaccine. However, in practice this has been quite difficult. As discussed above, one recent vaccine trial failed to protect against infection and in some cases appeared to facilitate infection.[135] A second trial showed a weak and transient but significant protective effect.[136] Understanding the basis for this protection could provide valuable leads for subsequent vaccine development.

Most currently used antiretroviral agents have been developed by rational design based on the three-dimensional structure of viral proteins and on functional inhibition detected by high throughput screening. The first class of antiretrovirals was nucleoside analog reverse transcriptase (RT) inhibitors such as AZT.[165] originating with studies in Broder's laboratory at the National Cancer Institute. This class was quickly followed by nonnucleoside RT inhibitors, including nevirapine.[166] Inhibitors of the viral protease,[167] such as ritonavir, saquinavir, and indinavir, were the next to be developed. Combinations of these agents with the two classes of RT inhibitors proved to be particularly potent.[168] This approach, called highly active anti-retroviral therapy (HAART), has been quite effective in reducing viral burden and delaying the development of AIDS. However, problems with toxicity, side effects, and the development of viral drug resistance occur commonly.

Recently, entry inhibitors have been introduced in the clinic. These include virus-cell fusion inhibitors such as T20 (Fuzeon)[169] and envelope-CCR5 binding inhibitors.[170] They are primarily used with people who are infected with HIV resistant to protease and RT inhibitors. Side effects and toxicities are still an issue, and Fuzeon must be injected regularly. Resistance to entry inhibitors also occurs, leading to fears that a shift from R5 to X4 usage would occur. X4 viruses are believed to be more pathogenic, although this has not been clearly established. This shift does not readily occur, however, and resistance instead appears to involve altered recognition and usage of CCR5.[171] Integrase inhibitors are also in the pipeline. One such integrase inhibitor, raltegravir, is now being used in patients with drug-resistant HIV,[172] but it only seems to be highly effective in combination with other drugs. Beviramat, a Chinese herb derivative, inhibits viral particle maturation[173] and has recently entered clinical trials.

The drugs described above primarily target viral proteins. However, HIV rapidly mutates, and, therefore, resistant variants tend to occur rapidly. As the interactions of viral proteins with cellular proteins and the contributions of those interactions to viral replication become identified and understood, it may become possible to target antiviral therapies against cellular proteins. The advantage of this approach is that cellular proteins do not mutate rapidly. If the cellular target were not critical for the host, this approach might be an effective antiviral strategy. An example of this kind of approach that has already been developed is CCR5 blockade. People who are homozygous for the Δ32 CCR5 mutation, as discussed above, are very resistant to infection, but have no obvious health abnormalities.[36–39] This gave some confidence that CCR5 could be safely targeted therapeutically. However, viruses resistant to these drugs do occur through selection of mutations in the envelope protein[171,174,175] This suggests that even if cellular proteins are successfully targeted, mutations in viral proteins could result in resistance. Moreover, some of the CCR5 blocking drugs have been associated with serious side effects, including cardiovascular problems. Drugs that target cell metabolism, such as hydroxyurea (which reduces intracellular DNA precursor levels)[176] and rapamycin (which affects mTOR-dependent signal transduction, blocks cell cycling, and reduces CCR5 expression)[177] synergize with other antiretrovirals (RT inhibitors with hydroxyurea, CCR5 inhibitors with rapamycin), but are associated wtih some toxicity.

In the future, gene therapy may yield useful antiviral therapies. Possible approaches include ribozymes, intracellular antibodies, antisense RNA, siRNA, and decoys for viral proteins. Gene therapy, although potentially highly promising, still has to overcome several serious technical obstacles. These problems include efficient delivery of genes to specific, appropriate cells and the maintenance of durable expression. Since infection with HIV or other retroviruses is effectively lifelong, expression of antiviral genetic constructs also needs to be lifelong. This requires a vector that can insert the appropriate gene into host DNA, which in turn raises the possibility of harmful insertional mutagenesis (for example, insertion near or within an oncogene). In fact, this possibility has been realized in otherwise partially successful gene therapy trials for patients with severe combined immunotherapy X1.[178] The only approach that would "cure" infected cells would be one that could specifically excise or destroy proviral DNA from host cell DNA. Excision of proviral DNA from infected cells without obvious cytotoxicity using an evolved recombinase has been reported,[179] but clinical use of this sort of approach is likely to be far in the future. Given that HIV can remain latent in long-lived T cells, it is not likely that a single therapy would provide safe, effective long-term treatment of HIV infection. Future progress will likely be incremental, and resistant mutants will probably occur with each new approach. Development of new approaches will thus continue to be needed.

References

1. Siegal FP, Lopez C, Hammer GS, et al. Severe acquired immunodeficiency in male homosexuals, manifested by chronic perianal ulcerative herpes simplex lesions. N Engl J Med 1981;305(24):1439–1444.

2. Masur H, Michelis MA, Greene JB, et al. An outbreak of community-acquired Pneumocystis carinii pneumonia: initial manifestation of cellular immune dysfunction. N Engl J Med 1981;305(24):1431–1438.

3. Hymes KB, Cheung T, Greene JB, et al. Kaposi's sarcoma in homosexual men-a report of eight cases. Lancet 1981;2(8247):598–600.

4. Gottlieb MS, Schroff R, Schanker HM, et al. Pneumocystis carinii pneumonia and mucosal candidiasis in previously healthy homosexual men: evidence of a new acquired cellular immunodeficiency. N Engl J Med 1981;305(24):1425–1431.

5. Friedman-Kien AE, Laubenstein LJ, Rubinstein P, et al. Disseminated Kaposi's sarcoma in homosexual men. Ann Intern Med 1982;96(6 Pt 1):693–700.

6. Gallo RC, Sarin PS, Gelmann EP, et al. Isolation of human T-cell leukemia virus in acquired immune deficiency syndrome (AIDS). Science 1983;220(4599):865–867.

7. Gelmann EP, Popovic M, Blayney D, et al. Proviral DNA of a retrovirus, human T-cell leukemia virus, in two patients with AIDS. Science 1983;220(4599):862–865.

8. Essex M, McLane MF, Lee TH, et al. Antibodies to cell membrane antigens associated with human T-cell leukemia virus in patients with AIDS. Science 1983;220(4599):859–862.

9. Barre-Sinoussi F, Chermann JC, Rey F, et al. Isolation of a T-lymphotropic retrovirus from a patient at risk for acquired immune deficiency syndrome (AIDS). Science 1983;220(4599):868–871.

10. Gallo RC, Salahuddin SZ, Popovic M, et al. Frequent detection and isolation of cytopathic retroviruses (HTLV-III) from patients with AIDS and at risk for AIDS. Science 1984;224:500–503.

11. Popovic M, Sarngadharan MG, Read E, Gallo RC. Detection, isolation, and continuous production of cytopathic retroviruses (HTLV-III) from patients with AIDS and pre-AIDS. Science 1984;224(4648):497–500.

12. Sarngadharan MG, Popovic M, Bruch L, Schupbach J, Gallo RC. Antibodies reactive with human T-lymphotropic retroviruses (HTLV-III) in the serum of patients with AIDS. Science 1984;224(4648):506–508.

13. Schupbach J, Sarngadharan MG, Gallo RC. Antigens on HTLV-infected cells recognized by leukemia and AIDS sera are related to HTLV viral glycoprotein. Science 1984;224(4649):607–610.

14. Kanki PJ, Barin F, M'Boup S, et al. New human T-lymphotropic retrovirus related to simian T-lymphotropic virus type III (STLV-IIIAGM). Science 1986;232(4747):238–243.

15. Barin F, M'Boup S, Denis F, et al. Serological evidence for virus related to simian T-lymphotropic retrovirus III in residents of west Africa. Lancet 1985;2(8469–70):1387–1389.

16. Kanki PJ, Alroy J, Essex M. Isolation of T-lymphotropic retrovirus related to HTLV-III/LAV from wild-caught African green monkeys. Science 1985;230(4728):951–954.

17. Chen Z, Telfier P, Gettie A, et al. Genetic characterization of new West African simian immunodeficiency virus SIVsm: geographic clustering of household-derived SIV strains with human immunodeficiency virus type 2 subtypes and genetically diverse viruses from a single feral sooty mangabey troop. J Virol 1996;70(6):3617–3627.

18. Sharp PM, Robertson DL, Hahn BH. Cross-species transmission and recombination of 'AIDS' viruses. Philos Trans R Soc Lond B Biol Sci 1995;349(1327):41–47.

19. Gao F, Bailes E, Robertson DL, et al. Origin of HIV-1 in the chimpanzee Pan troglodytes troglodytes. Nature 1999;397(6718):436–441.

20. Keele BF, Van HF, Li Y, et al. Chimpanzee reservoirs of pandemic and nonpandemic HIV-1. Science 2006;313(5786):523–526.

21. Bailes E, Gao F, Bibollet-Ruche F, et al. Hybrid origin of SIV in chimpanzees. Science 2003;300(5626):1713.

22. Gilbert MT, Rambaut A, Wlasiuk G, Spira TJ, Pitchenik AE, Worobey M. The emergence of HIV/AIDS in the Americas and beyond. Proc Natl Acad Sci U S A 2007;104(47):18566–18570.

23. Katzourakis A, Tristem M, Pybus OG, Gifford RJ. Discovery and analysis of the first endogenous lentivirus. Proc Natl Acad Sci U S A 2007;104(15):6261–6265.

24. Dalgleish AG, Beverley PC, Clapham PR, Crawford DH, Greaves MF, Weiss RA. The CD4 (T4) antigen is an essential component of the receptor for the AIDS retrovirus. Nature 1984;312(5996):763–767.

25. Klatzmann D, Champagne E, Chamaret S, et al. T-lymphocyte T4 molecule behaves as the receptor for human retrovirus LAV. Nature 1984;312(5996):767–768.

26. Gartner S, Markovits P, Markovitz DM, Betts RF, Popovic M. Virus isolation from and identification of HTLV-III/LAV-producing cells in brain tissue from a patient with AIDS. JAMA 1986;256(17):2365–2371.

27. Asjo B, Morfeldt-Manson L, Albert J, et al. Replicative capacity of human immunodeficiency virus from patients with varying severity of HIV infection. Lancet 1986;2(8508):660–662.

28. Cocchi F, DeVico AL, Garzino-Demo A, Arya SK, Gallo RC, Lusso P. Identification of RANTES, MIP-1 alpha, and MIP-1 beta as the major HIV-suppressive factors produced by CD8+ T cells. Science 1995;270:1811–1815.

29. Feng Y, Broder CC, Kennedy PE, Berger EA. HIV-1 entry cofactor: functional cDNA cloning of a seven-transmembrane, G protein-coupled receptor. Science 1996;272(5263):872–877.

30. Alkhatib G, Combadiere C, Broder CC, et al. CC CKR5: a RANTES, MIP-1alpha, MIP-1beta receptor as a fusion cofactor for macrophage-tropic HIV-1. Science 1996;272:1955–1958.

31. Berson JF, Long D, Doranz BJ, Rucker J, Jirik FR, Doms RW. A seven-transmembrane domain receptor involved in fusion and entry of T-cell-tropic human immunodeficiency virus type 1 strains. J Virol 1996;70:6288–6295.

32. Choe H, Farzan M, Sun Y, et al. The beta-chemokine receptors CCR3 and CCR5 facilitate infection by primary HIV-1 isolates. Cell 1996;85:1135–1148.

33. Deng H, Liu R, Ellmeier W, et al. Identification of a major co-receptor for primary isolates of HIV-1. Nature 1996;381:661–666.

34. Doranz BJ, Rucker J, Yi Y, et al. A dual-tropic primary HIV-1 isolate that uses fusin and the beta- chemokine receptors CKR-5, CKR-3, and CKR-2b as fusion cofactors. Cell 1996;85:1149–1158.

35. Dragic T, Litwin V, Allaway GP, et al. HIV-1 entry into CD4+ cells is mediated by the chemokine receptor CC-CKR-5. Nature 1996;381:667–673.

36. Dean M, Carrington M, Winkler C, et al. Genetic restriction of HIV-1 infection and progression to AIDS by a deletion allele of the CKR5 structural gene. Science 1996;273:1856–1862.

37. Huang Y, Paxton WA, Wolinsky SM, et al. The role of a mutant CCR5 allele in HIV-1 transmission and disease progression. Nat Med 1996;2:1240–1243.

38. Liu R, Paxton WA, Choe S, et al. Homozygous defect in HIV-1 coreceptor accounts for resistance of some multiply-exposed individuals to HIV-1 infection. Cell 1996;86:367–377.

39. Samson M, Libert F, Doranz BJ, et al. Resistance to HIV-1 infection in caucasian individuals bearing mutant alleles of the CCR-5 chemokine receptor gene. Nature 1996;382:722–725.

40. Bukrinsky MI, Sharova N, Dempsey MP, et al. Active nuclear import of human immunodeficiency virus type 1 preintegration complexes. Proc Natl Acad Sci U S A 1992;89(14):6580-6584.

41. Di Marzio P, Choe S, Ebright M, Knoblauch R, Landau NR. Mutational analysis of cell cycle arrest, nuclear localization and virion packaging of human immunodeficiency virus type 1 Vpr. J Virol 1995;69(12):7909–7916.

42. Mahalingam S, Ayyavoo V, Patel M, Kieber-Emmons T, Weiner DB. Nuclear import, virion incorporation, and cell cycle arrest/differentiation are mediated by distinct functional domains of human immunodeficiency virus type 1 Vpr. J Virol 1997;71(9):6339–6347.

43. Gallay P, Hope T, Chin D, Trono D. HIV-1 infection of nondividing cells through the recognition of integrase by the importin/karyopherin pathway. Proc Natl Acad Sci U S A 1997;94(18):9825–9830.

44. Bukrinsky MI, Haggerty S, Dempsey MP, et al. A nuclear localization signal within HIV-1 matrix protein that governs infection of non-dividing cells. Nature 1993;365(6447):666–669.

45. Muesing MA, Smith DH, Cabradilla CD, Benton CV, Lasky LA, Capon DJ. Nucleic acid structure and expression of the human AIDS/lymphadenopathy retrovirus. Nature 1985;313(6002):450–458.

46. Sanchez-Pescador R, Power MD, Barr PJ, et al. Nucleotide sequence and expression of an AIDS-associated retrovirus (ARV-2). Science 1985;227(4686):484–492.

47. Wain-Hobson S, Sonigo P, Danos O, Cole S, Alizon M. Nucleotide sequence of the AIDS virus, LAV. Cell 1985;40(1):9–17.

48. Ratner L, Haseltine W, Patarca R, et al. Complete nucleotide sequence of the AIDS virus, HTLV-III. Nature 1985;313(6000):277–284.

49. Muesing MA, Smith DH, Capon DJ. Regulation of mRNA accumulation by a human immunodeficiency virus trans-activator protein. Cell 1987;48(4):691–701.

50. Berkhout B, Jeang KT. trans activation of human immunodeficiency virus type 1 is sequence specific for both the single-stranded bulge and loop of the trans-acting-responsive hairpin: a quantitative analysis. J Virol 1989;63(12):5501–5504.

51. Hauber J, Cullen BR. Mutational analysis of the trans-activation-responsive region of the human immunodeficiency virus type I long terminal repeat. J Virol 1988;62(3):673–679.

52. Sodroski J, Patarca R, Rosen C, Wong-Staal F, Haseltine W. Location of the trans-activating region on the genome of human T-cell lymphotropic virus type III. Science 1985;229(4708):74–77.

53. Gowda SD, Stein BS, Engleman EG. Identification of protein intermediates in the processing of the p55 HIV-1 gag precursor in cells infected with recombinant vaccinia virus. J Biol Chem 1989;264(15):8459–8462.

54. Mervis RJ, Ahmad N, Lillehoj EP, et al. The gag gene products of human immunodeficiency virus type 1: alignment within the gag open reading frame, identification of posttranslational modifications, and evidence for alternative gag precursors. J Virol 1988;62(11):3993–4002.

55. Wilson W, Braddock M, Adams SE, Rathjen PD, Kingsman SM, Kingsman AJ. HIV expression strategies: ribosomal frameshifting is directed by a short sequence in both mammalian and yeast systems. Cell 1988;55(6):1159–1169.

56. Jacks T, Power MD, Masiarz FR, Luciw PA, Barr PJ, Varmus HE. Characterization of ribosomal frameshifting in HIV-1 gag-pol expression. Nature 1988;331(6153):280–283.

57. Schulze T, Nawrath M, Moelling K. Cleavage of the HIV-1 p66 reverse transcriptase/RNase H by the p9 protease in vitro generates active p15 RNase H. Arch Virol 1991;118(3–4):179–188.

58. Arrigo SJ, Weitsman S, Rosenblatt JD, Chen IS. Analysis of rev gene function on human immunodeficiency virus type 1 replication in lymphoid cells by using a quantitative polymerase chain reaction method. J Virol 1989;63(11):4875–4881.

59. Hammarskjold ML, Heimer J, Hammarskjold B, Sangwan I, Albert L, Rekosh D. Regulation of human immunodeficiency virus env expression by the rev gene product. J Virol 1989;63(5):1959–1966.

60. Schwartz S, Felber BK, Fenyo EM, Pavlakis GN. Env and Vpu proteins of human immunodeficiency virus type 1 are produced from multiple bicistronic mRNAs. J Virol 1990;64(11):5448–5456.

61. Hallenberger S, Bosch V, Angliker H, Shaw E, Klenk HD, Garten W. Inhibition of furin-mediated cleavage activation of HIV-1 glycoprotein gp160. Nature 1992;360(6402):358–361.

62. Schwartz S, Felber BK, Benko DM, Fenyo EM, Pavlakis GN. Cloning and functional analysis of multiply spliced mRNA species of human immunodeficiency virus type 1. J Virol 1990;64(6):2519–2529.

63. Robert-Guroff M, Popovic M, Gartner S, Markham P, Gallo RC, Reitz MS. Structure and expression of tat-, rev-, and nef-specific transcripts of human immunodeficiency virus type 1 in infected lymphocytes and macrophages. J Virol 1990;64:3391–3398.

64. Sodroski J, Rosen C, Wong-Staal F, et al. Trans-acting transcriptional regulation of human T-cell leukemia virus type III long terminal repeat. Science 1985;227(4683):171–173.

65. Kao SY, Calman AF, Luciw PA, Peterlin BM. Anti-termination of transcription within the long terminal repeat of HIV-1 by tat gene product. Nature 1987;330(6147):489–493.

66. Wei P, Garber ME, Fang SM, Fischer WH, Jones KA. A novel CDK9-associated C-type cyclin interacts directly with HIV-1 Tat and mediates its high-affinity, loop-specific binding to TAR RNA. Cell 1998;92(4):451–462.

67. Zhou Q, Chen D, Pierstorff E, Luo K. Transcription elongation factor P-TEFb mediates Tat activation of HIV-1 transcription at multiple stages. EMBO J 1998;17(13):3681–3691.

68. Raha T, Cheng SW, Green MR. HIV-1 Tat stimulates transcription complex assembly through recruitment of TBP in the absence of TAFs. PLoS Biol 2005;3(2):e44.

69. Chang HC, Samaniego F, Nair BC, Buonaguro L, Ensoli B. HIV-1 Tat protein exits from cells via a leaderless secretory pathway and binds to extracellular matrix-associated heparan sulfate proteoglycans through its basic region. AIDS 1997;11(12):1421–1431.

70. Ensoli B, Buonaguro L, Barillari G, et al. Release, uptake, and effects of extracellular human immunodeficiency virus type 1 Tat protein on cell growth and viral transactivation. J Virol 1993;67(1):277–287.

71. Frankel AD, Pabo CO. Cellular uptake of the tat protein from human immunodeficiency virus. Cell 1988;55(6):1189–1193.

72. Ensoli B, Barillari G, Salahuddin SZ, Gallo RC, Wong-Staal F. Tat protein of HIV-1 stimulates growth of cells derived from Kaposi's sarcoma lesions of AIDS patients. Nature 1990;345(6270):84–86.

73. Guo HG, Pati S, Sadowska M, Charurat M, Reitz M. Tumorigenesis by human herpesvirus 8 vGPCR is accelerated by human immunodeficiency virus type 1 Tat. J Virol 2004;78(17):9336–9342.

74. Buonaguro L, Barillari G, Chang HK, et al. Effects of the human immunodeficiency virus type 1 Tat protein on the expression of inflammatory cytokines. J Virol 1992;66(12):7159–7167.

75. Cohen SS, Li C, Ding L, et al. Pronounced acute immunosuppression in vivo mediated by HIV Tat challenge. Proc Natl Acad Sci U S A 1999;96(19):10842–10847.

76. Agwale SM, Shata MT, Reitz MS, et al. A Tat subunit vaccine confers protective immunity against the immune-modulating activity of the human immunodeficiency virus type-1 Tat protein in mice. Proc Natl Acad Sci U S A 2002;99(15):10037–10041.

77. Feinberg MB, Jarrett RF, Aldovini A, Gallo RC, Wong-Staal F. HTLV-III expression and production involve complex regulation at the levels of splicing and translation of viral RNA. Cell 1986;46(6):807–817.

78. Zapp ML, Green MR. Sequence-specific RNA binding by the HIV-1 Rev protein. Nature 1989;342(6250):714–716.

79. Felber BK, Derse D, Athanassopoulos A, Campbell M, Pavlakis GN. Cross-activation of the Rex proteins of HTLV-I and BLV and of the Rev protein of HIV-1 and nonreciprocal interactions with their RNA responsive elements. New Biol 1989;1(3):318–328.

80. Itoh M, Inoue J, Toyoshima H, Akizawa T, Higashi M, Yoshida M. HTLV-1 rex and HIV-1 rev act through similar mechanisms to relieve suppression of unspliced RNA expression. Oncogene 1989;4(11):1275–1279.

81. Daly TJ, Cook KS, Gray GS, Maione TE, Rusche JR. Specific binding of HIV-1 recombinant Rev protein to the Rev-responsive element in vitro. Nature 1989;342(6251):816–819.

82. Askjaer P, Jensen TH, Nilsson J, Englmeier L, Kjems J. The specificity of the CRM1-Rev nuclear export signal interaction is mediated by RanGTP. J Biol Chem 1998;273(50):33414–33422.

83. Pasquinelli AE, Powers MA, Lund E, Forbes D, Dahlberg JE. Inhibition of mRNA export in vertebrate cells by nuclear export signal conjugates. Proc Natl Acad Sci U S A 1997;94(26):14394–14399.

84. Henderson BR, Percipalle P. Interactions between HIV Rev and nuclear import and export factors: the Rev nuclear localisation signal mediates specific binding to human importin-beta. J Mol Biol 1997;274(5):693–707.

85. Neville M, Stutz F, Lee L, Davis LI, Rosbash M. The importin-beta family member Crm1p bridges the interaction between Rev and the nuclear pore complex during nuclear export. Curr Biol 1997;7(10):767–775.

86. Guy B, Kieny MP, Riviere Y, et al. HIV F/3' orf encodes a phosphorylated GTP-binding protein resembling an oncogene product. Nature 1987;330(6145):266–269.

87. Welker R, Kottler H, Kalbitzer HR, Krausslich HG. Human immunodeficiency virus type 1 Nef protein is incorporated into virus particles and specifically cleaved by the viral proteinase. Virology 1996;219(1):228–236.

88. Schwartz O, Marechal V, Danos O, Heard JM. Human immunodeficiency virus type 1 Nef increases the efficiency of reverse transcription in the infected cell. J Virol 1995;69(7):4053–4059.

89. Mariani R, Kirchhoff F, Greenough TC, Sullivan JL, Desrosiers RC, Skowronski J. High frequency of defective nef alleles in a long-term survivor with nonprogressive human immunodeficiency virus type 1 infection. J Virol 1996;70(11):7752–7764.

90. Kirchhoff F, Greenough TC, Brettler DB, Sullivan JL, Desrosiers RC. Brief report: absence of intact nef sequences in a long-term survivor with nonprogressive HIV-1 infection. N Engl J Med 1995;332(4):228–232.

91. Deacon NJ, Tsykin A, Solomon A, et al. Genomic structure of an attenuated quasi species of HIV-1 from a blood transfusion donor and recipients. Science 1995;270(5238):988–991.

92. Garcia JV, Miller AD. Serine phosphorylation-independent downregulation of cell-surface CD4 by nef. Nature 1991;350(6318):508–511.

93. Swigut T, Shohdy N, Skowronski J. Mechanism for down-regulation of CD28 by Nef. EMBO J 2001;20(7):1593–1604.

94. Stumptner-Cuvelette P, Morchoisne S, Dugast M, et al. HIV-1 Nef impairs MHC class II antigen presentation and surface expression. Proc Natl Acad Sci U S A 2001;98(21):12144–12149.

95. Schwartz O, Marechal V, Le GS, Lemonnier F, Heard JM. Endocytosis of major histocompatibility complex class I molecules is induced by the HIV-1 Nef protein. Nat Med 1996;2(3):338–342.

96. Rhee SS, Marsh JW. Human immunodeficiency virus type 1 Nef-induced down-modulation of CD4 is due to rapid internalization and degradation of surface CD4. J Virol 1994;68(8):5156–5163.

97. Anderson SJ, Lenburg M, Landau NR, Garcia JV. The cytoplasmic domain of CD4 is sufficient for its down-regulation from the cell surface by human immunodeficiency virus type 1 Nef. J Virol 1994;68(5):3092–3101.

150. Perron MJ, Stremlau M, Song B, Ulm W, Mulligan RC, Sodroski J. TRIM5alpha mediates the postentry block to N-tropic murine leukemia viruses in human cells. Proc Natl Acad Sci USA 2004;101(32):11827–11832.

151. Javanbakht H, An P, Gold B, et al. Effects of human TRIM5alpha polymorphisms on antiretroviral function and susceptibility to human immunodeficiency virus infection. Virology 2006;354(1):15–27.

152. Stremlau M, Perron M, Lee M, et al. Specific recognition and accelerated uncoating of retroviral capsids by the TRIM5alpha restriction factor. Proc Natl Acad Sci U S A 2006;103(14):5514–5519.

153. Yap MW, Dodding MP, Stoye JP. Trim-cyclophilin A fusion proteins can restrict human immunodeficiency virus type 1 infection at two distinct phases in the viral life cycle. J Virol 2006;80(8):4061–4067.

154. Javanbakht H, Yuan W, Yeung DF, et al. Characterization of TRIM5alpha trimerization and its contribution to human immunodeficiency virus capsid binding. Virology 2006;353(1):234–246.

155. Neil SJ, Zang T, Bieniasz PD. Tetherin inhibits retrovirus release and is antagonized by HIV-1 Vpu. Nature 2008;451(7177):425–430.

156. Goffinet C, Allespach I, Homann S, et al. HIV-1 antagonism of CD317 is species specific and involves Vpu-mediated proteasomal degradation of the restriction factor. Cell Host Microbe 2009;5(3):285–297.

157. Jia B, Serra-Moreno R, Neidermyer W, et al. Species-specific activity of SIV Nef and HIV-1 Vpu in overcoming restriction by tetherin/BST2. PLoS Pathog 2009;5(5):e1000429.

158. Sauter D, Schindler M, Specht A, et al. Tetherin-driven adaptation of Vpu and Nef function and the evolution of pandemic and nonpandemic HIV-1 strains. Cell Host Microbe 2009;6(5):409–421.

159. Smit-McBride Z, Mattapallil JJ, McChesney M, Ferrick D, Dandekar S. Gastrointestinal T lymphocytes retain high potential for cytokine responses but have severe CD4(+) T-cell depletion at all stages of simian immunodeficiency virus infection compared to peripheral lymphocytes. J Virol 1998;72(8):6646–6656.

160. Guadalupe M, Reay E, Sankaran S, et al. Severe CD4+ T-cell depletion in gut lymphoid tissue during primary human immunodeficiency virus type 1 infection and substantial delay in restoration following highly active antiretroviral therapy. J Virol 2003;77(21):11708–11717.

161. Brenchley JM, Price DA, Schacker TW, et al. Microbial translocation is a cause of systemic immune activation in chronic HIV infection. Nat Med 2006;12(12):1365–1371.

162. Blackburn SD, Wherry EJ. IL-10, T cell exhaustion and viral persistence. Trends Microbiol 2007;15(4):143–146.

163. Zagury D, Lachgar A, Chams V, et al. Interferon alpha and Tat involvement in the immunosuppression of uninfected T cells and C-C chemokine decline in AIDS. Proc Natl Acad Sci U S A 1998;95(7):3851–3856.

164. Finzi D, Hermankova M, Pierson T, et al. Identification of a reservoir for HIV-1 in patients on highly active antiretroviral therapy. Science 1997;278(5341):1295–1300.

165. Yarchoan R, Broder S. Development of antiretroviral therapy for the acquired immunodeficiency syndrome and related disorders. A progress report. N Engl J Med 1987;316(9):557–564.

166. Merluzzi VJ, Hargrave KD, Labadia M, et al. Inhibition of HIV-1 replication by a nonnucleoside reverse transcriptase inhibitor. Science 1990;250(4986):1411–1413.

167. Ashorn P, McQuade TJ, Thaisrivongs S, Tomasselli AG, Tarpley WG, Moss B. An inhibitor of the protease blocks maturation of human and simian immunodeficiency viruses and spread of infection. Proc Natl Acad Sci U S A 1990;87(19):7472–7476.

168. Collier AC, Coombs RW, Schoenfeld DA, et al. Treatment of human immunodeficiency virus infection with saquinavir, zidovudine, and zalcitabine. AIDS Clinical Trials Group. N Engl J Med 1996;334(16):1011–1017.

169. Wild C, Greenwell T, Matthews T. A synthetic peptide from HIV-1 gp41 is a potent inhibitor of virus-mediated cell–cell fusion. AIDS Res Hum Retroviruses 1993;9(11):1051–1053.

170. Baba M, Nishimura O, Kanzaki N, et al. A small-molecule, nonpeptide CCR5 antagonist with highly potent and selective anti-HIV-1 activity. Proc Natl Acad Sci U S A 1999;96(10):5698–5703.

171. Trkola A, Kuhmann SE, Strizki JM, et al. HIV-1 escape from a small molecule, CCR5-specific entry inhibitor does not involve CXCR4 use. Proc Natl Acad Sci U S A 2002;99(1):395–400.

172. Grinsztejn B, Nguyen BY, Katlama C, et al. Safety and efficacy of the HIV-1 integrase inhibitor raltegravir (MK-0518) in treatment-experienced patients with multidrug-resistant virus: a phase II randomised controlled trial. Lancet 2007;369(9569):1261–1269.

173. Li F, Goila-Gaur R, Salzwedel K, et al. PA-457: a potent HIV inhibitor that disrupts core condensation by targeting a late step in Gag processing. Proc Natl Acad Sci U S A 2003;100(23):13555–13560.

174. Marozsan AJ, Kuhmann SE, Morgan T, et al. Generation and properties of a human immunodeficiency virus type 1 isolate resistant to the small molecule CCR5 inhibitor, SCH-417690 (SCH-D). Virology 2005;338(1):182–199.

175. Kuhmann SE, Pugach P, Kunstman KJ, et al. Genetic and phenotypic analyses of human immunodeficiency virus type 1 escape from a small-molecule CCR5 inhibitor. J Virol 2004;78(6):2790–2807.

176. Lori F, Malykh A, Cara A, et al. Hydroxyurea as an inhibitor of human immunodeficiency virus-type 1 replication. Science 1994;266(5186):801–805.

177. Heredia A, Amoroso A, Davis C, et al. Rapamycin causes down-regulation of CCR5 and accumulation of anti-HIV beta-chemokines: an approach to suppress R5 strains of HIV-1. Proc Natl Acad Sci U S A 2003;100(18):10411–10416.

178. Hacein-Bey-Abina S, Von KC, Schmidt M, et al. LMO2-associated clonal T cell proliferation in two patients after gene therapy for SCID-X1. Science 2003;302(5644):415–419.

179. Sarkar I, Hauber I, Hauber J, Buchholz F. HIV-1 proviral DNA excision using an evolved recombinase. Science 2007;316(5833):1912–1915.

Chapter 7 LABORATORY TESTING FOR HIV/AIDS

YI-WEI TANG

*The three most important elements in practicing medicine are
diagnosis, diagnosis, and diagnosis.*

—Dr. William Osler,

*The Principles and Practice of Medicine:
Designed for the Use of Practitioners and Students of Medicine,*

D. Appleton & Company, 1892

Introduction

Diagnostic microbiology determines whether suspected pathogenic microorganisms are present in specimens collected from human beings, animals, and the environment. In medical practice, it is used to define infectious processes and elucidate treatment options through detection, quantification, and characterization of specific pathogens.[1] Therefore, diagnostic microbiology usually provides clinicians with antimicrobial susceptibility profiles of the identified microorganism. In the field of HIV diagnosis, laboratorians or clinical microbiologists determine whether a host is infected with HIV, evaluate the status of infections, and monitor antiretroviral therapy. The diagnostic capabilities for HIV infections have improved rapidly and have expanded greatly, thanks to the molecular technology revolution and profound HIV research. In particular, rapid techniques for nucleic acid amplification and characterization, combined with automation and user-friendly software, have significantly broadened the diagnostic arsenal used by the clinical microbiologist. Overall, an HIV infection can be diagnosed and monitored in any of five possible ways: (1) direct microscopic examination, such as visualization of an HIV virion by electronic microscopy, (2) cultivation and identification of HIV by suspension lymphocyte culture, (3), detection of HIV viral antigens, (4) measurement of HIV-specific immune responses, and (5) detection and quantification of HIV-specific nucleic acids.[1,2]

Positive culture provides direct evidence of HIV infection; however, the suspension lymphocyte culture procedure is labor-intensive and time-consuming. HIV cell culture, which was used to recover pathogenic agents, is now used primarily in research laboratories for pathogenesis studies and potential drug screening, but is no longer used for routine diagnosis.[3,4] Electron and confocal microscopes have played a critical role in classifying the pathogen, in characterizing the morphogenesis and viral gene products, and in elucidating the host cell targets and interactions in HIV research, but have never been used for routine diagnosis.[5,6] Several HIV antigen assays, including the Coulter HIV-1 p24 Ag assay (Coulter Co. Miami, FL), the VIDAS HIV P24 II (bioMérieux, Durham, NC), and the Elecsys HIV Ag (Roche Diagnostics, Indianapolis, IN), were approved by the U.S. Food and Drug Administration (FDA) for screening blood products and routine laboratory diagnosis.[7,8] However, the measurement of p24 antigen is less sensitive—but more specific—than nucleic acid amplification-based tests in documenting infection and is now rarely used alone for diagnosis.[9] Therefore, serology and molecular assays are now the state-of-the-art techniques used in the HIV diagnostic field. Current techniques used in laboratory diagnosis and monitoring of HIV infections are listed in **Table 7–1**.

Laboratory Diagnosis of HIV Infection

Primary diagnosis of HIV infection is commonly accomplished by serology via detection of HIV antibody using a screening enzyme immunoassay (EIA) or a rapid assay, followed by a subsequent confirmatory Western blot (WB) test. Infrequently, HIV antibody detection can be detected in immunofluoresence (*Fluorognost HIV-1, Sanochemia,* Stamford, CT)[2] or agglutination format (Capillus HIV-1/HIV-2, Trinity Biotech, Bray, Ireland)[10,11] In addition to serology assays, molecular methods are now routinely used to minimize the window period for diagnosis of acute or early infection in special populations. In newborns, the HIV proviral DNA detection method is used to rule out maternal antibody and confirm HIV infection.[12,13] Seronegative HIV-1 infected cases have been reported even for common HIV clades.[14,15] In immunocompromised hosts, serology may be limited, likely due to the inability to mount an effective immune response.

Enzyme Immunoassays (EIAs)

Since its introduction in the mid-1980s, HIV EIA testing has gradually improved both in terms of sensitivity and specificity, and remains the primary test used for diagnosis, screening, and surveillance of HIV infections.[16] Most commercially available EIA test kits used in the United States for detecting the presence of HIV-1 and/or HIV-2 antibodies incorporate recombinant antigens and synthetic peptides, and high sensitivity and specificity of these tests can be expected, with early detection of seroconverters. The most important limitation of HIV serodiagnostic tests is the "window period"—that is, the time between initial infection and the production of detectable antibody. Many assays approved by the FDA have a diagnostic window of 19–35 days for detection of a recent seroconversion or acute infection.

Four generations of HIV antibody EIA formats have been described. The first-generation assays relied on the detection of antibody to HIV viral protein lysates. The second-generation assays utilize HIV recombinant antigens as the source of antigen bound to the solid phase and include recombinant antigens for detection of HIV-2. Third-generation assays utilize solid phases coated with recombinant antigens and peptides, and HIV antibody in the patient's sample is detected with labeled recombinant antigens. Numerous diagnostic EIA devices are commercially available in the United States from Abbott Diagnostics (Abbott Park, IL), Bio-Rad (Hercules, CA), bioMérieux (Durham, NC), and Beckman Coulter (Brea, CA). The Genetic Systems HIV-1/HIV-2 PLUS O EIA (Bio-Rad), a third-generation EIA, detects the broadest range of antibodies to HIV-1 (groups M and O) and to HIV-2, thus minimizing the possibility of a false-negative in the detection of HIV-1 non-B subtypes or HIV-2 infection. This assay utilizes minimal

ciation of Public Health Laboratories/Center for Disease Control and Prevention.[53–55] The guidelines define as a positive result the presence of any two of the three essential bands (p24, glycoprotein gp41, and gp120/160). The gp24 band represents the core shell or capsid, whereas the gp41 band represents transmembrane glycoprotein. The gp120 band corresponds to the outer envelope or surface glycoproteins, and gp160 shows the presence of envelope protein precursors. The presence of gp120 and gp160 bands is considered as a single reaction for the purpose of interpreting the Western blot results. The presence of band/bands not meeting the criteria for being positive is defined as an "indeterminate" result. These bands include p17/18, p31/32, p51, p55, and p65/66. If no band is present, the test is defined as negative.[56] Interpretation of Western blot data should include risk factors. All indeterminate HIV-1 Western blots should be followed with a repeat screening test and Western blot after 2 weeks to 6 months, depending on the patient's risk factors.

There are no FDA-approved Western blot products for HIV-2; however, the format can be used to confirm positive HIV-2 EIA results. In general, an HIV-2 antibody will react to bands such as p17, p26, p31, gp36, p51, p55, gp58, p65/66, gp105, gp125, and gp140. Cross-reactivity between the HIV-2 antibody and the HIV-1 antigen bands in the HIV-1 Western blot devices has been observed.[57]

Qualitative Molecular Assays

Molecular technologies based on in vitro nucleic acid amplification can be utilized in the diagnosis of acute or primary infection when viral RNA can be detected earlier than the antibody or p24 antigen. Qualitative RNA molecular assays have been developed and are commercially available for blood donor screening in the blood bank.[58] The APTIMA HIV-1 RNA Qualitative Assay and the Procleix HIV-1/HCV assay (Gen-Probe), which incorporates transcription-mediated amplification technology, has been approved by the FDA for aid in diagnosis of HIV-1 infection, including acute or primary infection.[59] This assay has been evaluated recently as being a more sensitive screening tool for HIV-positive samples from a sexually transmitted disease clinic than typical antibody testing followed by pooled RNA testing. The data indicate that screening and confirmation of HIV infection by the qualitative molecular method alone may constitute an effective alternative HIV diagnostic algorithm in certain settings.[60] The qualitative format can detect a lower amount of viral RNA than quantitative tests—that is, less than 100 copies of HIV-1 RNA per mL.[61] Since HIV viral loads in patients with acute or primary infection are usually high, other HIV RNA quantification assays have been used for diagnostic purposes.[62–66]

In addition to blood donor screening, the qualitative molecular assays—especially those for the detection of HIV proviral DNA—have become the method of choice for establishing the diagnosis of infection in infants born to HIV-1–infected mothers.[12,13] The persistence of maternal antibodies against HIV in exposed infants up to 18 months of age prevents the use of antibody-based assays for the early diagnosis of HIV infection. However, because the effectiveness of HAART at an early age has been demonstrated, it is important to promptly establish the infection status of an HIV-exposed infant. Thus, approaches to the early diagnosis of infection in infants lean towards molecular techniques that amplify target HIV DNA,[67] RNA,[65] or total nucleic acid.[63,64,66] Detection of HIV-1 DNA can be used to differentiate primary infection during the diagnostic window period or in newborns of infected mothers. In the diagnosis of HIV in infants, the DNA polymerase chain reaction (PCR) assays possess sensitivities of 95% and even higher specificities[12,68,69] At this time, only one qualitative HIV-1 DNA PCR assay is commercially available from Roche and has not been approved by the FDA.[13,70]

Laboratory Monitoring of HIV Infection and Antiretroviral Therapy

HIV RNA Viral Load Assays

HIV-1 infection results in lifelong persistence of the virus, independent of antiretroviral treatment. In chronically infected patients, the HIV RNA viral load in plasma in conjunction with the CD4 T-lymphocyte cell numbers are the routine laboratory markers used to guide both initiation of the highly-active antiretroviral therapy (HAART) and to monitor treatment effectiveness and the feasibility of clinical progression.[71–7] Viral load assays, which measure the quantity of HIV-1 RNA present in plasma, are used as prognostic markers, to monitor response to therapy and to guide HIV treatment decisions.[75–77] Characterization of HIV-1 RNA levels as being below the limit of detection indicates HAART adherence and effectiveness.[71,78,79] Periodic monitoring of HIV-1 viral loads can be performed by either HIV RNA amplification or branched chain DNA (bDNA) tests. Technically, less than a 3-fold variation (0.5 $\log_{10}$ copies) is considered as intra-assay or biological variabilities; however, an over 10-fold (1 $\log_{10}$ copies) change is considered clinically significant.[80–83] In the clinical setting, one month after an effective regimen, viral load should fall by at least one log. By 4 to 6 months into therapy, viral load should have fallen below the detection limit of the test, usually less than 50–75 copies/mL.[75–77]

Sensitive measurement of viral load with broad dynamic range of detection, and enhanced ability to quantitate HIV-1 Group M subtypes A-G of the virus are two major requirements for the quantitative assay for HIV RNA. While HIV-1 subtype B continues to predominate in Western countries, studies now confirm that the incidence of HIV-1 non-B subtypes is increasing all over the world. The ability of a test to detect a broader range of these genetically diverse viruses is therefore crucial to HIV patient care on a global basis. In the US, five commercial assays are FDA approved for the quantification of HIV-1 RNA in plasma. All of these assays are licensed for monitoring HIV-1 infected patients; they are not proposed for use as HIV screening tests nor for confirmatory HIV testing, but have often been used in this context.[62–66,84] Most of these assays have not been optimized for Group O virus and, except for the Abbott RealTime TaqMan HIV-1 assay (which covers Group O virus as well), will likely underquantify HIV-1 RNA levels.[85] None of the assays detect HIV-2.

Plasma is the main specimen type for HIV-1 viral load testing. Plasma collected by plasma preparation tubes should be transferred to a secondary tube before freezing and transportation.[86–89] HIV viral RNA is relatively unstable and requires the blood samples (plasma) to be processed within 4–6 hours of collection and stored in a deep freezer. Nonplasma specimens—such as peripheral blood mononuclear cells (PBMCs), saliva, cerebrospinal fluid, seminal plasma, dried plasma, and dried blood spots—have been evaluated for HIV-1 viral load testing.[84,90–94] Dried blood spots have been used at rural and remote healthcare facilities to collect and transport specimens for HIV-1 RNA viral load monitoring.[95–98] When specimens are carefully processed, viral load results are stable and reproducible and cross-contamination is rare and avoidable.[99–101]

The Cobas Amplicor HIV-1 Monitor Assay (Roche Diagnostics) is a reverse transcription (RT)-PCR-based system targeting HIV-1 RNA.[80,82,102] Three variations of these assays exist: (1) the Amplicor HIV-1 Monitor assay, which is a manual test performed in microwell plates, (2) the Cobas Amplicor HIV-1 Monitor assay, in which amplicons are captured on magnetic beads, with the Cobas analyzer used to automate the amplification and detection steps, and (3) the Cobas AmpliPrep/Cobas TaqMan HIV-1 assay, which provides full automation of the nucleic acid extraction followed by real-time PCR amplification. Its first FDA-approved HIV viral load test in 1996 measures viral loads at levels as low as 400 HIV-1 RNA copies/mL. The Amplicor Ultra Sensitive test, approved in 1999, uses a slightly different sample processing protocol and measures viral loads down to 50 HIV-1 RNA copies/mL. The current Amplicor version 1.5, which can detect and quantify non-B HIV subtypes (Group M subtypes A–G), offers a detection range of 50–750,000 copies/mL of plasma, with a detection rate of greater than 95% at 50 copies/mL.[103] The fully automated version of the Roche Diagnostics COBAS AmpliPrep/COBAS TaqMan HIV-1 system has been in use in the United States with the reported upper limit of quantification and lower limit of detection of 1,000,000 and 50 RNA copies/mL, respectively.[104–106] The system targets the HIV-1 *gag* gene and has been designed to quantify all group M and N viruses and many circulating recombinant forms.[105,107]

The bDNA-based test known as VERSANT HIV-1 RNA 3.0 Assay (Siemens Healthcare Diagnostics) provides good reproducibility, because no amplification variation is expected due to its signal amplification technology.[108,109] Without extraction steps to isolate HIV-1 RNA, the reproducibility of the bDNA assay has been reported to be a superior test, particularly at the low end of the dynamic range.[80,109] The influence of inhibitory substances contained in a variety of clinical specimens is much lower compared to other methods, and the risk of contamination is reduced as well. This test has good precision across a wide reporting range and can distinguish three-fold ($0.5 \log_{10}$) changes across the entire assay range.[80,102,110] The bDNA test can also be used to determine quantification of the viral load down to 75 copies/mL.[103,111] The disadvantages from the intrinsic bDNA technique include the requirement for a large volume of plasma, the absence of an internal quantification standard for each sample tested, and lower specificity compared to target amplification methods. The recently available Bayer System 440 provides more extensive automation.

The NucliSens HIV-1 RNA QT assay (bioMérieux) incorporates three key technologies: silica-based nucleic acid extraction; nucleic acid sequence-based amplification (NASBA) for HIV RNA amplification; and electrochemiluminescence detection and quantification of the amplified RNA.[102,112] The NASBA technology is a sensitive, isothermal amplification method that does not require a thermocyler, so there is no need for heat-stable enzymes. The NucliSens assay is more sensitive in detecting HIV-1 RNA at lower concentrations than the standard Roche AMPLICOR test and reaches a broad linear dynamic ranging from 51 to 5,390,000 copies/mL.[113,114] The second-generation assay currently in use cannot reliably quantify subtypes A and G.[113] The assay can be used for measuring viral loads at other body sites because the RNA extraction procedure consistently generates RNA products that are free of interfering substances.[80,106,111,115] The isothermal process runs at 41°C, which is lower than the annealing temperature of the primers used, resulting in a lower specificity of the amplification process.

The RealTime HIV-1 assay in the *m*2000 system (Abbott Molecular) consists of two components: the m2000sp for nucleic acid extraction and loading of sample and master mix into the 96-well optical reaction plate, and the m2000rt for amplification and detection.[85,106,116,117] Incorporated with the TaqMan hydrolysis probes, these assays offers several advantages over conventional viral load assays, including a very broad linear, extensive automation, and decreased risk of carryover contamination. The system is fully automated, with wide coverage of HIV-1 genotypes, including groups M and N circulating recombinant forms, as well as Group O virus.[85,106,107,117] The assay possesses a wide linear dynamic range of between 40 and 10 million HIV-1 RNA copies/mL, and the limit of detection of the assay is 40 copies/mL for a 1.0 ml sample volume, 75 copies/mL for a 0.5 ml sample volume, and 150 copies/mL for a 0.2-mL sample volume.

CD4 Lymphocyte Identification and Counting

The CD4 lymphocyte count is another cornerstone test in HIV laboratory diagnostics. Early in the study of patients infected with HIV-1, it was determined that there was a significant and steady decline in CD4 cells that correlated with progression to disease, which led to guidelines for performance of CD4 cell determinations in peripheral leukocytes in persons with HIV infections.[118] Used for both staging and monitoring of patients for HIV antiretroviral therapy, CD4 testing has been used together with HIV viral loads as a predictor of disease progression, a criterion for treatment initiation, and as a marker of treatment outcome in both adults and children. CD4 testing is performed at multiple points during the course of patient care. After a positive HIV diagnosis, a CD4 count is used to stage the disease, so as to help determine whether the patient is eligible for antiretroviral therapy.

Flow cytometry remains the mainstay technique for CD4 identification and quantification in which absolute CD4 counts and percentages are reported. Available automated flow cytometry-based instruments fall into two main throughput categories. The low-throughput instruments, which can analyze 30–100 samples per day, include FACSCount (Becton Dickinson Bioscience), CyFlow Counter (Partex; Görlitz, Germany), Easy CD4 Analyzer (Guava Technologies), Point-Care (PointCare Technologies), and Apogee Auto40 (Apogee Flow Systems; Hemel Hempstead, Hertfordshire, UK). The high-throughput instruments include FACSCalibur (Becton Dickinson), EPICS XL (Beckman Coulter), and CyFlow SL 3 (Partec), which can analyze 250–350 samples per day under normal conditions. Manual and semiannual assays are available for laboratories with daily test volumes of less than 50. The procedures involve manual magnetic isolation of peripheral leukocytes and automated counts on a hematology analyzer or microscopic counter. Instruments including Sysmex (Sysmex; Norderstedt, Germany), Dynabeads (Invitrogen, Dynal SA, Oslo, Norway), and Cyto-spheres (Beckman Coulter) have been used for these manual and semimanual assays.[119] Companies that provide monoclonal antibodies for the immunophenotyping, including CD4 cells, include Amac (Westbrook, ME), Becton Dickinson (Mountain View, CA), and Coulter Immunology (Hialeah, FL).

Current guidelines recommend that, in the absence of an AIDS-defining illness, antiretroviral therapy should start in patients with blood CD4 cell counts under 200 or 350 cells/L and in infants under 5 years of age with CD4 cells less than 15% to 25%.[120] With the development of treatment regimens with lower toxicity and increasing evidence that HIV-associated morbidity and mortality develop at CD4 cell counts substantially higher than 200 cells/L, it might be time for the pendulum to swing once more toward earlier treatment. A recent study analyzed data from more than 45,000 patients from 18 observational HIV cohorts in Europe and North America. Frequency of death or combined AIDS and death in patients receiving and not receiving antiretroviral therapy was used to identify a minimum threshold for starting therapy of 350 cells/L.[121] In another smaller, subgroup analysis, therapy-naïve patients with CD4 counts higher than 350 cells/L were randomly assigned either to receive immediate or to defer therapy until counts were less than 250 cells/L. Those who deferred treatment had a far higher rate of major morbidity and all-cause mortality than did those treated immediately.[122] These data suggest that 350 cells/L should be the minimum threshold for initiation of antiretroviral therapy, and should help to guide physicians and patients in deciding when to start treatment. Asians, including Chinese, have approximately 100 fewer CD4 cells/L, on average, than Caucasians, indicating that lower CD4 cell cutoffs for classifying and monitoring HIV infection may be needed for different racial populations.[123,124]

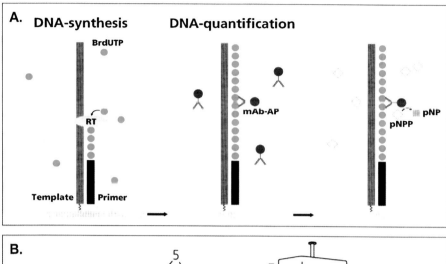

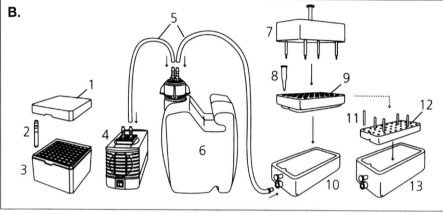

Figure 7–2. *The Version 3 ExaVir Load assay for measuring HIV-1 viral reverse transcriptase (RT) activity that correlates with plasma viral loads. (**A**) In a 96-well microtiter plate, the RNA template is bound to the bottom. A reaction mixture is added to the plate together with the lysates. If the lysates contain any RT, the enzyme will synthesize a DNA-strand. This product is detected with an alkaline phosphatase (AP) conjugated BrdUTP antibody. The product can then be quantified by addition of a colorimetric AP substrate. (**B**) Separation equipment for Version 3. 1, Sample Box Lid; 2, Plasma Processing Tube; 3, Sample Box; 4, Vacuum Pump; 5, Vacuum Tubing; 6, Waste Container; 7, Buffer Dispenser; 8, Column; 9, Column Holder; 10, Waste Collector; 11, Storage Tube; 12, Collector Tube Rack; and 13, Lysate Collector. Adapted from product insert of Cavidi, Sweden.*

study revealed that polymorphisms in toll-like receptors 4 and 9 influence viral load in a sero-incident cohort of HIV-1-infected individuals.[209]

Accordingly, detection of host polymorphisms in the HIV diagnostic field can help identify those at risk of rapid disease progression and help with timing the initiation of treatment. Allele frequencies and relative hazard values of CCR5-Δ32, CCR2 64I, CCR5 P1, IL-10 5'A, HLA-B*35, and HLA homozygosity were determined to generate a composite relative hazard of progression to AIDS.[210] Possession of a CCL3L1 copy number lower than the population average is associated with markedly enhanced HIV/AIDS susceptibility; which is enhanced in individuals who possess the CCR5-Δ32 genotype [211]. A model was defined that retained CCR5-Δ32, CCR2 64I, CCR5 59029AA, CCL3 495TT, SDF1 3'A, PML –225TT, PPIA 1650G, and TSG101–183C where the differences between carrying opposing genetic variants would translate into lengthening or shortening the time from 500 CD4 T cells/μl to <200 CD4 T cells/μl by up to 2.8 years.[212]

Genetically, polymorphic profiles in cytochrome P450s and transporters facilitate the optimal chemotherapy for HIV infections. An association between *CYP2D6* genetic variants and plasma levels of EFV and NVP in treatment-naïve individuals with HIV infection was observed, in which patients carrying a loss-of-function *CYP2D6* allele had higher median plasma levels of both drugs.[213] Polymorphisms in CYP2B6 correlates with high Efavirenz concentrations in plasma and the central nervous system. [214, 215]

Microarray has become a powerful technique to screen many genes for multiple polymorphisms on hundreds of samples.[192] With recent technological advances, it is now possible to genotype over one million polymorphisms for thousands of samples by using either the Illumina or Affymetrix system.[216,217] While more and more HIV infection resistance and disease progression-related host gene polymorphisms have been demonstrated, simple, user-friendly techniques for the detection of such known mutations will soon be adapted for the clinical diagnostic field. Currently used techniques include allele-specific nucleotide amplification,[218,219] single nucleotide primer extension,[220] and the oligonucleotide ligation assay.[221,222] PCR-led amplification technology has been important for these methods because it is either used for the generation of DNA fragments or is part of the detection method. Real-time PCR assays based on TaqMan hydrolysis probes have been used as confirmatory methods, which are very robust but less cost effective for larger scale studies.[223,224] DNA sequencing remains the gold standard and is enhanced by high-throughput processing and deep production scaling[225] and is now considered the most powerful procedure for polymorphism detection.

Host Response Testing for Therapy Efficacy and Side-Effect Monitoring

In addition to CD4 cell counting, other host responses can be used for monitoring therapy efficacy and side effects in HIV-infected patients receiving antiretroviral therapy. T-cell-receptor-chain rearrangement excision circles (TREC) are episomal circles which are generated during T cell maturation in the thymus. TREC are stable and persist in newly matured T cells, and, after entering the peripheral blood, they are diluted out during mitosis of these cells. Quantification of TREC present in naïve T cells is considered to be an accurate measure of thymic function. Although thymic function declines mainly with age, substantial output is maintained into late adulthood. HIV infection leads to a decrease in thymic function that can be measured in the peripheral blood and lymphoid tissues. In most adults treated with HAART, there is a rapid and sustained increase in thymic output, indicating that the adult thymus can contribute to immune reconstitution following antiretroviral therapy.[226–228] In addition to CD4 cell counts and HIV-1 viral loads, TREC has been described as another biomarker to monitor the treatment effectiveness and the feasibility of clinical progression.[226, 228–232]

Mitochondrial toxicity of antiretroviral drugs, particularly the nucleoside reverse transcriptase inhibitor (NRTI), has been postulated to be responsible for the etiopathogenesis of many secondary effects of HAART, including hyperlactatemia.[233,234] During HIV antiretroviral therapy, clinically symptomatic mitochondrial dysfunction has been associated with mitochondrial DNA depletion, and a real-time PCR was developed to determine a mitochondrial DNA versus nuclear DNA ratio as a biomarker of NRTI toxicity.[235] The observed increases in mitochondrial DNA and RNA content during the first year of treatment may represent a restorative trend resulting from suppression of HIV-1 infection, independent of the treatment used. Mitochondrial DNA and RNA content in individual cell subtypes rather than in peripheral leukocytes may be better markers of toxicity and deserve further investigation.[236] Other assays, which pigmented plaques, morbilliform eruptions, and palpable purpuric papules that frequently involve the perineal or genital areas. Because the clinical presentations are nonspecific, a diagnosis is based on biopsy findings, viral culture, or immunoglobulin titers. Diagnosis on a biopsy is definitive if characteristic basophilic intranuclear "owl-eye" inclusions and smaller basophilic cytoplasmic inclusions are identified. The treatment of choice for CMV infection is intravenous ganciclovir, 5 mg/kg every 12 hours. Vidarabine should be used if ganciclovir resistance is suspected. In patients with CD4 counts <100/mm³, valganciclovir prophylaxis can be given in doses of 900 mg by mouth every 24 hours.[45]

Epstein–Barr Virus

The vast majority of adults harbor latent Epstein-Barr virus (EBV) within B-lymphocytes after at some point contracting its primary infection, infectious mononucleosis. Infectious mononucleosis presents with common symptoms of fever, fatigue, loss of appetite, sore throat, headache, swollen lymph nodes, and cough. There is a risk of rupture of an enlarged spleen with trauma; however, many people endure the symptoms and recover without ever receiving a specific diagnosis. With advanced immunodeficiency, EBV reactivation occurs and may give rise to diverse illnesses, including recurrence of infectious mononucleosis and oral hairy leukoplakia (OHL).[46] EBV has also been implicated in the etiology of several malignancies, including nasopharyngeal carcinoma, Burkitt's lymphoma, Hodgkin's disease, and EBV-associated large cell lymphoma, all of which have increased incidence with immunosuppression.[47]

OHL manifests on the lateral margins of the tongue as single or multiple asymptomatic white plaques with a verrucous surface, which do not scrape off easily (**Figure 8–5**). The presence of OHL correlates with moderate to advanced immunosuppression and may be a harbinger of progression from HIV infection to AIDS. OHL responds to systemically administered acyclovir and valacyclovir, or topical podophyllin. However, many clinicians elect not to treat because the OHL is asymptomatic and recurrence is common following discontinuation of treatment. Treatment with HAART leading to improved immune status can be effective.[48]

Bacterial Infections

Bacillary Angiomatosis

Bacillary angiomatosis (BA) presents as red to violaceous nodules that clinically resemble a vascular neoplasm. The cutaneous lesions can occur anywhere on the body and may resemble a pyo-

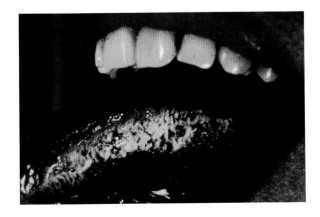

Figure 8–5. *Oral hairy leukoplakia is a distinctive condition characterized by thick white plaques on the lateral tongue. It is associated with EBV. More than one-third of AIDS patients have oral hairy leukoplakia.*

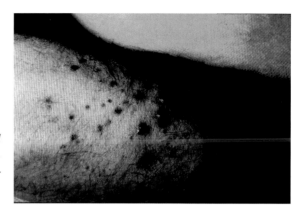

Figure 8–6. *Bacillary angiomatosis, which is caused by* Bartonella henselae *and* B. quintana, *was quite common before the advent of HAART. It presents as vascular papules that resemble pyogenic granulomas.*

genic granuloma or Kaposi's sarcoma. They typically range in size from millimeters to over a centimeter (**Figure 8–6**). BA may also present as subcutaneous nodules or as widespread erythematous plaques. The lesions may be tender, ulcerated, crusted, or have associated scale. Cutaneous manifestations are most common, but systemic and visceral disease may also occur. Systemic symptoms can include fever, chills, nausea, anorexia, lymphadenopathy, and generalized malaise. The most common extracutaneous manifestation is peliosis hepatis of the liver, but lymph node, soft tissue, and lytic bone lesions have also been described.[49]

Once considered a hallmark of HIV, with the advent of more effective treatments for HIV including HAART, this disease has now become quite uncommon. Several studies report an incidence of BA within the HIV population of approximately 0.1%. BA usually occurs in severely immunocompromised patients with CD4 cell counts of less than 200 cells/mm^3.[49]

BA is caused by infection with either of two species of Gram-negative bacteria in the genus *Bartonella*—namely, *Bartonella henselae*, the organism associated with cat scratch disease, and *Bartonella quintana*, the causative organism of trench fever. *B. henselae* is transmitted by cat fleas and *B. quintana* is transmitted by the human body louse. It is not known why *B. henselae* manifests as cat scratch disease in some patients and bacillary angiomatosis in others. Although each of these organisms may cause BA, soft tissue involvement and lytic bone disease is more commonly associated with *B. quintana,* whereas peliosis hepatitis and lymph node involvement is attributed to *B. henselae* infection.[50]

A biopsy will reveal an exophytic lobular capillary proliferation, with cuboidal endothelial cells and a mixed inflammatory infiltrate consisting of lymphocytes, neutrophils, and histiocytes. Within histiocytes and adjacent to venules, violaceous basophilic granular material may be seen that is composed of clumps of bacteria.[51] A Warthin-Starry stain may help to highlight the bacilli; immunohistochemical staining with antibodies directed to *Bartonella* can confirm the diagnosis.

Bacillary angiomatosis may be treated with a number of different antibiotics, including erythromycin, clarithromycin, azithromycin, or doxycycline. Courses of treatment lasting for 2 to 3 months may be required for cutaneous disease; even longer courses of therapy are required for patients with systemic symptoms. Some patients may develop a disseminated inflammatory reaction after antibiotic administration that requires the addition of an anti-inflammatory agent.[49]

Syphilis

Syphilis, in both active and latent forms, has a higher prevalence among HIV-positive populations than in HIV-negative individuals.[52] The overall incidence of the disease has been

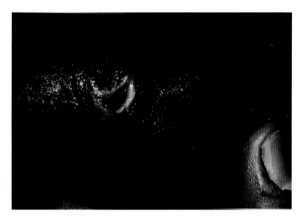

Figure 8–7. *The chancre is the first cutaneous manifestation of syphilis and presents 3 weeks after infection. It is a painless, indurated erosion. HIV patients share a similar clinical presentation to non-HIV patients, but they are more likely to have multiple chancres*

increasing over the past decade and has particularly increased among men who have sex with men. As these diseases share risk factors for transmission, coinfection is somewhat common.[53] Also, there is evidence that the occurrence of syphilis contributes to an increased risk for transmission of HIV, likely secondary to the presence of ulcers and other skin lesions that serve as portals of entry.[54] Therefore, it is recommended that all patients with syphilis should undergo screening for HIV.

The causative agent of syphilis is the spirochete *Treponema pallidum*. Syphilis is most commonly sexually transmitted and has a high transmission rate between sexual partners, in the range of 50% to 75%.[55] The clinical presentation of syphilis is usually similar in HIV-positive patients and HIV-negative individuals. However, the course of the disease may be more severe in immunocompromised patients. The primary lesions are painless, clean-based, 1- to 2-cm chancres with indurated borders that occur at the site of inoculation approximately 3 weeks after exposure (**Figure 8–7**). Regional lymphadenopathy is common. The chancre usually heals within 3 to 6 weeks, leaving an atrophic scar. In HIV-positive patients there may be multiple large chancres, or the chancres may take longer to heal.

Progression to secondary syphilis occurs within 4 to 10 weeks in more than 90% of cases.[56] Typical secondary syphilis is characterized by a papulosquamous eruption of numerous erythematous macules and papules presenting diffusely on the face, trunk, and genital region (**Figure 8–8**). Later, mucous membrane and palmoplantar involvement may be noted (**Figure 8–9**). Syphilis has been referred to as the "great masquerader" and may present with many morphologies, including macular, lichenoid, psoriaform, and follicular-based eruptions. In the setting of HIV infection, it may also manifest with atypical presentations, such as verrucous plaques, extensive oral ulcerations, alopecia, keratoderma, deep cutaneous nodules, or widespread gummata. Additional features that may be seen include condyloma lata and a "motheaten," patchy alopecia. Lues maligna is a rare, widespread aggressive form of secondary syphilis in which papulopustular lesions enlarge into sharply bordered ulcers that can be associated with fever, malaise, vasculitis, and ocular disease. Lues maligna most commonly affects patients with low CD4 cell counts.

Following resolution of secondary syphilis the infection may progress to an asymptomatic, quiescent period known as latent syphilis, which can persist indefinitely. Approximately one-third of untreated patients will progress to develop tertiary syphilis within 15 years, although it can also present many decades later. Tertiary syphilis is associated with significant neurologic and cardiovascular symptoms, as well as cutaneous manifestations of granulomas, psoriaform papules and plaques, and gummas, which are painless, indurated nodules with serpiginous

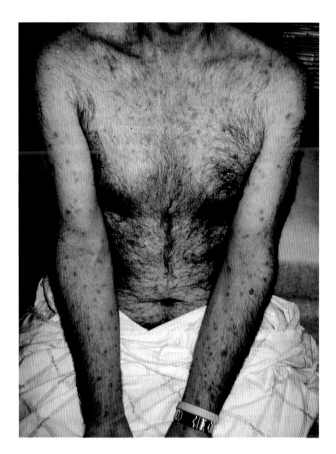

Figure 8–8. *Secondary syphilis presents as a symmetrical, generalized eruption. It may be macular or exanthematous, psoriaform, follicular, or lichenoid.*

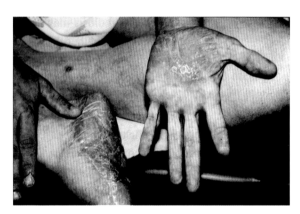

Figure 8–9. *Secondary syphilis often involves the palms and soles. This is a papulosquamous example.*

borders that may be ulcerated or locally destructive.[56] Syphilis may progress faster from secondary to tertiary disease in HIV-infected individuals, even despite appropriate treatment. Those with CD4 counts below 350 cells/mm^3 are four times more likely to develop neurosyphilis.

Serologic screening tests, including the rapid plasma reagin (RPR) test and Venereal Disease Research Laboratory (VDRL) test, are the initial studies that should be performed when syphilis is suspected. These tests have a sensitivity of approximately 80% in primary syphilis, and approach 95%–100% positivity in more advanced stages. The tests are not entirely specific, and false-positive results may occur due to many different causes, including HIV infection. Therefore, a positive result requires a confirmatory treponemal-specific test, such as *T. pallidum* particle agglutination (TPPA) or fluorescent treponemal antibodies (FTA-ABS) test. Serologic

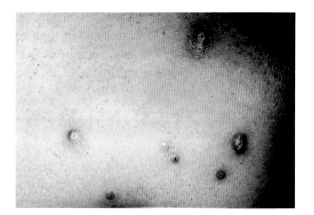

Figure 8–12. *Disseminated histoplasmosis is very rare, and the majority of disseminated infections occur in immunocompromised patients. The clinical appearance is variable and may present as umbilicated papules, as seen in this patient, or as nodules, ulcers, pustules, furuncles, and abscesses.*

with a broad spectrum of clinical manifestations that are partially determined by the magnitude of exposure and the patient's immune status. Cutaneous lesions occur in less than 10% of cases of histoplasmosis, and should prompt investigation for systemic disease.

The cutaneous lesions can have diverse morphologies including macules, papules, pustules, ulcers, subcutaneous nodules, a rosacealike eruption, a disseminated folliculitis-like pattern, or umbilicated papules resembling molluscum contagiosum[78] (**Figure 8–12**). The most common site for cutaneous involvement is the face, followed by the extremities and the trunk. Oropharyngeal plaques, nodules, and ulcers are also common, in addition to lesions involving the remainder of the gastrointestinal tract. [89]

Systemic infection can have a variety of appearances including asymptomatic infections, pulmonary histoplasmosis, mediastinal fibrosis, and granulomatous disease. Symptomatic pulmonary histoplasmosis presents with fever, dry cough, and fatigue. Disseminated disease, which is an AIDS-defining illness, occurs in 2 to 5 percent of HIV-positive individuals, most often in those with CD4 counts <150 cells/mm^3.[90] In patients with AIDS, 95% of cases of histoplasmosis presents as a disseminated infection that in some cases may be severe with an acute, rapidly fatal course. Signs and symptoms include fever, weight loss, pulmonary infiltrates, pancytopenia, hypergammaglobulinemia, respiratory distress, rhabdomyolysis, shock, hepatic and renal failure, obtundation, or coagulopathy.[91]

Histoplasma capsulatum is found in the soil, commonly in the vicinity of chicken coops, roosting places of birds, or bat caves. It is most common in endemic regions, including the river valleys of central and eastern U.S., South America, and the Caribbean.[92] At soil temperatures, *H. capsulatum* exists in the mycelial form, harboring macroconidia and microconidia. The microconidia, measuring 25 μm in diameter, readily aerosolize, and, on inhalation by a host, convert from the mycelial phase into a budding yeast that rapidly replicates within macrophages.[92] Immunocompetent individuals recruit immune cells that form granulomas, but failure of the immune response in immunocompromised individuals allows the organism to disseminate. [93]

The diagnosis of histoplasmosis can be made via biopsy, culture, or serologic testing for antibodies. A biopsy will show small intracellular budding yeasts and granulomatous inflammation. A silver stain such as the Gomori methenamine silver stain or periodic acid-Schiff stain may be useful in highlighting the small intracellular yeast forms, which are each only 2–3 μ in diameter (**Figure 8–13**). Cultures are positive in 85% of cases of disseminated or chronic pulmonary histoplasmosis but require 4 to 6 weeks for final results.[91] In patients with disseminated disease, serologic studies for detection of antibodies to *H. capsulatum* are positive in over 80% of cases.[94] Clinical correlation is required as prior infection can result in positive serologic results

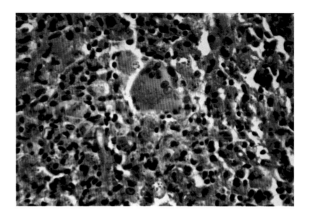

Figure 8–13. *On this PAS stain, the histoplasmosis organisms are highlighted as small pink inclusions within histiocytes that are surrounded by a clear halo or pseudocapsule. The organisms measure only 2-3 microns in diameter, and each is smaller than a red blood cell.*

and misleadingly suggest a diagnosis of active histoplasmosis. Antibody titers decrease and become undetectable after 2 to 5 years following disease resolution.

The treatment of choice in severe or disseminated histoplasmosis is amphotericin B.[90] Maintenance or prophylactic therapy with itraconazole is recommended in patients with CD4 counts below 150 cells/mm^3.[84, 95]

Coccidioidomycosis

Coccidioidomycosis is a fungal infection caused by inhalation of the spores, or arthroconidia, of *Coccidioides immitis*, a dimorphic fungus endemic to areas of the southwestern U.S. (particularly southern Arizona and the San Joaquin Valley in California), northern Mexico, and scattered regions of Central and South America.[96] A prospective study demonstrated that 10% of HIV-positive individuals in endemic areas will develop disease each year, either as a new manifestation or as recurrent disease.[97]

Coccidioidomycosis in HIV-positive individuals most frequently presents as an influenzalike illness, with symptoms of fever, night sweats, cough, pleuritic chest pain, fatigue, and anorexia. Patients with CD4 cell counts below 250 cells/mm^3 are more likely to develop disseminated disease involving extrapulmonary sites, including the skin, soft tissue, synovium, bones, meninges, or peritoneum.[98] Disseminated coccidioidomycosis in HIV-positive patients is associated with high mortality, estimated as greater than 40%, even despite appropriate antifungal therapy.[98]

Cutaneous manifestations are the most common signs of disseminated coccidioidomycosis and should prompt investigation for systemic infection. Cutaneous lesions are often either keratotic papules or verrucous lesions. Pustules, plaques, and granulomatous nodules with minimal surrounding erythema may also be seen and, in some cases, will expand to become confluent ulcers, abscesses, sinus tracts, or cellulitis. Erythema nodosum and erythema multiforme may also occur as associated conditions, and are often seen in combination with fever and arthralgias.

A diagnosis of coccidioidomycosis can be established by fungal culture, serologic studies, tissue biopsy, bronchoalveolar lavage, or sputum specimens. After the spores of *Coccidioides* are inhaled, the fungi convert to multinucleate, spherical structures (spherules), which undergo internal division to produce hundreds of uninucleate endospores.[97] The larger spherules are readily identifiable due to their distinct appearance in tissue biopsy or cytologic preparations. A biopsy will also show granulomatous inflammation and a suppurative response to the ruptured spherules. *Coccidioides* is a fast-growing fungus, and a fungal culture can yield results in 2 to 5 days. Once growth is noted on the plates, a DNA-specific probe can be used to identify the organism.

Serologic testing detecting IgM antibodies can identify 75% of patients with primary disease.[97] In addition, antibodies correlate with the disease course and may be helpful in following disease resolution.

HIV-positive patients with pulmonary or disseminated disease should be treated initially with amphotericin B, until resolution of signs and symptoms of infection. Once clinically improved, patients may be switched to oral azole therapy, which should be continued indefinitely. Coccidioidal meningitis should be treated with fluconazole, which has demonstrated an 80% response rate.[99]

Aspergillosis

Invasive aspergillosis is rare in AIDS, but when present, is associated with a mortality rate of over 90%. It usually begins as a pulmonary infection and occurs predominantly in patients with advanced HIV with neutropenia and CD4 cell counts less than 50 cells/mm^3. Cutaneous lesions occur in less than 10% of patients with disseminated aspergillosis and may consist of erythematous-to-violaceous plaques or papules with central areas of necrosis.[100] Localized primary cutaneous infections with aspergillus may occur at sites of trauma or burns. A biopsy will reveal a branching septate fungus, but culture is required for definitive identification. An enzyme-linked immunosorbent assay (ELISA) performed on serum can identify the fungal wall component galactomannan, but occasionally this assay can yield false-negative results.[101] Systemic antifungal therapy with amphotericin B or voriconazole is recommended and may be combined with other antifungal drugs.

Paracoccidioidomycosis

Paracoccidioides brasiliensis causes a chronic, progressive, systemic fungal infection, referred to as South American blastomycosis because it is endemic to South America. Painful violaceous, mucocutaneous lesions of the lips and oral mucosa are usually associated with systemic disease, which causes pulmonary symptoms and lymphadenitis. The diagnosis is made by serologic studies or by tissue biopsy demonstrating the diagnostic "mariner's wheel" morphology, caused by the presence of equally spaced buds around a central round yeast. Treatment is usually with sulfonamides.[102]

Penicilliosis

Penicilliosis, caused by infection with *Penicillium marneffei,* is rare in the U.S. but is the third most common opportunistic infection in HIV-infected individuals in southeast Asia and southern regions of China. The majority of cases of penicilliosis are seen in patients with CD4 counts <50 cells/mm^3. The most common clinical presentation includes fever, cough, lymphadenopathy, anemia, and disseminated umbilicated papular skin lesions, which tend to involve the face, pinnae, extremities, and, occasionally, the genitalia. The diagnosis can be established by biopsy or tissue scrapings that demonstrate the thin-walled oval yeasts, or by fungal cultures from tissue or blood. Treatment is with amphotericin B at 0.6 mg/kg/day IV for 2 weeks, followed by oral itraconazole. Simultaneous administration of treatment for penicilliosis and initiation of HAART may improve outcomes. On completion of initial therapy, secondary prophylaxis with oral itraconazole should be given for life.[103]

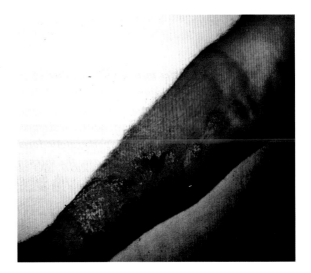

Figure 8–14. *This patient demonstrates a large thickened plaque on the forearm with many smaller ascending red patches along the lines of lymphatic drainage. This pattern is classic for cutaneous sprorotrichosis.*

Blastomycosis

Blastomycosis occurs infrequently in the HIV-positive population, but when it occurs in immunosuppressed patients, it may be disseminated, have an aggressive course, and may be fatal. Most cutaneous lesions of blastomycosis occur secondary to disseminated disease, although primary cutaneous inoculation may also occur. The lesions are usually crusted verrucous nodules, which may be ulcerated. A biopsy demonstrates suppurative granulomatous inflammation with marked pseudoepitheliomatous hyperplasia and the characteristic, broad-based, budding yeast of *Blastomyces dermatitides*. Treatment is usually with amphotericin B, fluconazole, or itraconazole.[100]

Sporotrichosis

Sporotrichosis occurs with infection by *Sporothrix schenckii* at sites of cutaneous inoculation. The organism frequently resides on rose thorns, but infections may also result from other environmental exposures or trauma such as a cat scratch. The typical lesion begins with a dermal or subcutaneous nodule that may ulcerate, followed by linear lymphangitic ascending spread with the development of satellite lesions (**Figure 8–14**). In the setting of HIV-associated immunosuppression patients may develop disseminated sporotrichosis that can also involve the eyes, joints, lungs, liver, spleen, intestines, and meninges. Definitive diagnosis at any site requires culture isolation of *Sporothrix schenckii* from a normally sterile body site. A biopsy may show suppurative granulomatous inflammation with rare yeast surrounded by structures resembling asteroid bodies. Treatment is usually with amphotericin B or itraconazole.[104]

Parasitic and Ectoparasitic Infestations

Scabies

Scabies is a pruritic eruption caused by the mite *Sarcoptes scabeii*, and is the most common ectoparasitic infection seen in patients with HIV. The clinical presentation can vary from discrete scattered erythematous papules to hyperkeratotic plaques present on the palms, wrists, web spaces between the fingers, trunk, genitals, nipples, and extremities, and can be associated with intense

The incidence of KS in homosexual or bisexual men skyrocketed during the first years of the epidemic, affecting 30% to 40% of HIV-infected patients in the early 1980s.[2] As a visible, easy-to-recognize and difficult-to-hide mark of HIV infection, KS betrayed its carrier's most private information about health, prognosis, and—rightly or wrongly—lifestyle. People commonly referred to KS as "gay cancer" and used this same phrase interchangeably with AIDS itself. The public regarded KS as a death sentence. Actually, it was more of a prognostic indicator as most AIDS patients were more likely to succumb to opportunistic infections than to KS itself. However, with the advent of HAART therapy, the presence of KS is no longer such a dire prognostic marker.

Early KS lesions appear as discrete, red-to-violaceous patches that may simulate bruises, arthropod bite reactions, or dermatofibromas.[109] Initially, there is unilateral involvement of the head (including the face, scalp and ears) and the trunk, where the patches often follow skin tension lines.[110] With time, bilateral involvement occurs, the patches develop into confluent papules or plaques, and nodules or tumors that may erode or ulcerate (**Figure 8–16**). The evolution generally progresses through patch, plaque, and nodular phases.

In addition to the skin, KS may involve the mucous membranes, especially the oral cavity, where 50% of intraoral lesions are located on the hard palate. Oral involvement with KS is a clue that CD4 T-cell counts have dropped below 200 cells/mm^3.[111] Extracutaneous KS also commonly occurs in the lymph nodes, the gastrointestinal tract, and the lungs. Lymphedema of the involved areas is a common complication secondary to involvement of lymphatics and lymph nodes.[112] Of note, extracutaneous KS may occur in the absence of cutaneous involvement.

The diagnosis is based on the finding of violaceous skin lesions in the appropriate clinical setting in conjunction with characteristic histologic findings. The histologic features of KS vary with the stage of the lesion. Early patch lesions manifest as proliferations of spindle-shaped endothelial cells forming subtle, vascular slits. Extravasated erythrocytes, siderophages, and plasma cells may be present. Plaque-stage lesions are characterized by a more diffuse proliferation of spindle cells, expanding the dermis and forming jagged, irregular, slit-like vascular channels. Small, pink, hyaline globules are commonly present, representing breakdown products of red blood cells. Tumor-stage KS appears as diffuse sheets of spindle-shaped cells with mild-to-moderate cytologic atypia, single-cell necrosis, and the presence of mitoses. Immunoperoxidase studies are often positive for vascular-associated antigens such as factor VIII, CD31, and *Ulex europaeus* antigen.[113] Immunohistochemical staining for HHH-8 also reveals positive nuclear staining.

Over the past 3 decades, substantial progress has been made in understanding KS. In 1994, Chang et al.[114] identified a new herpesvirus, designated as human herpesvirus type 8 (HHV-8) or

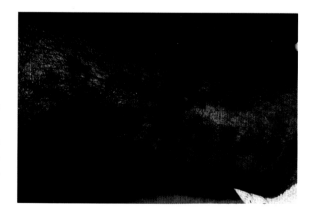

Figure 8–16. *The incidence of Kaposi's sarcoma, a well-know AIDS defining illness, has decreased dramatically with the advent of HAART therapy. Lesions begin as small dusky macules and progress and coalesce to form large violaceous plaques, nodules, and eventually raised tumors.*

KS-associated herpes virus (KSHV), as the possible causative agent of KS.[114] The virus has been identified in over 95% of the tumors and has been shown to be necessary but not sufficient to develop KS. Studies suggest that after the host acquires HHV-8, the virus subsequently enters a latent phase of infection. When the host becomes immunocompromised, HHV-8 activates and triggers cytokine and chemokine reactions that lead to cellular proliferation, angiogenesis, and inhibition of apoptosis.[115,116]

Discovery of the integral and defining role of HHV-8 has raised the interesting question of whether KS is best characterized as a multifocal and systemic infection or as a neoplasm. Depending on the characterization, distant disease could be considered multifocal emergence or metastasis. This debate is not yet settled.

Alongside our increasing understanding of the pathogenesis of KS, substantial strides have been made in prevention and treatment. The introduction of HAART has decreased the risk of developing KS by 90%.[117] HAART, which reduces the size and number of KS lesions, is the backbone of therapy for KS in HIV-positive patients.

Nevertheless, KS treatment is not standardized and treatment regimens should be tailored to the individual patient's clinical presentations.[118] Treatments for localized lesions include destructive methods such as cryosurgery, laser surgery, excisional surgery and electrocauterization, or localized radiation. Chemotherapy, radiotherapy, and immunotherapy can be used for those with visceral involvement or life-threatening disease. Newer cytotoxic agents, such as liposomal anthracyclines and paclitaxel, are highly effective and may be used as first- or second-line agents for advanced KS.[119,120] As our understanding of the biology of KS improves, research is ongoing to develop and approve novel antiangiogenesis and cytokine-inhibitor–based treatments.

Lymphomas

HIV-infected individuals have a 200-fold increased risk of developing lymphomas, particularly B cell lymphomas. It is estimated that 10% of HIV-positive individuals will develop a lymphoma at some point during the course of their disease. Lymphoma is the first AIDS-defining illness in 3% to 5% of patients.[121] Several lymphomas are AIDS-defining illness, including Burkitt's lymphoma, immunoblastic lymphoma, and primary lymphoma of the brain. In addition, lymphomas that are not AIDS-defining illnesses include Hodgkin's disease, lymphomatoid granulomatosis, and CD30 lymphoproliferative disorders. Lymphomas related to Epstein-Barr virus infection are also increased in HIV-positive patients. Notably, many of the lymphomas associated with HIV (for example, primary brain lymphoma) do not present with cutaneous lesions.

HIV-associated Burkitt's lymphoma is an aggressive lymphoma that tends to involve lymph nodes and bone marrow. It is more common in the setting of HIV infection than with other causes of immunodeficiency. When it involves the skin, it presents similarly to other lymphomas, as a cutaneous or subcutaneous nodule that may ulcerate. EBV can be detected in 25% to 40% of cases.

Immunoblastic lymphoma is a variant of diffuse large B cell lymphoma (DLBL) and has a distinct histologic morphology, composed of large cells with basophilic cytoplasm and a centrally located nucleus that may resemble plasmablasts. Cutaneous lesions often present as solitary or clustered cutaneous nodules or tumors. When associated with HIV, these tumors are more often EBV-positive than those in HIV-negative individuals.

CD30 lymphoproliferative disorders are T-cell disorders that comprise anaplastic large cell lymphoma (ALCL) and lymphomatoid papulosis (LyP). ALCL presents similarly to other large-cell lymphomas, such as immunoblastic lymphoma. Lymphomatoid papulosis is characterized by recurrent crops of pruritic papules that ulcerate and eventually resolve over several weeks. Histologically, LyP usually consists of a wedge-shaped infiltrate containing a variable number of large, atypical lymphocytes. One form of LyP appears histologically similar to anaplastic large cell lymphoma but is distinguished from ALCL by clinical history.[122]

The incidence of mycosis fungoides (MF), the most common type of skin lymphoma, is decreased in HIV positive patients.[123] Although the incidence of MF is decreased in the setting of HIV, if it does occur, it may follow a more aggressive course. Although survival in typical MF is measured in decades and may not be decreased at all in low-stage disease, the survival of HIV patients with MF ranges between 5 and 10 months.

A biopsy of MF reveals a bandlike infiltrate of lymphocytes, some of which display epidermotropism or extension into the epidermis, without spongiosis. The lymphocytes may be atypical and have convoluted nuclei displaying a cerebriform appearance. Treatments for mycosis fungoides are not standardized and include topical corticosteroids, topical nitrogen mustard, phototherapy, and chemotherapeutic agents, or radiation therapy for progressive or advanced disease.

Several inflammatory dermatoses, including eczema, psoriasis, or medication reactions, may mimic MF clinically or histologically. In the setting of HIV, one of these mimics, referred to as pseudo-CTCL, likely represents reactive cutaneous infiltration by HIV-specific cytotoxic T cells. Pseudo-CTCL demonstrates a predominance of CD8 T cells rather than the typical CD4 T cells of MF.[124] Pseudo-CTCL responds to treatments such with topical corticosteroids or psoralen with ultraviolet A (PUVA).

The diagnosis and evaluation of cutaneous lymphomas in HIV-positive patients is based on clinical and histologic findings, and typically includes ancillary tests such as immunohistochemical staining, gene rearrangement studies, flow cytometry, and the use of DNA probes. Further work-up to evaluate for concurrent systemic involvement should be undertaken with lymph node evaluations, imaging studies, and, possibly, bone marrow biopsy.

Treatment options must take into account the patient's clinical condition, prognosis, and quality of life. Isolated primary cutaneous lymphomas may be treated with surgical excision, radiation, or both. Systemic, multifocal, or clinically aggressive lymphomas may require multiagent chemotherapy or radiation therapy. Aggressive immunosuppressive therapies, such as multiagent chemotherapy, should be used cautiously, as this may lead to further immunocompromise and can result in higher mortality from other AIDS-related illnesses. Palliative therapy may be the most appropriate option in patients with advanced disease.

Basal Cell and Squamous Cell Carcinomas

In HIV-positive individuals, the incidence of nonmelanoma skin cancer—including basal cell carcinoma (BCC) and squamous cell carcinoma (SCC)—is three to five times that seen in HIV-negative individuals. SCC of oral and anogenital sites is even more markedly increased. Most SCC in situ in this population arises in the anogenital area and correlates strongly with the presence of oncogenic strains of human papillomavirus.[125]

BCC and SCC in HIV-positive patients usually demonstrate a typical clinical appearance, although in these individuals they occur more readily on areas of the skin that have not been sun-exposed. BCCs manifest as pearly papules or nodules with raised edges and telangiectatic vessels that slowly enlarge and may ulcerate[126] (**Figure 8–17**). SCCs present as erythematous, hyperkeratotic patches or plaques, or areas of persistent ulceration. Lesions of anogenital Bowen's disease are often brown, flat-topped papules or plaques, although other morphologies—

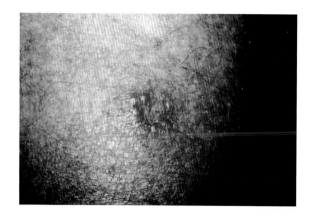

Figure 8–17. *This is a textbook example of a basal cell carcinoma in an individual with HIV. Note the pearly papule with the rolled border and prominent telangiectases. HIV-infected patients have 3 to 5 times the incidence of nonmelanoma skin cancer compared to the non-HIV population.*

such as erythematous shiny plaques or persistent ulceration—may also occur. Routine skin examination with early biopsy of suspicious lesions is important in these patients. In addition, patients should avoid excess ultraviolet radiation exposure and apply appropriate sun protection. Surgical excision with adequate surgical margins or Mohs micrographic surgery can provide control of early lesions and will decrease recurrence, as well as morbidity and mortality from these skin cancers.[127] Adjunctive local radiation, chemotherapy, or both should be considered for those with extensive tumor burden. Sentinel lymph node biopsies may also be useful in a subset of advanced cases of SCC.[128]

Melanoma

HIV-positive patients are also believed to have an increased incidence of melanoma. The development of multiple, primary melanomas and early nodular melanomas has been reported in the setting of HIV infection.[129,130] However, it is uncertain whether this finding is secondary to increased surveillance, detection, and reporting, or if it represents a true increase in the incidence of melanoma. The clinical presentation of melanoma is similar in HIV-infected and noninfected individuals. Melanomas often demonstrate asymmetry, irregular border, varied color, diameter greater than 6 mm, or a history of evolution or change, described by the mnemonic "ABCDE" (**Figure 8–18**).

Standard guidelines apply to all patients with melanoma, regardless of immune status. However, although there are no special guidelines for HIV positive patients, melanoma may have a more aggressive course in this population. Reports have shown that lower CD4 T cell counts

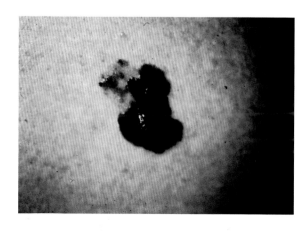

Figure 8–18. *This melanoma demonstrates classic features including asymmetry, variegated colors including brown, black and pink, and large size. Melanoma in HIV patients may have a more aggressive course, and sentinel lymph node biopsy should be considered even for thin melanomas in the HIV population.*

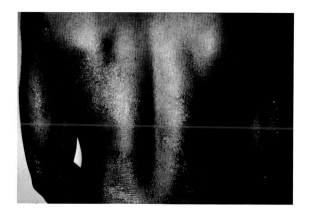

Figure 8–21. *Atopic dermatitis is a symmetrical, pruritic dermatitis. This patient has widespread lichenified papules and plaques.*

possible first-line treatments.[147] Other options include administration of systemic corticosteroids, antihistamines, itraconazole, isotretinoin, and metronidazole.

Xerosis

Approximately one-third of patients with HIV infection will develop diffuse xerosis or acquired ichthyosis, with development of fine to thick keratotic scale, secondary hyperpigmentation, or crusting. Fissures can develop and may become secondarily infected. The etiology is poorly understood, but xerosis may be secondary to the effects of chronic illness, immunosuppression, poor nutrition, or poor autonomic regulation with decreased sweating or sebum production. Treatment is with emollients or a lotions containing 12% lactic acid.[134,148]

Atopic Dermatitis

Atopic dermatitis (AD) is an extremely pruritic dermatitis characterized by increased sensitivity to irritating factors. It is common in patients without HIV infection, especially children, but its incidence is increased among individuals with HIV infection. [149] AD manifests as ill-defined, erythematous, eczematous patches and plaques. Lesions may be lichenified from scratching or secondarily impetiginized (**Figure 8–21**). Patients often give a history of other IgE-mediated diseases, including asthma, allergic rhinitis, urticaria, or food allergies. The diagnosis of AD is clinical. Biopsy is nonspecific and typically shows epidermal acanthosis with foci of spongiosis, along with a perivascular lymphocytic infiltrate and occasional eosinophils.[136]

AD is believed to be caused by immune dysfunction or an impaired barrier function of the skin that allows increased penetration by antigens. Treatments include emollients, topical corticosteroids, oral antihistamines, and avoidance of irritants. Phototherapy may also be helpful. HAART therapy to improve immune status may decrease the number and severity of flares.[150]

Psoriasis

HIV-infected patients clearly have a higher incidence and more severe manifestations of psoriasis through much of their HIV disease course.[151] Classically, psoriasis presents as sharply demarcated, erythematous, raised plaques with silvery scales (**Figure 8–22**). HIV-infected patients with psoriasis may show multiple coexisting morphologies, such as eruptive or guttate psoriasis, pustular psoriasis, and sebopsoriasis. Associated nail dystrophy may be seen in 10% to

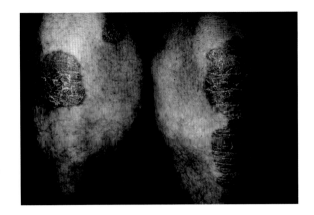

Figure 8–22. *This patient has classic plaque-type psoriasis on his knees. There are red, well-demarcated plaques with overlying silvery scales.*

55% of patients. In addition, patients with HIV infection are at increased risk for severe exfoliative or erythrodermic psoriasis and for psoriatic arthritis.

The diagnosis may be confirmed by biopsy, which demonstrates histologic features similar to those seen in HIV-negative individuals. However, in HIV-infected patients, the characteristic features may be somewhat less pronounced. The biopsy may show the usual psoriaform hyperplasia with somewhat more irregular acanthosis or with thicker suprapapillary plates.

Pathophysiologically, psoriasis in the setting of HIV raises interesting observations. We know that psoriasis is a T-cell–mediated disease that is associated with increased cytokines from T-helper type 1 cells (Th1). In patients with HIV, Th1 activity is diminished, and the predominant activity is from T-helper type 2 cells (Th2). Thus, it would be expected that the Th2 milieu in HIV would diminish the severity of psoriasis. Actually, however, psoriasis severity worsens as CD4 count decreases, and only diminishes with very advanced HIV disease. From a research standpoint, this conundrum has raised interesting questions regarding the pathophysiology of psoriasis and possible future therapies.[151,152]

Standard treatments include topical therapies such as corticosteroids and calcipotriene. Topical retinoids, anthralin derivatives, emollients, and tar have also been safely used. Phototherapy appears to be safe and effective, although there has been debate about the possible effect on viral loads. Systemic drugs such as acitretin can be used. Drugs that modulate immune response, such as biologic therapies, should be used with exceptional caution, as these may exacerbate immunodeficiency.[151] Methotrexate and cyclosporine are generally not recommended because of risk of immunodeficiency or toxicity.[153]

Reactive Arthritis Syndrome

The syndrome has been referred to as Reiter's syndrome, although this name has fallen out of favor, given Dr. Reiter's history of prisoner deaths due to unethical medical experimentation and his later conviction as a Nazi war criminal following World War II.[154,155] The reactive arthritis syndrome is an autoimmune condition that results from the body's response to an inciting infection, most commonly a genital or gastrointestinal infection. Following the inciting infection, typically 3 to 4 weeks later, the patient develops inflammation of the large joints (reactive arthritis), the eyes (conjunctivitis or uveitis), and urogenital area (dysuria, prostatitis in men, and cervicitis or salpingitis in women). This classic triad occurs in only one-third of patients. Patients with HIV are at increased risk for developing this syndrome, with an incidence of approximately 6% to 10%.[156,157]

Patients less commonly develop cutaneous manifestations. Associated skin lesions consist of circinate balanitis or vulvitis, small nodules of the palms and soles (keratoderma blennorrhagica), nail dystrophy, and erosive and pustular lesions of the digits. The psoriaform lesions begin as erythematous macules and rapidly evolve into hyperkeratotic plaques.

Establishing the diagnosis can be difficult and is based on clinical features in combination with supportive studies of affected systems, including radiologic studies, serologic studies demonstrating an HLA-B27 haplotype, and studies to evaluate for infectious urethritis. A skin biopsy shows features of psoriaform dermatitis, possibly occurring with subcorneal or intracorneal pustules.

Treatments for the cutaneous lesions include topical corticosteroids, phototherapy, and systemic acitretin. Treatments with immunosuppressive drugs such as methotrexate or cyclosporine are not routinely used in HIV-infected patients, as these medications may exacerbate immunosuppression.[158]

Lipodystrophy

HIV-infected patients frequently develop abnormalities of adipose distribution manifesting as lipoatrophy or hypertrophy. Lipoatrophy presents with fat wasting and decreased subcutaneous fat in the face, buttocks, and extremities. Lipohypertrophy presents with a diffuse increase in subcutaneous fat, resulting in a cervicodorsal fat pad or "buffalo hump," as well as enlarged breasts and increased abdominal fat. The diagnosis is based on characteristic clinical findings. Evaluation includes lipid studies, but clinicians typically forego biopsy and radiographic studies as these techniques do not provide much additional information.[159]

Although the causes of lipodystrophy are not well understood, some theories include decreased lipid uptake by cells, inducible insulin resistance, impaired lipid metabolism, and an altered cytokine environment. Lipodystrophy most often occurs secondary to treatment with specific drug classes, most commonly protease inhibitors or nucleoside reverse transcriptase inhibitors (NRTIs). Occasionally, lipodystrophy may be secondary to HIV infection itself. The degree of lipodystrophy correlates with length of disease or treatment.[159, 160]

Treatment involves discontinuing the responsible medication, if identified, and treatment of any hyperlipidemia or impaired glucose tolerance. Cosmetic fillers or procedures may be helpful.[161]

Hypersensitivity Diseases

Drug Reactions Associated with Highly Active Antiretroviral Therapy

Although no cure has been found for AIDS, there have been tremendous advances in understanding and treating this condition. Thirty years ago, there were no treatments available. Now there are five classes of drugs, more than 30 individual medications, and effective multiagent therapy. Since its introduction in the mid-1990s, the combination of multiple classes of antiretroviral drug therapy, referred to as highly active antiretroviral therapy (HAART), has produced dramatic decreases in the morbidity and mortality among patients infected with HIV. HAART has been effective in reducing viral replication and reconstituting CD4 T lymphocyte counts.[82]

HAART regimens are composed of drugs from five classes, based on their specific mechanism of action: nucleoside/nucleotide reverse transcriptase inhibitors (NRTIs), nonnucleoside reverse transcriptase inhibitors (NNRTIs), protease inhibitors (PIs), fusion or entry inhibitors, and integrase inhibitors. Despite their efficacy, these medications have been associated with numerous adverse side effects, many of which are dermatologic in nature.[162] It is important to be aware of the possible adverse reactions in order to accurately diagnose them and effectively manage treatments.

In 1987, the U.S. Food and Drug Administration (FDA) approved the first drug for the treatment of HIV. Zidovudine belongs to a class of drugs called nucleoside/nucleotide reverse transcriptase inhibitors (NRTIs), which are analogs of deoxynucleotides required for synthesis of viral DNA. They function by competing for incorporation into the viral DNA chain, but because of slight biochemical differences, they cause termination of the viral replication process. The list of currently approved NRTIs includes zidovudine, abacavir, didanosine, emtricitabine, lamivudine, stavudine, tenofovir, and zalcitabine. Although individual medications may have distinct adverse effects, NRTIs as a group are associated with the lipodystrophy syndrome manifested by hyperlipidemia, abnormal fat distribution, and glucose intolerance.[163]

Zidovudine commonly results in nail and mucocutaneous hyperpigmentation. Up to half of patients started on this drug experience this side effect.[164] Discoloration typically develops within 1 to 2 months of the initiation of therapy but may present up to a year later. It usually presents as multiple blue, brown or black-pigmented longitudinal bands beginning in the proximal nail fold and extending throughout the length of the nail plate (**Figure 8–23**). A biopsy taken at the nail matrix would show increased melanin in the nail bed epithelium with scattered subepithelial melanophages. The pigmentary changes are dose-dependent and reversible with discontinuation of therapy.[164] Other side effects include pruritus, urticaria, morbilliform eruptions, a lichenoid drug reaction resembling lichen planus, and leukocytoclastic vasculitis. Stevens-Johnson and toxic epidermal necrosis have also been reported with this drug.[165–167]

Other drugs in the NRTI class are associated with cutaneous side effects. In 2% to 3% of patients, abacavir may trigger a multisystem hypersensitivity reaction that is characterized by a morbilliform eruption with associated fever, nausea, diarrhea, hypotension, respiratory or musculoskeletal dysfunction, and—rarely—death.[168] Emtricitabine has been shown to induce xerosis and an associated cutaneous eruption in up to one-third of patients. Less frequently, it may cause palmoplantar hyperpigmentation.[169] Rare cases of Stevens-Johnson syndrome and leukocytoclastic vasculitis have been reported with didanosine administration.[170]

Protease inhibitors (PIs) were the second class of antiretroviral drugs approved by the FDA. The first drug in this class, saquinavir, was approved in 1995, some 8 years after zidovudine was

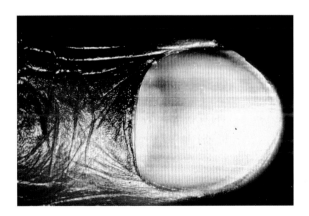

Figure 8–23. *Zidovudine causes nail pigmentation, usually within 1-2 months after starting therapy. This side effect is reversible with discontinuation of the drug.*

approved. Protease inhibitors function by binding HIV-1 viral protease, inactivating the enzyme, and preventing assembly of viral particles. Currently approved PIs include indinavir, nelfinavir, saquinavir, lopinavir, ritonavir, amprenavir, fosamprenavir, atazanavir, tipranavir, and darunavir. PIs are used frequently in combination with other drugs in HIV treatment protocols. When used in combination, there are increased risks of drug-drug interactions and cutaneous complications. These complications, in addition to increased antiviral drug resistance, have limited the utility of PIs.

In terms of cutaneous reactions, PIs most frequently cause morbilliform or urticarial hypersensitivity reactions. Other reactions include acute generalized eruptive pustulosis (AGEP), generalized pruritus, xerosis, desquamative cheilitis, striae formation, and angiolipomatosis.[171–174] Indinavir is associated with the greatest incidence of cutaneous complications, such as hypersensitivity eruptions, Stevens-Johnson syndrome, acute porphyria, progressive alopecia, and paronychia.[175–177] Indinavir-related alopecia typically presents as a patchy to diffuse alopecia of the scalp, lower extremities, axilla, thorax, or genital region in the first 6 months of treatment. Paronychia usually develops within several months following the initiation of therapy and commonly exhibits concurrent granulomatous lesions.[178] These adverse effects have been shown to resolve upon discontinuation of the medication. Indinavir is also associated with a higher incidence of lipodystrophy compared with other PIs.

In 1998, FDA approval of nevirapine established a third class of antiretroviral drugs: nonnucleoside reverse transcriptase inhibitors (NNRTIs). This class also includes delavirdine, efavirenz, and etravirine. NNRTIs terminate the HIV-replication cycle at the point of RNA-dependent DNA synthesis by selectively binding to and inactivating the viral reverse transcriptase enzyme. NNRTIs are only effective against the HIV-1 strain of the virus.

NNRTIs have the lowest incidence of side effects among the different classes of antiretroviral drugs. Nevertheless, the reported complications still include a number of cutaneous reactions. These range from mild to severe and typically appear within 2 to 3 weeks after implementation of therapy. Mild reactions include urticaria, morbilliform eruptions, and leukocytoclastic vasculitis. A small percentage of patients taking these drugs develop severe, life-threatening eruptions such as Stevens-Johnson syndrome or drug rash with eosinophilia and systemic symptoms (DRESS syndrome).[179,180] Nevirapine and efavirenz are associated with the highest incidence of cutaneous complications, with up to one–third of patients reporting an associated drug hypersensitivity reaction.[181]

In 2003, the FDA approved the fourth class of antiretroviral medication known as fusion inhibitors or entry inhibitors that prevent HIV from binding to, fusing with, or entering human cells. This class includes two medications, enfuvirtide and maraviroc. Enfuvirtide is administered via subcutaneous injection and is associated with a high frequency of injection site reactions, including induration, erythema, nodules, cysts, and tenderness at or around the site of administration.[182] The rotation of injection sites and smaller medication volumes may aide in minimizing this complication.[183] Maraviroc is an oral medication. The most serious cutaneous reaction is DRESS syndrome, which is associated with hepatotoxicity. Other reported adverse reactions include pruritus, erythema, and lipodystrophy.

Integrase inhibitors are the fifth and most recently approved class of antiretroviral drugs. The sole drug in use at this time is raltegravir, which was approved in 2007. Integrase inhibitors block the integration of viral DNA into the host's DNA by blocking the viral enzyme integrase. Cases of Stevens-Johnson syndrome have been reported with use of raltegravir.

The timing of the initiation of medications and the patient's clinical appearance are often sufficient to determine the etiology of the adverse reaction. However, isolating a specific agent may be more difficult when the patient is taking multiple medications, as in HAART. Discontinuation of the causative medication is the mainstay of treatment.

When the adverse reaction is mild and when withdrawal of a specific HAART medication would be detrimental, desensitization to the causative drug has also been shown to be effective in certain cases.[184] In addition, systemic corticosteroid administration during the period of immune reconstitution, generally the initial 8 weeks of HAART therapy, can prevent or decrease undesirable drug reactions.[185]

Photosensitivity Reactions

Photosensitivity reactions occur when there is an inflammatory response to sunlight. This may occur as a result of a reaction with an exogenous substance such as a systemic or topical drug or may occur without an exogenous trigger (representing an atypical idiopathic reaction). While initially present in sun-exposed areas, over time the reaction may become more widespread and occur independently of any photosensitizing agent. The mechanisms by which UV light produces cutaneous manifestations in the setting of HIV infection are not entirely known, but it is theorized that when UV light generates stress-induced damage to host cell DNA, subsequent cellular DNA repair processes then enable dormant HIV genes, already incorporated into the host genome, to become activated, resulting in cell damage or destruction.[186]

Photoeruptions can be classified as chronic actinic dermatitis (CAD), lichenoid photoeruptions, photosensitive hyperpigmentation, porphyria cutanea tarda (PCT), and photosensitive granuloma annulare (GA). Among these, CAD and lichenoid photoeruptions are the two categories most commonly seen in HIV-positive patients. The degree of immunosuppression and the viral load have been shown to correlate with the morphology and severity of cutaneous manifestations. Patients with lower CD4 T cells tend to demonstrate the more chronic and severe eruptions. Nonlichenoid reactions, which include spongiotic and hyperpigmentation reactions, are more common in severely immunocompromised patients rather than lichenoid eruptions. African American patients with HIV are more likely to develop photosensitivity eruptions than patients in other racial groups.[187]

There is significant variability in the clinical presentation of HIV-related photodermatoses, but evaluation of a patient with a photodistributed eruption benefits by following an algorithmic pattern. The patient should first be evaluated for exogenous photosensitizing agents, including a thorough review of medications, topical applications, and nutritional or herbal supplements. Laboratory studies to evaluate for lupus erythematosus and similar autoimmune conditions should be considered in the majority of patients. Additional evaluation may include photopatch testing to exclude photoallergic contact dermatitis or evaluation for a porphyria. In patients with a chronic unexplained course, pellagra should be excluded. A biopsy may add valuable information, as histologic features vary considerably among the common causes of photosensitivity reactions in HIV-positive patients.

Chronic actinic dermatitis (CAD) is a persistent photosensitivity disorder, which comprises a group of photosensitivity disorders previously referred to as photosensitive "eczema" or dermatitis (PD), actinic reticuloid (AR), and persistent light reaction (PLR). It may present as an end stage of several other photodermatitides. By definition, CAD excludes conditions with a known exogenous trigger. CAD presents as lichenified, pruritic plaques in a photodistributed pattern, affecting the face, neck, upper portion of the chest, and areas of limbs commonly exposed to the sun (**Figure 8–24**). Eruptions may be accompanied by edema, and some cases may progress to generalized erythroderma.[188,189] The incidence of CAD is increased in patients with

66. Popovich KJ, Weinstein RA, Aroutcheva A, Rice T, Hota B. Community-associated methicillin-resistant Staphylococcus aureus and HIV: intersecting epidemics. Clin Infect Dis. Apr 1 2010;50(7):979–987.

67. Becker BA, Frieden IJ, Odom RB, Berger TG. Atypical plaquelike staphylococcal folliculitis in human immunodeficiency virus-infected persons. J Am Acad Dermatol. Nov 1989;21(5 Pt 1):1024-1026.

68. Wu JJ, Huang DB, Pang KR, Tyring SK. Selected sexually transmitted diseases and their relationship to HIV. Clin Dermatol. Nov–Dec 2004;22(6):499–508.

69. Martin-Iguacel R, Llibre JM, Nielsen H, et al. Lymphogranuloma venereum proctocolitis: a silent endemic disease in men who have sex with men in industrialised countries. Eur J Clin Microbiol Infect Dis. May 28 2010.

70. White JA. Manifestations and management of lymphogranuloma venereum. Curr Opin Infect Dis. Feb 2009;22(1):57–66.

71. Johnson RA. Dermatophyte infections in human immune deficiency virus (HIV) disease. J Am Acad Dermatol. Nov 2000;43(5 Suppl):S135–142.

72. Kaviarasan PK, Jaisankar TJ, Thappa DM, Sujatha S. Clinical variations in dermatophytosis in HIV infected patients. Indian J Dermatol Venereol Leprol. Jul–Aug 2002;68(4):213–216.

73. Rodwell GE, Bayles CL, Towersey L, Aly R. The prevalence of dermatophyte infection in patients infected with human immunodeficiency virus. Int J Dermatol. Apr 2008;47(4):339–343.

74. Phelan JA. Oral manifestations of human immunodeficiency virus infection. Med Clin North Am. Mar 1997;81(2):511–531.

75. Greenspan D. Treatment of oral candidiasis in HIV infection. Oral Surg Oral Med Oral Pathol. Aug 1994;78(2):211–215.

76. McCreary C, Bergin C, Pilkington R, Kelly G, Mulcahy F. Clinical parameters associated with recalcitrant oral candidosis in HIV infection: a preliminary study. Int J STD AIDS. May–Jun 1995;6(3):204–207.

77. Sabetta JR, Andriole VT. Cryptococcal infection of the central nervous system. Med Clin North Am. Mar 1985;69(2):333–344.

78. Johnson RA. HIV disease: mucocutaneous fungal infections in HIV disease. Clin Dermatol. Jul–Aug 2000;18(4):411–422.

79. Dimino-Emme L, Gurevitch AW. Cutaneous manifestations of disseminated cryptococcosis. J Am Acad Dermatol. May 1995;32(5 Pt 2):844–850.

80. Perfect JR, Casadevall A. Cryptococcosis. Infect Dis Clin North Am. Dec 2002;16(4):837–874, v–vi.

81. Sorvillo F, Beall G, Turner PA, Beer VL, Kovacs AA, Kerndt PR. Incidence and factors associated with extrapulmonary cryptococcosis among persons with HIV infection in Los Angeles County. AIDS. Apr 1997;11(5):673–679.

82. Palella FJ, Jr., Delaney KM, Moorman AC, et al. Declining morbidity and mortality among patients with advanced human immunodeficiency virus infection. HIV Outpatient Study Investigators. N Engl J Med. Mar 26 1998;338(13):853–860.

83. Feldmesser M, Tucker S, Casadevall A. Intracellular parasitism of macrophages by Cryptococcus neoformans. Trends Microbiol. Jun 2001;9(6):273–278.

84. Hage CA, Goldman M, Wheat LJ. Mucosal and invasive fungal infections in HIV/AIDS. Eur J Med Res. May 31 2002;7(5):236–241.

85. Zuger A, Louie E, Holzman RS, Simberkoff MS, Rahal JJ. Cryptococcal disease in patients with the acquired immunodeficiency syndrome. Diagnostic features and outcome of treatment. Ann Intern Med. Feb 1986;104(2):234–240.

86. Powderly WG. Current approach to the acute management of cryptococcal infections. J Infect. Jul 2000;41(1):18–22.

87. Lortholary O, Fontanet A, Memain N, Martin A, Sitbon K, Dromer F. Incidence and risk factors of immune reconstitution inflammatory syndrome complicating HIV-associated cryptococcosis in France. AIDS. Jul 1 2005;19(10):1043–1049.

88. Ruhnke M. Mucosal and systemic fungal infections in patients with AIDS: prophylaxis and treatment. Drugs. 2004;64(11):1163–1180.

89. Wheat LJ, Kauffman CA. Histoplasmosis. Infect Dis Clin North Am. Mar 2003;17(1):1–19, vii.

90. Wheat J, Sarosi G, McKinsey D, et al. Practice guidelines for the management of patients with histoplasmosis. Infectious Diseases Society of America. Clin Infect Dis. Apr 2000;30(4):688–695.

91. Williams B, Fojtasek M, Connolly-Stringfield P, Wheat J. Diagnosis of histoplasmosis by antigen detection during an outbreak in Indianapolis, Ind. Arch Pathol Lab Med. Dec 1994;118(12):1205–1208.

92. Antinori S, Magni C, Nebuloni M, et al. Histoplasmosis among human immunodeficiency virus-infected people in Europe: report of 4 cases and review of the literature. Medicine (Baltimore). Jan 2006;85(1):22–36.

93. Woods JP. Histoplasma capsulatum molecular genetics, pathogenesis, and responsiveness to its environment. Fungal Genet Biol. Mar 2002;35(2):81–97.

94. Wheat LJ, Kohler RB, Tewari RP. Diagnosis of disseminated histoplasmosis by detection of Histoplasma capsulatum antigen in serum and urine specimens. N Engl J Med. Jan 9 1986;314(2):83–88.

95. McKinsey DS, Wheat LJ, Cloud GA, et al. Itraconazole prophylaxis for fungal infections in patients with advanced human immunodeficiency virus infection: randomized, placebo-controlled, double-blind study. National Institute of Allergy and Infectious Diseases Mycoses Study Group. Clin Infect Dis. May 1999;28(5):1049–1056.

96. Pappagianis D. Epidemiology of coccidioidomycosis. Curr Top Med Mycol. 1988;2:199–238.

97. Chiller TM, Galgiani JN, Stevens DA. Coccidioidomycosis. Infect Dis Clin North Am. Mar 2003;17(1):41–57, viii.

98. Ampel NM, Dols CL, Galgiani JN. Coccidioidomycosis during human immunodeficiency virus infection: results of a prospective study in a coccidioidal endemic area. Am J Med. Mar 1993;94(3):235–240.

99. Benson CA, Kaplan JE, Masur H, Pau A, Holmes KK. Treating opportunistic infections among HIV-infected adults and adolescents: recommendations from CDC, the National Institutes of Health, and the HIV Medicine Association/Infectious Diseases Society of America. MMWR Recomm Rep. Dec 17 2004;53(RR-15):1–112.

100. Minamoto GY, Rosenberg AS. Fungal infections in patients with acquired immunodeficiency syndrome. Med Clin North Am. Mar 1997;81(2):381–409.

101. Aquino VR, Goldani LZ, Pasqualotto AC. Update on the contribution of galactomannan for the diagnosis of invasive aspergillosis. Mycopathologia. Apr 2007;163(4):191–202.

102. Paniago AM, de Freitas AC, Aguiar ES, et al. Paracoccidioidomycosis in patients with human immunodeficiency virus: review of 12 cases observed in an endemic region in Brazil. J Infect. Oct 2005;51(3):248–252.

103. Sirisanthana T, Supparatpinyo K. Epidemiology and management of penicilliosis in human immunodeficiency virus-infected patients. Int J Infect Dis. Jul–Sep 1998;3(1):48–53.

104. Hardman S, Stephenson I, Jenkins DR, Wiselka MJ, Johnson EM. Disseminated Sporothix schenckii in a patient with AIDS. J Infect. Oct 2005;51(3):e73–77.

105. Giamarellou H. AIDS and the skin: parasitic diseases. Clin Dermatol. Jul–Aug 2000;18(4):433–439.

106. Clyti E, Sayavong K, Chanthavisouk K. [Demodecidosis in a patient infected by HIV: successful treatment with ivermectin]. Ann Dermatol Venereol. May 2005;132(5):459–461.

107. Galarza C, Ramos W, Gutierrez EL, et al. Cutaneous acanthamebiasis infection in immunocompetent and immunocompromised patients. Int J Dermatol. Dec 2009;48(12):1324–1329.

108. Alvar J, Aparicio P, Aseffa A, et al. The relationship between leishmaniasis and AIDS: the second 10 years. Clin Microbiol Rev. Apr 2008;21(2):334–359, table of contents.

109. Cheuk W, Wong KO, Wong CS, Dinkel JE, Ben-Dor D, Chan JK. Immunostaining for human herpesvirus 8 latent nuclear antigen-1 helps distinguish Kaposi sarcoma from its mimickers. Am J Clin Pathol. Mar 2004;121(3):335–342.

110. Schwartz RA. Kaposi's sarcoma: an update. J Surg Oncol. Sep 1 2004;87(3):146–151.

111. Crowe SM, Carlin JB, Stewart KI, Lucas CR, Hoy JF. Predictive value of CD4 lymphocyte numbers for the development of opportunistic infections and malignancies in HIV-infected persons. J Acquir Immune Defic Syndr. 1991;4(8):770–776.

112. Ruocco V, Schwartz RA, Ruocco E. Lymphedema: an immunologically vulnerable site for development of neoplasms. J Am Acad Dermatol. Jul 2002;47(1):124–127.

113. Gray MH, Trimble CL, Zirn J, McNutt NS, Smoller BR, Varghese M. Relationship of factor XIIIa-positive dermal dendrocytes to Kaposi's sarcoma. Arch Pathol Lab Med. Aug 1991;115(8):791–796.

114. Chang Y, Cesarman E, Pessin MS, et al. Identification of herpesvirus-like DNA sequences in AIDS-associated Kaposi's sarcoma. Science. Dec 16 1994;266(5192):1865–1869.

115. Koster R, Blatt LM, Streubert M, et al. Consensus-interferon and platelet-derived growth factor adversely regulate proliferation and migration of Kaposi's sarcoma cells by control of c-myc expression. Am J Pathol. Dec 1996;149(6):1871–1885.

116. Zimring JC, Goodbourn S, Offermann MK. Human herpesvirus 8 encodes an interferon regulatory factor (IRF) homolog that represses IRF-1-mediated transcription. J Virol. Jan 1998;72(1):701–707.

117. Biggar RJ, Rabkin CS. The epidemiology of AIDS--related neoplasms. Hematol Oncol Clin North Am. Oct 1996;10(5):997–1010.

118. Krown SE. Clinical overview: issues in Kaposi's sarcoma therapeutics. J Natl Cancer Inst Monogr. 1998(23):59–63.

119. Cattelan AM, Trevenzoli M, Aversa SM. Recent advances in the treatment of AIDS-related Kaposi's sarcoma. Am J Clin Dermatol. 2002;3(7):451–462.

120. Tulpule A, Groopman J, Saville MW, et al. Multicenter trial of low-dose paclitaxel in patients with advanced AIDS-related Kaposi sarcoma. Cancer. Jul 1 2002;95(1):147–154.

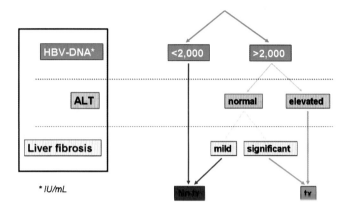

Figure 9–2. *Management of chronic hepatitis B in HIV/HBV coinfected patients: When to treat*

The benefits of inhibiting HBV replication have been well established, with the demonstration of a direct association between serum HBV-DNA levels and the risk for developing liver cirrhosis and hepatocellular carcinoma, regardless of HBeAg status and/or liver enzyme elevations.[10–12] The most recent HBV guidelines recommend starting anti-HBV treatment in individuals positive for the hepatitis B e antigen (HBeAg) when serum HBV-DNA is >2 x10^4 IU/mL. In contrast, in patients with negative serum HBeAg, the threshold above which therapy should be recommended is 2×10^3 IU/mL.[7–9] In view of the suppressive rather than curative nature of HBV therapeutics in most cases, the medication must be provided for long periods (and even indefinitely) to maintain its benefit through persistent HBV suppression. Treatment is most beneficial and effective when patients are in the immunoactive phase of HBV chronic disease.[7] Patient characteristics that contribute to treatment success have been identified, and include low serum HBV-DNA levels, HBeAg positivity, and elevated ALT levels[7–9]

Given the accelerated course of chronic hepatitis B in HIV-positive persons,[2] treatment should be considered more strongly than in their HIV-negative counterparts.[1,6] **Figure 9–2** shows an algorithm for anti-HBV treatment in HIV-positive patients; this is based on the following three parameters (listed in order of importance): serum HBV-DNA, ALT levels, and liver fibrosis staging. When viremia is above 2,000 IU/mL and/or ALT is elevated, significant liver damage must be expected and, therefore, anti-HBV treatment should be advised. Advanced liver fibrosis or cirrhosis is occasionally seen in patients with low serum HBV-DNA and/or normal ALT; accordingly, these patients may also benefit from antiviral treatment.

Antiviral Drugs for Chronic Hepatitis B in HIV-Positive Patients

Seven drugs have been approved so far for the treatment of chronic hepatitis B, and another, emtricitabine, is under final evaluation.

Interferon-α-2b. Interferon-α–2b (IFNα-2b) was the first drug approved for treating chronic hepatitis B. Standard interferon-α, however, has been replaced by pegylated IFNα in most instances. IFNα (or pegylated IFNα) is particularly effective for HBeAg+ chronic hepatitis B in the presence of elevated ALT, low serum HBV-DNA, and HBV genotypes A and B.[7–9] Frequent side effects of the drug (including flulike symptoms, psychiatric effects, bone marrow suppression, thyroid dysfunction) and the need for subcutaneous administration have limited its use. Moreover, it is contraindicated in decompensated cirrhotic patients because it may exacerbate decompensation events. Liver enzyme flares during IFNα treatment are more common in HIV-

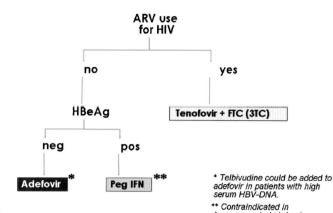

Figure 9–3. *Management of chronic hepatitis B in HIV/HBV coinfected patients: Which drugs to use*

positive persons than in HIV-negative counterparts for unclear reasons. Finally, the efficacy of IFNα is lower in HBV/HIV co-infection regardless CD4 counts most likely as result of underlying immune abnormalities[13] The recommended duration of therapy is 12 months.

Pegylated Interferon α-2a. Pegylated forms of IFNα have a longer half-life and higher potency than standard IFNα. In individuals with HBV monoinfection, pegylated IFNα is more effective than standard IFNα. Nearly one-third of patients who are HBeAg+ may lose serum HBeAg and normalize ALT with 12 months of therapy[14] Trials comparing pegylated IFNα and lamivudine have shown that rates of HBeAg seroconversion, serum HBV-DNA suppression, and ALT normalization are significantly higher with use of pegylated IFNα compared to lamivudine, but, interestingly, there is no additional benefit when both drugs are used in combination.

In HBV-HIV coinfection, IFN-based therapies are associated with lower rates of therapeutic success and increased toxicity,[13,14] so these agents should be used only in nondecompensated cirrhotic patients who have no need for antiretroviral therapy and who have a good chance of having a response to IFNα response—for example, such as in those with HBeAg+, elevated ALT, and low serum HBV-DNA.[1] Treatment is generally provided for 12 months. **Figure 9–3** summarizes the preferred antiviral agents to treat chronic hepatitis B in HIV/HBV coinfected patients, according to the need for antiretroviral therapy and HBeAg status.

When markers of response to either IFNα or pegylated IFNα are not achieved after 12 months of therapy (that is, HBeAg seroconversion, ALT normalization, or significant serum HBV-DNA decline), a therapeutic switch to nucleoside analogs must be considered. Given that these drugs are generally better tolerated, therapy for an indefinite period of time often is anticipated.

Lamivudine. Lamivudine (3TC) is an oral cytosine nucleoside analog with both anti-HIV and anti-HBV activity, although the doses needed to suppress HBV (100 mg/day) are much lower than those required for suppressing HIV (300 mg/day). The effectiveness of 3TC in the treatment of chronic hepatitis B is very well documented, providing significant reductions in serum HBV-DNA and ALT levels, improvement in liver histology, and an enhanced rate of serum HBeAg loss. However, a major problem with the long-term use of 3TC is selection of resistance, which is inherently associated with rebounds in serum HBV-DNA and liver enzyme flares. For treating HBV/HIV co-infection, the recommended dose of 3TC is 300 mg/day and the drug should always be given with at least two other anti-HIV agents; otherwise, HIV resistance mutations would rapidly emerge.

Given its oral administration, excellent tolerability and posology (one pill once daily), 3TC has been widely used as anti-HBV agent, including administration in patients coinfected with HIV, many of whom have received long-term 3TC therapy and, unfortunately, currently harbor 3TC-resistant HBV.[15,16] Overall, HBV resistance mutations can be recognized in more than 90% of viremic patients with HIV infection who have received antiretroviral therapy, including 3TC, for more than 4 years.[17]

Adefovir. Adefovir (ADV) was the first nucleotide analog approved for the treatment of HBV infection. The drug may also inhibit HIV at doses greater than those approved for treating HBV, but then is associated with a relatively high risk for nephrotoxicity. At doses of 10 mg/day, ADV suppress HBV replication and, interestingly, is associated with a relatively low rate of resistance (~30% at 5 years).[17]

In HBV-HIV coinfected individuals, the performance of ADV was examined in 35 patients with ongoing antiretroviral therapy, including 3TC. After 144 weeks of adding ADV, a decrease in serum HBV-DNA levels was observed in 45% of subjects, which is lower than the 56% observed in patients with HBV monoinfection.[18] Selection of mutation K65R in HIV using ADV monotherapy in HBV-HIV coinfected patients not taking antiretroviral therapy has been a matter of concern, but at least one study failed to demonstrate this possibility, even after examining minor virus populations using endpoint dilutions.[19]

It is noteworthy that about 10% of patients with chronic hepatitis B do not respond to ADV. Several reasons may explain this failure, and include pharmacokinetic/pharmacodynamic limitations of the low ADV dosing, presence of genetic polymorphisms (I233V and L217R), and cross-resistance with 3TC upon selection of changes at codon 181 (A→STV).[20] HBV genotype A2 could be particularly less susceptible to ADV due to natural polymorphisms, and this genotype is quite frequent among HIV-HBV coinfected men who have sex with men in Europe.[16]

Entecavir. Entecavir (ETV) is a guanosine analog that inhibits HBV replication at three different steps: priming, reverse transcriptase, and positive strand synthesis. ETV shows more potency in suppressing serum HBV-DNA than is seen with 3TC and ADV; ETV also is effective against wild-type and 3TC- and ADV-resistant HBV. ETV resistance generally results from the accumulation of multiple changes in the HBV polymerase, including 3TC resistance mutations.[21] For this reason, ETV doses of 0.5 mg/day are recommended for 3TC-naïve patients, but 1 mg/day is advised for patients with 3TC-resistant HBV.

Although the drug was originally not thought to be active against HIV, a report in early 2007 highlighted that it might produce significant reductions in plasma HIV-RNA and occasionally select for mutation M184V in HIV.[22] Similar cases were soon reported by others, suggesting that while the antiretroviral activity of ETV might be only residual, it is enough for selecting resistance changes in HIV. Recent in vitro findings have confirmed these results. Therefore, a warning has alerted against the use of ETV in the absence of antiretroviral therapy in HBV/HIV coinfected patients.

Telbivudine. Telbivudine (LdT) is a thymidine L-analog with significantly greater antiviral efficacy than either 3TC or ADV in patients with chronic hepatitis B. It selects for resistance mutations at intermediate rates. In studies used for the registration of the drug, up to 60% of HBeAg+ chronic hepatitis B individuals achieved undetectable serum HBV-DNA after 12 months of LdT treatment compared to 40% treated with 3TC.[23] In the second year of treatment, this rate decreased to 54% due to selection of LdT resistance. Characteristically, LdT selects for mutation M204I, which causes cross-resistance to 3TC; therefore, LdT should not be used following 3TC failure, and vice versa. Interestingly, there is no evidence so far of cross-resistance between LdT and ADV. Although no experimental evidence exists to support any anti-HIV activity of LdT, a recent clinical report has questioned this. Thus, it seems advisable to use LdT with great caution in HIV-HBV coinfected patients.

Emtricitabine. Like 3TC, emtricitabine (FTC) is a cytosine analog with antiviral activity against both HBV and HIV. It has a longer half-life than 3TC and similarly induces a rapid and sharp reduction in serum HBV-DNA at doses of 200 mg/day. Suppression of HBV replication is maintained over 48 weeks of treatment in more than half of patients.[24] No data are available on FTC monotherapy in HBV-HIV coinfection, although extensive experience already exists derived from using the drug in combination with tenofovir as a single-pill formulation (Truvada). In fact, the combination drug is the preferred agent for treating chronic hepatitis B in HBV-HIV coinfected patients in need of antiretroviral therapy (see **Figure 9–3**).[1] This combination provides potent anti-HBV activity along with a solid backbone for a triple combination antiretroviral regimen. Like 3TC, FTC should not be used as monotherapy in HBV-HIV coinfected persons due to the high risk of selection of the M184V resistance mutation in HIV. Because FTC and 3TC show almost total cross-resistance, FTC should not be prescribed after 3TC failure.

Tenofovir. Tenofovir (TDF) is an adenosine nucleotide analog, already approved for the treatment of HIV infection. It also shows potent activity against HBV in patients with and without 3TC resistance.[25] HBV resistance to TDF has occasionally been described in HBV-HIV coinfected patients with 3TC resistance mutations. In this subset of patients, selection of one additional change, A194T, resulted in more than a ten-fold loss of susceptibility to TDF.[26] Large clinical trials have proven the safety and efficacy of this drug in HBV-monoinfected patients, as well as potency greater than that seen with ADV.[27]

Treatment Choices for Chronic Hepatitis B in HIV-Positive Patients

When HBV infection requires treatment but HIV infection does not (generally based on elevated CD4 counts, >500 cells/mm^3), treatment options for HBV should include agents with no clinical activity against HIV, such as pegylated IFNα, ADV, or LdT (**Figure 9–3**). ETV should not be used, given its residual activity against HIV and potential for selection of the M184V resistance mutation. A 12-month course of pegylated IFNα may be advisable for patients with high CD4 counts and HBeAg+ status, elevated ALT, low serum HBV-DNA, and minimal liver fibrosis, particularly when infection is with HBV genotype A. Up to one-third of these patients may show sustained suppression of serum HBV-DNA on stopping therapy, a benefit that cannot be achieved with any other drug. The limitation of pegylated IFNα is its poor tolerability and lower efficacy in the HIV setting.[13] Moreover, the drug is contraindicated in patients with decompensated cirrhosis, although it can be used with caution in individuals with compensated cirrhosis.[4]

For the rest of HBV-HIV coinfected patients who do not need antiretroviral therapy, long-term nucleos(t)ide therapy is the only available option. At the moment, either ADV or LdT are possible options; however, given the risk of selecting drug resistance, an "early add-on" strategy should be considered for patients who do not reach undetectable serum HBV-DNA by week 24 of therapy (**Figure 9–4**). Adding a drug rather than replacing it is advisable because there is evidence for a protective activity against selection of resistance and less of a synergistic or additive

consistently effective or adequately studied in vaccine nonresponders. Currently, vaccination should be performed as previously recommended (0–1–6 months), with standard doses and testing for anti-HBs 1 month after completion. New controls of anti-HBs titers must be performed every 1 to 2 years, especially in patients with a weak initial response. When responses fall below protective titers, boosted doses should be administered. Conversely, if no response occurs, revaccination should be considered, up to three further standard or double doses that could be given 1 month apart. However, additional studies are needed to determine optimal HBV vaccination strategies in HIV-positive persons.

Patients positive for anti-HBc but negative for both HBsAg and anti-HBs are infrequently seen in the general population, but are not rare in the HIV-positive population and/or in persons with chronic hepatitis C.[38] Determining whether hepatitis B vaccine should be administered to patients with "isolated" anti-HBc is not clear because, in addition to a false-positive result, this pattern might suggest exposure in the distant past with subsequent loss of anti-HBs or, more rarely, occult HBV. The majority of HIV-positive patients with isolated anti-HBc are not immune to HBV infection and should be vaccinated with a complete course of hepatitis B vaccine. However, we recommend testing for HBV-DNA to rule out occult chronic HBV infection before administration of a complete course of hepatitis B vaccine.[1]

HIV-HBV Coinfection in Resource-Constrained Settings

In addition to the growing pandemic of HIV, there is an enormous burden of HBV infection in low-income countries, leading to very high rates of HIV-HBV coinfection, mainly in Sub-Saharan Africa and the Far East. With the advent of HAART and the resultant decline in AIDS-related opportunistic infections, liver disease will likely emerge as a significant cause of morbidity and mortality in those settings, similar to the trend already seen in the Western world.[39] There are many open issues and new challenges in the management of HIV-HBV coinfection for regions where chronic hepatitis B is highly endemic.

The management of HIV-HBV coinfection in high-income settings involves individualized therapy, usually from an expert provider, with the support of an array of diagnostic tests. The primary goal of this treatment is to reduce the risk of cirrhosis and hepatocellular carcinoma. Conversely, HIV programs in Africa and other resource-poor settings involve standardized treatment protocols and simplified monitoring to achieve the best possible use of available resources. Limited availability of diagnostic tools and antiviral agents to treat chronic hepatitis B, as well as lack of expertise among health care providers, may contribute to the mismanagement of hepatitis B in these settings.

Three of the agents used for treating HIV in the Western countries (lamivudine, emtricitabine, and tenofovir) also have activity against HBV, but only one—the nucleoside analog lamivudine—is widely available throughout most of Africa and Asia. Lamivudine has been and remains pivotal to all first-line HAART regimens in resource-limited settings. It has a favorable toxicity profile, is not teratogenic, is relatively inexpensive, and is widely available, including within fixed-dose combinations. Nevertheless, using HAART with lamivudine as the sole HBV active agent is a double-edged sword in patients with HIV-HBV coinfection. On one hand, its use as component of HAART has been associated with prevention of new HBV infections, histologic improvement, and prevention of liver disease progression toward cirrhosis and hepatocellular carcinoma.[40] On the other hand, the efficacy of lamivudine is limited by the occurrence of HBV resistance, which develops in 50% of patients after 2 years of 3TC monotherapy and in 90% of patients after 4 years of treatment.[41]

Selection of lamivudine-resistant HBV must be avoided for many reasons. First, the benefit of slowing the progression of liver disease disappears. Although lamivudine resistance usually leads to an asymptomatic rise in transaminases, there are reports of severe hepatitis B reactivation events leading to death after the appearance of lamivudine-resistant mutants.[40] Second, selection of lamivudine-resistant HBV causes cross-resistance; affected patients are prone to treatment failure with subsequent use of other anti-HBV agents (such as emtricitabine, telbivudine, and entecavir).[20] Third, from a public-health perspective, transmission of drug-resistant HBV could increase[42] and—even more alarming—selection of HBV vaccine escape mutants and HBV variants that can escape detection by standard HBsAg tests may be favored.[43] Finally, there is also a risk of HBV flares when HBV-active drugs are stopped. Fatal cases of acute HBV have been documented in HIV-HBV coinfected patients following discontinuation of 3TC therapy. Therefore, before lamivudine is discontinued in favor of another anti-HIV agent, HBV infection must always be discharged. Unless the replacement agent also has anti-HBV activity, 3TC should be continued.[44] Additional anti-HBV drugs with greater potency and less vulnerability to selection of HBV-resistant variants than lamivudine (particularly tenofovir) should be made available for the treatment of all HIV-HBV coinfected individuals in developing regions.

There are other important causes of liver enzyme elevations in HIV-HBV coinfected individuals on HAART. Antiretroviral therapy may cause liver injury through direct toxicity or through idiosyncratic reactions such as those that occur with nevirapine and abacavir. Tuberculosis therapy and other drugs are more likely to cause liver enzyme elevations in HIV-HBV coinfected patients. Infection with hepatitis D virus may cause acute hepatitis, and HAART may lead to a paradoxical flare of hepatitis during immune recovery, caused by the immune reconstitution syndrome. All of these causes of liver enzyme elevations in HIV-HBV infected populations must be distinguished from other, miscellaneous etiologies, which are more common in developing countries than in the Western world. They include acute hepatitis A, C, or E, *Schistosoma mansoni* infection, visceral leishmaniasis, malaria, infection with opportunistic fungi (*Histoplasma capsulatum, Penicillium marneffei*), and typhoid fever. These illnesses often are misdiagnosed in countries with a shortage of resources. The most devastating complication of HBV infection is the development of hepatocellular carcinoma, a disease that usually cannot correctly managed in resource-constrained settings. Thus, complicated clinical care is a pressing issue for providers of HIV treatment, and it will remain an immense challenge in the future.

Universal infant HBV vaccination, availability of screening for HBsAg in HIV-positive people, monitoring of liver enzymes in HIV-HBV coinfected individuals, availability of tenofovir for the treatment of those with elevated liver enzymes, and lamivudine-sparing strategies as anti-HIV treatment of inactive HBV carriers have all been recognized as main key issues for the management of HIV-HBV coinfected patients in resource-limited countries.[45] There are many other aspects regarding epidemiology, natural history, prevention and treatment of chronic hepatitis B that deserve further research in developing regions with high HBV endemicity.[39,43]

Hepatitis C and HIV

Of the nearly 34 million people currently living with HIV worldwide, about 20% (~7 million) have chronic hepatitis C (**Figure 9–1**). This population is mainly represented by individuals with a past history of intravenous drug use, hemophiliacs, and recipients of contaminated blood.

Outbreaks of Acute Hepatitis C Virus Infection in HIV-Positive Patients

Outbreaks of hepatitis C virus (HCV) infection among homosexual men have been reported in several large European and North American cities since the year 2000.[46,47] This observation is striking because HCV was not thought in the past to be efficiently transmitted by sexual contact, as HBV or HIV. High levels of sexual promiscuity, certain particularly traumatic sex practices, and concomitant ulcerative sexually transmitted diseases (such as syphilis) have all been associated with these HCV outbreaks. The increased level of HCV viremia characteristically seen in HIV-positive persons might further contribute to this enhanced infectivity.

In contrast to HIV-negative individuals, in whom acute HCV infection may show spontaneous viral clearance in 30% of cases within the first 12 weeks following initial exposure, HIV-positive patients experience chronicity more frequently. Therefore, early therapeutic intervention in acute hepatitis C is particularly indicated in HIV-positive individuals. Because some patients will have spontaneous HCV clearance, treatment of HIV-positive patients should not be instituted before 12 weeks of estimated exposure, but prolonged delays are discouraged since these may reduce treatment responses. Treatment of acute hepatitis C in HIV-positive patients seems to provide a lower rate of cure than in HIV-negative patients (60% vs. 80%, respectively). Since the antiviral activity of IFN may be mediated through the cytokine network, immunologic abnormalities in the HIV setting could negatively influence interferon efficacy. On the other hand, the rates of HCV clearance obtained in HIV-positive patients treated during the acute phase are much higher than in chronic hepatitis C. HCV genotypes 2 and 3 respond better than genotypes 1 and 4. Elevated ALT levels during the acute episode and rapid viral clearance while on therapy predict a higher chance viral elimination (SVR). In contrast, treatment response does not seem to be influenced by patient age, CD4 count, HIV or HCV load, or having symptomatic infection. At this time, it is unclear whether adding ribavirin to pegylated IFN would offer any advantage when treating acute hepatitis C in HIV-positive individuals. However, given the worse prognosis of HCV infection in HIV-positive persons, it seems worthwhile to provide ribavirin to maximally ensure the attainment of HCV clearance. Following what is advised in HIV-negative persons, 24 weeks of therapy is the recommended duration of treatment of acute hepatitis C in HIV-positive patients, regardless of HCV genotype.[48,49]

Natural History of HCV-Related Liver Disease in HIV-Positive Patients

Besides experiencing an increased risk for chronicity following initial HCV infection, HIV-positive individuals with chronic hepatitis C show a faster progression of liver fibrosis.[50,51] On average, 50% patients have developed liver cirrhosis after 25 years of HCV infection. Low CD4 counts enhance the hepatic fibrogenesis process in coinfected patients; therefore, early introduction of HAART in these patients is warranted.[28,29]

Treatment of Chronic Hepatitis C in HIV-Positive Patients

Treatment of HCV in HIV-coinfected patients become a priority for at least two reasons. First, progression to end-stage liver disease occurs more rapidly in this population.[50,51] Second, the tolerance of antiretroviral agents is much reduced in the presence of underlying chronic hepatitis C, with a greater risk of hepatotoxicity.[52,53] Successful treatment of chronic hepatitis C can

TABLE 9–1	Factors Associated With Sustained Virologic Response to HVC Therapy in HIV-Infected Patients		
	Host	**Virus**	**Treatment**
	• Genetic (white race; IL-28 polymorphisms) • Younger age • Minimal liver fibrosis • Low body mass index • Lack of insulin resistance • Lack of hepatic steatosis • Higher CD4 count • No polysubstance abuse • No psychiatric disease	• Genotypes 2/3 • Low baseline hepatitis C virus RNA • Undetectable hepatitis C virus RNA at week 4	• Adequate pegylated interferon dose • Weight-based ribavirin dose • Good adherence • No concurrent didanosine or zidovudine • Use of hematopoietic growth factors when needed

reverse these drawbacks. Indeed, clearance of HCV has been associated with a regression of liver fibrosis[54,55] as well as with a reduced risk of antiretroviral-related hepatotoxicity.[56]

Selection of HIV-Positive Candidates for HCV Therapy

Virologic features such as HCV genotype and HCV load largely influence the response to HCV therapy. However, viral factors rarely determine who should be considered a good candidate for HCV therapy. Host factors, including extent of liver fibrosis, CD4 counts, and a patient's motivation are the most important parameters that should determine who should receive HCV therapy (see **Table 9–1**).

The extent of hepatic fibrosis is the best prognostic factor for disease progression in patients with chronic hepatitis C and, therefore, its consideration is worthwhile before HCV therapy is initiated. For many years, liver biopsy was the only tool available to assess hepatic fibrosis. However, biopsy is invasive and is associated with occasional serious and even life-threatening complications, sampling error, and inherent heterogeneity of hepatic fibrosis, along with low acceptance by most patients and relatively high cost. These drawbacks have prompted the development of noninvasive tools for staging hepatic fibrosis: ultrasound techniques, such as elastometry (FibroScan), and serum biochemical indexes (including Fibrotest, APRI, SHASTA, FIB-4, and hyaluronic acid). Generally, these noninvasive tools can accurately distinguish between lack of fibrosis and advanced fibrosis, but are less precise for distinguishing among intermediate fibrosis stages. Their predictive value is particularly good for advanced hepatic fibrosis and cirrhosis. However, serum fibrosis markers are generally less reliable in coinfected patients, given the inflammatory nature of HIV disease and/or the frequent prescription of drugs in this population that may interfere with some fibrosis markers in the blood. This is the case for bilirubin elevations due to atazanavir, gamma-glutamyl transpeptidase (GGT) abnormalities with nonnucleoside reverse transcriptase inhibitors, or cholesterol elevations seen with most ritonavir-boosted protease inhibitors. In contrast, liver fibrosis staging using elastometry avoids such interference and seems to be more reliable in this setting.[57] Elastometric measurements can be made in 10 minutes, be repeated periodically, are inexpensive, and have more than 90% positive predictive value for advanced liver fibrosis.

When the diagnosis of another hepatic disease determined by other means—as occurs with chronic hepatitis C testing positive for serum HCV-RNA—the need for a liver biopsy to stage

Complete clinical and histologic remission is observed in patients with HIV/AIDS with immune reconstitution from HAART.[71] Boiling drinking water, hand washing, and avoiding potentially contaminated food are measures that may reduce the acquisition risk.

Microsporidial infection (microsporidiosis). Over the past 2 decades, microsporidial infection has assumed prominence as a heretofore unrecognized cause of diarrhea in humans. These unicellular, eukaryotic spore-forming parasites can infect a number of invertebrate and vertebrate hosts. Microsporidia have been identified in a variety of environmental sources, including water and domestic and farm animals, suggesting the possibility of waterborne, food-borne, or even zoonotic transmission. Several species of microsporidia have been identified, each with different histologic findings, and the manifestations of disease vary according to the specific infecting organism. *Enterocytozoon bieneusi* and *Encephalitozoon intestinalis* are the most common organisms found in humans. *E. bieneusi* most commonly infects the gut; *E. intestinalis* is associated with disseminated infection to other sites.[72]

Microsporidia were first described in AIDS patients when the organisms were observed on electron microscopy of small bowel biopsy specimens (**Figure 10–5a**). With more experience, the infection was seen on small bowel biopsy by routine H&E staining and, more recently, by Gram staining of small bowel biopsy specimens (**Figure 10–5b,c**). The prevalence of infection is likely worldwide.[73] In some series, microsporidia are the most common parasitic cause of diarrhea identified on stool examination.[74,75] Overall, the infection can be found in approximately 15% of patients with diarrheal.[74] Colonic involvement has not been described.[60] The clinical manifestations of these intestinal infections are diarrhea and weight loss, both of which are generally mild. Immunodeficiency is a characteristic setting.[74] Endoscopic findings are usually normal, but the tiny intracytoplasmic spores may be found on Gram, Giemsa, or periodic acid-Schiff (PAS) staining of duodenal biopsy specimens (**Figure 10–5c**). Spores can be found in the stool using a modified trichrome stain, Giemsa statin, or fluorescent dye. The anthelminthic agent albendazole has been shown to be effective in the treatment of *E. intestinalis*. *E. bieneusi* has been shown to respond to treatment with fumagillin.[76] As with cryptosporidial infections, HAART therapy results in clinical and histologic remission.[71]

Other parasitic infections. Other parasites that may infect the small bowel include *Cyclospora cayetanensis, Isospora belli,* and *Giardia lamblia.* These infections may have a higher prevalence in patients with AIDS, but even in this population, prevalance varies according to geographic location. Like cryptosporidiosis, cyclosporiasis and isosporiasis are transmitted via the fecal-oral route, through the ingestion of infective oocysts. Cyclosporiasis has been identified worldwide, whereas isosporiasis is endemic in Africa, Asia, and South America, with high rates of infection also seen in Haiti. Strongyloidiasis is acquired through contaminated water and soil. All of these infections can be identified on appropriate stool examination and staining. The pathogenicity of *Blastocystis hominis* remains controversial.

Mycobacterium avium *complex (MAC).* MAC is seen uncommonly in developing countries but is well recognized in patients with AIDS from the U.S. In the pre-HAART era, an incidence study from a metropolitan center in the southeast U.S. suggested that up to 23% of patients developed the infection.[77] Typical clinical manifestations include fever (which may be unrelenting), night sweats, and profound weight loss; abdominal pain may be prominent; and diarrhea, if present, is generally mild in nature. The small bowel is the most common luminal organ involved, and the presence of MAC infection is suggested by thickening on abdominal CT

Figure 10–5. *Microsporidia.*

Figure 10–5a. *Electron micrograph of* E. intestinalis, *showing the cytoplasmic septations.*

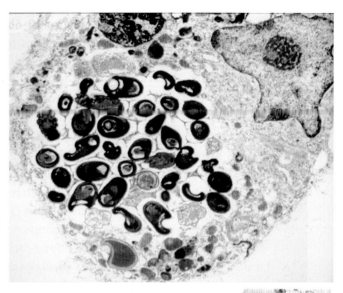

Figure 10–5b. *Paraffin-embedded thick section demonstrating multiple small structures of* E. bienusi *in the epithelium.*

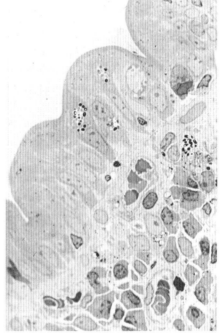

Figure 10–5c. *Gram stain showing small structures staining purple in the epithelium.*

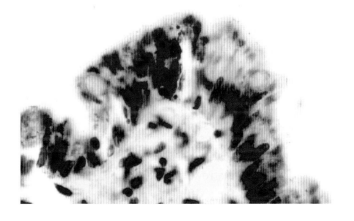

11. Sharma SK, Mohan A, Kadhiravan T. HIV-TB co-infection: epidemiology, diagnosis & management. Indian J Med Res 2005;121:550–567.

12. Devi SB, Devi TS, Ningshen R, Devi KhR, Singh TB, Singh NB. Penicillium marneffei, an emerging AIDS-related pathogen—a RIMS study. J Indian Med Assoc 2009;107:208–210.

13. Wilcox CM, Saag MS. Gastrointestinal complications of HIV infection: changing priorities in the HAART era. Gut. 2008;57:861–870.

14. Mönkemüller KE, Lazenby AJ, Lee DH, Loudon R, Wilcox CM. Occurrence of gastrointestinal opportunistic disorders in AIDS despite the use of highly active antiretroviral therapy. Dig Dis Science 2005;50:230–234.

15. Selik RM, Chu SY, Ward JW. Trends in infectious diseases and cancers among persons dying of HIV infection in the United States from 1987 to 1992. Ann Intern Med 1995;123:933–936.

16. HIV-CAUSAL Collaboration. The effect of combined antiretroviral therapy on the overall mortality of HIV-infected individuals. AIDS 2010;24:123–137.

17. Lubeck DP, Bennett CL, Mazonson PD, Fifer SK, Fries JF. Quality of life and health service use among HIV-infected patients with chronic diarrhea. J Acquir Immune Defic Syndr 1993;6:478–484.

18. Tramarin A, Parise N, Campostrini S, Yin DD, Postma MJ, Lyu R, et al. Association between diarrhea and quality of life in HIV-infected patients receiving highly active antiretroviral therapy. Qual Life Res 2004;13:243–250.

19. Wilcox CM, Straub RF, Alexander LN, Clark WS. Etiology of esophageal disease in human immunodeficiency virus-infected patients who fail antifungal therapy. Am J Med 1996;101:599–604.

20. Mofenson LM, Brady MT, Danner SP, Dominguez KL, Hazra R, Handelsman E, Havens P, Nesheim S, Read JS, et al. Guidelines for the prevention and treatment of opportunistic infections among HIV-exposed and HIV-infected children: recommendations from CDC, the National Institutes of Health, the HIV Medicine Association of the Infectious Diseases Society of America, the Pediatric Infections Diseases Society, and the American Academy of Pediatrics. MMWR Recomm Rep 2009;58:1–166.

21. Wilcox CM. A technique to examine the underlying mucosa in patients with AIDS and severe Candida esophagitis. Gastrointest Endosc 1995;42:360–363.

22. Wilcox CM, Straub RF, Clark WS. Prospective evaluation of oropharyngeal findings in human immunodeficiency virus-infected patients with esophageal ulcer. Am J Gastroenterol 1995;90:1938–1941.

23. Wilcox CM, Alexander LN, Clark WS, Thompson SE. Fluconazole compared with endoscopy for human immunodeficiency virus-infected patients with esophageal symptoms. Gastroenterology 1996; 110:1803–1809.

24. Wilcox CM, Schwartz DA. Endoscopic-pathologic correlates of Candida esophagitis in acquired immunodeficiency syndrome. Dig Dis Sci 1996;41:1337–1345.

25. Pappas PG, Kauffman CA, Andes D, Benjamin DK Jr., Calandra TF, Edwards JE Jr, Filler SG, et al. Clinical practice guidelines for the management of candidias 2009 update by the Infectious Diseases Society of America. Clin Infect Dis 2009;48:503–535.

26. Barbaro G, Barbarini G, Caladeron W et al. Fluconazole versus itraconazole for *Candida* esophagitis in acquired immunodeficiency syndrome. Gastroenterology 1996; 111:1169–1177.

27. Parente F, Ardizzone S, Cernuschi M, Antinori S, Esposito R, Moroni M, Lazzarin A, Bianchi Porro G. Prevention of symptomatic recurrences of esophageal Candidiasis in AIDS patients after the first episode: a prospective open study. Am J Gastroenterol 1994;89:416–420.

28. Wilcox CM, Straub RA, Schwartz DA. Prospective endoscopic characterization of cytomegalovirus esophagitis in patients with AIDS. Gastrointest Endosc. 1994;40:481–484.

29. Wilcox CM, Rodgers W, Lazenby A. Prospective comparison of brush cytology, viral culture, and histology for the diagnosis of ulcerative esophagitis in AIDS. Clin Gastroenterol Hepatol 2004;2:564–567.

30. Wohl DA, Kendall MA, Andersen J, Crumpacker C, Spector SA, Feinberg J, Alston-Smith B, Owens S, Chafey S, Marco M, Maxwell S, Lurain N, Jabs D, Benson C, Keiser P, Jacobson MA; A5030 Study Team. Low rate of CMV end-organ disease in HIV-infected patients despite low CD4+ cell counts and CMV viremia: results of a ACTG protocol A5030. HIV Clin Trials 2009;10:143–152.

31. Brantsaeter AB, Holberg-Petersen M, Jeansson S, Goplen AK, Bruun JN. CMV quantitative PCR in the diagnosis of CMV disease in patients with HIV-infection—a retrospective autopsy based study. BMC Infect Dis 2007;7:127.

32. Jang EY, Park SY, Lee EJ, Song EH, Chong YP, Lee SO, Choi SH, Woo JH, Kim YS, Kim SH. Diagnostic performance of the cytomegalovirus (CMV) antigenemia assay in patients with CMV gastrointestinal disease. Clin Infect Dis 2009;48:e121–124.

33. Wilcox CM, Straub RF, Schwartz DA. Cytomegalovirus esophageitis in AIDS: a prospective evaluation of clinical response to ganciclovir therapy, relapse rate, and long term outcome. Am J Med 1995;98:169–176.

34. Cvetkovi RS, Wellington K. Valganciclovir: a review of its use in the management of CMV infection and disease in immunocompromised patients. Drugs 2005;65:859–878.

35. Benmarzouk-Hidalgo OJ, Cordero E, Martín-Pea A, García-Prado E, Gentil MA, Gomez-Bravo MA, Barrera-Pulido L, Cisneros JM, Perez-Romero P. Prevention of cytomegalovirus disease using pre-emptive treatment after solid organ transplant in patients at high risk for cytomegalovirus infection. Antivir Ther 2009;14:641–647.

36. Len O, Gavaldà J, Aguado JM, Borrell N, Cervera C, Cisneros JM, Cuervas-Mons V, Gurgui M, Martin-Dávila P, Montejo M, Muoz P, Bou G, Carratalà J, Torre-Cisneros J, Pahissa A. Valganciclovir as treatment for cytomegalovirus disease in solid organ transplant recipients. Clin Infect Dis 2008;46:20–27.

37. Heiden D, Ford N, Wilson D, Rodriguez WR, Margolis T, Janssens B, Bedelu M, Tun N, Goemaere E, Saranchuk P, Sabapathy K, Smithuis F, Luyirika E, Drew WL. Cytomegalovirus retinitis: the neglected disease of the AIDS pandemic. PLoS Med 2007;4.e334.

38. Wilcox CM, Schwartz DA, Clark WS. Esophageal ulceration in human immunodeficiency virus infection-causes, response to therapy, and long-term outcome. Ann Intern Med. 1995;122:143–149.

39. Généreau T, Lortholary O, Bouchaud O et al. Herpes simplex esophagitis in patients with AIDS: Report of 34 cases. Clin Infect Dis. 1996;22: 926–931.

40. Lingappa JR, Celum C. Clinical and therapeutic issues for herpes simplex virus-2 and HIV co-infection. Drugs 2007;67:155–174.

41. Strohlein S, Posner G, Colby S et al. Giant esophageal ulcers in patients with AIDS-related complex. Dysphagia. 1986;1:84–187.

42. Wilcox CM, Schwartz DA. Comparison of two corticosteroid regimens for the treatment of idiopathic esophageal ulcerations associated with HIV infection. Am J Gastroenterol. 1994;89: 2163–2167.

43. Alexander LN, Wilcox CM. A prospective trial of thalidomide for the treatment of HIV-associated idiopathic esophageal ulcers. AIDS Res Hum Retroviruses 1997;13:301–304.

44. Villanueva JL, Torre-Cisneros J, Jurado R, Villar A, Montero M, López F, Sánchez-Guijo P, Kindelán JM. Leishmania esophagitis in an AIDS patient: an unusual form of visceral leishmaniasis. Am J Gastroenterol 1994;89:273–275.

45. Sharma SK, Mohan A. Extrapulmonary tuberculosis. Indian J Med Res 2004;120:316–353.

46. Wilcox CM. Esophagitis in the Immunocompromised Host. In: The Esophagus. Castell DO, Richter JE Editors. Lippincott Williams Wilkins 1999 Third Edition pgs 539–556.

47. Nagi B, Lal A, Kochhar R, Bhasin DK, Gulati M, Suri S, Singh K. Imaging of esophageal tuberculosis: a review of 23 cases. Acta Radiol 2003;44:329–333.

48. Bernal A, deI Junco GW. Endoscopic and pathologic features of esophageal lymphoma; a report of for cases in patients with acquired immunodeficiency syndrome. Gastrointest Endosc. 1986;96–99.

49. Bonnet F, Lewden C, May T, Heripret L, Jougla E, Bevilacqua S, et al. Malignancy-related causes of death in human immunodeficiency virus-infected patients in the era of highly active antiretroviral therapy. Cancer 2004;101:317–324.

50. Chiu HM, Wu MS, Hung CC, Shun CT, Lin JT. Low prevalence of Helicobacter pylori but high prevalence of cytomegalovirus-associated peptic ulcer disease in AIDS patients: Comparative study of symptomatic subjects evaluated by endoscopy and CD4 counts. J Gastroenterol Hepatol 2004;19:423–428.

51. Varsky CG, Correa MC, Sarmiento N, Bonfanti M, Peluffo G, Dutack A, et al. Prevalence and etiology of gastroduodenal ulcer in HIV-positive patients: a comparative study of 497 symptomatic subjects evaluated by endoscopy. Am J Gastroenterol 1998;93:935–940.

52. AliMohamed F, Lule GN, Nyong'o A, Bwayo J, Rana FS. Prevalence of Helicobacter pylori and endoscopic findings in HIV seropositive patients with upper gastrointestinal tract symptoms at Kenyatta National Hospital, Nairobi. East Afı Med J 2002;79.226–231.

53. Werneck-Silva AL, Prado IB. Gastroduodenal opportunistic infections and dyspepsia in HIV-infected patients in the era of Highly Active Antiretroviral Therapy. J Gastroenterol Hepatol 2009;24:135–139.

54. Lv FJ, Luo XL, Meng X, Jin R, Ding HG, Zhang ST. A low prevalence of H. Pylori and endoscopic findings in HIV-positive Chinese patients with gastrointestinal symptoms. World J Gastroenterol 2007;13:5492–5496.

55. Wilcox CM, Waites KB, Smith PD. No relationship between gastric pH, small bowel bacterial colonisation, and diarrhoea in HIV-1 infected patients. Gut 1999;44:101–105.

56. Walenda C, Kouakoussui A, Rouet F, Wemin L, Anaky MF. Msellati P. Morbidity in HIV-1-infected children treated or not treated with highly active antiretroviral therapy (HAART), Abidjan, Cote D'Ivoire, 2000-04. J Trop Pediatr 2009;55:170–176.

57. Miriam ZT, Abebe G, Mulu A. Opportunistic and other intestinal parasitic infections in AIDS patients, HIV seropositive healthy carriers and HIV seronegative individuals in southwest Ethiopia. East Afr J Public Health 2008;5:169–173.

58. Assefa S, Erko B, Medhin G, Assefa Z, Shimelis T. Intestinal parasitic infections in relation to HIV/AIDS status, diarrhea and CD4 T-cell count. BMC Infect Dis 2009;9:155.

59. Call SA, Heudebert G, Saag M, Wilcox CM. The changing etiology of chronic diarrhea in HIV-infected patients with CD4 cell counts less than 200 cells/mm^3. Am J Gastroenterol 2000; 95:3142–146.

60. Blanshard C, Francis N, Gazzard BG. Investigation of chronic diarrhea in acquired immunodeficiency syndrome. A prospective study of 155 patients. Gut 1996;39:824–832.

61. Weber R, Ledergerber B, Zbinden R, Altwegg M, Pfyffer GE, Spycher MA, et al. Enteric infections and diarrhea in human immunodeficiency virus-infected persons. Arch Intern Med 1999;159:1473–1480.

62. Datta D, Gazzard B, Stebbing J. The diagnostic yield of stool analysis in 525 HIV-1-infected individuals. AIDS 2003;17:1711–1712.

63. Rene E, Marché C, Regnier B et al. Intestinal infections in patients with acquired immunodeficiency syndrome: A prospective study in 132 patients. Dig Dis Sci. 1989;34:773–780.

64. Brink AK, Mahe C, Watera C, Lugada E, Gilks C, Whitworth J, et al. Diarrhea, CD4 counts and enteric infections in a community-based cohort of HIV-infected adults in Uganda. J Infect 2002;45:99–106.

65. Sarfati C, Bourgeois A, Menotti J, Liegeois F, Moyou-Somo R, Delaporte E, et al. Prevalence of intestinal parasites including microsporidia in human immunodeficiency virus-infected adults in Cameroon:a cross-sectional study. Am J Trop Med Hyg 2006;74:162–164.

66. Kulkarni SV, Kairon R, Sane SS, Padmawar PS, Kale VA, Thakar MR, Mehendale SM, Risbud AR. Opportunistic parasitic infections in HIV/AIDS patients presenting with diarrhoea by the level of immunesuppression. Indian J Med Res 2009;130:63–66.

67. Manabe YC, Clark DP, Moore RD et al. Cryptosporidiosis in patients with AIDS: correlates of disease and survival. Clin Infect Dis 1998; 27:536–542.

68. Abubakar I, Aliyu SH, Arumugam C, Hunter PR, Usman NK. Prevention and treatment of cryptosporidiosis in immunocompromised patients. Cochrane Database Syst Rev 2007;24:CD004932.

69. Anderson VR, Curran MP. Nitazoxanide: a review of its use in the treatment of gastrointestinal infections. Drugs 2007;67:1947–1967.

70. Abraham DR, Rabie H, Cotton MF. Nitazoxanide for severe cryptosporidial diarrhea in human immunodeficiency virus infected children. Pediatr Infect Dis J 2008;27:1040–1041.

71. Carr A, Marriott D, Field A et al.Treatment of HIV-1-associated microsporidiosis and cryptosporidiosis with combination antiretroviral therapy. Lancet 1998; 351:256–261.

72. Didier ES. Microsporidiosis: an emerging and opportunistic infection in humans and animals. Acta Trop 2005;94:61–76.

73. Viriyavejakul P, Nintasen R, Punsawad C, Chaisri U, Punpoowong B, Riganti M. High prevalence of Microsporidium infection in HIV-infected patients. Southeast Asian J Trop Med Public Health 2009;40:223–228.

74. Endeshaw T, Kebede A, Verweij JJ, Zewide A, Tsige K, Abraham Y, Wolday D, Woldemichael T, Messele T, Polderman AM, Petros B. Intestinal microsporidiosis in diarrheal patients infected with human immunodeficiency virus-1 in Addis Ababa, Ethiopia. Jpn J Infect Dis 2006;59:306–310.

75. Sobottka I, Schwartz DA, Schottelius J, Visvesvara GS, Pieniazek NJ, Schmetz C, Kock NP, Laufs R, Albrecht H. Prevalence and clinical significance of intestinal microsporidiosis in human immunodeficiency virus-infected patients with and without diarrhea in Germany: a prospective coprodiagnostic study. Clin Infect Dis 1998;26:475–480.

76. Molina JM, Tourneur M, Sarfati C, Chevret S, de Gouvello A, Gobert JG, Balkan S, Derouin F; Agence Nationale Recherches sur le SIDA 909 Study Group. Fumagillin treatment of intestinal microsporidiosis. N Engl J Med 2002;346:1963–1969.

77. Havlik JA, Horsburgh CR, Metchock B et al. Disseminated *Mycobacterium avium* complex infection: clinical identification and epidemiologic trends. J Infect Dis 1992; 165:577–580.

78. Gray JR, Rabeneck L. Atypical mycobacterial infection of the gastrointestinal tract in AIDS patients. Am J Gastroenterol. 1989;84:1521–1524.

79. Shafran SD, Singer J, Zarowny DP et al. A comparision of two regimens for the treatment of *Mycobacterium avium* complex bacteremia in AIDS: Rifabutin, ethambutol, and clarithromycin versus rifampin, ethambutol, clofazimine, and ciprofloxacin. N Engl J Med 1996; 335:377–383.

80. Brooks JT, Song R, Hanson DL, Wolfe M, Swerdlow DL; Adult and Adolescent Spectrum of Disease Working Group. Discontinuation of primary prophylaxis against *Mycobacterium avium* complex infection in HIV-infected persons receiving antiretroviral therapy: observations from a large national cohort in the United States, 1992-2002. Clin Infect Dis 2005;41:549–553.

81. API Consensus Expert Committee. API TB consensus guidelines 2006: Management of pulmonary tuberculosis, extra-pulmonary tuberculosis and tuberculosis special situations. J Assoc Physicians India 2006;54:219–234.

82. Wilcox CM, Chalasani N, Lazenby A, Schwartz DA. Cytomegalovirus colitis in acquired mmunodeficiency syndrome: a clinical and endoscopic study. Gastrointest Endosc 1998;48:39–43.

83. Cello JP, Day LW. Idiopathic AIDS enteropathy and treatment of gastrointestinal opportunistic pathogens. Gastroenterology 2009;136:1952–1965.

84. Keating J, Bjarnason I, Somasundaram S et al. Intestinal absorptive capacity, intestinal permeability and jejunal histology in HIV and their relation to diarrhoea. Gut 1995; 37:623–629.

85. Kotler DP. Intestinal disease associated with HIV infection: characterization and response to antiretroviral therapy. Pathobiology 1998;66:183–8.

86. Knox TA, Spiegelman D, Skinner SC, Gorbach S. Diarrhea and abnormalities of gastrointestinal function in a cohort of men and women with HIV infection. Am J Gastroenterol 2000;95:3482–3489.

87. Batman PA, Kotler DP, Kapembwa MS, Booth D, Potten CS, Orenstein JM, et al. HIV enteropathy: crypt stem and transit cell hyperproliferation induces villous atrophy in HIV/Microsporidia-infected jejunal mucosa. AIDS 2007;21:433–439.

88. Foudraine NA, Weverling GJ, van Gool T, Roos MT, de Wolf F, Koopmans PP, et al. Improvement of chronic diarrhea in patients with advanced HIV-1 infection during potent antiretroviral therapy. AIDS 1998;12:35 41.

89. Smith PD, Lane HC, Gill VJ et al. Intestinal infections in patients with the acquired immunodeficiency syndrome (AIDS): aetiology and response to therapy. Ann Intern Med. 1988;108:328–333.

90. Sanchez TH, Brooks JT, Sullivan PS, Juhasz M, Mintz E, Dworkin MS, et al. Bacterial diarrhea in persons with HIV infection, United States, 1992-2002. Clin Infect Dis 2005;41:1621–1627.

91. Pulvirenti JJ, Mehra T, Hafiz I, DeMarais P, Marsh D, Kocka F, Meyer PM, Fischer SA, Goodman L, Gerding DN, Weinstein RA. Epidemiology and outcome of Clostridium difficile infection and diarrhea in HIV infected inpatients. Diagn Microbiol Infect Dis 2002;44:325–330.

92. Wilcox CM. Etiology and evaluation of diarrhea in AIDS: a global perspective at the millennium. World J Gastroenterol 2000;6:177–186.

93. Bini EJ, Weinshel EH. Endoscopic evaluation of chronic human immunodeficiency virus-related diarrhea: is colonoscopy superior to flexible sigmoidoscopy? Am J Gastroenterol 1998;93:56–60.

94. Bini EJ, Gorelick SM, Weinshel EH. Outcome of AIDS-associated cytomegalovirus colitis in the era of potent antiretroviral therapy. J Clin Gastroenterol 2000;30:414–419.

95. Wei SC, Hung CC, Chen MY, Wang CY, Chuang CY, Wong JM. Endoscopy in acquired immunodeficiency syndrome patients with diarrhea and negative stool studies. Gastrointest Endosc 2000;51:427–432.

96. Martin Relloso MJ, Sanchez-Fayos P, Gonzalez Guirado A, Rico L, Porres JC. Colonic histoplasmosis in AIDS. Endoscopy 2005;37:1036.

97. Bini EJ, Green B, Poles MA. Screening colonoscopy for the detection of neoplastic lesions in asymptomatic HIV-infected subjects. Gut 2009;58:1129–1134.

98. Chapman C, Aboulafia DM, Dezube BJ, Pantanowitz L. Human immunodeficiency virus-associated adenocarcinoma of the colon: clinicopathologic findings and outcome. Clin Colorectal Cancer 2009;8:215–219.

99. Barrett WL, Callahan TD, Orkin BA. Perianal manifestations of human immunodeficiency virus infection: experience with 260 patients. Dis Colon Rectum 1998;41:606–611.

100. Burke EC, Orloff SL, Freise CE, Macho JR, Schecter WP. Wound healing after anorectal surgery in human immunodeficiency virus-infected patients. Arch Surg 1991;126:1267–1270.

101. Goldstone SE, Winkler B, Ufford LJ, Alt E, Palefsky JM. High prevalence of anal squamous intraepithelial lesions and squamous-cell carcinoma in men who have sex with men as seen in a surgical practice. Dis Colon Rectum 2001;44:690–698.

102. Etienney I, Vuong S, Daniel F, Mory B, Taouk M, Sultan S, Thomas C, Bourguignon J, de Parades V, Méary N, Balaton A, Atienza P, Bauer P. Prevalence of anal cytologic abnormalities in a French referral population: a prospective study with special emphasis on HIV, HPV, and smoking. Dis Colon Rectum 2008;51:67–72.

103. Forti RL, Medwell SJ, Aboulafia DM, Surawicz CM, Spach DH. Clinical presentation of minimally invasive and in situ squamous cell carcinoma of the anus in homosexual men. Clin Infect Dis 1995;21:603–607.

104. Friedlander MA, Stier E, Lin O. Anorectal cytology as a screening tool for anal squamous lesions: cytologic, anoscopic, and histologic correlation. Cancer 2004;102:19–26.

105. Berry JM, Palefsky JM, Jay N, Cheng SC, Darragh TM, Chin-Hong PV. Performance characteristics of anal cytology and human papillomavirus testing in patients with high-resolution anoscopy-guided biopsy of high-grade anal intraepithelial neoplasia. Dis Colon Rectum 2009;52:239–247.

106. Fox P. Anal cancer screening in men who have sex with men. Curr Opin HIV AIDS 2009;4:64–67.

107. Sulkowski MS, Thomas DL, Chaisson RE, Moore RD. Hepatotoxicity associated with antiretroviral therapy in adults infected with human immunodeficiency virus and the role of hepatitis C or B virus infection. JAMA 2000;283:74–80.

108. Ratnam I, Chiu C, Kandala NB, Easterbrook PJ. Incidence and risk factors for immune reconstitution inflammatory syndrome in an ethnically diverse HIV type 1-infected cohort. Clin Infect Dis 2006;42:418–427.

109. Torti C, Lapadula G, Maggiolo F, Casari S, Suter F, Minoli L, Pezzoli C, Pictro MD, Migliorino G, Quiros-Roldan EN, Sighinolfi L, Gatti F, Carosi G; Italian MASTER Cohort. HIV Clin Trials 2007;8:112–120.

Chapter 11 CARDIOVASCULAR MANIFESTATIONS OF HIV/AIDS

GIUSEPPE BARBARO

Life becomes harder for us when we live for others,
but it also becomes richer and happier.

—ALBERT SCHWEITZER

Introduction

The introduction of highly active antiretroviral therapy (HAART) has significantly improved the clinical evolution of human immunodeficiency virus (HIV) disease, with the increased survival of HIV-infected patients. However, the introduction of HAART has also generated the double clinical face of cardiology in acquired immunodeficiency syndrome (AIDS). In developed countries, we have observed a reduction in the prevalence of HIV-associated cardiomyopathy, possibly related to the reduction in the incidence of opportunistic infections and myocarditis. On the other hand, in developing countries, where HAART is not widely available and the pathogenetic impact of nutritional factors is significant, we have also observed an increase in the prevalence of HIV-associated cardiomyopathy, along with a high mortality rate for congestive heart failure. In the context of these new clinical findings, we have observed in developed countries that some HAART regimens, especially those including protease inhibitors (PIs), may cause an iatrogenic metabolic syndrome (HIV-lipodystrophy syndrome) that is associated with an increased risk for cardiovascular disease. At the same time, in HIV-infected patients receiving HAART, and in the context of the recently described immune reconstitution inflammatory syndrome, the relapse of some opportunistic infections with possible myocardial involvement has yielded an intriguing and complex profile of this double face of cardiology in AIDS in the HAART era.[1]

HIV-Associated Cardiomyopathy

HIV disease is recognized as an important cause of dilated cardiomyopathy, with an estimated annual incidence of 15.9/1,000 before the introduction of HAART.[2] The importance of cardiac dysfunction is demonstrated by its effect on survival in AIDS. Median survival to AIDS-related death is 101 days in patients with left ventricular dysfunction and 472 days in patients with a normal heart by echocardiography at a similar infection stage. The unadjusted hazard ratio for death in HIV-associated cardiomyopathy compared to idiopathic cardiomyopathy is 4.0; the ratio adjusted after multivariate analysis is 5.86. Since the introduction of HAART, the prevention of opportunistic infections and the associated reduction in the incidence of myocarditis has resulted in reduction of about 30% in the prevalence of HIV-associated cardiomyopathy in developed countries. However, the median prevalence of HIV-associated cardiomyopathy is increasing in developing countries (about 32%), where the availability of HAART is poor and the pathogenetic impact of nutritional factors is greater.

Pathologic Features

The pathologic features of HIV-associated cardiomyopathy are similar to those observed in HIV-uninfected patients.[3] At autopsy, the heart shape is modified, because of ventricular dilation and apical rounding. Heart weight is generally increased, owing to fibrosis and myocyte hypertrophy. On average, long-term survivors have significantly heavier hearts than those who die after a brief disease course. The epicardium is usually normal, and coronary arteries do not show significant atherosclerosis. The myocardium is rather flabby and the ventricular wall usually collapses on sectioning. On cut surface, the ventricles show an eccentric hypertrophy—that is, a mass increase with chamber volume enlargement. Although hypertrophy is demonstrated by the increase in cardiac weight, this is not always grossly evident owing to ventricular dilation. The free wall width may be normal, or even thinner than normal, as happens in short-term survivors. Endocardial fibrosis is a common finding, as well as mural thrombi, mainly located at the apex. Dilated cardiomyopathy can be associated with pericardial effusion or infective endocarditis, especially in intravenous drug abusers. On histology, myocytes show variable degrees of hypertrophy and degenerative changes, such as myofibril loss, causing hydropic changes within the myocardial cells. An increase in interstitial and endocardial fibrillar collagen is a constant feature in HIV-associated cardiomyopathy.

Pathogenesis

Myocarditis. Myocarditis and HIV-1 myocardial infection are still the best studied causes of dilated cardiomyopathy in HIV disease. It may be defined as a process characterized by a lymphocytic infiltrate of the myocardium, with necrosis and/or degeneration of adjacent myocytes which is not typical of the ischemic damage associated with coronary artery disease seen in subjects infected by HIV (with or without evidence of opportunistic infective agents).[4] Histologic findings in HIV-infected patients with myocarditis do not substantially differ from those observed in uninfected patients. Lymphocytes, along with fewer macrophages, are distributed diffusely as single cells or in small clusters. HIV-1 virions appear to infect myocardial cells in patchy distributions, without a clear, direct association between HIV-1 and cardiac myocyte dysfunction (**Figure 11–1**). It is unclear how HIV-1 may enter CD4-receptor-negative cells such as myocytes. Reservoir cells—that is, myocardial dendritic cells—may play a pathogenic role in the interaction between HIV-1 and the myocyte, as well as in the activation of multifunctional cytokines—tumor necrosis factor-α (TNF-α), interleukin (IL)-1, IL-6, and IL-10—that contribute to progressive and late tissue damage.

Autoimmunity. Cardiac-specific autoantibodies (anti-α myosin autoantibodies) have been reported in up to 30% of patients with HIV-associated cardiomyopathy. This finding supports the theory that cardiac autoimmunity plays a role in the pathogenesis of HIV-related heart disease and suggests that cardiac autoantibodies may be markers of left ventricular dysfunction in HIV-positive patients with previously normal echocardiographic findings.

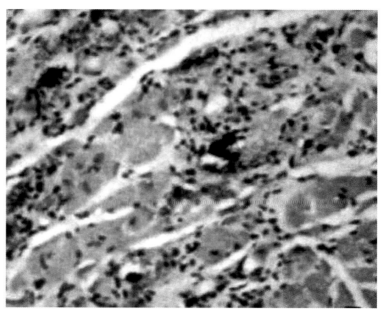

Figure 11–1. *In situ hybridization from endomyocardial biopsy sample in HIV-infected subject with echocardiographic diagnosis of dilated cardiomyopathy (ejection fraction: 28%; left ventricular end-diastolic volume index: 97.5 mL/m³) and histologic diagnosis of active myocarditis. It is possible to observe two myocytes showing a positive signal for nucleic sequences of HIV-1. Source: Reproduced with permission from Barbaro G.[1]*

Myocardial cytokine expression. Myocardial dendritic cells may play a role in the interaction between HIV-1 and the cardiac myocyte, as well as in the activation of cytotoxic cytokines. It has been demonstrated that HIV-1 invades the myocardium through endothelial cells by micropinocytosis and infects perivascular macrophages, which produce additional virus and cytokines such as TNF-α. The virus produces cardiomyocyte apoptosis, either by signaling through CCR3, CCR5 or CXCR4, by entry into cardiomyocytes (after binding to ganglioside GM1), or through TNF-α. It is also possible that HIV-1–associated protein gp 120 (envelope glycoprotein) may induce myocyte apoptosis through a mitochondrion-controlled pathway by activation of inflammatory cytokines. In HIV infection, dendritic cells can initiate the primary immunologic response and present the antigen to T lymphocytes. The interaction between dendritic cells and T lymphocytes—particularly CD8 cells—could promote a local elevation in the multifunctional cytokine TNF-α, which can also be produced and secreted by infected macrophages. TNF-α produces a negative inotropic effect by altering intracellular calcium homeostasis, possibly by inducing nitric oxide (NO) synthesis, which also reduces myocyte contractility.[5]

Relationship with encephalopathy. Several studies have reported that patients with encephalopathy were more likely to die of congestive heart failure than were patients without encephalopathy (hazard ratio after multivariate analysis: 3.4). The reservoir cells in the myocardium and the cerebral cortex—which are not susceptible to treatment—may hold HIV-1 on their surfaces for extended periods of time and may chronically release cytotoxic cytokines, contributing to progressive and late tissue damage in both systems, independently of HAART regimens.[6]

Autonomic dysfunction. There is evidence that an altered autonomic function is present in HIV-infected patients. Left ventricular asynergy may develop due to regional differences in the distribution of cardiac sympathetic nerve endings, even in the context of acute myocarditis. In fact, an alteration of catecholamine dynamics (or autonomic function) has been associated with a transient extensive akinesis of the apical and middle portions of the left ventricle, with hypercontraction of the basal segment (*takotsubo*-like dysfunction) in HIV-infected patients with myocarditis.[7]

Nutritional deficiencies. Nutritional deficiencies are common in HIV infection, particularly in patients with late-stage disease and in those in developing countries, and may contribute in inducing ventricular dysfunction independently of HAART regimens. Deficiencies of trace elements have been associated directly or indirectly with cardiomyopathy. Selenium replacement may reverse cardiomyopathy and restore left ventricular function in nutritionally depleted patients. Levels of vitamin B_{12}, carnitine, and growth and thyroid hormone may also be altered in HIV disease. All have been associated with left ventricular dysfunction.

Drug cardiotoxicity. Studies in transgenic mice suggest that zidovudine is associated with diffuse destruction of cardiac mitochondrial ultrastructure and inhibition of mitochondrial DNA replication. This mitochondrial dysfunction may result in lactic acidosis, which could also contribute to myocardial cell dysfunction. Other nucleoside reverse transcriptase inhibitors, such as didanosine, zalcitabine, and lamivudine, do not seem to either promote or prevent dilated cardiomyopathy. In AIDS patients with Kaposi's sarcoma, reversible cardiac dysfunction was associated with prolonged, high-dose therapy with interferon-α. High-dose interferon alpha treatment is not associated with myocardial dysfunction in other patient populations, so it has been proposed that it may have a synergistic effect with HIV-1 infection. Doxorubicin (adriamycin), which is used to treat AIDS-associated Kaposi's sarcoma and non-Hodgkin's lymphoma, has a dose-related effect on dilated cardiomyopathy, as does foscarnet sodium when used to treat cytomegalovirus esophagitis.

Treatment

No prospective studies have investigated the efficacy of specific therapeutic regimens on HIV-associated cardiomyopathy other than intravenous immunoglobulins. The apparent efficacy of immunoglobulin therapy may be the result of immunoglobulins inhibiting cardiac autoantibodies by competing for Fc receptors or dampening the secretion or effects of cytokines and cellular growth factors. There is no evidence from prospective studies to suggest that HAART has a beneficial effect on HIV-associated cardiomyopathy. However, some retrospective studies suggest that by preventing opportunistic infections and reducing the incidence of encephalopathy, HAART might reduce the incidence of HIV-associated heart disease and improve its course.

HIV Infection, Opportunistic Infections, and Vascular Disease

Endothelial Dysfunction

Endothelial dysfunction and injury have been described in HIV infection. Endothelial activation in HIV-1 infection may also be caused by cytokines (e.g., tumor necrosis factor [TNF]-α) secreted in response to mononuclear or adventitial cell activation by the virus, or may be a direct effect of the secreted HIV-1-associated proteins gp 120 and tat (transactivator of viral replication) on the endothelium, with possible induction of the apoptosis signaling pathway. Opportunistic agents, such as cytomegalovirus, as well as human herpesvirus-8 (a virus that is involved in the development of AIDS-associated Kaposi's sarcoma), frequently coinfect HIV-infected patients and may contribute to the development of endothelial damage. Circulating markers of endothelial activation, such as soluble adhesion molecules and procoagulant proteins, are elaborated in HIV infection. HIV-1 may enter the endothelium via CD4 or galactosyl-ceramide receptors. Other possible mechanisms of entry include chemokine receptors—for example, coronary endothelium strongly expresses CXCR4 and CCR2A coreceptors, whereas CCR5 is expressed at a lower level. The HIV-1 entry inhibitor TAK-799 is an antagonist for the chemokine receptors CCR5 and CXCR3, which are expressed on leukocytes, especially T-helper-1 cells, and these receptors may be involved in the recruitment of these cells to atherosclerotic vascular lesions. TAK-779 not only suppresses HIV-1 entry via blockade of CCR5 but also attenuates atherosclerotic lesion formation by blocking the influx of T-helper-1 in the atherosclerotic plaque. Since TAK-799 impairs atherogenesis, treatment with TAK-799 could be beneficial for young HIV-infected patients facing lifelong HAART regimens.

Vasculitis

A wide range of inflammatory vascular diseases—including polyarteritis nodosa, Henoch-Schonlein purpura, and drug-induced hypersensitivity vasculitis—may develop in HIV-infected individuals. Kawasaki-like syndrome and Takayasu's arteritis have also been described.[8] The incidence of vasculitis (excluding adverse drug reactions) in HIV infection is estimated to be about 1%. Some HIV-infected patients have a clinical presentation resembling systemic lupus erythematosus, including vasculitis, arthralgias, myalgias, and autoimmune phenomena with a low titer positive antinuclear antibody, coagulopathy with lupus anticoagulant, hemolytic anemia, and thrombocytopenic purpura. Hypergammaglobulinemia from polyclonal B-cell activation may be present, but often diminishes in the late stages of AIDS. Specific autoantibodies to double-stranded DNA, Sm antigen, RNP antigen, SSA, SSB, and other histones may be found in a majority of HIV-infected persons, but their significance is unclear.

HIV Infection and Coronary Arteries

The association between viral infection (cytomegalovirus or HIV-1 itself) and coronary artery lesions is not clear. HIV-1 sequences have been detected by in situ hybridization in the coronary vessels of an HIV-infected patient who died from acute myocardial infarction.[9] Potential mechanisms through which HIV-1 may damage coronary arteries include activation of cytokines and cell-adhesion molecules and alteration of major-histocompatibility-complex class I molecules on the surface of smooth-muscle cells. It is possible also that HIV-1-associated protein gp 120 may induce smooth-muscle cell apoptosis through a mitochondrion-controlled pathway by activation of inflammatory cytokines.

Pericardial Effusion

The prevalence of pericardial effusion in asymptomatic HIV-infected patients has been estimated at 11% before the introduction of HAART. According to some retrospective data, the prevalence of pericardial effusion in HIV-infected patients is reduced by about 30% to 35% after the introduction of HAART, with a trend similar to that observed for HIV-associated cardiomyopathy. In developing countries, the prevalence of pericardial effusion is increased by about 35% to 40%, mostly related to mycobacterial infection. HIV infection should be included in the differential diagnosis of unexplained pericardial effusion or tamponade.[10] Pericardial effusion in HIV disease may be related to opportunistic infections (for example, *Mycobacterium tuberculosis*, *Mycobacterium avium* complex infection) (**Figure 11–2**) or to malignancy (for example, non-

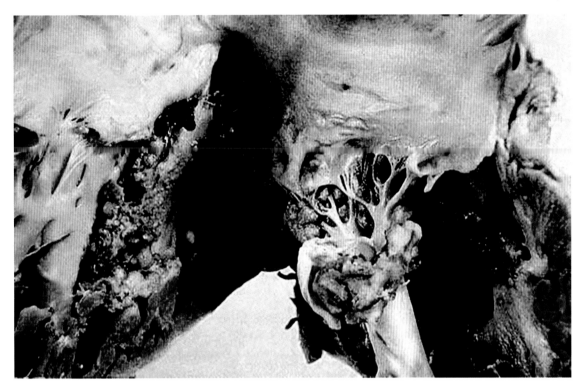

Figure 11–2. *Staphylococcus aureus endocarditis in HIV-infected drug addict who died of cardiogenic shock. The mitral valve shows numerous, large, greyish and friable vegetations. Involvement of the atrial endocardium is also shown. (Courtesy of Prof. D. Scevola, Department of Infectious and Parasitic Disease, University of Pavia, Italy.)*

Hodgkin's lymphoma), but most often a clear etiology is not found. The effusion may be part of a generalized serous effusive process also involving pleural and peritoneal surfaces. This "capillary leak" syndrome is likely related to enhanced cytokine expression (e.g., TNF-α) in the later stages of HIV disease and correlates with the immunodeficiency state of the patient.

Endocarditis

The prevalence of infective endocarditis did not vary in HIV-infected patients who use intravenous drugs after the introduction of HAART, even in the developed countries, being similar to that observed in HIV-uninfected intravenous drug users. Estimates of infective endocarditis prevalence vary from 6.3% to 34% of HIV-infected patients who use intravenous drugs, independently of HAART. Among intravenous drug users, the tricuspid valve is most frequently affected, and the most frequent infecting agents are *Staphylococcus aureus* (>75% of cases) **(Figure 11–3)**, *Streptococcus pneumoniae, Haemophilus influenzae, Candida albicans, Aspergillus fumigatus,* and *Cryptococcus neoformans*. Virulent bacteria known as the HACEK group (*Haemophilus* species, *Actinobacillus actinomycetemcomitans, Cardiobacterium hominis, Eikenella corrodens,* and *Kingella kingae*), which are often part of the endogenous flora of the mouth, can cause endocarditis in HIV-infected patients. Vegetation may form on the tricuspid or pulmonary valves with resultant pulmonary embolism and consequent septic pulmonary infarcts, which appear as multiple opacities on chest radiograms. Systemic emboli often involve coronary

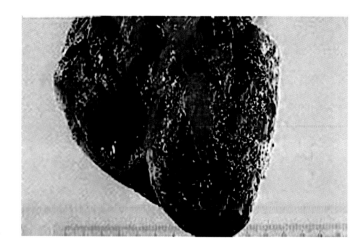

Figure 11–3. *Fibrinous pericarditis by Mycobacterium avium intracellulare in HIV-infected subject with dilated cardiomyopathy who died of congestive heart failure.*

arteries, spleen, bowel, extremities and the central nervous system. Cardiac rhythm alterations (i.e, atrioventricular block) may suggest the presence of an abscess in proximity to the atrioventricular node. Peripheral pulses should be examined for signs of embolic occlusion or a pulsating mass suggesting mycotic aneurysm. Mycotic aneurysms may occur in the intracranial arteries potentially leading to intracranial hemorrhage. Patients with HIV infection generally have similar presentations and survival (85% vs. 93%) from infective endocarditis as those without HIV. However, patients with late-stage HIV disease have about 30% higher mortality with endocarditis than asymptomatic HIV-infected patients, which may be related to the degree of immunodeficiency. Nonbacterial thrombotic endocarditis, also known as marantic endocarditis, had a prevalence of 3% to 5% in AIDS patients, mostly in those with HIV-wasting syndrome, before the introduction of HAART. Marantic endocarditis is characterized by friable endocardial vegetation, affecting predominantly the left-sided valves, consisting of platelets within a fibrin mesh with few inflammatory cells. It is now more frequently observed in developing countries with a high incidence (about 10% to 15%) and mortality for systemic embolization.

HIV-Associated Pulmonary Hypertension

The incidence of HIV-associated pulmonary hypertension has been estimated at 1/200, much higher than 1/200,000 found in the general population, and it is increased after the introduction of HAART.[11] The histopathology of HIV-associated pulmonary hypertension is similar to that of primary pulmonary hypertension.The most common alteration in HIV-associated pulmonary hypertension is plexogenic pulmonary arteriopathy; thrombotic pulmonary arteriopathy and pulmonary veno-occlusive disease are more rare histologic findings. The pathogenesis of primary pulmonary hypertension in HIV infection is multifactorial and poorly understood. Primary pulmonary hypertension has been found in hemophiliacs receiving lipophilized factor VIII, intravenous drug users, and patients with left ventricular dysfunction, obscuring any relationship with HIV-1. HIV-1 is frequently identified in alveolar macrophages on histology. These macrophages release TNF-α, oxide anions, and proteolytic enzymes in response to infection. Clinical symptoms and outcome of patients with right ventricular dysfunction are related to the degree of pulmonary hypertension, varying from a mild asymptomatic condition to severe cardiac impairment with cor pulmonale and death. Activation of alpha-1 receptors and genetic factors (increased frequency of HLA-DR6 and DR52) have also been hypothesized in the pathogenesis of HIV-associated pulmonary hypertension. Effects of HAART regimens on the clinical course of HIV-associated pulmonary hypertension are unknown. Encouraging results have been reported with the administration of endothelin-1 receptor antagonists (such as bosentan), especially in the early stages of the disease.[12]

Cardiac Involvement in AIDS-Associated Neoplasms

In retropsective autopsy studies performed in the pre-HAART era, the prevalence of cardiac Kaposi's sarcoma in AIDS patients ranged from 12% to 28%.[13] Cardiac involvement with Kaposi's sarcoma usually occurs when widespread visceral organ involvement is present. The lesions are typically less than 1 cm in size and may be pericardial or, less frequently, myocardial, and are only rarely associated with obstruction, dysfunction, morbidity, or mortality. Microscopically, there are atypical spindle cells lining slit-like vascular spaces. Non-Hodgkin's lymphoma involving the heart is infrequent in AIDS. Most are high-grade B cell (small, non-leaved) Burkitt-like lymphomas, with the rest classified as diffuse large B cell lymphomas (according to the the Revised European-American Lymphoma [REAL] classification system). Lymphomatous lesions may appear grossly as either discrete localized or more diffuse, nodular to polypoid masses. Most involve the pericardium, with variable myocardial infiltration. There is little or no accompanying inflammation and necrosis. The prognosis of patients with HIV-associated cardiac lymphoma is generally poor because of widespread organ involvement, although some patients treated with combination chemotherapy have experienced clinical remission. The introduction of HAART led to a reduction of about 50% in the overall incidence of cardiac involvement by Kaposi's sarcoma and non-Hodgkin's lymphomas. The decrease may be attributable to the improved immunologic state of the patients and the prevention of opportunistic infections (human herpesvirus-8 and Epstein-Barr virus) known to play an etiologic role in these neoplasms. In contrast, an increased prevalence of cardiac involvement of AIDS-associated tumors may be observed in developing countries in relation to the scant availability of HAART.

HAART-Associated Lipodystrophy and Metabolic Syndrome

HIV-associated lipodystrophy or lipoatrophy, unreported before the introduction of HAART, was first described in 1998. It is characterized by the presence of a dorsocervical fat pad (also known as *buffalo hump*), increased abdominal girth and breast size, lipoatrophy of subcutaneous fat of the face, buttocks and limbs, and prominence of veins on the limbs. The overall prevalence of at least one physical abnormality is thought to be about 50% in otherwise healthy HIV-infected patients receiving HAART, although reported rates range from 18% to 83%. As in genetic lipodystrophy syndromes, fat redistribution may precede the development of metabolic complications in HIV-infected patients receiving HAART. Among HIV-infected patients with lipodystrophy, increased serum total and low-density lipoprotein cholesterol and triglyceride levels have been observed in about 70%, whereas insulin resistance (elevated C-peptide and insulin) and type 2 diabetes mellitus have been observed in 8% to 10%. The severity of these metabolic abnormalities increases with increasing severity of lipodystrophy, and they are associated with an increased risk for cardiovascular events—approximately 1.4 cardiac events per 1000 years of therapy, according to the Framingham score.[14,15]

Pathogenesis

PI-Associated Lipodystrophy and Metabolic Alterations. Protease inhibitors target the catalytic region of HIV-1 protease. This region is homologous, with regions of two human proteins that regulate lipid metabolism—cytoplasmic retinoic-acid binding protein-1 (CRABP-1) and low-density lipoprotein-receptor–related protein (LRP). It has been hypothesized, although without strong experimental support, that this homology may allow PIs to interfere with these proteins, which may be the cause of the metabolic and somatic alterations that develop in PI-treated patients. The hypothesis is that PIs inhibit CRABP-1-modified and cytochrome P450-3A–mediated synthesis of cis-9-retinoic acid and peroxisome proliferator-activated receptor type-γ heterodimer. The inhibition increases the rate of apoptosis of adipocytes and reduces the rate at which preadipocytes differentiate into adipocytes, with the final effect of reducing triglyceride storage and increasing lipid release. The binding of PIs to LRP would impair hepatic chylomicron uptake and endothelial triglyceride clearance, resulting in hyperlipidemia and insulin resistance. Some data indicate that PI-associated dyslipidemia may be caused, at least in part, either by PI-mediated inhibition of proteasome activity and accumulation of the active portion of sterol regulatory element-binding protein (SREBP)-1c in liver cells and adipocytes, or by apo-CIII polymorphisms in HIV-infected patients. Sequence homologies have been described between HIV-1 protease and human site-1 protease (S1P), which activates SREBP-1c and SREBP-2 pathways. A polymorphism in the S1P/SREBP-1c gene confers a difference in risk for development of an increase in total cholesterol with PI therapy. This suggests the presence of a genetic predisposition to hyperlipoproteinemia in PI-treated patients. There is also evidence that PIs directly inhibit the uptake of glucose in insulin-sensitive tissues such as fat and skeletal muscle by selectively inhibiting the glucose transporter Glut4.

TNF-α and Lipodystrophy. The relationship between the degree of insulin resistance and levels of soluble type 2 TNF-α receptor suggests that an inflammatory stimulus may contribute to the development of HIV-associated lipodystrophy. TNF-α activates 11-beta-hydroxysteroid dehydrogenase type 1, which converts inactive cortisone to active cortisol. The activity of this enzyme is higher in visceral fat compared to subcutaneous fat. Visceral fat is able to locally produce cortisol, which could act inside adipocytes and increase lipid accumulation.

Mitochondrial Dysfunction and Lipodystrophy. There is evidence for nucleoside-induced mitochondrial dysfunction in HIV-infected patients treated with nucleoside-containing HAART because lipodystrophy with peripheral fat wasting is associated with a decrease in subcutaneous adipose tissue mitochondrial DNA content. Disrupted pools of nucleotide precursors and inhibition of DNA polymerase-γ (DNA pol-γ) by specific nucleoside reverse transcriptase inhibitors are mechanistically important in mitochondrial toxicity. This effect has been especially described with the use of stavudine and was correlated with the length of exposure to this drug.

Adipocytokines and Lipodystrophy. Adipocytes secrete a range of adipocytokines that control insulin sensitivity. There is evidence that an adipocytokine, adiponectin, a protein product of the apM1 gene, which is expressed exclusively in adipocytes, plays a role in the development of HIV-associated lipodystrophy as well as in congenital and acquired lipodystrophies in non-HIV infected subjects. *In vitro* and animal studies and cross-sectional studies in humans have shown that adiponectin is inversely correlated with features of HAART-associated metabolic syndrome. This syndrome has recently been linked to a quantitative trait locus on chromosome 3q27, the location of the apM1 gene. These studies have shown that both adiponectin levels and the adiponectin-to-leptin ratio are positively correlated with features of HAART associated metabolic syndrome. According to these studies, this ratio could be used to predict insulin sensitivity and potential cardiovascular risk in HIV-infected patients receiving HAART.

HAART and Cardiovascular Disease

HAART-Associated Endothelial Dysfunction. Along with the alterations associated with visceral fat accumulation in lipodystrophy syndrome, and related metabolic disorders (e.g., insulin resistance), endothelial dysfunction and injury have been associated also with a direct action of drugs included in HAART regimens. In vitro data suggest that some HAART regimens—such as those including zidovudine, some non-nucleoside reverse transcriptase inhibitors (e.g., efavirenz), and PIs—disrupt endothelial cell junctions and cytoskeleton actin of the endothelial cells leading to endothelial dysfunction.[16] A reduced endothelial NO synthase expression and increased levels of superoxide anion have been reported by in vivo and in vitro studies as an expression of increased endothelial oxidative stress, which could facilitate the process of accelerated atherosclerosis in HIV-infected patients receiving HAART that includes a PI.

HAART-Associated Vasculitis. Drug-induced hypersensitivity vasculitis is common in HIV-infected patients receiving HAART. The vasculitis associated with drug reactions typically involves small vessels and has a lymphocytic or leukocytoclastic histopathology. The pathologic mechanisms include T-cell recognition of haptenated proteins or the deposition of immune complexes in blood-vessel walls. Medical practitioners need to be especially aware of abacavir hypersensitivity reactions because of the potential for fatal outcomes. Hypersensitivity reactions of this type should always be considered as a possible etiology for a vasculitic syndrome in an HIV-infected patient.

HAART-Associated Coagulation Disorders. HIV-infected patients receiving HAART, especially those with fat redistribution and insulin resistance, might develop coagulation abnormalities, including increased levels of fibrinogen, D-dimer, plasminogen activator inhibitor-1, and tissue-type plasminogen activator antigen, or deficiency of protein S. For instance, protein S deficiency has been reported in up to 73% of HIV-infected men. These abnormalities have been associated with thromboses involving veins and arteries and seem to be related to HAART regimens that include a PI. Thrombocytosis has been reported in 9% of patients receiving HAART, with cardiovascular complications in up to 25% of cases.

HAART-Associated Arterial Hypertension and Coronary Artery Disease. HIV-associated endothelial dysfunction and injury, autoimmune reaction to viral infection (vasculitis), and renal disease have been hypothesized in the etiopathogenesis of HIV-associated hypertension. HIV-associated renal impairment can present as acute or chronic kidney disease. It can be caused directly or indirectly by HIV-1 and/or by drug-related effects that are directly nephrotoxic or lead to changes in renal function by inducing metabolic vasculopathy and renal damage. Chronic renal disease can be caused by multiple pathophysiologic mechanisms, leading to HIV-associated nephropathy, a form of collapsing focal glomerulosclerosis, thrombotic microangiopathy, and various forms of immune complex glomerulonephritis. Antiretroviral agents such as indinavir and tenofovir have been associated with nephrotoxic effects that have been shown to be reversible in most cases.

Systemic arterial hypertension, even in agreement with the Adult Treatment Panel-III guidelines, is currently considered part of HAART-associated metabolic syndrome with a median prevalence of 30%. It appears to be related to PI-induced lipodystrophy and metabolic disorders, especially to elevated fasting triglyceride and insulin resistance. HIV-infected patients receiving HAART with pre-existing additional risk factors (e.g., hypertension, diabetes, or increased plasma homocysteine levels) might be at an increased risk for developing coronary artery disease because of accelerated atherosclerosis.

Conflicting data exist, however, on the relationship between HAART and the incidence of acute coronary syndromes—such as unstable angina or myocardial infarction—among HIV-infected patients receiving PI-containing HAART. Differences in the study design, selection of the patients, definition of clinical endpoints, and statistical analyses might explain this disparity. However, longer exposure to HAART and/or PIs seems to increase the risk of myocardial infarction. The results of the Data Collection on Adverse Events of Anti-HIV Drugs study showed that HAART therapy is associated with a 26% relative risk increase in the rate of myocardial infarction per year of HAART exposure.[17]

HAART-Associated Peripheral Vascular Disease and Stroke. The risk for peripheral vascular disease in HIV-infected patients receiving HAART has been evaluated by surrogate markers of atherosclerosis, such as the measurement of intima-media thickness (IMT). There is a unanimous consensus on the increased prevalence of subclinical atherosclerosis in HIV-infected patients compared to the general population. Presumably, both HIV infection and HAART may promote atherosclerosis through mechanisms involving endothelial cells, either directly or indirectly via metabolic disorders. According to most controlled clinical studies, HAART should be considered a strong, independent predictor for the development of subclinical atherosclerosis in HIV-infected patients, regardless of known major cardiovascular risk factors and atherogenic metabolic abnormalities induced by this therapy. These studies have addressed the impact of individual measures to reduce the cardiovascular risk and the progression of atherosclerosis. The increased use of lipid-lowering agents, of PI-free HAART regimens, and the reduction of smoking may decrease the IMT in HIV-infected patients over time. Markers of subclinical atherosclerosis should be carefully assessed in HIV-infected patients receiving HAART, especially in those with lipodystrophy.

Cerebrovascular hemodynamic function is impaired in HIV-infected patients with evidence of abnormal vasoreactivity, even in otherwise healthy individuals. When stroke occurs in patients with HIV infection, it is almost always due to cerebral infarction and infrequently due to intracerebral hemorrhage. Underlying causes for infarction include coagulopathies, meningitis, and thromboembolism. Many thromboemboli arise from nonbacterial thrombotic endocarditis. Underlying causes for hemorrhage include thrombocytopenia, neoplasms, and hypertension. In the absence of these underlying causes, in about 5% of AIDS cases, infarctions may be due to vasculopathy similar to arteriosclerosis, with findings of small-vessel thickening and perivascular space dilatation, rarefaction, hemosiderin deposition, vessel wall mineralization, and perivascular inflammatory cell infiltrates (but not vasculitis). The most common location for infarctions is the basal ganglia region, with the middle cerebral artery territory and the vertebrobasilar territory also involved, in some cases.

New Markers Defining Cardiovascular Risk in Patients Receiving HAART

New insights in defining the cardiometabolic risk in patients with HAART-associated metabolic syndrome have been provided recently by the echocardiographic measurement of the epicardial adipose tissue. Epicardial adipose tissue is the true visceral fat of the heart and is significantly correlated with abdominal visceral fat measured by magnetic resonance imaging. Given its potential as an easy and reliable marker of visceral fat, epicardial fat has been recently evaluated in patients with HIV-lipodystrophy syndrome. In these patients, echocardiographic epicardial fat correlates with intra-abdominal visceral fat, carotid IMT, and clinical parameters of the metabolic syndrome (especially waist circumference, blood pressure, fasting glucose, insulin, and markers of fatty liver disease).[18–20] Taken together, these findings suggest that echocardiographic assessment of epicardial fat may have the potential to be a simple and reliable marker of visceral adiposity and increased cardiovascular risk in patients with HIV-lipodystrophy syndrome.

Cardiovascular Risk Stratification and Management for HIV-Infected Patients on HAART

For patients on HAART, it may be important to evaluate the traditional vascular risk factors and to try to intervene on those that can be modified. Existing guidelines for the management of dyslipidemias in the general population, such as those of the National Cholesterol Education Program, currently represent the basis for therapeutic recommendations in HIV-infected individuals as well, such as those reported by the HIV Medicine Association of the Infectious Disease Society of America and Adult AIDS Clinical Trial Groups[21] and by the Pavia Consensus Statement.[22] In the absence of specific trial data, HIV patients presenting with acute coronary syndromes should be treated according to the international guidelines. Diet and exercise should not be overlooked, because both can be effective in managing these complications without causing further side effects. Fibric acid derivatives and statins can lower HIV-associated cholesterol and triglyceride levels, although further data are needed on interactions between statins and PIs. Most statins are metabolized through the CYP3A4 pathway, raising concern over the potential interactions with PIs. The inhibition of CYP3A4 by PIs could potentially increase by several-fold the concentrations of statins, thus increasing the risk for skeletal muscle toxicity or hepatic toxicity. Pravastatin, fluvastatin, and rosuvastatin appear to be the safest agents at this time, since they are least influenced by the CYP3A4 metabolic pathway. Although further controlled clinical trials are needed, promising results have been reported with the administration of ezetimibe and omega-3 fatty acids. These do not interact with PIs and may be safely administered in combination with low-dose statins. An approach to the treatment of dyslipidemia in patients treated with PI is to switch to PI-free combination regimens. Although large randomized trials are lacking, some favorable effects have been shown. In treating hypertension in HIV-infected patients with metabolic syndrome, it may be important to remember that beta-blockers and diuretics may worsen the metabolic profile in these patients. Calcium channel blockers should be used with caution, as they may interact with PIs. ACE-inhibitors and angiotensin II receptor blockers may be recommended, but controlled clinical trials are still lacking in this subset of patients. Hypoglycemic agents may have some role in managing glucose abnormalities. Glitazones can be administered in combination with metformin, but glitazones may interact with PIs and cannot be recommended for fat abnormalities alone, and metformin may cause lactic acidosis.

Conclusions

Cardiac and pulmonary complications of HIV disease are generally late manifestations and may be related to prolonged effects of immunosuppression and a complex interplay of mediator effects from opportunistic infections, viral infections, autoimmune response to viral infection, drug-related cardiotoxicity, nutritional deficiencies, and prolonged immunosuppression. In developed countries, HAART has significantly reduced the prevalence of HIV-associated cardiomyopathy, which heavily influenced the prognosis of HIV-infected patients living in these countries in the pre-HAART period, and still influences the prognosis of HIV-infected patients living in developing countries. However, HAART-associated lipodystrophy syndrome in developed countries is an increasingly recognized clinical entity. The atherogenic effects of PI-containing HAART may synergistically promote the acceleration of coronary and cerebrovascular disease and increase the risk of death from myocardial infarction and stroke, even in young HIV-infected people. The multifactorial pathogenesis of HIV-associated lipodystrophy syndrome represents an intriguing field of future basic and clinical research. A better understanding of the molecular mechanisms responsible for this syndrome will lead to the discovery of new drugs that will reduce the incidence of lipodystrophy and related metabolic disorders in HIV-infected patients receiving HAART. Careful cardiac screening is warranted for patients who are being evaluated for, or who are receiving, HAART regimens, particularly for those with known underlying cardiovascular risk factors. A close collaboration between cardiologists and infectious disease specialists is needed for decisions regarding the use of antiretrovirals, for a careful stratification of cardiovascular risk factors, and for cardiovascular monitoring of HIV-infected patients receiving HAART, according to the most recent clinical guidelines, such as those reported by the HIV Medicine Association of the Infectious Disease Society of America and Adult AIDS Clinical Trial Groups and by the Pavia Consensus Statement.

References

1. Barbaro G. Evolution and pathogenesis of the involvement of the cardiovascular system in HIV infection. In: Barbaro G, Boccara F, editors. Cardiovascular Disease in AIDS. Milan-Berlin-Heidelberg-New York: Springer-Verlag; 2009 (pp.15–31).

2. Barbaro G. HIV-associated cardiomyopathy: etiopathogenesis and clinical aspects. Herz 2005;30:486–492.

3. Barbaro G. Pathology of cardiac complications in HIV infection. In: Barbaro G, Boccara F, editors. Cardiovascular Disease in AIDS. Milan-Berlin-Heidelberg-New York: Springer-Verlag; 2009:55–64.

4. Barbaro G. HIV-associated myocarditis. Heart Failure Clin 2005;1:439–448.

5. Barbaro G, Di Lorenzo G, Soldini M et al. Intensity of myocardial expression of inducible nitric oxide synthase influences the clinical course of human immunodeficiency virus-associated cardiomyopathy. Circulation 1999;100:933–939.

6. Barbaro G. Cardiovascular manifestations of HIV infection. Circulation 2002;106:1420–1425.

7. Barbaro G, Pellicelli A, Barbarini G, Akashi YI. Takotsubo-like left ventricular dysfunction in HIV-infected patient. Curr HIV Res 2006;4:239–241.

8. Johnson RM, Barbarini G, Barbaro G. Kawasaki-like syndromes and other vasculitic syndromes in HIV-infected patients. AIDS 2003;17 (S1):S77–S82.

9. Barbaro G, Barbarini G, Pellicelli AM. HIV-associated coronary arteritis in a patient with fatal myocardial infarction. N Engl J Med 2001;344:1799–1800.

10. Barbaro G, Fisher SD, Giancaspro G, Lipshultz SE. HIV-associated cardiovascular complications: a new challenge for emergency physicians. Am J Emerg Med 2001;19:566–574.

11. Barbaro G. Reviewing the clinical aspects of HIV-associated pulmonary hypertension. J Respir Dis 2004;25:289–293.

12. Barbaro G, Lucchini A, Pellicelli AM, Grisorio B, Giancaspro G, Barbarini G. Highly Active Antiretroviral Therapy compared with HAART and bosentan in combination in patients with HIV-associated pulmonary hypertension. Heart 2006;92:1164–1166.

13. Barbaro G, Barbarini G. HIV infection and cancer in the era of highly active antiretroviral therapy. Oncol Rep 2007;17:1121–1126.

14. Barbaro G. Highly Active Antiretroviral Therapy associated metabolic syndrome. pathogenesis and cardiovascular risk. Am J Ther 2006;13:248–260.

15. Barbaro G. Visceral fat as target of highly active antiretroviral therapy associated metabolic syndrome. Curr Pharm Des 2007;13:2208–2213.

16. Fiala M, Murphy T, MacDougall J et al. HAART drugs induces mitochondrial damage and intercellular gaps and gp120 causes apoptosis. Cardiovascular Toxicol 2005;4:327–337.

17. Friis-Moller N, Weber R, Reiss P et al. Cardiovascular risk factors in HIV patients-association with antiretroviral therapy. Results from DAD study. AIDS 2003; 17:1179–1193.

18. Iacobellis G, Sharma AM, Pellicelli AM, Grisorio B, Barbarini G, Barbaro G. Epicardial adipose tissue is related to carotid intima-media thickness and visceral adiposity in HIV-infected patients with highly active antiretroviral therapy-associated metabolic syndrome. Curr HIV Res 2007;5:275–279.

19. Iacobellis G, Pellicelli AM, Sharma AM, Grisorio B, Barbarini G, Barbaro G. Relation of subepicardial adipose tissue to carotid intima-media thickness in patients with human immunodeficiency virus. Am J Cardiol 2007;99:1470–1472.

20. Iacobellis G, Pellicelli AM, Grisorio B et al. Relation of epicardial fat and alanine aminotransferase in subjects with increased visceral fat. Obesity 2008;16:179–183

21. HIV Medicine Association of the Infectious Disease Society of America and the Adult AIDS Clinical Trial Groups. Guidelines for the Evaluation and Management of Dyslipidemia in Human Immunodeficiency Virus (HIV)-Infected Adults Receiving Antiretroviral Therapy: Recommendations of the HIV Medicine Association of the Infectious Disease Society of America and the Adult AIDS Clinical Trial Groups. Clin Infect Dis 2004;37:613–627.

22. Volberding P, Murphy R, Barbaro G et al. The Pavia Consensus Statement. AIDS 2003;17 (S1):S170–S179.

Chapter 12 PULMONARY MANIFESTATIONS OF HIV/AIDS

MARK HULL, PETER PHILLIPS, DON SIN, PAUL MAN, AND JULIO S.G. MONTANER

> On December 17, 1984, I had surgery to remove
> two inches of my left lung due to pneumonia.
> After two hours of surgery the doctors told my mother I had AIDS.
>
> —RYAN WHITE

Introduction

It has been almost 30 years since unusual cases of *Pneumocystis* pneumonia and Kaposi's sarcoma in previously healthy gay men heralded the onset of the AIDS epidemic in North America and led to the identification of the human immunodeficiency virus (HIV).[1–3] Despite tremendous advancement in the management of HIV/AIDS in the developed world with the advent of highly active antiretroviral therapy (HAART),[4,5] respiratory diseases remain a major cause of morbidity amongst HIV-infected individuals. The epidemic has shifted in large part to the developing world and this has led to differences in presentations of HIV-related pulmonary disease worldwide.[6] In the developed world, opportunistic infections secondary to infectious causes have decreased among individuals receiving HAART, while there is growing recognition of the importance of chronic obstructive lung disease (COPD) and pulmonary neoplasms as causes of pulmonary morbidity (**Table 12–1**).[7,8] More recently, with the increased use of HAART, unusual manifestations of pulmonary disease have been recognized as a result of immune reconstitution syndromes (see Chapter 17). In contrast, opportunistic infections remain frequent in other settings where there is limited access to HAART and, in particular, the interlinked epidemics of HIV and tuberculosis (TB) have had significant consequences in resource-limited settings (see Chapters 22 and 23).[9,10] This chapter will review both infectious and noninfectious manifestations of HIV infection.

Pulmonary Infections

Bacterial Infections

Epidemiology and Microbiology of Community-Acquired Bacterial Pulmonary Infections. Bacterial pneumonias remain one of the most common causes of pulmonary infection and are a cause of considerable morbidity and mortality worldwide.[11,12] Rates of pneumonia were markedly elevated in the pre-HAART era in the developed world. In a prospective

TABLE 12–1	Common Causes of Pulmonary Disease in HIV-Infected Individuals
	Bacterial Infections
	Streptococcus pneumoniae
	Haemophilus influenzae
	Pseudomonas aeruginosa
	Legionella pneumonia
	Rhodococcus equi
	Mycobacterial Infections
	Mycobacterium tuberculosis
	Mycobacterium avium complex
	Fungal Infections
	Pneumocystis jiroveci
	Cryptococcus neoformans
	Histoplasma capsulatum
	Coccidioides immitis
	Aspergillus fumigatus
	Malignancy
	Carcinoma of the lung
	Lymphoma—non-Hodgkin's lymphoma
	Human herpesvirus-8–associated conditions
	Kaposi's sarcoma
	Multicentric Castleman's disease
	Primary effusion lymphoma
	Other Conditions
	Chronic obstructive pulmonary disease
	Pulmonary hypertension
	Bronchiectasis
	Lymphocytic interstitial pneumonia

study in North America, rates of pneumonia during the period 1988–1990 were 5.5/100 person-years in HIV-infected individuals compared to 0.9/100 person-years in uninfected individuals.[11] Data derived from a large cohort of HIV-infected women in the HIV Epidemiologic Research Study (HER) found similar rates of bacterial pneumonia of 8.5/100 person-years compared to 0.7/100 person-years in HIV-negative women over the period 1993 to 2000.[13] Risk of pneumonia in both studies was clearly associated with decreasing CD4 counts, and rates were as high as 10.8/100 person-years, and 17.9/100 person-years for patients with CD4 counts below 200 cells/mm^3 in the two respective studies.[11,13]

The use of effective antiretroviral therapy has led to a substantial reduction of the risk of bacterial pneumonia in the U.S. and Europe.[13–15] The HER study found that each month of HAART decreased the risk for bacterial pneumonia by 10% in those not on trimethoprim-sulfamethoxazole (TMP-SMX) prophylaxis.[13] Results from a single clinic cohort in Baltimore found that rates of bacterial pneumonia decreased from 22.7 cases/100 person-years to 9.1 cases/100 person-years following the introduction of HAART in 1997.[14] Population-based national data from Denmark demonstrated that hospitalization rates for pneumonia among HIV-infected individuals have decreased in the HAART era.[15] Incidence rates of pneumonia decreased from 50.6 hospitalizations/1000 person-years during the period 1995–1996 to 19.7 hospitalizations/

1000 person-years during 2005–2007.[15] Similar decreases in hospitalization for pneumonia in patients receiving HAART were noted in a cohort in France, where over a median follow-up period of 43 months, the incidence of bacterial pneumonia was only 0.8/100 person-years.[16]

The most common etiology of bacterial pneumonia in HIV-infected individuals is *Streptococcus pneumoniae*, followed by *Haemophilus influenzae*.[11,17,18] Other bacterial agents identified in the setting of HIV-related bacterial pneumonia include *Pseudomonas aeruginosa*, *Staphylococcus aureus*, and, less commonly, *Legionella pneumophila*.[16,17,19,20] An investigation into the etiology of acid-fast bacillus, smear-negative pneumonia in Asian and African sites found that *Pseudomonas* species, *Klebsiella pneumoniae*, and *S. aureus* are also possible causes of disease.[21] Infections due to *Pseudomonas* occur predominantly in the setting of advanced HIV infection, with CD4 cell counts lower than 50 cells/mm^3.[22]

Streptococcus Pneumoniae and Invasive Pneumococcal Disease.

Bacteremia and invasive disease in the setting of pneumococcal pneumonia is common among HIV-infected individuals, both in the developing world and in resource-limited settings. Rates of invasive pneumococcal disease (IPD) were seen to climb with the emergence of the HIV epidemic in North America and, similarly, have now been seen to be elevated in HIV-infected individuals in Africa (**Table 12–1**).[23–27] Population-based surveillance of pneumococcal bacteremia in the U.S. and Spain found that the rates of disease dropped substantially after the introduction of HAART (**Table 12–1**), although rates remain higher than in the general population.[28,29]

HIV infection has been associated with increased nasopharyngeal colonization, which is an important precursor to invasive disease.[30] Other risk factors for pneumococcal pneumonia, such as cigarette smoking, crowding, or malnutrition, are common in HIV-infected populations. Cigarette smoking, which has long been linked to IPD,[31] occurs at higher rates among HIV-infected individuals than in the general population. Almost 75% of patients report a prior smoking history, and 40% to 50% are current smokers.[32,33] In a retrospective review of bacterial pneumonia among hospitalized HIV-infected patients in Sardinia, Italy, from 1999–2004, 88% were found to be smokers.[34] Similarly, the Strategies for Management of Antiretroviral Therapy (SMART) trial, evaluating treatment interruption of antiretroviral therapy, found that smoking was a significant risk factor for those who developed bacterial pneumonia, with current smokers having more than an 80% higher risk of pneumonia compared to people who never smoked.[35]

IPD in the setting of HIV infection has also been associated with an increased risk of antibiotic resistance. An analysis of IPD isolates in Soweto, South Africa, identified higher rates of penicillin resistance among HIV-infected patients compared to HIV-uninfected adults (19% vs. 4.3%).[36] This has been attributed, in part, to the increase in pediatric serotypes (6, 14, 19 and 23), particularly in women.[37] Similarly, the use of TMP-SMX has been associated with increased colonization with resistant strains in Zambian infants.[38]

Although early studies found similar outcomes for IPD among HIV-infected and uninfected patients, a recent multicenter observational study of 768 episodes of IPD found that, after adjustment for age and severity of illness, HIV-infected cases had a higher 14-day mortality.[39]

Clinical Presentation and Management of Community-Acquired Pneumonia.

HIV-infected patients with bacterial pneumonia have clinical features similar to those seen in HIV-uninfected patients. Patients present with symptoms of fever, chills, dyspnea, and dry or productive cough. Pleuritic chest pain may also be reported. Examination may reveal evidence of rales or frank consolidation. Radiographic imaging may reveal unilateral or bilateral infiltrates or lobar consolidation.[39]

TABLE 12–2	Summary of Selected Studies of HIV and AIDS-Associated Invasive Pneumococcal Disease Rates[a]				
Location	**Study Period**	**Incidence Rate**	**Population studied**	**Comment**	**Ref.**
North America—Pre-HAART					
Ohio	1991–1994	940 cases/ 100,000	10 acute care hospitals, Franklin County, OH	Prospective case ascertainment; relative risk (RR) of bacteremia 41.8 (95% CI, 19.0–92.0) that of general population 18–64 years old	23
California	1994–1998	802.9 cases/ 100,000	San Francisco county, CA	Population-based laboratory surveillance; incidence rate for patients with AIDS	24
North America—Post-HAART					
Multiple Centers	1999/2000	467 cases/ 100,000	San Francisco County; Baltimore metropolitan area; CT	Population-based surveillance; incidence rate of patients with AIDS 18–64 years old	28
Europe					
Spain Pre-HAART Post-HAART	1986–1996 1997–2002	24.1 cases 8.2 cases/ per 1,000 person-years	Single site tertiary care hospital, Barcelona	Prospective cohort study; nested cohort study found use of HAART protective with adjusted odds ratio of 0.37 (95% CI, 0.15–0.88)	29
France Pre-HAART Post-HAART	1993–1996 1996–2004	10.6 cases 2.5 cases/ 1,000 person-years	Multi-site, university hospitals, Lyon	Lyon section of the French Hospital database, a prospective cohort; factors associated with decreased risk included lower age, and baseline CD4 cell count >200 cells/mm^3	27
Sub-Saharan Africa—Pre-HAART					
South Africa	1996	197 cases/ 100,000	Single site tertiary care hospital, Soweto	Prospective laboratory-based surveillance of bacteremic cases only	26
Kenya	1989–1992	42.5 cases/ 1000 person-years	Single site out-patient clinic, Nairobi	Prospective cohort of female sex-trade workers; HIV associated with RR of 17.8 (95% CI, 2.5–126.5)	25

[a]Unless otherwise specified, rates are for invasive pneumococcal disease (defined as isolation of *S. pneumoniae* from a normally sterile site).
Source: Adapted from Hull et al.[190]

Patients may present with more significant burden of disease, with evidence of hypoxemic respiratory failure or hypotension. Clinical stratification of disease severity or prognosis is important to ensure appropriate management of patients identified to be at high risk for poor outcomes. The use of differing classification scoring algorithms is recommended by international guidelines.[40] One of the common algorithms, the Pneumonia Severity Index, has been evaluated in the setting of HIV-infected patients with pneumonia and remains a useful tool to predict mortality and, hence, to guide appropriate decision-making for patient care.[20]

Laboratory diagnosis may include the use of sputum cultures (if a satisfactory specimen is obtained) and blood cultures in hospitalized patients. Severely ill patients, particularly those who require ventilatory support, may require bronchoscopy for evaluation for the presence of other pathogens.

Antibiotic management should be based on local susceptibility patterns and national guidelines[40] and would follow similar recommendations for HIV-uninfected patients. In general, the combination of a β-lactam agent such as a third-generation cephalosporin plus a macrolide would be sufficient. This combination would offer broad coverage for bacterial pathogens (excluding *Pseudomonas*) and atypical agents such as *Mycoplasma* and *Legionella*. The use of combination macrolide and β-lactam therapy also appears to offer additional benefit for patients with pneumococcal pneumonia and IPD, particularly older patients or those with more severe disease.[41,42] The use of a respiratory fluoroquinolone may be an alternative therapy.[40] If *Pseudomonas* is suspected, coverage with antipseudomonal agents such as a carbapenem or combination of ceftazidime and tobramycin or ciprofloxacin is indicated.

Antimicrobial Prophylaxis and Pneumococcal Vaccination. Interventions such as antimicrobial prophylaxis have been shown to decrease overall rates for bacterial pneumonia. TMP-SMX use was associated with a 67% reduction in rates of pneumonia in a large U.S. retrospective cohort study, and similarly was found to be protective in the prospective U.S. women's cohort.[11,13] However, the benefits of TMP-SMX wane in the setting of effective antiretroviral use.[14]

TMP-SMX prophylaxis has been shown to reduce morbidity and mortality in resource-limited settings on the African continent in the absence of HAART.[43,44] Two randomized trials conducted in Cote D'Ivoire (Ivory Coast) examined the impact of TMP-SMX on bacterial respiratory disease. One study conducted in patients with no major underlying co-morbid illnesses, and the other was conducted in patients with underlying tuberculosis.[43,44] Bacterial pneumonia occurred at a lower rate amongst those without tuberculosis receiving TMP-SMX, while the use of TMP-SMX reduced overall hospitalizations.[43,44]

Administration of the 23-valent pneumococcal polysaccharide vaccine elicits capsule-specific antibodies; however, response may be reduced compared to HIV-uninfected individuals.[45,46] Studies in the developed world have suggested that pneumococcal vaccine may prevent invasive disease, but a randomized clinical trial conducted in Uganda failed to confirm a protective effect.[47–49] More recently, an analysis conducted within the Veterans Aging Cohort also found that pneumococcal vaccination also reduced the risk of pneumonia.[50] The polysaccharide vaccine continues to be recommended for all HIV-infected patients, preferably before the CD4 cell count falls below 200 cells/mm^3.[51] Revaccination is recommended for patients who initially received the vaccine with a CD4 cell count below 200 cells/mm^3. A repeat vaccination 5 years apart may also be considered.[51]

Due to the poor immunogenicity of the polysaccharide vaccine in children, particularly those less than 2 years of age, protein-conjugated pneumococcal vaccine series have been developed. These vaccines offer 7- or 9-valent coverage, and have been shown to be effective at reducing IPD in children (with and without HIV infection).[52,53] Widespread uptake of the conjugate vaccine in pediatric populations has also been shown to indirectly reduce IPD in adults.[53] The 7-valent vaccine was assessed in HIV-infected adults in Malawi and was shown to reduce recurrent pneumonia due to vaccine serotypes.[54] The use of sequential vaccination with both polysaccharide and conjugate vaccination has not been demonstrated to increase immunoglobulin G levels compared to the polysaccharide vaccine.[55]

Rhodococcus equi and Nocardia Infections. *Rhodococcus equi* is an aerobic gram-positive bacillus that is usually seen in the setting of zoonotic infections.[56] *R. equi* is an opportunistic infection, predominantly causing infection in the setting of advanced immune suppression with CD4 cell counts <100 cells/mm[3.57] *R. equi* presents subacutely with symptoms of cough, sputum production, and even hemoptysis. Radiography is abnormal with evidence of pulmonary cavitations, effusion, or pulmonary nodules. *R. equi* has been reported to cause disseminated infection with involvement of other organs and the formation of cerebral abscess.[58] Culture of sputum or bronchoscopy specimens may confirm the diagnosis and blood cultures are frequently positive.[59] *R. equi* is susceptible to vancomycin, gentamicin, rifampin, imipenem, macrolides, and fluoroquinolones and usually requires a combination of two or three drugs for an extended duration of therapy—at least 6 months. In the pre-HAART era, *R. equi* infections were associated with high mortality rates.[59]

Nocardia are filamentous, gram-positive bacilli found ubiquitously within the environment. The lungs are the most frequently infected organ, but disseminated infection is possible. Clinical presentation is nonspecific and typically includes fevers, night sweats, and cough. Radiographic imaging reveals evidence of lung nodules, cavitary disease, and pleural effusions.[60] Nocardia species are slow-growing, and the laboratory should be notified if a nocardial infection is clinically suspected. Nocardia may be differentiated using a modified acid-fast stain, but can be mistaken for mycobacterial infections, particularly in regions with high prevalence of tuberculosis.[61] An autopsy series in West Africa found 4% of cases had pulmonary nocardiosis while 35% had evidence of pulmonary tuberculosis.[62] Nocardia species are usually susceptible to TMP-SMX, amikacin, third-generation cephalosporins, and imipenem. A prolonged course of therapy for up to 12 months is usually recommended.

Fungal Infections

Pneumocystis Pneumonia

Microbiology. The causative agent of *Pneumocystis* pneumonia was originally discovered more than 100 years ago by Carlos Chagas and subsequently identified in rat lung tissue by Antonio Carini.[63] Initially classified as a protozoan based on its morphologic appearance, the agent was named *Pneumocystis carinii*. The organism has recently been reclassified as a fungus based on ribosomal RNA sequences and cell wall composition.[64] Moreover, it is now clear that the organism causes infection in a species-specific manner, and that *Pneumocystis carinii*, which infects rats is different than *Pneumocystis jirovecii*, which infects humans. As a result, the infection previously referred to as *Pneumocystis carinii* pneumonia (PCP) is currently called *Pneumocystis jirovecii* pneumonia (PJP) (**Figure 12–1**).[65] *Pneumocystis* has a complex life cycle, consisting of trophic, precystic, and cystic forms, and cannot be cultured in vitro.

Epidemiology. PJP was one of the first documented opportunistic infections that heralded the beginning of the HIV epidemic and remains a major opportunistic infection today. PJP was the presenting AIDS-defining illness for a majority of HIV-infected individuals prior to the introduction of prophylactic strategies and HAART. It was originally estimated that up to 75% of HIV-infected individuals in the developed world would develop PJP during their lifetime.[66] The

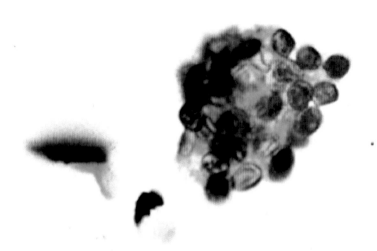

Figure 12–1. Pneumocystis
jirovecii *toluidine blue stain.*

recognition of a CD4 cell count of 200 cells/mm^3 as a critical threshold at which risk of PJP
infection increases was a major landmark in the management of HIV/AIDS, as it allowed formulation of guidelines for the use of specific PJP prophylaxis.[66] Incidence rates of 20 cases of PJP/
100 person-years in those with CD4 cell counts below 200 cells/mm^3 have been reported in the
early days of the epidemic.[66] However, the incidence of PJP has declined dramatically over time,
initially as a result of the introduction of TMP-SMX prophylaxis, and more recently with the
introduction of HAART. Rates in the U.S. decreased 3.4% per year during 1992–1995 and thereafter declined 21.5% per year from 1996–1998.[67] Similarly, in the EuroSIDA cohort, the incidence declined from 4.9 cases per 100 person-years prior to the introduction of HAART to
0.3 cases/100 person-years in 1998.[68]

PJP has been identified as a common opportunistic infection among untreated HIV-infected
individuals globally. PJP was the second most common opportunistic infection in a surveillance
program conducted between 1993–2002 in Rio de Janiero, Brazil.[69] and was also the second
most common AIDS defining illness in a hospital-based study in Kuala Lumpur.[70] Studies in
sub-Saharan Africa originally found low rates of PJP with prevalence rates of 0%–11% in differing geographic locales.[71] However, more recent studies in East Africa have found rates of 33%–
37% in patients undergoing bronchoscopy for acid-fast bacilli smear-negative pulmonary
infiltrates.[72,73]

Mortality secondary to PJP has remained stable despite the introduction of HAART. In the
pre-HAART era, mortality due to PJP was 10%–24%,[74,75] and 9%–12% in the period 1996–
2003.[74,76] Mortality in patients requiring intensive care support is significantly higher, ranging
from 60%–76% in the pre-HAART era, with lower rates of 29% documented in the late HAART
era.[76,77]

Clinical Presentation and Management. PJP presents commonly as a subacute deterioration in respiratory status, with a history of progressive exertional dyspnea accompanied by
fever and cough. Occasionally, a more acute illness with progression over the span of a several

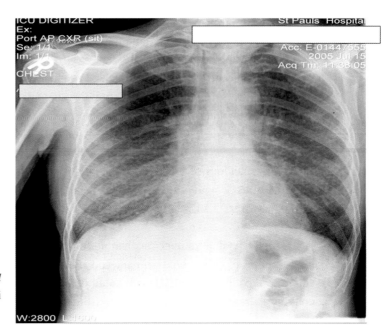

Figure 12–2. *Diffuse interstitial infiltrates of* Pneumocystis jirovecii *pneumonia.*

days may be seen. Acute dyspnea with chest pain may be indicative of a pneumothorax. Radiographic findings suggestive of PJP include bilateral interstitial infiltrates (**Figure 12–2**). Less common findings include nodular disease, pneumatoceles, or pneumothorax. Extrapulmonary manifestations involving the eyes, brain, or liver are rare.

Laboratory abnormalities may include an elevated lactate dehydrogenase and hypoxemia on arterial blood gases. Diagnosis requires visualization of the organism from respiratory tissue. Bronchoscopy with bronchial brushings and bronchoalveolar lavage (BAL) can be used to establish the diagnosis. Organisms can be demonstrated by staining with either toluidine blue (**Figure 12–1**), methenamine silver, or Giemsa stain.

Patients with mild to moderate PJP may be treated on an ambulatory basis. This decision is based on clinical status, including the degree of dyspnea, oxygen saturation, and the ability to tolerate and comply with oral therapy. TMP-SMX is the preferred treatment for the ambulatory treatment of PJP. If this regimen is not well tolerated, then dapsone/trimethoprim or clindamycin/primaquine are reasonable alternatives. Atovaquone may be an option in those who cannot tolerate these preferred regimens. Screening for G6-PD deficiency is recommended prior to the use of primaquine. Dapsone should be used with caution, as it can cause methemoglobinemia in the presence of another oxidizing agent (such as primaquine) or with overdoses.[78] Intravenous therapy is indicated if the patient is experiencing gastrointestinal intolerance or if there is evidence of borderline respiratory status ($PaO_2 < 70$ mm Hg, A-a gradient > 45 mm Hg). The optimal duration of therapy is 21 days.

Adjunctive corticosteroids are recommended for the treatment of patients with moderate to severe PJP (defined by PaO2 < 70mmHg) and have been shown to reduce mortality and morbidity in acute, moderate to severe PJP.[79–81] Prednisone therapy should be continued until discontinuation of the treatment phase of antimicrobial therapy. Early discontinuation of prednisone therapy has been associated with rebound of signs and symptoms.

Patients may worsen clinically during the first 2–3 days of treatment but usually show signs of improvement by about the fifth day. Failed therapy is defined as lack of improvement or worsening lung function after 5 to 8 days of therapy. A meta-analysis of salvage therapy suggested that clindamycin in combination with primaquine was the most effective alternative to the initially prescribed regimen.[82]

Primary prophylaxis is recommended in individuals with CD4 cell counts <200 cells/mm^3, CD4 percentages <15%, or recurrent oral thrush, and secondary prophylaxis (long-term suppressive therapy) should be continued in patients treated fore PJP but with ongoing immune suppression.[83] First line regimens for prophylaxis include TMP-SMX one double-strength tablet daily. Alternate but less effective strategies include single-strength dosage or intermittent dosing. Alternative methods of prophylaxis include dapsone or atovaquone therapy. Intermittent aerosol or intravenous pentamidine was used as an alternative to TMP-SMX in the early days of the epidemic, however, this is rarely needed today as simpler and highly effective oral alternatives have emerged.

HAART-related immune reconstitution leads to long-term protection from PJP, and as such, long-term prophylaxis, both primary and secondary, can be safely discontinued in virologically suppressed patients if the CD4 cell count is higher than 200 cells/mm^3.[68,84,85] Nonetheless, PJP continues to be a common presenting illness in HIV-infected individuals. This reflects both incomplete coverage and adherence to HAART, as well as poor adherence to PJP prophylaxis guidelines by physicians and patients.[71] This is also a reflection of the large burden of undiagnosed HIV in patients not accessing medical care.[71] Exposure to TMP-SMX as PJP prophylaxis has been associated with the development of dihydropteroate synthase gene mutations in the developed world, and genotypic studies have reported similar mutations in isolates from Southern Africa.[86–88] The presence of these mutations has been associated with decreased response to TMP-SMX therapy for PJP infection in some studies but not others.[86,89]

The optimal timing of initiation of antiretroviral therapy of HAART in the setting of acute PJP was a matter of some controversy until recently. Earlier case reports had documented deterioration of pulmonary status following early initiation of HAART, the result of an inflammatory response to persisting antigen: an exaggerated response known as immune reconstitution inflammatory syndrome (IRIS).[90] This suggested that initiation of HAART should be delayed in the setting of acute PJP. However, a recent randomized clinical trial has now provided definitive evidence in favor of early initiation of HAART in this setting.[91] In this study, early initiation of HAART begun within 2 weeks of starting therapy for an opportunistic infection was compared to deferred therapy begun after completion of therapy for the opportunistic infection. The most common infection documented was PJP. The final results of the study showed that early initiation of HAART resulted in less AIDS progression or deaths, with no increase in IRIS incidence.[91]

Aspergillosis. Aspergillosis is caused by species of the environmental mold *Aspergillus*, usually *Aspergillus fumigatus*. These are ubiquitous fungi found in soil and other environmental sources. *Aspergillus* is most commonly seen in patients with immune defects related to chemotherapy or transplantation, in whom prolonged neutropenia is observed. Aspergillosis is a rare infection in the setting of HIV, developing in the setting of advanced AIDS with CD4 cell counts <500 cells/mm^3 and often in conjunction with neutropenia.[92,93] Differing presentations of *Aspergillus* infection have been described in the setting of HIV, including an obstructive picture with mucus plugging of the airways and little evidence of invasion, tracheobronchitis with focal invasion of the tracheal mucosa, and a more aggressive, invasive presentation with extensive inflammation of the tracheobronchial structures.[94,95] Patients present with dyspnea, cough, and wheezing. Radiographic imaging may reveal upper lobe cavities, or unilateral or diffuse infiltrates.[96] Because *Aspergillus* colonization is a common finding in sputum samples, diagnosis of aspergillosis usually requires demonstration of invasion in a tissue sample, although presence of *Aspergillus* on bronchoalveolar lavage correlates with risk of invasive disease.[97] Therapeutic options would include the use of voriconazole or liposomal amphotericin as an alternate.

Histoplasmosis. The dimorphic fungus *Histoplasma capsulatum* is an endemic fungus found along large river valleys of North America and is common in tropical climates worldwide. Patients with advanced HIV are at risk of both primary infection and reactivation of old disease, and disseminated infection is a common presentation. Patients have nonspecific symptoms, including fever, weight loss, splenomegaly, and cytopenias. Respiratory symptoms were the most common presentation after persisting fever in patients admitted for histoplasmosis infection in Panama.[98] Radiographic changes include diffuse nodular infiltrates. Diagnosis can be made from bone marrow culture, blood cultures with lysis-centrifugation, or detection of antigen in urine or blood. Treatment of histoplasmosis consists of an induction phase, often initially with liposomal amphotericin for 14 days, and subsequently itraconazole twice daily to complete a 12-week course.[99,100] Maintenance therapy with once-daily itraconazole is required for 12 months, and can be discontinued at that point if HAART-induced immune reconstitution has occurred, and CD4 cell counts have increased to > 150 cells/mm^3 for 6 months.[101]

Viral Infections

Cytomegalovirus. Cytomegalovirus (CMV) is commonly isolated from cultures from BAL samples in patients with underlying PJP, but is not typically thought to be a pathogen in this setting.[102] In the setting of advanced HIV infection, CMV can occasionally lead to an interstitial pneumonitis. However, this diagnosis is only confirmed by tissue biopsy and the absence of other respiratory pathogens. Presentation is similar to that of PJP, with dry cough, dyspnea, and diffuse infiltrates on chest imaging.[103] Appropriate therapy for CMV is required in this setting: the use of intravenous ganciclovir with consideration of step down to oral valganciclovir.

Influenza. HIV infection is associated with increased risk for hospitalizations and cardiopulmonary events due to influenza.[104] In an analysis of women aged 15–64 enrolled in the Tennessee Medicaid program 1974–1993, women with underlying HIV were found to have higher influenza-attributable risk of hospitalization than women with other chronic conditions such as chronic lung disease.[104] Influenza was estimated to result in approximately 300 admissions/10,000 HIV-infected women.[104] Influenza has been identified as a common respiratory infection in HIV-infected patients receiving HAART. In prospective surveillance of patients presenting with signs of respiratory infection to an outpatient HIV clinic in Montreal, Canada, influenza was identified in 20/50 (40%) cases with an identifiable pathogen.[105] Influenza-associated hospitalizations were noted to decline after the introduction of HAART.[106] In an analysis of HIV-infected patients aged 15–50 years, the influenza-attributable hospitalization rate was 48/1,000 persons (95% CI, 16–91) in 1995, and declined to 5/1,000 persons/year (95% CI, 0.5–11) r during 1996–1999.[106]

HIV may affect response to vaccination, with lower antibody production being documented in some studies.[107,108] Nonetheless, annual influenza vaccination is strongly recommended in all HIV-infected patients.[51]

Mycobacterial Infections

Mycobacterium tuberculosis. HIV has fuelled a rampant expansion of the global tuberculosis epidemic (*see* Chapters 22, 23). HIV leads to increased risk of reactivation of latent tuberculosis as well as the development of active disease in recently acquired infections. Tuberculosis is now seen in many centers as the major pulmonary infection in HIV-infected patients.[109]

The clinical presentation, radiographic findings, and utility of sputum-based diagnostic modalities may differ between HIV-infected and HIV-negative cases, and may differ in HIV-infected individuals as immunosuppression progresses.[110,111] These factors increase the complexity in management of coinfected patients.

HIV-infected patients with tuberculosis should be managed the same way as HIV-uninfected patients are treated, as the two populations have similar treatment responses to a standard 6-month course of antituberculosis therapy. In addition, as in other infectious complications of HIV, the introduction of antiretroviral therapy has played a significant role in improving mortality rates in coinfected patients.[112–114] Furthermore, HAART has been shown to have a powerful secondary preventive effect on tuberculosis and, as such, it has led to decreases in the incidence of tuberculosis in the developed world and in resource-limited settings. This is particularly important as expansion of HAART coverage is now regarded as an essential tool to curb AIDS- and non-AIDS–related morbidity and mortality, the spread of HIV infection, and also to decrease TB (including drug-resistant TB variants) related morbidity, mortality, and incidence.[115–118]

Treatment of HIV-Associated TB. Current therapeutic guidelines recommend a standard approach to tuberculosis therapy in the setting of HIV infection.[119,120] Due to concerns regarding increased risk of rifampin resistance, the use of daily treatment (as opposed to twice- or thrice-weekly dosing schedules) is recommended, particularly in patients with CD4 cell counts under 100 cells/mm^3.[119,120]

Drug interactions between antiretroviral agents and rifampin-based regimens limit options for possible antiretroviral regimens. Drug interactions occur predominantly due to rifampin-related induction of the cytochrome p450 isoenzyme 3A4. Concomitant use of rifampin leads to reductions in concentrations of the non-nucleoside reverse transcriptase inhibitors, namely efavirenz and nevirapine.[121,122] This effect is greater for nevirapine, leading to a recommendation for the preferential use of efavirenz use in HAART regimens in coinfected patients on rifampin-based regimens.[120] However, the widespread use of nevirapine as a component of standard HAART in resource-limited settings and concerns regarding potential teratogenicity of efavirenz make this recommendation difficult to implement. The use of protease inhibitors (PIs) is contraindicated in patients receiving rifampin-based regimens because of profound decreases in plasma concentrations of these agents and, as such, alternatives such as rifabutin are recommended in patients who require PI-based HAART.

In addition, there is a remaining debate regarding optimal timing for initiation of anti-retroviral therapy in patients with TB. The risks of toxicities must be assessed with consideration of the risk of increased mortality if HAART is delayed. The recent Starting Antiretroviral Therapy at Three Points in Tuberculosis (SAPIT) study was a randomized prospective clinical trial that demonstrated significantly improved survival for HIV/TB coinfected patients who received concurrent HAART with antituberculous therapy compared to postponing HAART until completion of TB treatment, for individuals with CD4 cell count <500 cells/mm^3.[123] Outcomes are improved if HAART is initiated prior to the completion of TB therapy, regardless of CD4 cell count.[123] In individuals with CD4 cell counts between 100 and 200 cells/mm^3, it may be best to delay HAART for 2–8 weeks after initiation of tuberculosis therapy.[113] Additional clinical trials to assess optimal timing of HAART in this setting are under way. Additional mathematical modelling supports early initiation of HAART unless rates of immune-reconstitution related mortality rates are high (>4.6%).[124] The high rate of observed AIDS events and death during the 8-week induction phase of antituberculous therapy among patients with CD4 counts <200 cells/mm^3 argues for earlier initiation of HAART once there has been a clinical response to antituberculous therapy.[114]

Multidrug-Resistant and Extensively Drug-Resistant Tuberculosis and HIV. Multidrug resistant tuberculosis (MDR-TB), defined as TB resistant to both isoniazid and rifampin, represents nearly 5% of global annual cases of tuberculosis.[125] The recent report of extensively drug resistant tuberculosis (XDR-TB)—that is, MDR-TB resistant to fluoroquinolones and at least one second-line injectable agent—in rural South Africa has focused attention on HIV co-infection and tuberculosis drug resistance. In one study, the prevalence of XDR-TB was found to be 6% among 475 patients with culture-confirmed tuberculosis. All patients with XDR-TB tested for HIV were positive, and mortality was 98%, including all patients receiving concurrent HAART.[126] HIV-positive patients coinfected with MDR-TB represent complex management issues related to drug interactions and overlapping toxicities; this population also has been shown to have higher mortality compared to HIV-negative patients with MDR-TB.[127,128]

Mycobacterium Avium Complex (MAC). Disease due to MAC in the pre-HAART era was mainly disseminated, with constitutional symptoms, hepatosplenomegaly, cytopenias, and mycobacteremia, but usually without pulmonary infiltrates. Since the introduction of HAART, various pulmonary and extrapulmonary MAC immune reconstitution inflammatory syndromes have been described.[129] Pulmonary lesions have included cavitary lesions, infiltrates, endobronchial modules, and mediastinal or hilar lymphadenophathy.

Noninfectious Pulmonary Manifestations

Chronic Obstructive Pulmonary Disease (COPD). In the pre-HAART era, the most common form of COPD in HIV-infected patients was emphysema, but it is unclear if this condition has the same pathogenesis as smoking-related emphysema. Currently, HIV-infected individuals in the developed world have higher rates of smoking than the general population. Almost 75% of patients report a prior smoking history, and 40% to 50% are current smokers.[32,33] Smoking history, inhaled illegal drug use, and sequelae of other pulmonary insults—particularly, repeated infection—place patients with HIV infection at risk for development of emphysema, bronchial hyperresponsiveness, and, subsequently, COPD.[33,130–135] Furthermore, there is some evidence that HIV itself may be a risk factor for the development of COPD. In a study of 1,014 HIV-infected and 713 controls based on self-reporting and ICD-9 codes, HIV-infected individuals were 50%–60% more likely to have COPD.[7] The mechanisms by which COPD develops in HIV-infected patients and how HIV contributes to COPD are not fully understood. In addition, the long-term effects of HAART-related immune reconstitution on COPD development and prognosis are not yet known.

The management of COPD in the setting of HIV infection should follow the same principles as in other patient populations.[33] However, it is now clear that there is a significant drug interaction between commonly used inhaled corticosteroids and the protease inhibitor ritonavir. Under normal circumstances, the inhaled or nasal corticosteroids (including, for example, fluticasone propionate, beclomethasone, and budesonide) have little systemic absorption due to clearance by the cytochrome P450 (CYP3A4) enzyme system. Fluticasone, in particular, is highly potent, lipophilic, and has a greater volume of distribution and a longer elimination half-life.[136] The inhibition of the CYP3A4 system by ritonavir is thought to increase corticosteroid bioavailability and lead to the subsequent inhibition of the hypothalamic-pituitary-adrenal axis.[137–139] As a result, patients who have been on high-potency inhaled corticosteroids may present with clinical features of Cushing's syndrome and evidence of adrenal suppression based on basal morning cortisol values and abnormal ACTH stimulation tests. Patients requiring the use of inhaled corticosteroids for management of COPD should be managed with the lowest potency agent capable of maintaining control of their symptoms. Patients using corticosteroids concomitantly with ritonavir should be screened intermittently for adrenal suppression. Of note, the interaction between topical corticosteroids and ritonavir leading to adrenal suppression has now been documented in patients extensively exposed to corticosteroid cream, as well as in those who have received a single intra-articular or intraocular corticosteroid injection.

Bronchiectasis. A common complication of repeated pulmonary infections in the setting of HIV-related immune deficiency is bronchiectasis. These patients present with chronic cough and sputum production. With readily available CT scanning, distortion and dilatation of the airways with bronchial thickening is regularly seen; these were common radiographic findings in the pre-HAART era[140,141] or early HAART era. In these earlier studies, patients had CD4 cell counts <100 cells/mm^3, and a prior history of recurrent pulmonary infection was common.[142] Risk factors among pediatric patients with bronchiectasis are similar, with recurrent pneumonia, advanced immune suppression, or history of lymphocytic interstitial pneumonitis (LIP) being reported.[143] Secondary infection due to *Pseudomonas aeruginosa* is a complication of HIV-related bronchiectasis, and antibiotic management of patients presenting with acute deterioration of symptoms should be tailored to include appropriate coverage.[144]

HIV-Associated Pulmonary Arterial Hypertension. Pulmonary arterial hypertension (PAH) associated with HIV infection was initially described in 1987, and HIV infection remains an identifiable risk factor for PAH.[145–147] This is a rare condition that is associated with significant morbidity and mortality, even in the present era when HAART is commonly used. In a recently published systemic review, the average CD4 count at the time of diagnosis of PAH was 352 +/– 304 cells/μL, and the average time from diagnosis to HIV to diagnosis of PAH was 4.3 +/– 4.0 years.[148] Data from the French PAH Registry identified HIV as a risk factor in 7% of cases diagnosed in 2002–2003.[147] A recent analysis of more than 7,000 HIV-infected patients showed a prevalence of PAH of 0.46% (95% CI, 0.32–0.64), which is similar to pre-HAART estimates.[149] In contrast, analysis of the Swiss HIV Cohort Study showed a drop in incidence of PAH during the HAART era, from 0.21% in 1995 to 0.03% in 2006.[150]

The pathology of PAH in HIV-infected patients is not distinguishable from that in HIV-negative subjects; however, HIV-related proteins such as the *Nef* antigen have been implicated as directly affecting endothelial cells, leading ultimately to uncontrolled endothelial proliferation.[151,152] HIV *Nef* has been shown to significantly decrease eNOS expression and to induce oxidative stress in both porcine pulmonary arteries and human pulmonary artery endothelial cells; these findings would explain a reduction in endothelium-dependent vasorelaxation in vitro.[153] Alternatively, HIV infection may alter endothelin-1 production through effects on the inflammatory cascade.[154] Human herpesvirus-8 (HHV-8) has also been linked to risk of PAH in HIV-uninfected patients in some series.[155]

Patients present with symptoms related to right ventricular dysfunction, with progressive dyspnea, pedal edema, and fatigue. Examination may reveal evidence of increased jugular venous pressure, peripheral edema, and possible tricuspid regurgitation murmur.[156] Radiologically, cardiomegaly is present in 80% and pulmonary arterial enlargement in 75% of patients.[153] Diagnosis ultimately requires right heart catheterization, as well as assessment for other conditions leading to PAH.

Therapy is based on treatment algorithms for patients with idiopathic PAH, but HAART therapy is recommended regardless of CD4 cell count value.[157] Treatment with intravenous epoprostenol has shown to be associated with hemodynamic improvement, although long-term intravenous therapy is limited by risks of intravenous line complications.[157] The use of bosentan, an endothelin-1 receptor antagonist, has also been shown to improve hemodynamic outcomes and may be better tolerated in the long term.[156,157] Oral sildenafil has been used in the general PAH population; however, there is a significant drug interaction with protease inhibitors due to inhibition of cytochrome P450 and resulting increased sildenafil levels.[157]

Lymphocytic Interstitial Pneumonitis. Lymphocytic interstitial pneumonitis (LIP) in children and lymphocytic alveolitis in adults fall within the spectrum of lymphocytic infiltrative disorders.[158] LIP was common among HIV-infected children in the pre-HAART era, and was seen in 16%–50% of children infected perinatally.[159] LIP would occur early, often within the second year of life, and was associated with progression to AIDS. Lymphocytic alveolitis is relatively common in HIV-infected adults and can be seen in patients with no evidence of respiratory symptoms.[160] Affected patients show evidence of increased infiltration of CD8+ T lymphocytes within the interstitium and alveoli.[161] Association with certain major histocompatibility antigens have been demonstrated, including HLA-DR 5 and 7.[162,163] Evidence of Epstein- Barr virus from pediatric cases of LIP has also been demonstrated, although the significance of this finding is less clear.[164] Patients present with progressive dyspnea and cough.[158,165] The presence of systemic features such as fever has also been reported. Pediatric patients may present with failure to thrive, and may have evidence of clubbing on clinical examination.[158] Presence of bilateral bibasilar crackles is common.

Diagnosis is best undertaken with high-resolution chest computer tomography (CT), and pulmonary function tests may demonstrate a restrictive pattern.[158] Initiation of HAART therapy is associated with clinical and radiologic improvement.[166] Alternatively, the use of corticosteroid therapy has been described.[158,165]

HIV and Pulmonary Neoplasms

Primary Lung Cancers. Rates of non-AIDS–defining malignancies are climbing among HIV-infected patients in the HAART era.[8,167,168] In the modern post-HAART era, lung cancer is the most common solid tumor malignancy among HIV/AIDs patients,[169] accounting for 44% of all solid tumor malignancies. An analysis of an HIV-positive cohort in England found rates of lung cancer of 6.7/10,000 person-years post-HAART, compared to 0.8/10,000 person-years pre-HAART. Compared to the general population, the relative risk in this cohort was 8.93 (95% CI, 4.92–19.98).[8] Similarly, a cohort study in France found that rates of lung cancer were two-fold higher in the post-HAART era, with higher increased risk in injection drug users.[167] Confounders such as smoking have made interpretation of these data difficult. Recently, data from a large cohort of injection drug users in the U.S. showed that rates of lung cancer deaths had increased in the post-HAART era, and that after adjustment for smoking (which was comprehensively recorded within the cohort), HIV remained associated with increased lung cancer risk (hazard ratio 3.6; 95% CI, 1.6–7.9).[170] Finally, in a recent meta-analysis, which included 625,716 HIV-infected individuals, the standardized incidence ratio for lung cancer was 2.6 (95% CI, 2.1–3.1).[171] Importantly, the risk of lung cancer increases rapidly with aging in the HIV/AIDS population. The relative risk of lung cancer, for example, is nearly fifteen-fold higher in patients between 50 and 60 years of age compared to those who are less than 30 years of age. The risk increases to thirty-fold higher levels beyond 60 years of age.[169] Women with HIV/AIDS have a greater risk for developing lung cancer than do men with HIV/AIDS.[171] Unfortunately, HAART therapy does not appear to mitigate the risk for lung cancer, unlike other malignancies such as lymphoma and Kaposi's sarcoma.[171]

Postulated mechanisms include possible direct oncogenic effects of HIV, genetic instability due to HIV integration leading to increased susceptibility for carcinogens such as tobacco, or possible decreased immune surveillance for malignant cells.[168,170] Primary lung cancers appear to be predominantly non-small–cell lung cancers, including adenocarcinoma, squamous cell carcinoma, and large-cell carcinoma.[168] Patients present with symptoms similar to those seen in HIV-uninfected populations, with cough, hemoptysis, or symptoms related to pulmonary obstruction or metastatic disease. Patients with HIV present at a stage similar to that seen in individuals without HIV infection.[168] Therapeutic modalities such as chemotherapy or surgery follow protocols for HIV-uninfected patients, although prognosis appears worse for patients with HIV/AIDS compared to the general population. Antiretroviral agents, particularly protease inhibitors through their inhibition of the cytochrome P450 system, have the potential for drug interactions with certain chemotherapeutic agents.[168]

HHV-8-Associated Pulmonary Diseases: Kaposi's Sarcoma, Primary Effusion Lymphoma, and Multicentric Castleman's Disease. Kaposi's sarcoma, an HHV-8 associated malignancy, may present with pleuropulmonary disease. Most patients will have concomitant evidence of cutaneous lesions; however, in one series, up to 15.5% of patients had isolated pulmonary involvement.[172] Postmortem examinations have found evidence of pulmonary involvement in up to 75% of patients with cutaneous disease.[173] Patients with pulmonary Kaposi's sarcoma tend to have lower CD4 cell counts at the time of KS diagnosis.[174] Despite improved outcomes with the use of HAART therapy and chemotherapeutic regimens such as liposomal doxorubicin, mortality remains higher in patients with KS with pulmonary involvement compared to patients without pulmonary involvement.[174,175]

Patients present with symptoms of dyspnea and cough, although chest pain and hemoptysis are not uncommon.[176] Radiographic findings include the presence of pulmonary nodules, interstitial infiltrates, pleural effusion, or hilar lymphadenopathy.[176] The presence of vascular-appearing endobronchial lesions on bronchoscopy is often diagnostic. Transbronchial biopsy may help to confirm the diagnosis, but the procedure carries risk of hemorrhage or other complications and may not be necessary if radiographic and clinical features are suggestive of pulmonary Kaposi's sarcoma.[177]

Additional manifestations of HHV-8-related malignancies include primary effusion lymphoma and multicentric Castleman's disease. Primary effusion lymphoma is an uncommon body cavity B cell lymphoma. It accounts for approximately 4% of all non-Hodgkin's lymphomas seen in the setting of HIV infection.[178] Patients present with symptoms related to the accumulation of fluid within pleural spaces, pericardium, or peritoneum. Radiographic imaging reveals the presence of effusions with no other significant pulmonary disease. Diagnosis requires sampling of the effusion for cytology/flow cytometry and immunohistochemistry to document the presence of B cell lineage markers and the detection of HHV-8 in the nuclei of malignant cells.[178] Chemotherapy includes the use of CHOP regimens (cyclophosphamide, hydroxydaunorubicin [doxorubicin], Oncovin [vincristine], and prednisone/prednisolone), with or without rituximab.[179,180] Overall outcomes are poor, despite the use of HAART.[178]

Multicentric Castleman's disease is another HHV-8 associated lymphoproliferative disorder, but presenting with more protean manifestations, including fevers, lymphadenopathy, and hepatosplenomegaly. Patients may not have evidence of immune suppression, with relatively well-preserved CD4 cell counts at diagnosis.[181] Pulmonary symptoms are common, with fever, cough, and dyspnea being reported. Imaging may show interstitial infiltrates or hilar lymphadenopathy.[182,183] Diagnosis may be difficult, and tissue is required from lymph node excision or bone marrow biopsy. Lymph node biopsies may show coexistent Kaposi's sarcoma in up to 40% of cases.[184] Treatment with a variety of chemotherapeutic agents, thalidomide, and interleukin-6 receptor antibody therapies have been attempted, with unclear results.[185,186] Antiviral therapy targeting HHV-8 replication with the use of ganciclovir may be promising.[187]

Non-Hodgkin's Lymphoma. Pulmonary involvement of non-Hodgkin's lymphoma is common, although primary pulmonary lymphoma remains rare.[188,189] Symptoms include dyspnea and cough, while radiographic findings again demonstrate nodular disease, pleural effusion, or lymphadenopathy.[188] Cavitary lesions have been reported in patients with primary pulmonary lymphoma.[189] Diagnosis requires pulmonary tissue or fluid for cytologic analysis, and open-lung biopsy may be required. Chemotherapy is required, following protocols used for systemic lymphoma management.

Conclusions

Pulmonary manifestations of HIV disease have been among the most prominent presenting complaints since the first days of the HIV epidemic. Manifestations include both infectious and non-infectious etiologies, and overall trends have shown decreases in infectious etiologies with the advent of HAART. As such, current manifestations differ globally due to differences in the availability of HAART. In resource-limited settings, infectious complications such as PJP and pulmonary TB still predominate. In comparison, in patients accessing HAART, further attention to long-term consequences such as COPD and neoplasms is necessary.

Suggested Readings

Aberg JA, Kaplan JE, Libman H, Emmanuel P, Anderson JR, Stone VE, et al. Primary care guidelines for the management of persons infected with human immunodeficiency virus: 2009 update by the HIV medicine Association of the Infectious Diseases Society of America. Clin Infect Dis 2009,49:651–681.

Crothers K. Chronic Obstructive Pulmonary Disease in Patients Who Have HIV Infection. Clin Chest Med 2007,28:575–587.

Feikin DR, Feldman C, Schuchat A, Janoff EN. Global strategies to prevent bacterial pneumonia in adults with HIV disease. Lancet Infect Dis 2004,4:445–455.

Thomas CF, Jr., Limper AH. Pneumocystis pneumonia. N Engl J Med 2004,350:2487–2498.

References

1. Kaposi's sarcoma and Pneumocystis pneumonia among homosexual men--New York City and California. MMWR Morb Mortal Wkly Rep 1981;30:305–308.

2. Barre-Sinoussi F, Chermann JC, Rey F, Nugeyre MT, Chamaret S, Gruest J, et al. Isolation of a T-lymphotropic retrovirus from a patient at risk for acquired immune deficiency syndrome (AIDS). Science 1983;220:868–871.

3. Gallo RC, Sarin PS, Gelmann EP, Robert-Guroff M, Richardson E, Kalyanaraman VS, et al. Isolation of human T-cell leukemia virus in acquired immune deficiency syndrome (AIDS). Science 1983;220:865–867.

4. Hammer SM, Squires KE, Hughes MD, Grimes JM, Demeter LM, Currier JS, et al. A controlled trial of two nucleoside analogues plus indinavir in persons with human immunodeficiency virus infection and CD4 cell counts of 200 per cubic millimeter or less. AIDS Clinical Trials Group 320 Study Team. N Engl J Med 1997;337:725–733.

5. Montaner JS, Reiss P, Cooper D, Vella S, Harris M, Conway B, et al. A randomized, double-blind trial comparing combinations of nevirapine, didanosine, and zidovudine for HIV-infected patients: the INCAS Trial. Italy, The Netherlands, Canada and Australia Study. JAMA 1998;279:930–937.

6. UNAIDS/WHO. AIDS Epidemic Update. In; 2007.

7. Crothers K, Butt AA, Gibert CL, Rodriguez-Barradas MC, Crystal S, Justice AC. Increased COPD among HIV-positive compared to HIV-negative veterans. Chest 2006;130:1326–1333.

8. Bower M, Powles T, Nelson M, Shah P, Cox S, Mandelia S, Gazzard B. HIV-related lung cancer in the era of highly active antiretroviral therapy. AIDS 2003;17:371–375.

9. Dye C, Scheele S, Dolin P, Pathania V, Raviglione MC. Consensus statement. Global burden of tuberculosis: estimated incidence, prevalence, and mortality by country. WHO Global Surveillance and Monitoring Project. JAMA 1999;282:677–686.

10. Corbett EL, Steketee RW, ter Kuile FO, Latif AS, Kamali A, Hayes RJ. HIV-1/AIDS and the control of other infectious diseases in Africa. Lancet 2002;359:2177–2187.

11. Hirschtick RE, Glassroth J, Jordan MC, Wilcosky TC, Wallace JM, Kvale PA, et al. Bacterial pneumonia in persons infected with the human immunodeficiency virus. Pulmonary Complications of HIV Infection Study Group. N Engl J Med 1995;333:845–851.

12. Mayaud C, Parrot A, Cadranel J. Pyogenic bacterial lower respiratory tract infection in human immunodeficiency virus-infected patients. Eur Respir J Suppl 2002;36:28s–39s.

13. Kohli R, Lo Y, Homel P, Flanigan TP, Gardner LI, Howard AA, et al. Bacterial pneumonia, HIV therapy, and disease progression among HIV-infected women in the HIV epidemiologic research (HER) study. Clin Infect Dis 2006;43:90–98.

14. Sullivan JH, Moore RD, Keruly JC, Chaisson RE. Effect of antiretroviral therapy on the incidence of bacterial pneumonia in patients with advanced HIV infection. Am J Respir Crit Care Med 2000;162:64–67.

15. Sogaard OS, Lohse N, Gerstoft J, Kronborg G, Ostergaard L, Pedersen C, et al. Hospitalization for pneumonia among individuals with and without HIV infection, 1995–2007: a Danish population-based, nationwide cohort study. Clin Infect Dis 2008;47:1345–1353.

16. Le Moing V, Rabaud C, Journot V, Duval X, Cuzin L, Cassuto JP, et al. Incidence and risk factors of bacterial pneumonia requiring hospitalization in HIV-infected patients started on a protease inhibitor-containing regimen. HIV Med 2006;7:261–267.

17. Park DR, Sherbin VL, Goodman MS, Pacifico AD, Rubenfeld GD, Polissar NL, Root RK. The etiology of community-acquired pneumonia at an urban public hospital: influence of human immunodeficiency virus infection and initial severity of illness. J Infect Dis 2001;184:268–277.

18. Rimland D, Navin TR, Lennox JL, Jernigan JA, Kaplan J, Erdman D, et al. Prospective study of etiologic agents of community-acquired pneumonia in patients with HIV infection. AIDS 2002;16:85–95.

19. Allen SH, Brennan-Benson P, Nelson M, Asboe D, Bower M, Azadian B, et al. Pneumonia due to antibiotic resistant Streptococcus pneumoniae and Pseudomonas aeruginosa in the HAART era. Postgrad Med J 2003;79:691–694.

20. Curran A, Falco V, Crespo M, Martinez X, Ribera E, Villar del Saz S, et al. Bacterial pneumonia in HIV-infected patients: use of the pneumonia severity index and impact of current management on incidence, aetiology and outcome. HIV Med 2008;9:609–615.

21. Vray M, Germani Y, Chan S, Duc NH, Sar B, Sarr FD, et al. Clinical features and etiology of pneumonia in acid-fast bacillus sputum smear-negative HIV-infected patients hospitalized in Asia and Africa. AIDS 2008;22:1323–1332.

22. Baron AD, Hollander H. Pseudomonas aeruginosa bronchopulmonary infection in late human immunodeficiency virus disease. Am Rev Respir Dis 1993;148:992–996.

23. Plouffe JF, Breiman RF, Facklam RR. Bacteremia with Streptococcus pneumoniae. Implications for therapy and prevention. Franklin County Pneumonia Study Group. JAMA 1996;275:194–198.

24. Nuorti JP, Butler JC, Gelling L, Kool JL, Reingold AL, Vugia DJ. Epidemiologic relation between HIV and invasive pneumococcal disease in San Francisco County, California. Ann Intern Med 2000;132:182–190.

25. Gilks CF, Ojoo SA, Ojoo JC, Brindle RJ, Paul J, Batchelor BI, et al. Invasive pneumococcal disease in a cohort of predominantly HIV-1 infected female sex-workers in Nairobi, Kenya. Lancet 1996;347:718–723.

26. Jones N, Huebner R, Khoosal M, Crewe-Brown H, Klugman K. The impact of HIV on Streptococcus pneumoniae bacteraemia in a South African population. AIDS 1998;12:2177–2184.

27. Saindou M, Chidiac C, Miailhes P, Voirin N, Baratin D, Amiri M, et al. Pneumococcal pneumonia in HIV-infected patients by antiretroviral therapy periods. HIV Med 2008;9:203–207.

28. Heffernan RT, Barrett NL, Gallagher KM, Hadler JL, Harrison LH, Reingold AL, et al. Declining incidence of invasive Streptococcus pneumoniae infections among persons with AIDS in an era of highly active antiretroviral therapy, 1995–2000. J Infect Dis 2005;191:2038–2045.

29. Grau I, Pallares R, Tubau F, Schulze MH, Llopis F, Podzamczer D, et al. Epidemiologic changes in bacteremic pneumococcal disease in patients with human immunodeficiency virus in the era of highly active antiretroviral therapy. Arch Intern Med 2005;165:1533–1540.

30. Gill CJ, Mwanakasale V, Fox MP, Chilengi R, Tembo M, Nsofwa M, et al. Impact of human immunodeficiency virus infection on Streptococcus pneumoniae colonization and seroepidemiology among Zambian women. J Infect Dis 2008;197:1000–1005.

31. Nuorti JP, Butler JC, Farley MM, Harrison LH, McGeer A, Kolczak MS, Breiman RF. Cigarette smoking and invasive pneumococcal disease. Active Bacterial Core Surveillance Team. N Engl J Med 2000;342:681–689.

32. Niaura R, Shadel WG, Morrow K, Tashima K, Flanigan T, Abrams DB. Human immunodeficiency virus infection, AIDS, and smoking cessation: the time is now. Clin Infect Dis 2000;31:808–812.

33. Crothers K. Chronic Obstructive Pulmonary Disease in Patients Who Have HIV Infection. Clin Chest Med 2007;28:575–587.

34. Madeddu G, Porqueddu EM, Cambosu F, Saba F, Fois AG, Pirina P, Mura MS. Bacterial community acquired pneumonia in HIV-infected inpatients in the highly active antiretroviral therapy era. Infection 2008;36:231–236.

35. Gordin FM, Roediger MP, Girard PM, Lundgren JD, Miro JM, Palfreeman A, et al. Pneumonia in HIV-infected persons: increased risk with cigarette smoking and treatment interruption. Am J Respir Crit Care Med 2008;178:630–636.

36. Crewe-Brown HH, Karstaedt AS, Saunders GL, Khoosal M, Jones N, Wasas A, Klugman KP. Streptococcus pneumoniae blood culture isolates from patients with and without human immunodeficiency virus infection: alterations in penicillin susceptibilities and in serogroups or serotypes. Clin Infect Dis 1997;25:1165–1172.

37. Buie KA, Klugman KP, von Gottberg A, Perovic O, Karstaedt A, Crewe-Brown HH, et al. Gender as a risk factor for both antibiotic resistance and infection with pediatric serogroups/serotypes, in HIV-infected and -uninfected adults with pneumococcal bacteremia. J Infect Dis 2004;189:1996–2000.

38. Gill CJ, Mwanakasale V, Fox MP, Chilengi R, Tembo M, Nsofwa M, et al. Effect of presumptive co-trimoxazole prophylaxis on pneumococcal colonization rates, seroepidemiology and antibiotic resistance in Zambian infants: a longitudinal cohort study. Bull World Health Organ 2008;86:929–938.

39. Feldman C, Klugman KP, Yu VL, Ortqvist A, Choiu CC, Chedid MB, et al. Bacteraemic pneumococcal pneumonia: impact of HIV on clinical presentation and outcome. J Infect 2007;55:125–135.

40. Mandell LA, Wunderink RG, Anzueto A, Bartlett JG, Campbell GD, Dean NC, et al. Infectious Diseases Society of America/American Thoracic Society consensus guidelines on the management of community-acquired pneumonia in adults. Clin Infect Dis 2007;44 Suppl 2:S27–72.

41. Martinez JA, Horcajada JP, Almela M, Marco F, Soriano A, Garcia E, et al. Addition of a macrolide to a beta-lactam-based empirical antibiotic regimen is associated with lower in-hospital mortality for patients with bacteremic pneumococcal pneumonia. Clin Infect Dis 2003;36:389–395.

42. Baddour LM, Yu VL, Klugman KP, Feldman C, Ortqvist A, Rello J, et al. Combination antibiotic therapy lowers mortality among severely ill patients with pneumococcal bacteremia. Am J Respir Crit Care Med 2004;170:440–444.

43. Anglaret X, Chene G, Attia A, Toure S, Lafont S, Combe P, et al. Early chemoprophylaxis with trimethoprim-sulphamethoxazole for HIV-1-infected adults in Abidjan, Cote d'Ivoire: a randomised trial. Cotrimo-CI Study Group. Lancet 1999;353:1463–1468.

44. Wiktor SZ, Sassan-Morokro M, Grant AD, Abouya L, Karon JM, Maurice C, et al. Efficacy of trimethoprim-sulphamethoxazole prophylaxis to decrease morbidity and mortality in HIV-1-infected patients with tuberculosis in Abidjan, Cote d'Ivoire: a randomised controlled trial. Lancet 1999;353:1469–1475.

Chapter 13 HIV-1 AND THE NERVOUS SYSTEM: PAST, PRESENT, AND FUTURE

RICHARD W. PRICE

To array a man's will against his sickness
is the supreme art of medicine.

—HENRY WARD BEECHER

Introduction

The direct and indirect pathological effects of human immunodeficiency virus type 1 (HIV-1) infection on the nervous system are common, varied, and frequently associated with high morbidity and mortality.[1,2] They range from major central nervous system (CNS) opportunistic infections (OIs) to more fundamental consequences of HIV, and can affect all levels of the neuraxis.[3] Fortunately, as with other complications of HIV infection, the incidence and severity of these nervous system diseases have been markedly reduced by combination antiretroviral therapy (cART) (also referred to as highly active antiretroviral therapy [HAART]).[4,5]

The aim of this chapter is to provide a broad but succinct overview of these neurologic complications from an historical perspective, divided into three epochs: (1) the early years of disease recognition and symptomatic management, in which morbidity and mortality were little altered by medical intervention; (2) the current era of cART, with its potent prevention and treatment effects on all neurologic complications; and (3) the coming years, with their prospects for further refinements in prevention and therapy. I focus disproportionately on the CNS complications, and, more particularly, on the disease initially called the AIDS dementia complex (ADC)[6] and now more commonly referred to as HIV-associated dementia (HAD).[7] This is a unique aspect of HIV infection not explained simply by immunosuppression and opportunistic infection, but rather as a more essential interaction of HIV, the immune system, and the CNS. This focus relates in part to the author's interest, but also to the clinical importance and pathogenetic uniqueness of this condition. Additionally, its residual effects or its low-grade extension despite treatment may continue to affect patients. Furthermore, while I confine this discussion to the disease in adults—reflecting my own experience—the reader should be aware that these same conditions afflict children. Indeed, if anything, the childhood counterpart of ADC, commonly referred to as HIV encephalitis (HIVE), was even more common and often more devastating in children in the absence of treatment.[8,9]

TABLE 13–1	Major Neurologic Complications of Untreated HIV Infection in the U.S.		
	Anatomic Location	Diseases	
		Common	Uncommon/Rare
	Brain		
	Nonfocal	ADC (now HAD) CMV encephalitis Metabolic encephalopathies	Herpes simplex virus encephalitis
	Focal	Cerebral toxoplasmosis Primary CNS lymphoma (PCNSL) Progressive multifocal leukoencephalopathy (PML)	Tuberculous brain abscess/tuberculoma, cryptococcoma, varicella-zoster virus (VZV) encephalitis, aspergillosis
	Spinal Cord	Vacuolar myelopathy	VZV myelitis (complicating herpes zoster), spinal epidural lymphoma
	Meninges	Cryptococcal meningitis Aseptic meningitis (HIV)	Lymphomatous meningitis (metastatic), tuberculous meningitis
	Peripheral Nerves		
	Polyneuropathy	HIV-related distal sensory polyneuropathy (DSPN) Acute demyelinating polyneuropathy (Guillain-Barré)	
	Polyradiculopathy		CMV ascending polyradiculomyelopathy
	Focal or multifocal		CMV mononeuritis multiplex Early (benign) mononeuritis multiplex
	Muscle		Polymyositis, noninflammatory myopathies

The Early Years (1981–1995) of Recognition and Treatment of Complications

When AIDS was first recognized and the range of its clinical manifestations began to be categorized in the 1980s, it was clear that the nervous system was among its common targets. **Table 13–1** lists the neurologic disorders that emerged as most important, particularly in the setting of more advanced systemic infection. Major CNS diseases included a group of opportunistic infections, ADC, aseptic meningitis, peripheral neuropathies, and, less commonly, myopathies.

Opportunistic CNS Diseases

As with systemic complications, the CNS was subject to opportunistic diseases, and although the full spectrum of reported diseases was large, the list of *common* OIs was relatively small due to the circumscribed susceptibility conferred by the characteristic profile of altered T cell–

macrophage defenses in AIDS. Indeed, the high probabilities of this limited differential usually allowed accurate diagnosis following relatively simple algorithms.[10] Thus, in the presence of focal symptoms and signs a diagnosis of one of three major focal CNS conditions—cerebral toxoplasmosis, primary CNS lymphoma (PCNSL), or progressive multifocal leukoencephalopathy (PML)—was most likely in those with low blood CD4+ T cell counts. The first two of these were accompanied by mass effect and variable contrast enhancement, whereas in PML, these imaging characteristics were absent. Response to therapy (of toxoplasmosis) or cerebral biopsy (identifying PCNSL) was usually relied upon for more definitive diagnosis. PML was usually suspected by focal loss of white matter without mass effect or contrast enhancement; the definitive diagnosis was established by identification of the etiologic agent (JC virus) by PCR in CSF or by viral antigen or DNA detection in biopsied brain tissue.[11]

In this same way, *Cryptococcus neoformans* was by far the most common cause of meningitis complicating AIDS, presenting somewhat differently from infection in more immunocompetent individuals.[12] CMV encephalitis and ventriculitis were more subtle diseases, with less focal features and a more insidious presentation. Indeed, in the era when it was common, CMV encephalitis was often recognized because of its association with CMV retinitis.[13,14] Definitive diagnosis was by CSF PCR.[15,16]

These early AIDS years were accompanied by advances in diagnostics that helped refine the approach to disease management. Two conspicuous methodologies have already been cited in this regard, neuroimaging and nucleic acid hybridization. Neuroimaging technology, using computed tomography (CT) and, later, magnetic resonance imaging (MRI), evolved independently of HIV studies, but contributed enormously to refining diagnosis based on imaging features, including mass effect, tissue density, and contrast enhancement. In the case of nucleic acid diagnosis by PCR and related methods, it is likely that their early and day-to-day implementation in HIV infection accelerated their broader diagnostic use. As noted, CSF PCR analysis for JC virus and CMV are now the standard approach to PML and CMV encephalitis, while Epstein-Barr virus (EBV) PCR has been of value in PCNSL, although with less precision.[17]

In the early years of the epidemic, the main emphasis was on the treatment of these opportunistic conditions with specific therapies. Although this focus often resulted in reduced morbidity and delayed mortality, the persistent underlying immune compromise allowed such treatment to have only a limited overall impact, and CNS diseases carried a very poor prognosis, often resulting in death within a few months despite treatment.

Aseptic Meningitis and Early CNS Infection

Once HIV infection was identified, aseptic meningitis was reported as one of its common complications. Although aseptic meningitis was first described in association with headache and dementia, subsequent studies made it clear that mild CSF pleocytosis—usually with up to 20 cells/μL, but at times higher—is both common and characteristically asymptomatic.[18] This pleocytosis can be found throughout the full spectrum of HIV infection, although less frequently when blood CD4 counts fall below 50 cells/μL.

In fact, this CSF cell response proved to be an indicator of the early and almost ubiquitous invasion of the nervous system, or at least the meninges, by HIV.[18–20] While this may confound the diagnosis of neurosyphilis, it otherwise appears to be clinically benign and has not been shown to have prognostic significance. However, it remains uncertain whether this early asymptomatic invasion may be associated with subclinical, chronic brain injury. In fact, one of the overall mysteries of HIV neuropathogenesis relates to the question of how a virus that invades

TABLE 13–2	ADC Staging	
	ADC Stage	**Characteristics**
	Stage 0 (Normal)	Normal mental and motor function
	Stage 0.5 (Equivocal/subclinical)	Either minimal or equivocal *symptoms* of cognitive or motor dysfunction characteristic of ADC, or mild *signs* (snout response, slowed extremity movements), but *without impairment of work or capacity to perform activities of daily living (ADLs)*; gait and strength are normal
	Stage 1 (Mild)	Unequivocal evidence (symptoms, signs, neuropsychological test performance) of functional intellectual or motor impairment characteristic of ADC, but able to perform *all but the more demanding aspects of work or ADLs*; can walk without assistance
	Stage 2 (Moderate)	Cannot work or maintain the more demanding aspects of daily life, but able to perform *basic activities of self-care*; ambulatory, but may require a single prop
	Stage 3 (Severe)	*Major intellectual incapacity* (cannot follow news or personal events, cannot sustain complex conversation, considerable slowing of all output), *or motor disability* (cannot walk unassisted, requiring walker or personal support, usually with slowing and clumsiness of arms as well)
	Stage 4 (End stage)	Nearly vegetative; intellectual and social comprehension and responses are at a rudimentary level; nearly or absolutely mute; paraparetic or paraplegic, with double incontinence

the brain early, without apparent sequelae, can subsequently cause a more invasive disease, HIV encephalitis (HIVE), with devastating clinical consequences. Is it due to changes in the virus or alterations in the host that determines this switch from meningitis to encephalitis?

AIDS Dementia Complex (ADC)

Unlike the OIs, which had precedent as unusual conditions complicating other immunosuppressed states, ADC presented as a novel clinical-pathological entity and was noted early in a number of centers (albeit under different names.)[21,22] Although suspected by some to be a subacute encephalitis caused by CMV,[22] analysis of accumulating cases provided definition of a consistent constellation of symptoms and signs and distinct underlying pathology.[6,23] The discovery of HIV was followed by its clinical and pathologic association of ADC and HIVE.[24,25]

Clinical Features. While variable from case to case, ADC was noted to involve a cohesive pattern of dysfunction in three areas—cognition, motor performance, and behavior—which allowed definition of a core clinical phenotype.[6] Of these, cognitive and motor dysfunction were most helpful in characterizing patients and defining diagnosis. Patients with early or milder disease presented with a variable pattern of inattention, reduced concentration, slowing of processing, and difficulty changing mental sets, along with slowed movements, clumsiness, and ataxia. Behaviorally, they manifested apathy, dulled personality, and—in a subgroup—agitation and mania. With progression, patients went on to show a more global dementia and paraplegia with urinary and fecal incontinence. The final stage was one of mutism and quadriparesis. On the basis of these clinical features, ADC was classified as a "subcortical dementia."

In order to provide a vocabulary for describing the level of functional impairment, an empiric ADC staging system was also based on these features [26,27] (**Table 13–2**). This was derived from a review of the cognitive, motor, and behavioral features seen in patients encountered at Memorial Sloan-Kettering Cancer Center in the pretreatment era (Sidtis, Brew, and Price, unpublished) and has also been referred to as MSK staging. This staging only categorizes the level of dysfunction in activities of daily living, as obtained by the patient's history or as witnessed on direct examination, but does not directly incorporate diagnostic criteria; rather, it assumes an ADC diagnosis based on the clinical phenotype and setting. A research case definition that followed a similar vocabulary was introduced by a task force of the American Academy of Neurology. [28] Notably, this case definition and other diagnostic schemes have been imprecise regarding specific clinical features. More importantly, they do not incorporate any more objective laboratory criteria. For example, while neuroimaging is an essential component of evaluation, most often it is used to rule out other conditions rather than provide a definitive ADC diagnosis. Although cerebral atrophy and diffuse, "fluffy" or "ground glass" white matter abnormalities commonly accompany ADC and distinguish it from PML, these findings have not been sensitive and specific enough to be formally incorporated into diagnostic criteria. Likewise, routine CSF examination does not distinguish HIV encephalitis, since elevations in cell count and protein are often seen in patients without this disorder.[18] While CSF HIV RNA levels may be high, they also cannot be used to establish a certain diagnosis because of the nearly universal presence of HIV in the CSF in asymptomatic patients. Several inflammatory and neural biomarkers are characteristically altered in ADC, but none have yet seen broad clinical application.[29] Overall, the lack of diagnostic criteria related to either clinical phenotype or laboratory findings has remained a limitation in dealing with this disorder.

Neuropathology. Early descriptions noted that pathological changes were most prominent in subcortical structures and included: (1) Diffuse white matter pallor and associated gliosis, (2) multinucleated-cell encephalitis, and (3) vacuolar myelopathy.[30–33] Less common findings were diffuse or focal spongiform changes in the white matter and small areas of necrosis. The most common of these abnormalities was diffuse astrocytosis and white matter pallor that, in isolation, was associated with milder ADC. Inflammation was characteristically scant and consisted of a few perivascular lymphocytes and pigmented macrophages. Multinucleated cell encephalitis was a characteristic but not invariant finding. The term HIV encephalitis (HIVE) was supported by immunohistochemical and in situ hybridization studies showing that these multinucleated cells were infected by HIV.[34–36] However, infection of macrophages and microglia was not always accompanied by cell fusion; thus, the term HIVE can be applied more broadly.

Productive HIV infection was confined to cells of the monocyte-macrophage lineage, including microglia, and, therefore, these cells play a pivotal role in pathogenesis. Although astrocytes have also been reported to be infected, they characteristically do not produce progeny virus.[37] Subsequently, more detailed pathologic studies have elaborated on the cellular abnormalities, which include increased amyloid precursor protein (APP) staining of neurons and axons, dendritic and synaptic changes.[38] Vacuolar myelopathy was an overlapping but perhaps independent pathology that resembled subacute combined degeneration associated with vitamin B_{12} deficiency, and was clinically associated with spastic-ataxic gait. However, because the clinical findings in patients with vacuolar myelopathy merged with those exhibiting multinucleated-cell encephalitis, clinically these patients were included within the broader clinical term, ADC.[23,39]

Pathogenesis. The correlation of HIVE with ADC has led to the generally accepted concept that CNS HIV infection drives brain injury in this condition. However, because productive CNS HIV infection is supported in macrophages and related cells while the "functional elements" of the brain—particularly neurons—are not similarly infected, it seems that neuronal injury is the result of "indirect" processes. It appears that macrophages and related cells play a central role, both in supporting HIV replication and serving as key sources of virus- and cell-coded signals and toxins that lead to brain dysfunction. Research during the ensuing years has elaborated on these indirect injury pathways, but it remains uncertain which particular neurotoxic pathways are most important in human disease. Indeed, it is likely that multiple overlapping and interacting processes are involved.[40]

Peripheral Nervous System (PNS) and Muscle Diseases

Afflictions of peripheral nerves and muscle were also noted early in the epidemic.[22] Early reports characterized a subacute demyelination neuropathy clinically indistinguishable from Guillain-Barré syndrome in the general population,[41] except for the more frequent occurrence of pleocytosis (which might simply relate to the underlying HIV infection). Occasionally, this evolved to a more chronic form. These neuropathies were thought to have an autoimmune basis and provided early evidence that immunopathology could also be involved in HIV-related disease. These neuropathies were described mainly as complications of early systemic infection rather than of its late stage (AIDS). Their decline in the era of cART (below) now suggests that active HIV infection likely was an important component in their pathogenesis, perhaps by driving immune activation and autoimmunity as part of broader immune dysregulation.

Even more common was an axonal distal sensory peripheral neuropathy (DSPN) that may be related to HIV itself and a peripheral nervous system (PNS) pathogenetic analog of ADC/HIVE (although this has not been clearly established).[42-44] This was a distal, predominantly sensory, axonal neuropathy in which characteristically, sensory symptoms exceeded both sensory and motor dysfunction. While often mild, in some patients the sensory symptoms become severe, and painful paresthesias ("burning feet") were disabling.

CMV infection was associated with two types of neuropathy. One was an uncommon but severe and therapeutically important polyradiculopathy that was usually subacute in onset and associated with pain and sacral sensory loss, followed by ascending progression to flaccid paralysis.[45] The CSF revealed a characteristic pleocytosis, with polymorphonuclear cell predominance (nearly unique in HIV infection, except in rare bacterial meningitis). Early diagnosis and prompt institution of anti-CMV therapy can arrest progression and lead to clinical improvement. CMV was also associated with a mononeuritis multiplex, also developing in late HIV infection; this also had a severe course, leading to progressive weakness.[46] A second type of mononeuritis multiplex that followed a more benign course and was thought to relate to an immunopathological vasculitic process was reported to afflict patients in the earlier stages of HIV infection.

Several types of myopathy were also reported in HIV infection.[47,48] Classification and characterization of these conditions were imprecise, but both inflammatory and noninflammatory

myopathies were described. These ranged in severity from asymptomatic creatinine kinase elevation to severe proximal weakness. Improvement of patients with an inflammatory, polymyositis-
like illness was reported with corticosteroid therapy.

The Present (1996–2010): The Era of Combination Antiretroviral Therapy

Just as with systemic disease, combination antiretroviral therapy (cART) has had a profound
effect on all aspects of the neurologic complications of HIV infection. In the developed world,
where cART is widely available, the severe neurologic complications have markedly
decreased.[5,49] Indeed, these complications are now seen principally in population segments not
being treated, either because of difficulty adhering to treatment or outside of the umbrella of
medical care, including individuals with severe psychiatric disease, drug abusers, the homeless,
and those in socioeconomic settings isolated from therapeutic opportunity. Additionally, in cele-
brating this profound effect of antiretroviral therapy, it is important to remember that this is not
yet the case in many resource-poor parts of the world that continue to bear the brunt of the
expanding epidemic, including its effect on the nervous system.[50]

CNS Opportunistic Infections. The incidences of all of the CNS opportunistic infections discussed above have been reduced by cART.[5] Cerebral toxoplasmosis, PCNSL, cryptococcal meningitis, and CMV encephalitis are now all uncommon in patients on cART in the
developed world. This change in incidence has been well documented to have begun near 1996,
with the introduction of protease inhibitors and triple-combination drug therapy, and to have continued in the ensuing years as earlier and broader implementation of this therapy spread. PML,
which differs from the other major CNS OIs in developing at higher blood CD4+ T cell counts in
some patients, has probably been less affected, although it too has diminished.[11]

Not only is this incidence reduced, but the prognosis of the major OIs has also improved.
Specific therapies, as earlier, reduce neurologic deficits and delay the initial mortality, while antiretroviral therapy then sustains longer-term benefit by restoring host defenses against the opportunistic organisms. Of note, in the case of PML, for which no specific therapy yet exists, disease
remission follows institution of cART in about half of those cases that develop while patients are
off cART.[11]

ADC and Related Conditions. Combination treatment has had a similar impact on
ADC, and its incidence has decreased in parallel with that of the major OIs.[5] Individual case
examples have documented that treatment can halt progression and, in many cases, substantially
reverse the disease.[51–53] In fact, this response to therapy was clearly demonstrated in earlier case
reports and in a controlled clinical trial showing that the zidovudine monotherapy had a salutary
effect on this condition.[52] Despite the compartmentalized CNS infection underlying ADC/
HIVE[54] and the blood-brain barriers that restrict full entry of many drugs, it is largely prevented
by standard cART regimens and appears to respond therapeutically to these regimens.[55] While it
might seem advantageous to more clearly target this CNS infection in treating ADC, it has
proved difficult to assess either individual drugs or particular drug combinations in this setting.[56]
Nonetheless, there are arguments for including in the treatment regimens drugs that are known to
achieve therapeutic concentrations within the CNS. In the absence of clear evidence from

clinical trials, we generally recommend a potent combination regimen that includes at least two drugs that achieve such therapeutic levels.

With this marked success of prevention and therapy for more severe ADC, attention has now turned to milder CNS dysfunction, found in both untreated and treated patients, that can be detected using extensive psychological testing. These milder afflictions are integrated into the new HIV-associated neurocognitive disorder (HAND) nomenclature, which includes not only HAD, but defines criteria for symptomatic mild neurocognitive disorder (MND) and asymptom atic neurocognitive impairment (ANI).[1] These have been reported to have a relatively high prev alence.[57,58] Because these are lumped under the broad definition of HAND, at times this prevalence obscures the profound effect of cART on more severe disease. The issue of the patho-genetic basis and treatment strategies for this milder disease is discussed below.

CNS Immune Reconstitution Inflammatory Syndromes. A rare but notable compli-cation of antiretroviral therapy is the development of immune reconstitution inflammatory syn-drome (IRIS), complicating the treatment of CNS diseases.[59,60] This is perhaps the most clearly delineated in the case of progressive multifocal leukoencephalopathy (PML), in which inflam-mation, cerebral edema, and clinical deterioration may follow the institution of the cART. Indeed, institution of therapy can even precipitate the clinical presentation of PML, which is thought to be the result of unmasking of existing subclinical disease, although a provocative effect on JC virus has also been suggested.[11] This can also be an issue with cryptococcal menin-gitis[61,62] and individual cases have also been reported in which HIV encephalitis may also have provoked an IRIS response. This does not mean that antiretroviral therapy should not be started in these settings, but rather that these unusual adverse reactions should be monitored.

Neuropathies. The epidemiology of the peripheral neuropathies in the treatment era is less well established. However, it is likely that the incidence of Guillain-Barré syndrome is con-siderably reduced. In my own experience, this once common disease is now rare. The incidence and severity of DSPN in the treatment era is not yet clear. While certainly it persists as a problem in many treated patients, it is not yet clear how common it will prove to be in patients treated early in the course of infection. Initial reports are conflicting on this issue. The various myopa-thies reported early in the epidemic now seem rare, and likely are prevented by cART.

Non-AIDS Complications. The SMART study, which compared viral control to drug-sparing treatment regimens, established the importance of "non-AIDS" complications of HIV and the effect of therapy on reducing these complications.[63] This included cardiovascular dis-ease, although the number of strokes in this study was low. However, if one extends the general lesson of this trial to the CNS, it may suggest that cART for patients with between 350 and 500 CD4+ positive T cells/mL will have a salutary effect on preventing neurologic complications not traditionally associated with late HIV infection, particularly since other studies have shown that neuropsychological impairment in HIV-infected patients with higher CD4+ cell counts may associate with cardiovascular rather than "traditional" HIV-related risk factors.[64,65]

Antiviral Drug Neurotoxicities. Neurotoxicity has also been noted with several of the anti-HIV drugs. Myopathy related to zidovudine was, in fact, noted in the earlier era of mono-therapy, when doses were higher than those used in contemporary combination therapy. The "AZT-myopathy" was associated with proximal weakness, "ragged red fibers," and mitochon-drial abnormalities. It was largely reversible on dose reduction or discontinuation of the drug.[66,67] The deoxynucleosides d4T, ddI, and ddC also had toxic effects on mitochondrial DNA polymerase, but neurotoxicity manifested in an axonal polyneuropathy virtually indistinguishable from the HIV-related DSPN.[68,69] Efavirenz has CNS toxicity that includes vivid dreams, and although this may resolve after several weeks, in some patients it is dose-limiting.[70,71] The mechanism of this CNS toxicity is unknown.

More recently, at least one study has raised the question of whether cART more broadly might exert an adverse effect on cognitive performance in neuropsychological testing.[72] This remains a controversial finding and is under study.

The Future (2010–): Treatment Refinement and Prevention of Neurologic Morbidity

As one reflects on the extraordinary progress that has been made in reducing the neurologic morbidity and mortality of HIV infection, it seems evident that most of this progress has been achieved through advances in systemic therapy rather than as a result of more focused efforts to target the nervous system. The CNS OIs are, of course, exceptions. Morbidity associated with these infections has been reduced through advances in diagnostics and specific therapies, as discussed. Similarly, the characterizations of drug neurotoxicities have involved important neurologic contributions. However, even with the OIs, the great advance has been achieved by the advances in the development and use of potent cART, with its profound effect on systemic infection and immune preservation.

Future improvements will likely follow the same path. In the last few years, treatment has been improved by the introduction of simplified and less toxic regimens, resulting in better patient tolerance and adherence and reduced treatment failure. As these improvements unfold, it is reasonable to ask whether neurologic treatment requires special consideration, and, if so, what.

Dissemination of Treatment

As with other aspects of HIV disease, one of the most important tasks is now to more broadly implement these successful measures to affected populations. This, of course, includes the enormous number of infected individuals in resource-poor areas of the world that now bear the brunt of the continuing epidemic. However, even in the developed world, there remain populations that need to be brought under the therapeutic umbrella. These include people with limited access to treatment or with difficulty in adhering to treatment related to socioeconomic factors, substance abuse, psychiatric conditions, and the like. Since these are broad issues of healthcare delivery and not specific to neurologic diseases, I will not discuss them further, but only emphasize the great need in this area. Clearly, broader treatment delivery measures can greatly reduce the overall neurologic impact of HIV.

For those individuals out of reach of or who manage to slip through delivery systems and present with the late neurologic complications of HIV, the diagnostic and therapeutic methods of earlier times still hold, although they may be made more difficult for a number of reasons. First, as time has passed, many clinicians are now less familiar with the clinical presentations of these disorders and need to retrace the lessons of the past. Second, diagnosis may actually be more challenging now, even for the experienced clinician, because of the confounding background diseases and competing risks for neurologic diseases in those patients most likely to progress to AIDS. The odds of AIDS-related neurologic diagnoses may now be skewed away from the common disorders defined in the past. Therefore, the need continues for education and improving the precision of these diagnoses using contemporary tools.

Continuing CNS Morbidity Despite Treatment

As the major CNS opportunistic diseases and ADC have disappeared in well-treated patient populations, attention of the community of neuro-HIV investigators has now turned to the less severe causes of neurologic morbidity in HIV-infected patients—to the milder "neurocognitive impairments" embedded in two of the subcategories of HAND: asymptomatic neurocognitive impairment (ANI) and symptomatic minor neurocognitive disorder (MND).[7] As set out in the Frascati "consensus" definitions, these individuals are identified largely by performance on neuropsychological testing that is below established "norms," with the two designations separated by the absence or presence of symptoms (although the MND group also notes minor difficulty in daily living). Unlike ADC/HAD, these disorders do not have a consistent clinical phenotype beyond their testing failure in two or more cognitive domains, and both subcortical and cortical features have been reported[73]. In fact, this case definition is inclusive and may encompass individuals with HIV infection who suffer other causes of poor test performance. The diagnoses are independent of treatment, although as more and more patients are successfully treated and live longer, the greatest interest is in treated patients with this impairment and strategies to prevent or ameliorate this impaired performance.

Pathogenesis of Mild Neurocognitive Impairment. While inclusion of these milder disorders within the broad designation, HAND carries an implicit association with HAD and perhaps with CNS HIV infection. However, in addition to an undefined clinical phenotype, such disorders do not yet have a defined pathologic or pathogenetic basis. Indeed, even after eliminating the patients with non-HIV–related impaired performance, it is not yet clear that these diagnoses are a milder form of HAD/HIVE. Before considering the ways to ameliorate these milder disorders, it is thus reasonable to pose a number of fundamental questions, including:

1. What are the major causes of CNS injury in patients on treatment?
2. In that portion of patients in which CNS dysfunction is due to HIV, when did the injury occur?
3. If injury has continued on treatment, what are the mechanisms?

Causes of CNS Injury. There is likely to be a number of causes underlying the neuropsychological testing impairment in HIV-infected patients. Some of these will reflect the age susceptibilities of the normal population, others may relate to the risk behaviors of HIV (particularly drug abuse), and others may be more directly related to HIV infection. Importantly, some HIV-infected populations have a higher prevalence of smoking, hypertension, and other cardiovascular risk factors, accounting for impairment in some patients, as discussed above. Hepatitis C may also contribute to CNS injury or dysfunction, and, clearly, late stage hepatic failure can have an impact, as noted at autopsy in some series.[74] However, in some, the higher incidence or prevalence of impairment may indeed relate more directly to HIV infection. In these, the critical questions relate to when and how this injury occurs.

Timing of Injury. For the clinician caring for the patient with neurologic impairment, a critical questions is, When did the underlying injury occur? And, importantly, is it continuing at the time of evaluation? Hence, it is critical to know whether brain injury is *static* and due to past

70. van Luin M, Bannister WP, Mocroft A, et al. Absence of a relation between efavirenz plasma concentrations and toxicity-driven efavirenz discontinuations in the EuroSIDA study. Antivir Ther 2009;14(1):75–83.

71. Clifford DB, Evans S, Yang Y, et al. Impact of efavirenz on neuropsychological performance and symptoms in HIV-infected individuals. Ann Intern Med 2005 Nov 15;143(10):714–721.

72. Robertson KR, Su Z, Margolis DM, et al. Neurocognitive effects of treatment interruption in stable HIV-positive patients in an observational cohort. Neurology Apr 20;74(16):1260–1266.

73. Brew BJ. Evidence for a change in AIDS dementia complex in the era of highly active antiretroviral therapy and the possibility of new forms of AIDS dementia complex. AIDS 2004 Jan 1;18 Suppl 1:S75–78.

74. Everall I, Vaida F, Khanlou N, et al. Cliniconeuropathologic correlates of human immunodeficiency virus in the era of antiretroviral therapy. J Neurovirol 2009 Sep 8:1–11.

75. Price RW, Spudich S. Antiretroviral therapy and central nervous system HIV type 1 infection. J Infect Dis 2008 May 15;197 Suppl 3:S294–306.

76. Canestri A, Lescure FX, Jaureguiberry S, et al. Discordance between cerebral spinal fluid and plasma HIV replication in patients with neurological symptoms who are receiving suppressive antiretroviral therapy. Clin Infect Dis Mar 1;50(5):773–778.

Chapter 14 OPHTHALMIC MANIFESTATIONS OF HIV/AIDS

JYOTIRMAY BISWAS AND S. SUDHARSHAN

My lovers and my friends stand aloof from my sore;
and my kinsmen stand after off
My heart panteth, my strength faileth me;
as for the light of mine eyes, it is also gone from me.

—PSALM 38:10–16

This quote from Bible is, in fact, more appropriate now for patients with HIV/AIDS, who can have devastating and permanently crippling ocular manifestations of their disease.

Introduction

Since the report of an unusual occurrence of *Pneumocystis carinii* pneumonia in five cases on June 5, 1981 by Gottlieb and colleagues[1] (Pneumocystis pneumonia—Los Angeles), which was probably the first publication on this infection, a great body of literature has accumulated regarding this devastating disease. In the 30 years since the appearance of that article, the human immunodeficiency virus (HIV), the causative agent of acquired immune deficiency syndrome (AIDS), has been identified and has reached virtually every corner of the globe, emerging as the most challenging pandemic of our time. It appears to be omnipresent, with the manifestations sparing no organ.

Among HIV-positive individuals, the lifetime cumulative risk for developing at least one abnormal ocular lesion ranges from 52% to 100% in various studies.[2] Such lesions are varied and affect almost any structure of the eye. Ocular lesions usually occur in the late phase of HIV infection, but can also be the presenting manifestation of the disease.

Various ocular manifestations—including cytomegalovirus (CMV) retinitis, toxoplasma retinochoroiditis, and ocular tuberculosis—are considered to be AIDS-defining conditions.

CD4 T cell counts determine the immune status of a patient with HIV infection, and various case studies published since 1982 demonstrate that a definite pattern of ocular complications is associated with each level of CD4 cell counts (**Table 14–1**).

Although there are no confirmed reports of transmission of the infection through ocular fluids such as tears,[3] it is very important to understand that transmission can occur through corneal transplantation[4] or contact with other intraocular fluids such as aqueous or vitreous fluids.[5]

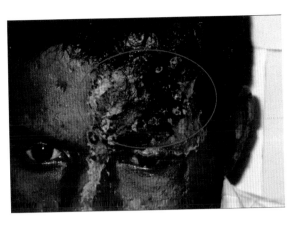

Figure 14–1. *External photograph showing herpes zoster ophthalmicus.*

Herpes zoster eventually occurs in 10% to 20% of all individuals, and reactivation in the ophthalmic division of the trigeminal nerve gives rise to HZO. The infection is characterized by typical clinical features such as a vesiculobullous rash over the distribution of the ophthalmic branch of the trigeminal nerve (**Figure 14–1**). It may be associated with dendritiform and stromal keratitis, conjunctivitis, blepharitis, uveitis (with secondary glaucoma), hemorrhagic hypopyon,[18] scleritis, retinitis,[19] or encephalitis. Tissue damage can be mediated through a necrotizing vasculitis.

The incidence of HZO is greater in HIV-infected patients than in noninfected, age-adjusted populations. Approximately 5% to 15% of HIV-positive patients are coinfected with herpes zoster, but only half of these individuals are at risk for ocular involvement (which can be an initial manifestation of HIV infection). Hodge and associates[2] found that HIV-infected individuals had a relative incident risk ratio for HZO of 6.6:1 when compared to individuals who are HIV-negative.

In immunosuppressed individuals, herpes zoster is more likely to be severe and prolonged, and may be systemic. Viremia may result in visceral or neurologic infection, leading to increased morbidity and mortality. The occurrence of HZO in an apparently healthy, young individual suggests that the patient may be immunosuppressed, and HIV should be ruled out.

The diagnosis of HZO is made on the basis of clinical features. Confirmation of a clinical diagnosis is available from a variety of laboratory tests, including viral cultures, Tzanck smears, polymerase chain reaction (PCR) techniques for VZV DNA, fluorescent antibody testing, and antigen detection by direct immunofluoresence.

In immunocompetent hosts, the virus has not been recovered by culture beyond the first 48 hours of the disease. VZV DNA has been detected on the ocular surface for as long as 34 days after the onset of rash and in excised corneal buttons obtained during penetrating keratoplasty up to 8 years after active disease.[20]

Treatment of HZO with in patients with HIV infection must be aggressive, with systemic acyclovir administered for 3 to 6 weeks followed by a prolonged course of maintenance therapy to prevent recurrence. Early initiation of systemic antiviral therapy can reduce the duration of skin lesions and ocular complications by about 50%. The most appropriate duration of treatment for HZO has not been determined for the general population, although the virus has been recovered from skin lesions up to 14 days after the onset of infection. In resistant cases, famciclovir can be used as well, 500 mg three times daily. In cases of resistance to thymidine kinase-dependent acyclovir or famciclovir, IV foscarnet may be used.[21]

A recent study[22] showed that in HIV-positive patients, infection with herpes zoster is more severe, of longer duration, and is associated with a higher rate of complications, increased need

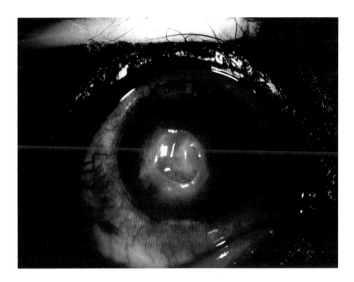

Figure 14–2. *Slit-lamp photograph showing viral keratitis in a patient with HIV.*

for hospitalization, and higher rates of recurrence than in HIV-negative patients. Although postherpetic neuralgia is a very frequent complication for both HIV-positive and -negative individuals, its duration is longer in those with HIV/AIDS. There was no significant difference in the severity, duration, or complications of the disease among male and female patients. To monitor for retinal infection, HIV-infected individuals with HZO should have regular fundus evaluation until skin vesicles are completely resolved.

There has also been a reported increase in the incidence of herpes zoster in patients with AIDS immediately after therapy with protease inhibitors. Martinez and colleagues[23] noted that the risk of zoster was independent of age, sex, type of protease inhibitor, and CD4 T cell counts and viral loads at baseline and 1 month. However, a significant increase in CD8 lymphocyte proportion at 1 month was independently associated with the risk for herpes zoster; this finding may help identify persons at risk so that prophylactic antiviral therapy can be instituted.

In our series of patients on HAART seen in the last 5 years, 18 patients had HZO; in 12 of these patients, the CD4 counts were >200 cells/mm^3 (unpublished data) and in 2 patients, the counts were between 150 and 200 cells/mm^3. HZO seems to occur with improvement in immune status in patients on HAART. In a previous study reported from our institute in the pre-HAART era, there was only one patient with HZO out of a series of 100 patients.[10]

Some patients develop severe debilitating pain and may need treatment with amitriptyline, opioids, or the more recently available gabapentin.[17]

Viral keratitis. Although CMV can cause infectious keratitis, VZV and herpes simplex virus (HSV) are the most common etiologic agents. HSV-1 is more common, but documented cases of HSV-2 ocular infection have also been reported.[24] Herpetic keratitis can cause painful and often recurrent corneal ulcerations, with varied manifestations. The characteristic presentation is the branching or dendritic pattern. Other presentations include epithelial keratitis with follicular conjunctivitis, vesicular eyelid lesions, stromal **(Figure 14–2),** and interstitial keratitis. HSV keratitis is usually associated with corneal scarring, iritis, and raised intraocular pressure and is known to recur frequently.

VZV keratitis may also be seen in 65% of individuals with HZO, and dendritiform lesions occur in up to 51% cases.[12] Among those with corneal involvement, neurotrophic keratitis occurs in 25% and, rarely, superadded bacterial infection can occur. Both epithelial and stromal disease have been described in the absence of skin lesions, a condition known as herpetic zoster sine herpete.[24,25]

HIV-infected patients with HZO are more likely to experience corneal involvement than their non-infected counterparts (89% vs. 65%), and the incidence of corneal perforation is also higher.[3] Individuals with AIDS can develop a chronic pleomorphic VZV infection of the corneal epithelium which tend to be more delicate and lacy in appearance than the discrete dendrites of HSV epithelial keratitis.[26] Peripheral ulcerative keratitis can occur in HIV-infected patients with HZO. Larger and more peripheral punctate corneal dendritic lesions are also seen, and the bulb-tipped branching pattern seen on slit-lamp examination is pathognomonic and is clinically confirmatory. Corneal stromal involvement is infrequent in individuals with AIDS or other immunosuppressed states, possibly as a result of protection due to T-lymphocyte dysfunction.

Young and associates[27] emphasized atypical clinical features of HSV keratitis, such as marginal lesions, a relative resistance to treatment, and more frequent and lengthier recurrences.[28] Overall recurrence rates are higher and, after the first episode, a site of chronic latent infection is established in the cornea. HIV-associated immunosuppression impairs those mechanisms that are normally responsible for containing such an infection in the cornea.[29]

The diagnosis of HSV infection is primarily clinical; laboratory studies (such as viral culture, direct fluorescent antibody tests for HSV antigens, and PCR techniques for HSV DNA) are rarely needed to confirm the diagnosis. Most commonly, treatment is with topical agents, such as acyclovir eye ointment five times daily or vidarabine 3% ointment five times daily, and cycloplegics. Debridement of the ulcer using a cotton-tipped applicator may increase the healing rate. Due to the increased recurrence rates of HSV keratitis in the HIV-infected population, long-term suppressive oral acyclovir therapy may benefit those with a history of HSV eye disease.

Famciclovir, 125 to 500 mg three times daily, or foscarnet are alternatives in resistant cases. Bodaghi et al[30] described the case of a young HIV-positive woman with chronic keratitis resistant to acyclovir. Conventional virologic methods remained inconclusive and in situ hybridization and PCR rapidly confirmed the diagnosis of HSV-1 keratitis. The thymidine kinase gene sequence revealed the presence of five variations, and the investigators postulated that this gene may be associated with acyclovir resistance.

VZV-mediated stromal keratitis is reported to be T-cell–mediated.[31] HAART with a protease inhibitor may potentially double the incidence of herpes zoster and related ocular involvement in patients with AIDS, although treatment with nucleoside analogue reverse transcriptase inhibitors does not pose the same risk. Thus, the risk of recurrence of stromal keratitis is increased in HIV-infected individuals as part of the immune recovery inflammatory syndrome (IRIS).

Cytomegalovirus keratitis. Cytomegalovirus (CMV) retinitis is the most common AIDS-related opportunistic eye infection, but rarely involves the anterior-segment tissues. CMV infection of the iris has been reported in a patient with CMV retinitis.[32]

CMV has been reported to be associated with both epithelial and/or stromal keratitis, although both conditions are uncommon. Asymptomatic corneal endothelial deposits, appearing as linear or stellate lesions forming a reticular pattern,[33] have been described in about 80% of eyes affected by CMV retinitis.[34] For immunocompromised patients of any age, restoring immunity prevents herpesvirus disease, as is seen in the cases of CMV in AIDS patients on HAART.

Molluscum contagiosum. Molluscum contagiosum, is a highly contagious infection caused by a large DNA poxvirus. It is typically seen in children and young adults, but also affects

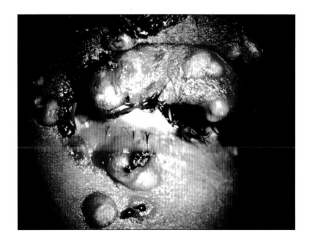

Figure 14–3. *External photograph showing multiple molluscum contagiosum lesions.*

up to 5% of HIV-infected patients. The face, trunk, and genitalia are commonly affected. In HIV-infected patients, distribution in the chin-strap region is common.

In immunocompetent patients, molluscum contagiosum is typically self-limiting, although treatment may be considered to hasten resolution of the lesions. In HIV-positive individuals, such lesions can occur on the eyelid and conjunctiva and are characteristically larger in number and size, often confluent, bilateral, and resistant to therapy (**Figure 14–3**). To avoid missing the diagnosis, clinicians should carefully examine the lash line in all HIV-positive patients wtih chronic conjunctivitis.

Molluscum contagiosum lesions of the eyelid have even been reported as the initial clinical manifestation of HIV disease.[35,36] It is characterized by pink or pearly-white, wartlike nodules on the skin. Sections of the lesions show large (20- to 30-μ) eosinophilic hyaline inclusion bodies which displace the nuclei to the margin. These bodies are composed of large numbers of virus particles embedded in a protein matrix. Rarely, conjunctival involvement in patients with AIDS can also result in nodular pink lesions.

Treatment options include topical application of phenol and trichloroacetic acid or serial applications of liquid nitrogen. Incision with or without curettage, excision, and cryotherapy are equally effective. Lesions may recur within 6 to 8 weeks, corresponding to the incubation period of the virus. In HIV-infected patients, administration of HAART with restoration of immunity leads to complete resolution of disseminated molluscum contagiosum and limitation of the infection.

Although HIV-infected individuals can experience an aggressive form of the infection, a severe inflammatory reaction is not seen, even in those patients with coexistent conjunctivitis. Paradoxically, the phenomenon of IRIS after treatment with HAART can also cause new presentations of molluscum contagiosum in patients without a history of the disease.[37] Severe conjunctival inflammation may be noted until the lesions regress. Although immune reconstitution does not prevent recurrence of molluscum contagiosum, when new lesions do develop, the manifestations are less severe and are similar to those seen in immunocompetent individuals.

Bacterial Diseases

Bacterial keratitis. Several studies comparing ocular flora in immunocompromised and immunocompetent individuals have yielded varied results.[12] Ocular flora in HIV-infected individuals is not very different from that in the general population, but the risk of infection with this "normal" flora may be greater for severely immunosuppressed individuals. *Staphylococcus aureus, Staphylococcus epidermidis,* and *Pseudomonas aeruginosa* are most frequently implicated.[38] *Klebsiella oxytoca, Streptococcus, Bacillus, Micrococcus, Capnocytophaga,* and *Acanthamoeba* species have also been shown to cause disease, with some cases of recalcitrant infection requiring keratoplasty and even evisceration of the globe.[39-41] HIV-infected hosts may be predisposed toward these spontaneous bacterial keratitides because of pre-existing keratoconjunctivitis sicca (KCS) and viral keratitis, which create corneal epithelial erosions and facilitate subsequent bacterial entry. Unlike the clinical presentation in the general population, bacterial keratitis in immunosuppressed individuals is usually bilateral, involves multiple pathogens, and carries a higher risk for perforation. There have been reports of eventual enucleation despite intensive appropriate antibiotic therapy for more than 2 weeks.[14] A low incidence of inflammation in immunosuppressed patients also contributes to a delay in diagnosis and treatment.

Neisseria gonorrheae infection can be unilateral or bilateral and is usually transmitted to the eye by accidental autoinoculation. Such infections cause membranous or pseudomembranous conjunctivitis with ulceration, scarring, and perforation, as the organism can penetrate even normal corneal epithelium. HIV infection can modify the typical host response to gonococci, resulting in more severe ocular signs and symptoms. Gram-staining and culture help in the identification of the etiologic agent. Topical therapy alone is ineffective; systemic treatment with ceftriaxone or other appropriate antibiotics is required.

Protozoal Disease[12-14, 42]

AIDS-associated microsporidial keratoconjunctivitis is characterized by a bilateral, superficial punctate epithelial keratitis, white intraepithelial infiltrates (**Figure 14–4**), mild anterior chamber reactions, and conjunctivitis in the form of mild conjunctival follicular hypertrophy. Patients may complain of photophobia and grittiness. Vision loss is secondary to keratitis.

Diagnosis is by Gram or Giemsa stain, and spores from conjunctival scrapings or corneal biopsies can be easily seen with Masson trichrome or Giemsa stain. Immunofluorescence and electron microscopy can help confirm the diagnosis.[3] Ocular microsporidiasis should be suspected in all HIV-positive patients with persistently negative cultures for epithelial keratitis. Although HAART has been shown to alleviate and resolve microsporidial keratoconjunctivitis in

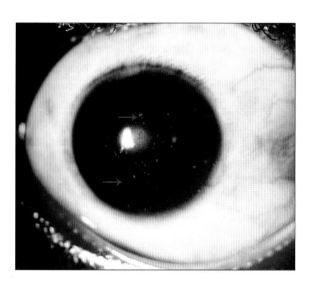

Figure 14–4. *Slit lamp photograph showing multiple corneal lesions due to microsporidiasis.*

HIV-positive hosts, postimmune recovery-mediated microsporidial keratoconjunctivitis reactivation has also been reported.[43]

Fumagillin eye drops, 70 mg/mL, should be used indefinitely in HIV-positive individuals. Oral albendazole, 400 mg twice daily, should be used as an adjunct for the management of systemic infection. Other protozoa, such as toxoplasma, can also rarely cause a granulomatous type of anterior uveitis.

Mycobacterial Disease

Mycobacterium tuberculosis is the most common systemic opportunistic infection associated with AIDS even though ocular TB is not as common.[44] It is important to consider it as a differential diagnosis, especially in developing nations like India. Mycobacterium can cause varied manifestations in the eye and can be vision threatening.

M. avium was reported to be the cause of endophthalmitis[45] with an intense inflammatory reaction and hypopyon in an individual with AIDS who had a history of disseminated *M. avium* infection. Prominent iris nodules caused by *M. avium complex* (MAC) has also been observed as the initial manifestation of panophthalmitis in an individual with AIDS.[45]

Clinical manifestations include ulcers, tubercles, granular masses, and pedunculated polypoid tumors. Patients may present with a localized nodule in the eyelid, simulating chalazion. Orbital and lacrimal gland involvement by *M. tuberculosis* leads to localized granuloma,[46] although, unusually, they can present as a conjunctival mass.[44,47] TB also may cause interstitial keratitis with stromal infiltration. Interstitial keratitis secondary to TB may be associated with uveitis and/or scleritis.

Tuberculous conjunctivitis is a very rare condition in the developed world and may require the identification of *M. tuberculosis* organisms in conjunctival biopsy specimens, either through microscopic detection of acid-fast bacilli or through more sensitive culture techniques. Keratoconjunctivitis may occur in association with cutaneous TB.[48] While intraocular disease is mostly a secondary infection, cutaneous TB is almost always primary.[49]

Tuberculosis can present as a granulomatous type of anterior uveitis, even in HIV-infected individuals and the inflammatory reaction correlates with the level of CD4 cell counts. Infection of the iris can present either with or without iris nodules.

Appropriate systemic anti-tuberculous therapy (ATT) is the primary treatment. Specific ocular treatment should be instituted along with ATT. There have been reports of scleral TB responding favorably to additional streptomycin sulfate topical (every 2 hours) and subconjunctival (every 3 days), along with ATT.[9] In individuals with HIV infection, therapy may require longer duration and additional drugs.

Fungal Infections

In the general population, fungal corneal ulcers are rare in the absence of preceding trauma, ocular surface disease, or corticosteroid therapy, but individuals with HIV/AIDS can develop spontaneous fungal infections. *Candida* and cryptococci are the most common organisms. *Candida* causes anterior segment keratitis; cryptococci commonly trigger posterior-segment pathology, although they can sometimes cause conjunctivitis, limbal infection, and iris granulomas.[50] *Cryptococcus albidus,* causing scleral ulceration, has been reported.[51] *Histoplasma* and *Pneumocystis* can also cause anterior-segment manifestations, but are not as commonly reported in India. Fungal keratitides have a more acute and protracted course in the HIV/AIDS population, and are more likely to result in bilateral disease with corneal perforation. Hence, culture or biopsy of lesions is important for HIV-infected patients with ocular surface infections, to differentiate between bacterial and fungal etiology.

Spirochaetal Infections

Ocular syphilis caused by *Treponema pallidum* tends to present with more aggressive, severe, and relapsing manifestations in HIV-positive hosts than in immunocompetent hosts.[52–54]

Anterior-segment manifestations of syphilis include chancres of the conjunctiva (primary syphilis), conjunctivitis (secondary syphilis), and gummata (late syphilis). Conjunctivitis can be granulomatous and histologically similar to sarcoidosis.

T. pallidum is the most common bacterial cause of uveitis in HIV-positive hosts, with an incidence of 0.6%. It tends to be more severe and consists of panuveitis in conjunction with anterior uveitis.[53,54] Eighty-five percent of HIV-positive patients with ophthalmic syphilis have coexisting neurosyphilis, and so all patients must undergo CSF analysis to rule out neurosyphilis when syphilitic uveitis is first diagnosed.[55] The diagnosis of syphilis involves a good clinical history in addition to serologic screening and confirmatory tests (such as the rapid plasma reagin or fluorescent treponemal antibody absorbent tests, respectively). Direct examination using dark-field microscopy or biopsy of suspicious lesions can be performed if results are uncertain. Isolated episcleritis and scleritis are uncommon during any stage of the disease, but when present, are usually features of secondary or late syphilis.[56]

Treatment of ocular syphilis is similar to that of neurosyphilis. The most effective treatment involves high-dose IV penicillin G, 12 to 24 million units/day for 14 days. Because of the high rate of relapse, HIV-positive patients should have extensive follow-up for at least 2 years.

Other Adnexal Infectious Lesions[12–14]

Preseptal cellulitis. *Staphylococcus aureus* is the most common cause of cutaneous and systemic bacterial infection in HIV-positive patients. It is found in the nasal mucosa in more than twice the number of HIV patients when compared to normal individuals. Treatment is similar to that in immunocompetent individuals.

Eyelid abscess. Infections of the eyelid and conjunctiva are rare in patients with AIDS. Dermal abscesses due to *staphylococci*, acid-fast bacilli, and CMV have been reported in molluscum lesions in patients with AIDS indicating the tendency of such lesions to acquire secondary infection.[35,36] Diagnosis is by smear and culture. Topical and systemic antibiotics are indicated for treatment.

Bacillary angiomatosis. Bacillary angiomatosis (BA)[57] is the vascular proliferative form of infection with *Bartonella* organisms. Bacillary angiomatosis was first described in 1983 and, subsequently, has been described in patients following organ transplantation and in other immunocompromised persons. Patients with HIV disease are at increased risk for developing BA when their CD4 T cell count is ≤200 cells/mm^3. BA can mimic the more lethal KS, so it is important to differentiate this entity from KS.

Other Manifestations

Keratoconjunctivitis sicca (KCS).[12–14,58] Dry eye occurs in 20%–38.8% of HIV-positive hosts in the later stages of AIDS.[3] It is thought to be due to lymphocytic infiltration of the lacrimal gland. Afflicted individuals are more susceptible to bacterial keratitis, and abnormalities in the composition of the tear film are typically present. Etiology is multifactorial and is due to the combined effects of HIV-mediated inflammatory destruction of primary and accessory lacrimal glands and to direct conjunctival damage due to the HIV itself. The virus is also postulated to play a role in spontaneous corneal thinning and perforation observed in some infected patients. Contrary to its effect on many other ocular HIV/AIDS-related diseases, HAART has not significantly reduced the prevalence of KCS. Management options include the use of artificial tears and long-acting lubricants, and, in severe cases, punctal occlusion.

Conjunctivitis. Nonspecific, culture-negative conjunctivitis has been reported in less than 1% of patients with HIV. Rarely, cytomegalovirus or cryptococcus can be the causative organism. Gram-stain and culture are required before conjunctivitis is labeled as noninfective. In nonresponsive cases, biopsy is indicated.

Trichomegaly. Acquired trichomegaly or hypertrichosis have been described, especially in the late stages of HIV infection. The exact cause is not known, although drug toxicity[58] or elevated viral loads have been suggested to play a role. Treatment is indicated if the condition is annoying or if cosmetically unacceptable.

Conjunctival microvasculopathy. Seventy to eighty percent of patients have some form of asymptomatic conjunctival microvascular changes. These include segmental vascular dilatation and narrowing, microaneurysm formation, and comma-shaped vascular and visible granularity to the flowing blood column (sludging). These are seen more commonly near the inferior limbus and have a good correlation with the occurrence of retinal microvasculopathy. The exact cause is not known, but this condition has been postulated to be due to increased plasma viscosity, endothelitis, or immune complex deposition. No treatment is required.

Anterior uveitis. Symptomatic anterior uveitis is rare in HIV-positive patients.[60] Uveitis associated with CMV retinitis is seen rarely. More severe anterior chamber inflammation may be seen with toxoplasmic or syphilitic retinochoroiditis/panuveitis, or, rarely, in other infectious retinitis such as acute retinal necrosis.

HIV itself has been isolated from tears, vitreous and aqueous humor, and from the conjunctiva, cornea, iris, sclera, and retina, and occasionally has been suspected as a cause of intraocular inflammation in the absence of other pathogens.

Diagnosis requires slit-lamp examination, and therapy is primarily directed at identifying an infectious etiology. Topical steroids are often employed but must be used with caution and in combination with appropriate antimicrobial therapy.

Angle-closure glaucoma.[12–14] Acute angle-closure glaucoma has been described in association with uveal effusion syndrome[61] in patients infected with HIV. The cause of angle-closure glaucoma is not known. Intraocular inflammation is usually minimal, but can be severe in cases of primary choroidal inflammation with secondary exudative retinal detachment. B-scan ultrasonography and ultrasound biomicroscopy (UBM) helps in confirming the diagnosis.

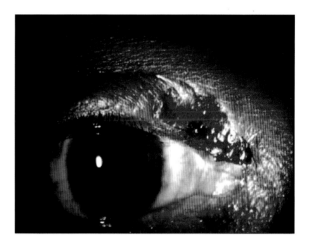

Figure 14–5. *External photograph showing squamous blepharitis.*

Treatment includes cycloplegics, corticosteroids, aqueous suppressants, hyperosmolar agents, and surgical drainage of suprachoroidal fluid.

Atopic dermatitis and blepharitis. Atopic dermatitis can be the first ocular manifestation of HIV infection in some individuals. Blepharitis is more serious in HIV-infected individuals and its presentation with an eyelid ulcer has been reported as an initial manifestation of HIV disease[92] (**Figure 14–5**). New-onset chronic, relapsing episodes of blepharitis, which begin months to years after initiation of indinavir therapy, have also been reported. These patients present with retinoid effects such as desquamative or erosive cheilitis, mucocutaneous xerosis, alopecia, asteatotic eczema, paronychia, and ingrown nails.

Posterior-Segment Lesions

Posterior-segment lesions can lead to severe ocular morbidity. Cytomegalovirus retinitis is still the most common ocular opportunistic infection in patients with HIV and, if left untreated, can lead to irreversible blindness. CMV retinitis usually occurs when the CD4 counts are low but can also be seen at higher counts.

HIV Retinopathy: Systemic Significance
• HIV vasculopathy is an indication of an ischemic process
• HIV can cause endothelitis. Patients with significant HIV retinopathy changes may have associated significant endothelitis of the vasculature of other organs such as the brain and can lead to life-threatening, multiple cerebral infarcts
• Such patients need to be treated with additional anticoagulants/vasodilators

HIV-Related Microangiopathy of the Retina

This is the most common ocular finding in patients with AIDS, occurring in about 50% to 70% of cases.[62] It is characterized by retinal hemorrhages, microaneurysms, and cotton wool spots **(Figure 14–6)**, usually distributed along the vascular arcades. These are probably the result of both an underlying microvasculopathy and hematologic abnormalities such as increased leukocyte activation and rigidity. These findings generally regress spontaneously in 6 to 9 weeks.

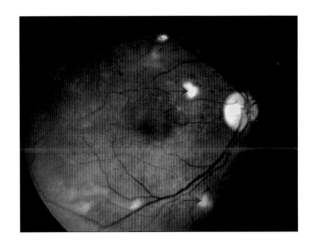

Figure 14–6. *Color fundus photograph showing multiple cotton wool spots in a patient with HIV retinopathy.*

The white and fluffy appearance of a cotton wool spot is caused by a circulatory disturbance in a tiny area of the retina. The condition may mimic diabetic and hypertensive retinopathy. However, the hard exudates typically observed in diabetic retinopathy are not seen in HIV retinopathy. Cotton wool spots in hypertensive retinopathy have associated vascular changes such as arteriolar narrowing, which is not present in HIV retinopathy. Periodic fundus examinations are mandatory to differentiate this condition from early CMV retinitis.

Opportunistic Infections of the Posterior Segment[62]

Cytomegalovirus retinitis.[38,62–64] Cytomegalovirus is the most common infectious agent affecting the retina, the optic nerve, or both in patients with AIDS and is seen in 15% to 40% of these patients.[38,65] CMV retinitis is usually seen when the CD4 count is <50 cells /mm^3. If the infection does not involve the posterior pole, patients may be asymptomatic or may present with diminished vision. Although vitritis occurs only occasionally, floaters could be an early warning sign of vitritis. Well established CMV retinitis is easily recognized as a full-thickness retinal opacification associated with hard exudates and hemorrhages, which are often perivascular in distribution. This appearance is sometimes described as "cottage cheese with tomato ketchup" or "pizza pie" (**Figure 14–7**). There may be a yellow-white margin of slowly advancing retinitis at the border of an atrophic retina (brushfire pattern), and a granular pattern, which is seen in the periphery as focal white granular lesions without associated hemorrhage. In 6% of cases, CMV retinitis can have a frosted branch appearance (**Figure 14–8**). Vitritis is typically absent or minimal. Retinal detachment is seen in the healed stage in 30% of cases (**Figure 14–9**). Prior to the HAART era, CMV retinitis was known to occur in 15% to 40% of patients with AIDS, and the median elapsed time between the diagnosis of AIDS and development of CMV retinitis was about 9 months. However, more recent studies have shown that this infection can occur as long as 3 to 5 years after the diagnosis of AIDS and usually develops when CD4 cell counts are <50 cells/mm^3.

Prior to the introduction of HAART, the median survival time following the diagnosis of CMV retinitis was 6 weeks in patients receiving no treatment. Anti-CMV treatment increased the survival time to 10 months in patients who responded partially to therapy. In the era of HAART, CMV retinitis is associated with a substantial risk of incident vision loss. Those with HAART-induced immune recovery have been found to be at an approximately 50% lower risk for visual acuity loss. Studies have shown that the presence of immune recovery uveitis at baseline attenuated the protective effect of immune recovery for moderate vision loss, but not for blindness.

Patterns of Posterior Segment Infections
• Retinitis is more common than choroiditis
• CD4 counts are helpful in making the diagnosis
• Low CD4 counts are seen in CMV retinitis and progressive outer retinal necrosis
• Retinitis in inflamed eyes is associated with high CD4 counts

CMV Retinitis: Systemic Significance
• Very early CMV retinitis lesions resemble cotton wool spots
• CMV can cause esophagitis, which can be confirmed endoscopically by esophageal biopsy
• Any patient with complaints of dysphagia with CMV retinitis can be presumed to also have CMV-related systemic infection

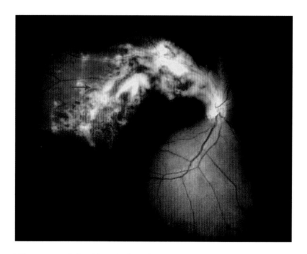

Figure 14–7. *Color fundus photograph showing the typical "pizza pie" appearance in a patient with active CMV retinitis.*

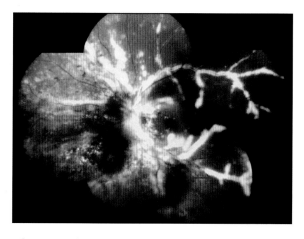

Figure 14–8. *Color fundus photograph showing "frosted branch" appearance in a patient with CMV retinitis.*

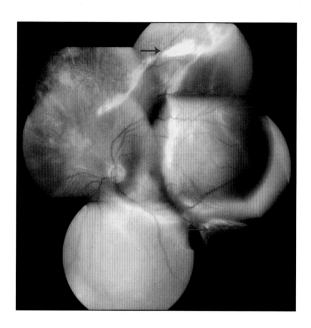

Figure 14–9. *Montage color fundus photograph showing retinal detachment due to a complication of CMV retinitis in a patient with HIV.*

Currently 5 medications are approved for treatment of CMV retinitis in USA. These are ganciclovir, foscarnet, cidofovir, fomiversen, and valganciclovir. CMV retinitis is an ocular manifestation of a systemic CMV infection and needs to be treated with systemic anti CMV medication. Recent studies have also shown the beneficial effect of anti CMV therapy in the reduction of overall mortality in these patients.

Ganciclovir, a nucleoside analogue that acts as a competitive inhibitor and faulty substrate for CMV DNA polymerase, is the most common drug used. Activation of ganciclovir requires monophosphorylation by the CMV enzyme, protein kinase. Ganciclovir is virustatic, and thus, viral replication will resume when the drug is removed. Ganciclovir has been shown to be initially effective in 90% to 100% of cases of newly diagnosed retinitis. A clinical effect is apparent in 2 to 3 weeks, and an inactive border is achieved in 3 to 6 weeks. Without maintenance treatment, the disease will relapse, usually within 3 weeks of cessation of induction treatment. Resistance to the drug is very common after prolonged use.

Ganciclovir may be given via three modes of administration: intravenous, oral, or intravitreal, in the form of injection or implant. The treatment of choice is intravenous ganciclovir, administered at a dosage of 5–7 mg/kg/day in 2 divided doses for 2 weeks of induction therapy, followed by a once-daily maintenance dose, which is continued until the lesions are completely resolved and the patient's immune status is improved.

Oral valganciclovir[66] is the valine ester of ganciclovir and is rapidly converted to ganciclovir in the intestinal wall. Oral valganciclovir, 900 mg twice daily as induction therapy followed by and 900 mg once daily as a maintenance dose, has the additional advantage of being a nonparenteral mode of treatment and avoiding complications related to indwelling catheters, especially in immunocompromised individuals. Appropriate management of underlying systemic disease promotes early resolution of ocular lesions.

Intravitreal injections of either ganciclovir or foscarnet may be considered, especially in cases where the macula is threatened; this mode of administration delivers the greatest concentration of the drug to the affected area immediately. The dose of intravitreal injection of ganciclovir is about 2 mg/0.1 mL.[67] This drug is usually well tolerated, highly effective, and relatively inexpensive. The primary risks are endophthalmitis, retinal detachment, and vitreous hemorrhage.

Ganciclovir implant (Vitrasert) can be implanted in the eye for long-term, controlled drug delivery.[68] This mode of administration may be especially useful in patients who are not available for regular opthalmic follow-up and who have systemic side-effect–related contradications to system anti-CMV drugs.

Foscarnet is a pyrophosphate analogue that inhibits DNA polymerase and reverse transcriptase by directly affecting the pyrophosphate binding site (it does not have to be phosphorylated to become active). This agent is also virustatic and has an intrinsic anti-HIV effect. Foscarnet, 90 mg/kg, is administered twice daily for 14 to 21 days as induction therapy, followed by once-daily administration as maintenance therapy. Viral replication will resume on cessation of therapy. Ganciclovir-resistant retinitis can be treated with foscarnet because the mechanism of action differs. Combined therapy with ganciclovir and foscarnet has been shown to decrease emergence of resistance.

Finally, treatment with cidofovir can be considered. Cidofovir is a nucleotide analog and phosphorylation by viral-encoded enzymes is not required for its activity. CMV-DNA polymerase is the drug's target. Cidofovir is eliminated primarily by glomerular filtration and partially by tubular secretion. Increased proteinuria and elevations in serum creatinine are the major dose-limiting toxicities. Saline hydration and concomitant administration of probenecid were candidal infection in HIV positive patients. The majority of patients have indwelling venous catheters or are intravenous drug abusers. The eye can also be part of disseminated candidal infection. Fluffy-white chorioretinal lesions along with snowball like masses are usually seen. Other lesions are creamy-white multiple chorioretinal masses with overlying vitreous inflammation. Cryptococcus neoformans is the most common fungal infective agent in AIDS. It usually causes chronic meningitis, which usually results in papilloedema, optic neuropathy, and chiasmal involvement[74]. It can involve each part of the eye, most commonly causing chorioretinitis. Cranial nerve palsies indicate a poor prognosis.

Treatment: Systemic and intravitreal antifungal agents.

Mycobacterial Infection. HIV/tuberculosis coinfection is of special concern especially in developing nations where background rates of TB are among the highest in the world. Ocular TB can present with protean manifestations, including choroiditis, choroidal granulomas **(Figure 14–11)**, chorioretinitis, endophthalmitis, subretinal abscess, and panophthalmitis.

Choroidal tuberculosis has not been found to be as common as systemic tuberculosis in patients with AIDS. No definite correlation of the occurrence of ocular tuberculosis with CD4 counts was found in a recent study.[44] Unlike cyrptococcal meningitis, toxoplasmosis, or other opportunistic infections, which occur at very low CD4 counts, ocular TB occurs in all ranges of CD4 counts.

Polymerase chain reaction (PCR) and histopathologic examination are very helpful in the diagnosis of ocular TB. Ocular course may not coincide with systemic TB. Patients with AIDS can have aggressive manifestations of ocular TB, which sometimes may not resolve with anti-TB therapy, even in the context of improving systemic infection.[44] Initiation of HAART before anti-TB therapy can lead to florid inflammation and paradoxical worsening of tuberculosis due immune reconstitution inflammatory syndrome (IRIS). Regular ophthalmic screening for ocular TB is imperative in all HIV cases in India, in spite of relatively preserved CD4 counts and regular HAART.

While mycobacterial infection (such as *Mycobacterium avium intracellulare*) is atypical, it can occur in about 15% to 20% of patients with AIDS; such organisms have been demonstrated in autopsies in the choroids in 1% to 6% of these patients.[75]

Toxoplasmic Retinochoroiditis.[76] *Toxoplasma gondii*, a protozoan, affects about 10% of patients wtih AIDS, but toxoplasmic retinochoroiditis is relatively rare and accounts for only

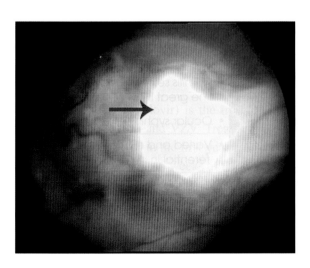

Figure 14–11. *Color fundus photograph showing a choroidal tubercle/subretinal abcess.*

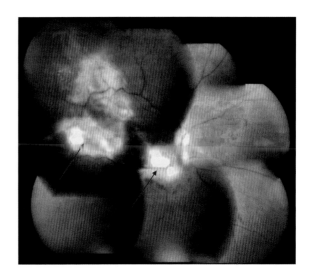

Figure 14–12. *Color fundus picture showing atypical toxoplasmic necrotizing retinochoroiditis.*

1% of AIDS-related retinal infections. In HIV-infected patients, ocular toxoplasmosis is much less common than toxoplasmic encephalitis, probably due to the difference in parasite load in the eye and the CNS. There can be a single lesion or multifocal lesions in one or both eyes, with broad areas of retinal necrosis (**Figure 14–12**). The retina appears to have a hard, "indurated" appearance, with sharply demarcated borders and little retinal hemorrhage. When patients with AIDS develop necrotizing retinitis, toxoplasmosis must be considered in the differential diagnosis, along with cytomegalovirus retinitis, progressive outer retinal necrosis, and syphilitic retinitis. Unlike the other infections, however, toxoplasmosis can cause a progressive intraocular infection, panophthalmitis, and orbital cellulitis in patients with AIDS.[25] It is usually caused by a newly acquired infection. CNS lesions are seen in 29% to 50% of HIV-infected patients with ocular toxoplasmosis. Serologic diagnosis is often difficult due to a depressed antibody response, in which IgM and IgG titre may not be of much use. Nested PCR testing of aqueous fluid may help in confirmation of the diagnosis.

Systemic anti-toxoplasma therapy is required. Pyrimethamine, in combination with a sulfonamide or clindamycin, or both, is the treatment of choice. Long-term or repeated therapy is often necessary. Atovaquone has been used successfully, but is expensive and has yet to be shown to be superior to standard therapy.[77]

Orbital Lesions[5, 12–14]

Fungal lesions involving the orbit have been reported. Kaposi's sarcoma and lymphoma can also involve the orbit. Optic nerve toxoplasmosis and orbital inflammation as an initial presentation of AIDS have also been reported.[78]

Neurophthalmic Lesions

Papilledema and Optic Atrophy

Ocular involvement secondary to intracranial infections may manifest as papilledema, optic atrophy, and ophthalmoplegias.[79] Patients may present with headache, vomiting, or diplopia. The

21. Biswas J, Fogla R, Gopal L, Narayana KM, Banker AS, Kumarasamy N, et al . Current approaches to diagnosis and management of ocular lesions in human immunodeficiency virus positive patients. Indian J Ophthalmol 2002;50:83–96

22. Sharvadze L, Tsertsvadze T, Gochitashvili N, Bolokadze N, Dolmazashvili E. Peculiarities of herpes zoster in immunocompetent and immunocompromised hosts. Georgian Med News 2006;141:50–53

23. Martinez E, Gatell J, Moran Y, Aznar E, Buira E, Guelar A, et al . High incidence of herpes zoster in patients with AIDS soon after therapy with protease inhibitors. Clin Infect Dis 1998;27:1510–1513.

24. Basic and clinical science course. Intraocular inflammation and uveitis. USA: American Academy of Ophthalmology; 2005–2006 (p. 241–262).

25. Silverstein BE, Chandler D, Neger R, Margolis TP. Disciform keratitis: A case of herpes zoster sine herpete. Am J Ophthalmol 1997;123:254–255.

26. Engstrom RE, Holland GN. Chronic herpes zoster virus keratitis associated with the acquired immunodeficiency syndrome. Am J Ophthalmology 1988;105:556–558

27. Young IL, Robin JB, Holland GN, Hendricks RL, Paschal JF, Engstrom RE Jr, et al. Herpes simplex keratitis in patients with acquired immune deficiency syndrome. Ophthalmology 1989;96:1476–1479

28. Hodge WG, Margolis TP. Herpes simplex virus keratitis among patients who are positive or negative for human immunodeficiency virus: An epidemiologic study. Ophthalmology 1997;104:120–124.

29. Hendricks RL. An immunologist's view of the herpes simplex keratitis. Cornea 1997;16:503–506

30. Bodaghi B, Mougin C, Michelson S, Agut H, Dighiero P, Offret H, et al. Acyclovir-resistant bilateral keratitis associated with mutations in the HSV-1 thymidine kinase gene. xp Eye Res 2000;71:353–359

31. Naseri A, Margolis TP. Varicella zoster virus immune recovery stromal keratitis in a patient with AIDS. Br J Ophthalmol 2001;85:1390–1391

32. Cheng L, Rao NA, Keefe KS, Avila CP Jr, Macdonald JC, Freeman WR. Cytomegalovirus iritis. Ophthalmic Surg Lasers 1998;29:930–932

33. Brody JM, Butrus SI, Laby DM, Ashraf MF, Rabinowitz AI, Parenti DM. Anterior segment findings in AIDS patients with cytomegalovirus retinitis. Graefes Arch Clin Exp Ophthalmol 1995;233:374–376.

34. Walter KA, Coulter VL, Palay DA, Taravella MJ, Grossniklaus HE, Edelhauser HF. Corneal endothelial deposits in patients with cytomegalovirus retinitis. Am J Ophthalmol 1996;121:391–396.

35. Biswas J, Lily Therese, Kumarasamy N, Solomon S: Lid abscess with extensive molluscum contagiosum in a patient with acquired immunodeficiency syndrome (AIDS). Ind. J. Ophthalmol. December, 1997;45:234–236.

36. Biswas J, Madhavan HN, Kumarasamy N, Solomon S: Blepharitis and lid ulcer as initial ocular manifestations in acquired immunodeficiency syndrome (AIDS) patients. Ind. J. Ophthalmol. December, 1997;45:233-234,

37. Ratnam I, Chiu C, Kandala NB, Easterbrook PJ. Incidence and risk factors for immune reconstitution inflammatory syndrome in an ethnically diverse HIV type 1-infected cohort. Clin Infect Dis 2006;42:418–427.

38. Moraes HV Jr. Ocular manifestations of HIV-AIDS. Curr Opin Ophthalmol 2002;13:397–403.

39. Aristimuno B, Nirankari VS, Hemady RK, Rodrigues MM. Spontaneous ulcerative keratitis in immunocompromised patients. Am J Ophthalmol 1993;115:202–208.

40. Hansen B, Kronborg G. Acanthamoeba keratitis in a non-contact lens wearer with human immunodeficiency virus. Scand J Infect Dis 2003;35:207–209.

41. Tandon R, Vajpayee RB, Gupta V, Vajpayee M, Satpathy G, Dada T. Polymicrobial keratitis in an HIV-positive patient. Indian J Ophthalmol 2003;51:87-8.

42. Bryan RT. Microsporidiosis as an AIDS-related opportunistic infection. Clin Infect Dis 1995;21:S62–65.

43. Gajdatsy AD, Tay-Kearney ML. Microsporidial keratoconjunctivitis after HAART. Clin Exp Ophthalmol 2001;29:327–329

44. Babu RB, Sudharshan S, Kumarasamy N, Therese KL, Biswas J. Ocular tuberculosis in acquired immunodeficiency syndrome. Am J Ophthalmol 2006;142:413–418

45. Cohen JI, Saragas SJ. Endophthalmitis due to Mycobacterium avium in a patient with AIDS. Ann Ophthalmol 1990;22:47–51

46. Gopal L, Rao SK, Biswas J, Madhavan HN, Agarwal S. Tuberculous granuloma managed by full thickness eye wall resection. Am J Ophthalmol 2003;135:93–94.

47. Valentina C, Mircla C. Phlyctenular keratoconjunctivitis and lymph node tuberculosis. Ophthalmologia 1999;48:15–18

48. Singal A, Aggarwal P, Pandhi D, Rohatgi J. Cutaneous tuberculosis and phlyctenular keratoconjunctivitis: A forgotten association. Indian J Dermatol Venereol Leprol 2006;72:290–292.

49. Dinning WJ, Marston S. Cutaneous and ocular tuberculosis: A review. J Royal Soc Med 1985;78:576-81.

50. Muccioli C, Belfort Junior R, Neves R, Rao N. Limbal and choroidal Cryptococcus infection in the acquired immunodeficiency syndrome. Am J Ophthalmol 1995;120:539–540

51. Garelick JM, Khodabakhsh AJ, Lopez Y, Bamji M, Lister M. Scleral ulceration caused by cryptococcus albidus in a patient with acquired immune deficiency syndrome. Cornea 2004;23:730–731.

52. McLeish WM, Pulido JS, Holland S, Culbertson WW, Winward K. The ocular manifestations of syphilis in the human immunodeficiency virus type 1-infected host. Ophthalmology 1990;97:196–203.

53. Becerra LI, Ksiazek SM, Savino PJ, Marcus DK, Buckley RM, Sergott RC, et al. Syphilitic uveitis in human immunodeficiency virus-infected and non infected patients. Ophthalmology 1989;96:1727–1730.

54. Musher DM, Hamill RJ, Baughn RE. Effect of human immunodeficiency virus (HIV) infection on the course of syphilis and on the response to treatment. Ann Intern Med 1990;113:872–881.

55. Aldave AJ, King JA, Cunningham ET Jr. Ocular syphilis. Curr Opin Ophthalmol 2001;12:433–441.

56. Moloney G, Branley M, Kotsiou G, Rhodes D. Syphilis presenting as scleritis in an HIV-positive man undergoing immune reconstitution. Clin Experiment Ophthalmol 2004;32:526–528

57. Batard ML, Cheret A, Muller P, Sarrouy J, Mareel A, Lamaury I. Bacillary angiomatosis associated with AIDS. Ann Dermatol Venereol 2006;133:498–499.

58. Matui R, Nussenblatt R, de Smet MD. Prevalence of tear hyposecretion and vitamin A deficiency in patients with AIDS. Invest Ophthalmol Vis Sci 1994;35:1308.

59. Graham DA, Sires BS. Acquired trichomegaly associated with acquired immunodeficiency syndrome. Arch Ophthalmol 1997;115:557-8

60. Rosberger DF, Heinemann MH, Friedberg DN, Holland GN, Uveitis associated with human immunodeficiency virus infection. Am J Ophthalmol 1998;125:301-5.

61. Nash RW, Lindquist TD. Bilateral angle-closure glaucoma associated with uveal effusion: Presenting sign of HIV infection. Surv Ophthalmol 1992;36:255-8

62. Basic and clinical science course. Intraocular inflammation and uveitis. 2005–2006. American Academy of Ophthalmology. (pp .24–262).

63. Gross JG, et al. Longitudinal study of CMV retinitis in AIDS. Ophthalmology'90; 97:681-6

64. Roarty DJ, et al. Long term visual morbidity of CMV retinitis in patients with AIDS. Ophthalmology '93.100;1685–1688

65. Thorne JE, Jabs DA, Kempen JH, Holbrook JT, Nichols C, Meinert CL; Studies of Ocular Complications of AIDS Research Group. Incidence of and risk factors for visual acuity loss among patients with AIDS and cytomegalovirus retinitis in the era of highly active antiretroviral therapy. Ophthalmology 2006;113(8):1432–1440

66. Martin DF, Sierra-Madero J, Walmsley S, Wolitz RA, Macey K, Georgiou P, Robinson CA, Stempien MJ; Valganciclovir Study Group. A controlled trial of valganciclovir as induction therapy for cytomegalovirus retinitis. N Engl J Med. 2002;346(15):1119–1926

67. Young S et al. High dose intravitreous ganciclovir in the treatment of CMV retinitis. Ophthalmology 98;105:1404–1410

68. Dhillon B, Kamal A, Leen C. Intravitreal sustained-release ganciclovir implantation to control cytomegalovirus retinitis in AIDS. Int J STD AIDS 1998 9:227–230.

69. Akler ME, Johnson DW, Burman WJ et al. Anterior Uveitis and hypotony after intravenous cidofovir for treatment of cytomegalovirus retinitis. Ophthalmology 1998;105:651–657

70. Vrabec TR. Posterior segment manifestations of HIV/AIDS. Surv Ophthalmol 2004 ;49:131–157

71. Yoser SL, Forster DJ, Rao NA. Systemic viral infections and their retinal and choroidal manifestations. Surv Ophthalmol 1993;37:313–352

72. Biswas J, Choudhry S, Priya K, Gopal L Detection of cytomegalovirus from vitreous humor in a patient with progressive outer retinal necrosis. Indian J Ophthalmol. 2002;50:319–321.

73. Rao NA, Zimmerman PL,Boyer D, Biswas J Causey D, Beniz J, Nichols PW. A clinical, histopathologic, and electron microscopic study of Pneumocystis carinii choroiditis. Am J Ophthalmol 1989; 15;107:218–228

74. Battu RR, Biswas J, Jayakumar N, Madhavan HN, Kumarasamy N, Solomon S: Papilloedema with peripapillary retinal hemorrhage in an AIDS patient with cryptococcal meningitis. Ind J Ophthalmol. 2000 Mar;48(1):47–49.

75. Zamir E, Hudson H, Ober RR et al. Massive mycobacterial choroiditis during highly active antiretroviral therapy, another immune-recovery uveitis? Ophthalmology 2002;109:2144–2148

76. Moorthy RS, Smith RE, Rao NA. Progressive ocular toxoplasmosis in patients with acquired immunodeficiency syndrome.Am J Ophthalmol. 1993 ;15;115:742-7

77. Schimkat M, Althaus C, Armbrecht C, Jablonowski H, Sundmacher R. Treatment of toxoplasmosis retinochoroiditis with atovaquone in an AIDS patient Klin Monatsbl Augenheilkd. 1995;206:173–177.

78. Lee MW, Fong KS, Hsu LY, Lim WK. Optic nerve toxoplasmosis and orbital inflammation as initial presentation of AIDS.Graefes Arch Clin Exp Ophthalmol 2006;244:1542–1544.

79. Karna S, Biswas J, Kumarasamy N, Sharma P, Solomon S. Multiple cranial nerve palsy in an HIV-positive patient. Ind J Ophthalmol 2001;49:118–120.

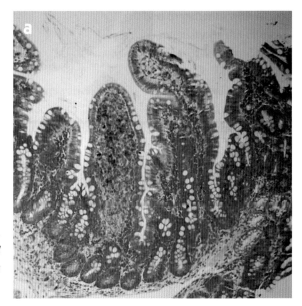

Figure 15–4a. Mycobacterium avium *complex.*
Low-power photomicrograph of a Ziehl Neilson–stained
small intestinal biopsy demonstrating a single villus
stuffed with acid-fast bacilli.

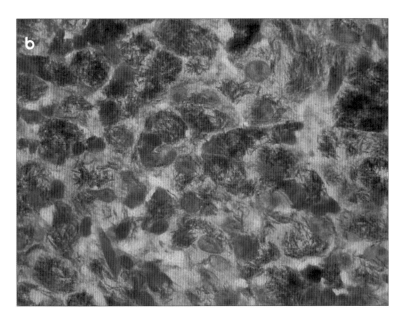

Figure 15–4b. *High-power view*
demonstrating acid-fast bacilli within
macrophages.

malabsorption. *Mycobacterium avium* complex infection (**Figure 15–4**) of the small intestine promotes malabsorption, particularly of fats, because of lymphatic obstruction and exudative enteropathy. Pathogenic strains of *Escherichia coli* may cause ileal dysfunction due to a chronic bacterial enteropathy and result in malabsorption of fats and bile acids. Cytomegalovirus is a common cause of diarrhea and weight loss in severely immunodeficient patients, but in patients with AIDS, the major site of infection is the colon, so that malabsorption is not present.

Metabolic alterations in HIV-infected individuals include elevated resting energy expenditure, hypertriglyceridemia, and decreased serum cholesterol concentrations.[8] Hypertriglyceridemia is associated both with decreased clearance of chylomicrons and with increased *de novo* fatty acid synthesis and elevated serum concentrations of bioactive interferon-α. Endocrine alterations include elevations in serum cortisol concentration, with loss of its normal diurnal periodicity. Deficiencies in testosterone and other endogenous anabolic factors may occur and promote protein depletion. In some cases, testosterone deficiency is associated with sexual dysfunction.

Alterations in Energy Balance

Weight loss ultimately is a consequence of negative caloric balance, regardless of cause. Studies found that food intake was the most important predictor of short-term weight change in HIV-infected patients. Macallan and colleagues,[9] using the technique of doubly labelled water measurement, found that total energy expenditure was decreased in the weight-losing patients. The decrease was confined largely to voluntary energy expenditure, as average resting energy expenditure was elevated. The decrease in caloric intake exceeded the decrease in voluntary energy expenditure and, thus, promoted weight loss. However, simply maintaining caloric intake does not lead to repletion of body cell mass (see below).

Nutritional Management

The workup of malnutrition in an HIV-infected patient should begin with a thorough history and physical examination, with special emphasis on changes in body weight and habitus, as well as changes in appetite, eating habits, and physical activity. An initial determination and frequent measures of body weight should be standard of care for primary providers. Alterations in body weight and nutritional status may provide the earliest clues to the presence of an opportunistic infection.

Dietitian assistance in the determination of caloric intake can be helpful, as clinical history may be inaccurate. The clinical evaluation of malabsorption is confounded by the possibility of diarrheal illnesses that are not associated with malabsorption, as well as by moderation of diarrhea due to reduced food intake. Malabsorption can be assessed starting with a careful history, stool examinations, and noninvasive tests such as the D-xylose absorption test and/or qualitative fecal fat analysis. Quantitative fat analysis rarely is necessary for the detection of malabsorption. Stool analyses for enteric pathogens are important adjuncts to the evaluation and endoscopic biopsies may be required to provide an etiologic diagnosis.

The rationale for nutritional therapy to an AIDS patient is straightforward: malnutrition may have adverse consequences which may be prevented by improving the nutritional status of the patient by appropriate therapy. Concepts guiding the decisions to provide nutritional support in an HIV infected patient should be the same as in anyone with a chronic illness.

Food Based Therapies and Oral Supplements. There are no data to support the standard use of oral nutrient supplements in HIV infected individuals, whether normally nourished or malnourished, although they are usually prescribed in patients complaining of fatigue and lassitude. In patients with severe malabsorption, either elemental or semielemental oral formulas may be beneficial. There is little consensus about the use of micronutrient supplements, such as antioxidant and vitamins, and studies in the United States have had mixed results. However, a study of micronutrient supplementation from Africa showed that vitamin A supplementation in mothers led to a significant decrease in the transmission of HIV to their infants.[10] Obviously, micronutrient therapies will have the most impact in patients with micronutrient deficiencies at baseline. However, micronutrient supplementation may not be helpful if protein and caloric deficiencies persist. It also is not clear that specific nutritional therapy beyond a normal diet is necessary if HAART is provided.

Appetite Stimulants. Numerous appetite stimulants have been studied or used in HIV-infected patients. The synthetic progestin megestrol acetate increases caloric intake and

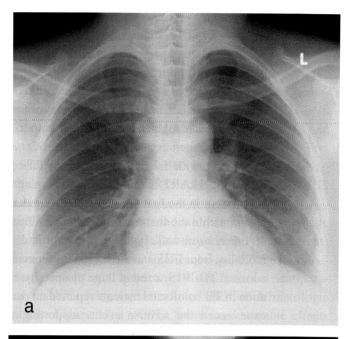

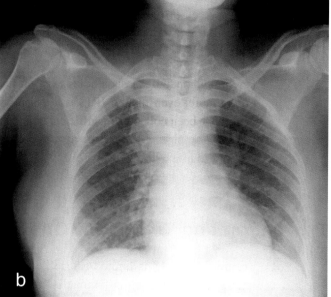

Figure 17–2. *Illustrative chest radiographs of pulmonary TB-IRIS. Normal baseline chest radiograph in a patient prior to the initiation of antiretroviral therapy* (**a**) *is followed by abrupt onset of bilateral airspace disease* (**b**) *and conversion to positive acid-fast bacilli on sputum smears.*

initiation of HAART monotherapy, long before the widespread availability and use of HAART.[15] With the emergence of HAART, increasing reports of clinical deterioration occurred, mainly in the form of worsening chest radiographs. In one of the few prospective TB-IRIS trials, Narita and colleagues examined paradoxical responses in three groups: 33 HIV-infected TB patients treated with anti-TB therapy and HAART, 55 HIV-negative TB patients treated with anti-TB therapy alone, and 28 HIV-infected TB patients treated with anti-TB therapy but no HAART. In the dual-therapy group, paradoxical responses were seen in 12/33 (36%) of patients, compared to only three such cases in the other two groups combined. Compatible with the first documented mycobacterial IRIS case, paradoxical responses were strongly associated with PPD skin conversions.[4] Documented symptoms are those that HIV clinicians can expect from the syndrome: high fevers; intrathoracic lymphadenopathy, with or without worsening pulmonary infiltrates or

Mortality

All available data suggest the mortality directly attributable to IRIS is low. Study differences, including the application of various IRIS case definitions, methods for ascertaining IRIS cases, and retrospective versus prospective designs make mortality comparisons difficult. In addition, concerns have been expressed over rates of loss to follow-up in some studies.[40] Mortality among such patients is high and significant loss to follow-up rates can result in underestimation of mortality by as much as 80%.[41] This concern is valid, given loss to follow-up rates ranging from 0% to 44% in a wide range of African HAART cohorts.[42,43] Additionally, mortality in the first year following HAART initiation is high, ranging from 8% to 26%.[43] Most of these deaths (50% to 87%) occur in the first 6 months following the introduction of HAART,[24,43] and, as IRIS usually occurs within the first 6 months of HAART and commonly involves common pathogens such as *M. tuberculosis* and cryptococci, it is difficult, if not impossible, to distinguish between the early mortality from IRIS and the mortality caused by any of the other events. Although limited to paradoxical TB-IRIS, a recent large prospective cohort study examining the timing of HAART initiation in TB coinfected patients reported no deaths directly attributable to IRIS in 61 patients who experienced the adverse event, supporting the observation that IRIS mortality is generally low.[24,44]

Immunopathogenesis

Few immunopathogenesis studies exist on the underlying causative immune response in IRIS. Furthermore, even though IRIS is a tissue-specific process, even fewer histopathologic specimens have been collected in sufficient quantity to make any firm immunopathologic conclusions. Since the specific etiologies may each precipitate a different immunologic response responsible for the syndrome—that is, bacterial versus viral causes—the pathogenesis of IRIS, where available, is presented for each IRIS pathogen in the rest of this chapter.

Prevention and Treatment Options

Treatment of IRIS is limited to anecdotal reports involving therapies aimed at suppressing or relieving the exuberant inflammation that characterizes the syndrome. Because of the different IRIS pathogens that make up the spectrum of the syndrome, therapies involving specific infectious IRIS etiologies are discussed within respective disease-specific sections. However, in general, therapies have focused on the inflammatory nature of the disease, and often involve anti-inflammatory medications, such as corticosteroids and nonsteroidal anti-inflammatory drugs (NSAIDs). Underlying most IRIS treatment strategies is the continuation of HAART, the reasons for which will be discussed in pertinent sections.

Mycobacterial IRIS

Mycobacterium tuberculosis IRIS (TB-IRIS)

The first reported case of IRIS in HIV-infected patients arguably involved the reporting of restored mycobacterial responses to purified protein derivative (PPD) antigen following

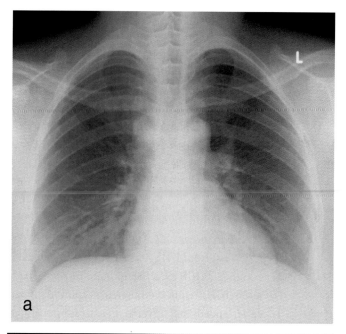

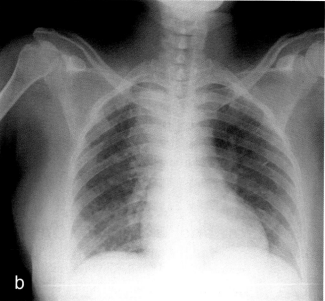

Figure 17–2. *Illustrative chest radiographs of pulmonary TB-IRIS. Normal baseline chest radiograph in a patient prior to the initiation of antiretroviral therapy (**a**) is followed by abrupt onset of bilateral airspace disease (**b**) and conversion to positive acid-fast bacilli on sputum smears.*

initiation of HAART monotherapy, long before the widespread availability and use of HAART.[15] With the emergence of HAART, increasing reports of clinical deterioration occurred, mainly in the form of worsening chest radiographs. In one of the few prospective TB-IRIS trials, Narita and colleagues examined paradoxical responses in three groups: 33 HIV-infected TB patients treated with anti-TB therapy and HAART, 55 HIV-negative TB patients treated with anti-TB therapy alone, and 28 HIV-infected TB patients treated with anti-TB therapy but no HAART. In the dual-therapy group, paradoxical responses were seen in 12/33 (36%) of patients, compared to only three such cases in the other two groups combined. Compatible with the first documented mycobacterial IRIS case, paradoxical responses were strongly associated with PPD skin conversions.[4] Documented symptoms are those that HIV clinicians can expect from the syndrome: high fevers; intrathoracic lymphadenopathy, with or without worsening pulmonary infiltrates or

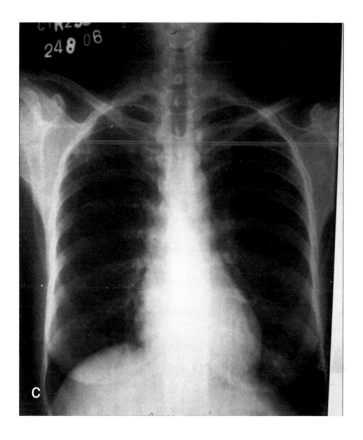

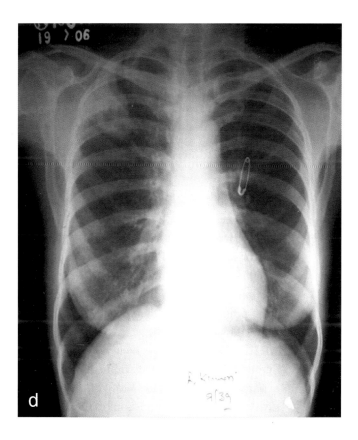

Figure 17–2—continued. This (c) is a baseline chest radiograph from a patient who subsequently developed pulmonary TB-IRIS, manifested as focal consolidation with cavity formation (d). Figures 2c and 2d courtesy of Upasna Agarwal, LRS Institute of Tuberculosis and Respiratory Diseases, New Delhi, India.

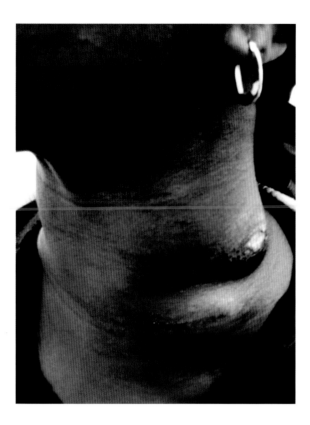

Figure 17–3. *Classic TB-IRIS cervical suppurative lymphadenitis in a patient who had recently initiated antiretroviral therapy. Photo courtesy of Graeme Meintjes, Infectious Diseases Unit, GF Jooste Hospital, Cape Town, South Africa.*

pleural effusions (**Figure 17-2**); cervical or axillary lymphadenopathy (**Figure 17–3**); cutaneous TB; and disseminated TB, most often manifested as peritoneal symptoms.

Epidemiology

Retrospective and prospective studies indicate that 7% to 43% of patients will develop paradoxical TB-IRIS following initiation of HAART, with most of these estimates falling in the 20% to 30% range in cohorts in which paradoxical TB-IRIS was the primary focus. TB-IRIS incidences are difficult to estimate, given the variability of TB screening and TB prevalence within a population. Although not reproducible between studies, TB-IRIS risk factors include lower baseline CD4 cell count, coexisting extrapulmonary TB, a more rapid fall in HIV RNA levels, and significant increases in CD4 cell count or CD4 percentages following initiation of HAART.[4,45-55] Importantly, specific risk may be associated with disseminated TB.[46,55,56]

As early as 2002, TB-IRIS was recognized to be potentially associated with a shorter interval between TB diagnosis and therapy and HAART initiation,[57] replicated in subsequent investigations and disputed by others.[45,53,57] A decision analysis of the timing of HAART in HIV/TB coinfected patients reported the highest rates of IRIS occurred in those who began HAART within 2 months of TB therapy. However, withholding or deferring HAART until completion of 2 to 6 months of TB therapy was associated with higher mortality.[58] This model has been confirmed by a recent prospective trial (the SAPIT trial) examining the timing of HAART initiation in HIV/TB coinfected patients. In this study, 53/429 (12.3%) of patients in the integrated therapy group (HAART initiated within 12 weeks of TB treatment) experienced paradoxical TB-IRIS, compared to only 8/213 (3.8%) of the patients in the sequential therapy group (HAART initiated within 4 weeks of completion of TB therapy).[59]

TABLE 17–2	Summary Table of Infectious and Noninfectious IRIS Manifestations[a]

Central nervous system

Infectious

Cryptococcus neoformans meningitis[12,35–38,53]
PML[17111,113,117,182]
Toxoplasmosis[17,191,192]
Expanding intracranial tuberculomas[193,194]
Intracranial cryptococcoma[91,102]
Tuberculous meningitis[196]
Parvovirus B19 meningitis[197]
CMV ventriculitis[198]
VZV myelitis and encephalitis[133,199,200]

Dermatologic

Infectious

HSV labialis[33,173,183]
Cutaneous bacterial abscesses[19]
Dermatomal VZV[17,18,27,129,131,132,173,183,184]
Folliculitis[19,137]
Tinea capitis[19]
Acne vulgaris and acne rosacea[209]
Cryptococcus neoformans abscess[93,102]
Mycobacterium leprae leprosy and Hansen's disease[211–215]
MAI cutaneous abscess and extremity pyomyositis[88]

Noninfectious

Intradermal granulomatous tattoo ink reaction[168]
Seborrheic dermatitis[33]
Erythema nodosum[219]

Gastrointestinal

Infectious

Kaposi's sarcoma with GI hemorrhage[19]
Hepatitis C virus[151,152]
Hepatitis B virus[17,18,156]
TB hepatitis[48]
Strongyloides stercoralis infection[27,223–225]
Diffuse abdominal microsporidiosis IRIS[226]
Oral candidiasis and recurrent oral ulcers[227,228]

Noninfectious

IRIS-induced ulcerative colitis[138,229]
Autoimmune hepatitis IRIS[230]
Sarcoidosis hepatitis and duodenitis[217]

Ophthalmologic

Infectious

CMV retinitis and uveitis[140–143,145,149,150]

Cardiovascular

Infectious

Streptococcus pneumoniae sepsis[33]
TB pericarditis and pericardial effusion[190]

Noninfectious

Onset of subclinical atheromatous lesions[195]

Pulmonary

Infectious

Tuberculous pleural effusions[4,19,53,60]
TB-SIRS and -ARDS[201,202]
TB cystic lung disease[203]
Streptococcus pneumoniae empyema[33]
Mycobacterium celatum disease[204]
Cryptococcus neoformans cavitary pneumonia and pneumonitis, mediastinal lymphadenopathy[36,92,94]
Mycobacterium kansasii pneumonitis and respiratory failure[205]
Mycobacterium xenopi pneumonia and pulmonary cavitation[206]
CMV pneumonitis[33]
Necrotizing pulmonary aspergillosis[207,208]
MAI pleural effusion[210]

Noninfectious

Pulmonary sarcoidosis[216,217]
Interstitial lymphoid pneumonitis[218]

Hematologic/Lymphatic

Infectious

Parvovirus B-19 red cell aplasia[220]
Cryptococcus neoformans lymphadenitis[30,36,94,95]
MAI osteomyelitis[89]
TB splenic infarction[221]
Visceral leishmaniasis and hemophagocytic syndrome[51]

Noninfectious

Hemophagocytic syndrome[222]

Genitourinary

Infectious

Molluscum contagiosum and genital warts[18,19]
Anogenital herpes[16,18,19,27]

Noninfectious

Sarcoidosis interstitial nephritis[217]

Rheumatologic/Autoimmune

Noninfectious

SLE[163]
Rheumatoid arthritis[167]
Graves disease and autoimmune thyroid disease[161,162,231,232]
Still's disease[165,166]
Polymyositis[164]

ARDS=adult respiratory distress syndrome; CMV=cytomegalivirus; GI=gastrointestinal; HSV=herpes simplex virus; IRIS=immune reconstitution inflammatory syndrome; MAI=Mycobacterium avium-intracellulare; PML=progressive multifocal leukoencephalopathy; SIRS=systemic inflammatory response; SLE=systemic lupus erythematosus; TB=tuberculosis; VZV=varicella zoster virus.

Clinical Signs and Symptoms

TB-IRIS is capable of manifesting a wide spectrum of disease (see **Table 17–2**). Pathology most commonly involves the lung, where additional radiographic changes such as thoracic lymphadenopathy, pleural effusions, and parenchymal disease with or without consolidation and cavitation are possible.[60] Some manifestations may be severe, and include tracheal compression and stridor with possible respiratory failure.[61]

The timing of both paradoxical and unmasking TB-IRIS is important in the diagnosis of the syndrome. By definition, paradoxical or unmasking symptoms should occur within the first 3 months of HAART. Although it is possible for TB-IRIS cases to occur outside of this time, the vast majority of cases occur within 90 days. For cases outside of this period, increasing difficulty occurs in discerning TB-IRIS from new exogenous incident TB infections or opportunistic infections secondary to delayed or impaired immune reconstitution following HAART. Additional complexities such as drug toxicities and medication compliance can cloud the diagnosis. In a prospective study of 100 TB-IRIS patients, the median time to onset to symptoms was 14 days (IQR 7-25).[34]

Paradoxical TB-IRIS in HIV-infected patients often presents with new lesions at distant sites from the original site of infection,[48] suggesting that disseminated disease is present in patients believed to have localized disease. In addition, the similar presentation in HIV-uninfected patients may suggest the immunology of IRIS is, in part, independent of HIV infection itself.

Pathogenesis

In a small, early longitudinal immunologic study, responses to mycobacterial antigens were assessed in 10 HAART-naïve HIV patients initiating HAART and 11 HIV-negative controls through the measurement of interferon (IFN)-γ, interleukin (IL)-2, IL-10, and IL-12. Following HAART initiation, HIV-infected patients demonstrated significant increases in IFN-γ production; however, this increase peaked at a delayed 8 months following HAART initiation and did not reach IFN-γ production levels of the HIV-negative controls.[62]

The hypothesis currently gaining the most attention is that IRIS results from a redistribution of antigen-specific memory T-lymphocytes from peripheral lymphoid tissues following HAART initiation.[63-65] Such a response could favor a T helper cell type 1 (Th1) response in the presence of appropriate antigenic stimulus, a mechanism that is supported by a study that found a sharp amplification of PPD-specific IFN-γ T cells with Th1 cytokine production (IL-2, IL-10, IFN-γ). No increase in Th2 cytokines occurred, and these results were independent of CD4 cell counts, HIV RNA levels, and the timing of HAART initiation.[66]

Other small investigations have suggest additional immunologic mechanisms, such as increased PPD-specific IFN-γ–producing T cells following HAART initiation in patients with TB-IRIS, with no differences in FoxP3+ T regulatory cells (Tregs) between groups.[67] These observations of increased IFN-γ production in response to PPD antigen have been replicated in another small longitudinal IRIS study.[68] Others have reported significant increases in Tregs in patients with *Mycobacterium avium-intracellulare* IRIS (MAI-IRIS); however, this population possessed decreased suppressive function, suggesting that IRIS may be due, in part, to qualitative dysfunction of this T cell population.[69] Expanding the spectrum of possible lymphocyte populations potentially involved in the syndrome, another study again reported an increase in activated PPD-specific effector memory CD4+ T cells and $\gamma\delta$ T cells in TB-IRIS patients.[70] $\gamma\delta$ T cells play a role in host defense against bacterial ligands, including TB. The finding of increased activation on more effector-type memory T cells has also been reported by a small, prospective immunologic study in IRIS, though significant activation (as defined by CD38+ HLA-DR+ cells) was most pronounced in CD8+ T cells.[71] All of these small studies contribute to our understanding of the immunopathogenesis of the syndrome, but provide only a glimpse into the full immunopathogenesis of TB-IRIS.

TB-IRIS definitions have often included known drug-resistant TB as an exclusionary criterion for the diagnosis, primarily because the routine testing of TB isolates is not available or routinely performed. Such criteria sought to clarify the diagnosis of an already confusing clinical diagnosis. However, in terms of the immunopathogenesis of TB-IRIS, an immunologic difference between sensitive and resistant strains in cases of TB-IRIS seems unlikely. A recent study in South Africa reported rifampin resistance in 10.1% of patients who presented with TB-IRIS.[72] This finding argues that drug-resistant TB should not be an exclusion criterion for TB-IRIS and that investigations into the susceptibility of TB isolates in TB-IRIS should be considered in the appropriate settings.

The public health implications for these various proposed immunologic mechanisms is the observation that some cases of TB "reactivation" are associated with positive smears, occurring in 4/6 patients in an early TB-IRIS series.[57] These findings were followed by observations that TB-IRIS occurred in a distinct "early TB" group with a median onset of 41 days (IQR: 7–109 days).[73] Although the incidence of TB disease prior to HAART is variable, depending on the setting and degree of pre-HAART screening, these small observations may be reflected in larger cohorts documenting high TB incidences in the immediate period following HAART, at least partially due to TB-IRIS.[74–76] It is possible that such observations may be secondary to increased localized pulmonary inflammation with resulting communication of localized or contained TB infection with larger airways, resulting in increased sputum positivity. However, pathologic correlations of such mechanisms do not yet exist to support this hypothesis.

Prevention and Therapy

Perhaps the best method to prevent the occurrence of TB-IRIS or minimize its morbidity is to adequately screen patients for signs and symptoms (fever, night sweats, weight loss, close contact with an active TB case) and systemically employ the diagnostic means available to diagnose TB. This should include two to three quality sputum specimens for TB staining and, where available, mycobacterial culture. Additional diagnostic modalities, such as chest radiographs and mycobacterial blood cultures, should be employed where available and suspicion for TB is moderate to high. That said, the combined sensitivities of these diagnostics are relatively poor (often less than 70%), and many patients manifest unmasking TB-IRIS even after being screened for TB in relatively resource-intense clinical settings.[19,27] Until the diagnosis of TB improves, this scenario will likely persist.

Although cessation of HAART may be considered in severe, rare, life-threatening presentations––for example, airway compromise due to extrinsic lymphadenopathy compression or severe expanding central nervous system (CNS) tuberculomas—HAART can safely be continued in the majority of cases. Evidence for this arises from the aforementioned SAPIT trial.[59] Although paradoxical TB-IRIS incidence was higher in the integrated HIV/TB arms (12.3%), a lower mortality was observed compared to the sequential treatment arm (hazard ratio in integrated therapy group 0.44; 95% CI, 0.25–0.79; $p = 0.003$). These results indicate that HAART should be initiated earlier in the TB treatment course despite a higher risk for TB-IRIS, and also support similar conclusions regarding early initiation of HAART even in patients with recently diagnosed non-TB opportunistic infections.[77]

Although NSAID use is anecdotally reported in TB-IRIS, the use of corticosteroids has received the most attention, given their more potent and rapid immunomodulatory effects. The strongest evidence for corticosteroid therapy arises from the first randomized controlled trial in TB-IRIS. In this South African study, 110 patients with mild to moderate TB-IRIS restricted to lymph node enlargement, cold abscesses, serous effusion, or radiographic pulmonary infiltrate were randomized to either corticosteroids (prednisone, 1.5mg/kg for 2 weeks, followed by 0.75mg/kg for 2 weeks) or to no corticosteroid therapy. Clinical endpoints included cumulative hospitalization days and outpatient therapeutic procedures. No difference in mortality between groups was observed. For the cumulative primary endpoints, treatment with prednisone favored a better response: the median hospitalization days in the placebo group was 3 days (range, 0–9 days) versus 1 day (range, 0–3 days) for the prednisone group ($p = 0.046$). Symptom scores, pulmonary infiltrate improvement at weeks 2 and 4r, and reduction in CRP levels all favored prednisone therapy.[78]

For CNS TB-IRIS, the use of corticosteroids in HIV-negative patients experiencing tuberculous meningitis is associated with improved survival and decreased neurologic sequelae[79,80]; however, care should be taken to exclude other concurrent CNS infections prior to their initiation. Corticosteroids were used in 91% of patients with paradoxical CNS TB-IRIS in a large, single center setting.[34] These results lend support to the widespread anecdotal evidence that corticosteroid therapy may be beneficial in some patients with paradoxical TB-IRIS. However, in the setting of unmasking IRIS due to TB or other infectious organisms, these results should be considered with caution, as the effects of corticosteroids in the setting of many active opportunistic infections is not as clear.

Nontuberculous Mycobacterial IRIS

The diversity of mycobacterial species yields a diversity of IRIS manifestations. Rare reports of various mycobacterial species involved in IRIS include *Mycobacterium leprae*, *M. xenopi*, and other rare species, and are summarized in **Table 17–2**. Of the nontuberculous mycobacteria, *Mycobacterium avium-intracellulare* (MAI) deserves special mention, as it was the most frequently reported IRIS organism early in the history of IRIS.[16,53,81] This is largely reflected by the fact that its prevalence outweighed that of TB in cohorts in developed countries, which first reported much of the IRIS literature.

Clinically, MAI-IRIS typically presents as lymphadenitis, with or without suppuration and abscess formation. Sites of lymphadenopathy include the mesenteric, abdominal, axillary, and supraclavicular regions, with the latter two being the most common presentation sites. The lymphadenitis is often painful and a source of complaint from patients.[16,82] Common systemic symptoms include high fever, malaise, and leukocytosis,[82] which likely reflect the systemic inflammatory component of IRIS. However, less dramatic presentations, without marked systemic symptoms, can also occur.[83] Suppurative lesions are often MAI culture-positive, although cases describing similar paradoxical reactions in patients on MAI therapy support the clinical conclusion that a paradoxical form of MAI-IRIS to dead but immunologically reactive antigens is also possible.[84] Although two case studies report MAI-IRIS occurring 5 to 9 weeks after HAART initiation,[85,86] cumulative data suggest that most cases of MAI-IRIS, like TB-IRIS, occur within the first 3 months of HAART (range, 6–50 days).[82–84,87] Other, less common MAI-IRIS presentations include cutaneous ulcerative lesions,[87] pyomyositis,[88] osteomyelitis,[89] and disseminated disease.[16,90]

A case series of MAI-IRIS provides some of the only histopathologic insight into mycobacterial IRIS at the site of tissue involvement. In this investigation, excisional lymph nodes and lymph node aspirates were analyzed by flow cytometry to reveal a dominance of memory T cells (CD45RA- CD62L-), representing 92% to 95% of CD4+ T cells in these tissue specimens.[82] Although no baseline immunophenotyping was available on these limited samples, these findings provide important insight and support for the hypothesis that IRIS is caused, in part, by restoration of antigen-specific memory T cells in immune reconstituted patients. Importantly, these investigations emphasize the importance of performing such immunopathologic IRIS investigations at the site of disease rather than confined to the peripheral blood compartment, where immune responses may not reflect those found at the tissue level.

The treatment of MAI-IRIS primarily involves initiation or continuation of MAI therapy and continuation of HAART. In severe cases or in non-resolving suppurative lymphadenopathy, surgical debridement or repeated lymph node aspirations may be warranted.[88,89] Such aspirations may leave scarring and fistula tracts; however, these results may still outweigh the pain and physical disfigurement that may persist otherwise. The use of corticosteroids in MAI-IRIS is untested. However, evaluation of their use may be inferred from randomized trials of their use in mild to moderate TB-IRIS,[78] where the clinical situation and severity of illness are similar.

Cryptococcal IRIS

Following mycobacterial IRIS and dermatologic presentations of the syndrome, cryptococcal IRIS is the next most common manifestation of IRIS. Although it may present as a lymphadenitis, cutaneous abscess, pulmonary cavitations and mediastinitis, and CNS cryptococcoma,[91–95] most presentations of the syndrome are cryptococcal meningitis IRIS (CM-IRIS). CM-IRIS may present as a paradoxical reaction to previously treated or partially treated CM.[30,94,96–99] Such cases occur despite completed or ongoing amphotericin B and/or fluconazole treatment and are often culture-negative,[99] supporting the hypothesis that residual cryptococcal antigen is the precipitating factor. The unmasking form is secondary to subclinical cryptococcal disease present at the time of HAART initiation and is often culture-positive at CM-IRIS diagnosis.[100, 101]

Few studies exist to estimate the incidence of the unmasking form of CM-IRIS. Unmasking CM-IRIS is noticeably absent from large case series and cohorts from developed countries, which may reflect differences in antifungal prophylaxis practices, underlying environmental OI burden, or access to diagnostics.[16–18] However, the unmasking form accounts for the minority of CM-IRIS cases, representing only 3/17 (17.6%) of CM-IRIS cases in one series.[30] Studies from both resource-limited and developed countries estimate that 8% to 42% of patients with previously diagnosed CM will develop CM-IRIS, with three of the studies yielding consistent estimates of 17% to 21.4%.[12,30,35–38,102]

Although the incidence of CM-IRIS in patients with previously diagnosed CM is high (approximately 20%), the overall occurrence of CM-IRIS in large, prospective, all-cause IRIS cohorts is low. In three prospective South African cohorts initiating HAART, CM-IRIS occurred in 3/423 (0.7%), 9/434 (2.1%), and 4/498 (0.8%).[19,27,100] Thus, even in resource-limited settings, the occurrence of CM-IRIS is low overall, despite a relatively high associated morbidity.

Although about 20% of patients with previously diagnosed CM will develop IRIS, this is an overall estimate, and some studies suggest certain risk factors may be associated with an increased risk for CM-IRIS. Although studies vary in their findings, these include a shorter interval between CM diagnosis and HAART initiation (usually less than 2 months), a more rapid fall in HIV RNA, a greater increase in CD4 cell count at 6 months, and the presence of fungemia at baseline. One study found no such associations for the development of CM-IRIS.[38] For the clinician, the timing of CM-IRIS following HAART is generally soon after HAART, with three studies reporting estimates ranging from 29 to 63 days (IQR 19–129 days).[30,35,37] Although it is possible for CM-IRIS to occur several months from HAART initiation,[12,38] CM-IRIS generally occurs within 3 months following initiation of HAART. Symptoms include those classic for CM, including fever, neck stiffness, photophobia, vomiting, and headache. In addition, focal neurologic symptoms, such as facial nerve palsies and hemiparesis, are possible. Other symptoms of nonmeningitis cryptococcal IRIS include hypercalcemia.[35,37,94]

A distinct feature of CM-IRIS is its association with substantial morbidity and mortality arising from involvement of the CNS. Although low mortality is reported in some cohorts,[12,38] associated morbidities are significant and include seizures, hemiparesis, and dysarthria. In other cohorts, mortality ranges from 9% to as high as 66%, illustrating the severity of this form of IRIS.[30,35,36,100] Despite the wide mortality estimates, CM-IRIS requires a high level of care, reflected in high hospitalization rates for its management with 7/11 (63.6%) of patients requiring hospitalization.[35]

Despite this, in general, HAART should not be withheld from severely immunosuppressed patients in need of HAART. Overall, cryptococcal mortality rates have decreased from 63.8 to 15.3/100 person-years in the HAART era in one developed country cohort,[103] and the prevalence of CM as an AIDS diagnosis has decreased in another European cohort.[102] Lastly, recent data support the use of early HAART after the diagnosis of an "acute" opportunistic infection, resulting in decreased AIDS progression and death.[77]

Insights into the pathogenesis of CM-IRIS have largely centered on the analysis of cerebrospinal fluid (CSF) profiles and CSF opening pressures, as these are the most obtainable data in CM-IRIS. With the exception of increased neutrophils, no differences in CSF profiles (IFN-γ, TNF-α, IL-6, lymphocyte percentage, glucose levels) were noted between pre-HAART CM and CM-IRIS episodes.[35] The finding of increased neutrophils at CM-IRIS compared to baseline (16% versus 0%, respectively; $p<0.01$) has also been noted in another study,[37] and suggests a possible unique immunologic response in the resolution phase of CM, possibly to residual cryptococcal antigens. However, another study with limited pathologic specimens revealed lesions containing lymphocytes, plasma cells, macrophages, and histiocytes forming granulomas with or without necrosis.[12] Higher opening CSF pressures are observed in CM-IRIS patients.[30,36] These may reflect delayed clearance of residual antigen from the leptomeninges and the precipitating inflammation induced by a Th1 response following HAART. Another possible explanation for the often dramatic inflammatory presentation of CM-IRIS and elevated CSF pressures may be partially explained by the organisms' polysaccharide capsule, which is known to influence *Cryptococcus neoformans* strain-specific virulence.[104] Coupled with the severe immunodeficiency of HIV disease, it may be plausible that glucuronoxylomannan (GXM) polysaccharide is poised to maintain high antigen loads in the CSF compartment and mediate local immune responses. Following HAART and restoration of antigen-specific immunity, this may result in exaggerated immune responses within the confined CNS compartment. Limited immunologic data from peripheral blood lymphocyte responses to *C. neoformans* antigens suggest an increase in IFN-γ responses in patients experiencing the syndrome.[68] Until larger numbers of CM-IRIS patients are recruited in prospective trials obtaining adequate CSF, peripheral blood, and tissue samples, much of the pathogenesis of CM-IRIS will remain speculative.

No randomized trials of the treatment of CM-IRIS exist. Since paradoxical CM-IRIS is usually associated with culture-negative CSF findings and higher CSF opening pressures,[30,36–38] treatment should focus on the management of elevated CSF pressures. In HIV-infected patients experiencing non-IRIS cryptococcal meningitis, high pretreatment opening pressure (>25 cm H_2O) or an increase in CSF pressure of >1 cm H_2O after 2 weeks of treatment are associated with a poorer clinical outcome.[105] Therefore, as for non-IRIS patients, therapeutic CSF drainage can be recommended in these cases.[106] Continuation of HAART in the setting of paradoxical cryptococcal IRIS is usually associated with favorable outcomes.[38,53] However, profound CSF inflammation is manifested by sustained high CSF pressures, and a poor clinical response to antifungal therapy occurs in some cases. The administration of corticosteroids and discontinuation of HAART to reduce meningeal inflammation and neurologic symptoms may assist in cases of aseptic paradoxical cryptococcal meningitis.[35] In addition, initiation or continuation of antifungal therapy is important, because sterilization of CSF ranges from 21 to 64 days, depending on the antifungal regimen.[107] Treatment options remain conventional until studies optimizing the timing and dosages of antifungal therapy in patients initiating HAART become available.

Progressive Multifocal Leukoencephalopathy (PML)

With the introduction of HAART in the mid-1990s and before the large recognition of IRIS as a frequent complication of HAART, early case series suggested the initiation of antiretroviral therapy had beneficial effects on survival in patients with PML.[108] Of those who received HAART, median survival was markedly increased (median survival, >500 days) compared to those patients who received nucleoside analogs alone or no antiretroviral therapy (median survival, 123 and 127 days, respectively; $p<0.0002$ for difference between HAART and non-HAART groups). Interestingly, this analysis included a description of one patient initiated on HAART who suffered from expansion of his pre-existing lesions after an initial clinical improvement; this is perhaps one of the first descriptions of PML-IRIS. Additional cohort studies supported this observation of improved survival in the HAART era.[109,110]

However, soon thereafter, reports of contrast-enhancing PML lesions following HAART were reported, which was hypothesized to be secondary to an increased inflammatory immune response against the JC virus.[111] This report was followed by a detailed analysis of 28 PML patients treated with HAART and included brain biopsy descriptions. In four of nine patients with brain biopsies, a predominantly perivascular lymphomonocytic infiltrative pattern was noted, with the infiltrate to be predominately CD8 suppressor T cells, accompanied by some B cells and no associated CD4 T cells. In 3/28 patients (10.7%), clinical deterioration directly attributable to the initiation of HAART was noted, each of which exhibited this characteristic inflammatory reaction within the PML lesions.[112]

These observations of inflammatory reactions in patients with PML soon led to the first descriptions of fatal cases of IRIS involving PML. In two cases, initiation of HAART was abruptly followed by new onset quadriplegia, hemiplegia, worsened cognitive function, and dysphonia. In both cases, stereotactic brain biopsies and repeated imaging revealed expansion of PML lesions, characterized by prominent, enlarged, multinucleated glial cells with perivascular lymphocytic infiltrates.[113]

The characteristic noninflammatory lesions in PML provide a unique insight into the pathogenesis of PML-IRIS. With the availability of well-characterized brain biopsies, it appears that the lymphocytic infiltrate consistently observed in such lesions is central to the pathogenesis of the syndrome. Specifically, cytotoxic CD8 T cells are thought to be primarily involved, outnumbering CD4 T cells in biopsied PML IRIS lesions. This has led to the hypothesis that an imbalance of CD8/CD4 T cells plays a role developing the syndrome.[114] JC virus-specific CD4 T cells are central to controlling JC virus infection,[115] and a paucity of such cells in some PML patients could explain the detectable JC virus in two of the fatal cases of PML-IRIS.[113] Coupled with the predominant perivascular cytotoxic CD8 T cell inflammatory response, these findings provide some of the most convincing insight into the pathogenesis of this form of IRIS.

Nevertheless, despite this immunopathogenic insight, no specific therapy for PML IRIS exists. The initiation of HAART is still the treatment of choice, given the evidence for improved survival, despite the fact that some PML patients continue to progress despite beginning HAART, and up to 23% of patients with PML will develop PML-IRIS. Survival did not differ between IRIS and non-IRIS PML patients, and other than contrast enhancement on MRI (observed in only 4/14 (29%) of the IRIS cases), no statistical differences in clinical factors were observed between groups.[116]

Given these discouraging observations, a recent analysis examined the possible role of corticosteroid therapy in the management of PML IRIS. It included a total of 54 patients who met criteria for PML-IRIS, of which 36 had an "unmasking" PML-IRIS and who were asymptomatic at baseline and 18 of which who had pre-existing PML at HAART initiation but who experienced a "paradoxical" PML-IRIS event. A total of only 12 patients received corticosteroids, and no difference in survival was noted between those who received corticosteroids and those who did not. For some corticosteroid cases, the therapy was administered late, when the patient was moribund. When analyzed separately, those who received corticosteroids earlier in their PML IRIS event, and for a longer duration, tended to have better outcomes. An additional caveat to this study is the fact that only 21/37 (57%) of patients had contrast-enhancing lesions at the time of IRIS. Of those who received corticosteroids and who survived, 6/7 (86%) exhibited such contrast enhancement, whereas only 1/5 (20%) with a poor corticosteroid outcome exhibited such a finding.[117] Thus, corticosteroids could arguably have a role in the treatment of PML-IRIS in those patients who exhibit contrast enhancement on CT or MRI, suggesting an excessive inflammatory component possibly due to cytotoxic CD8 T cell infiltration. However, such enhancement could be a sign of a beneficial immune response,[111,118] and the challenge, as with all manifestations of IRIS, is balancing the beneficial and harmful effects of immune reconstitution through the use of such immunomodulatory therapy.

Kaposi's Sarcoma (KS)

The introduction of HAART led to improved survival even in patients with advanced Kaposi's sarcoma (KS) and has been associated with complete resolution of KS lesions.[119,120] However, as with other opportunistic infections, the introduction of HAART led to the recognition that some KS lesions could undergo expansion despite ongoing treatment.[121–123] The primary concern regarding KS-IRIS is the potential for life-threatening dramatic presentations of the syndrome. Such cases include explosive growth of oral lesions with severe epistaxis and lesion bleeding requiring tracheostomy for airway compromise and massive gastrointestinal bleeding from KS-IRIS lesions.[19,124] Even in the absence of bleeding and hemorrhage from the lesions, the associated edema can be severe or disfiguring.[123] The propensity for bleeding and hemorrhage may be related to the irregular vascular lesions observed in the histology of these KS specimens. With immune reconstitution, intra-lesion infiltrates of CD4 and/or CD8 T lymphocytes may precipitate significant inflammation with disruption of these vascular spaces within these lesions with resulting edema and hemorrhage.

In a large, prospective cohort of patients initiating HAART at a single center, 10/150 (6.7%) experienced rapid expansion of existing KS lesions and the appearance of new KS lesions within 2 months of HAART initiation. The primary difference between KS-IRIS and non-IRIS groups was a significantly higher median CD4 count at HAART initiation (335 versus 121 cells/mm^3, respectively; p=0.028). Interestingly, non-IRIS patients demonstrated a significant increase in CD4 cell count compared to baseline during the 2-year follow-up. This difference may be a result of the higher baseline CD4 counts in KS-IRIS patients, or may be secondary to the fact that 5 of the 10 KS-IRIS patients received chemotherapy or radiotherapy within the first year of HAART. Lastly, KS-IRIS patients exhibited significantly more KS-associated edema (p=0.013). In a review of KS-IRIS, cases were noted to occur as early as 3 weeks following HAART initiation, with most cases occurring within 2 months of initiation.[122]

In general, IRIS-associated KS lesions are clinically similar to those that are not IRIS-associated. This is supported by an analysis of pulmonary KS-IRIS lesions in four HIV-infected patients experiencing the syndrome. Characteristics included those similar to non-IRIS pulmonary KS (reticular and reticulonodular opacities, consolidation, lymphadenopathy, interlobular septal thickening, and pleural effusions), but the severity of lymphadenopathy and pleural effusions noted in the IRIS patients was greater.[125] Cutaneous KS-IRIS lesions may appear darker in color or may be associated with peripheral redness, indicative of possible increased localized inflammation, with or without signs of edema.[123,124] This observation, coupled with the increased severity of pulmonary manifestations, is the strongest clinical evidence for an exaggerated inflammatory response that characterizes IRIS.

Once diagnosed, the treatment of KS-IRIS follows that for non-IRIS KS disease and involves continuation of HAART and initiation of single or combination chemotherapy with agents such as vinblastine, vincristine, etoposide, adriamycin, paclitaxel, or bleomycin. Thalidomide is also used, given its propensity to block angioneogenesis.[126] Other novel therapies specific to treatment of KS-IRIS involve intramuscular injections of interferon-∝ administered with HAART, which resulted in total resolution of KS-IRIS lesions in one patient.[127] Although the overall prognosis for disseminated KS is poor, no difference in time to chemotherapy or radiotherapy was noted in one cohort.[128] Thus, although occasionally dramatic and severe, the expansion of KS-IRIS lesions are transient, and collective case series data suggest KS-IRIS lesions are just as responsive to appropriate therapy as are non-IRIS KS.

Dermatologic IRIS

A wide array of other dermatologic IRIS manifestations may occur. Some of these manifestations are described in disease-specific sections and will not be discussed in detail here. The proportion of patients developing dermatologic IRIS depends on the study population and on the level of vigilance for subtle dermatologic manifestations. In both developed and resource-limited settings, dermatologic or orogenital diseases account for a significant proportion of IRIS events. These presentations can be divided into those secondary to common cutaneous virus eruptions —for example, varicella zoster virus (VZV) and herpes simplex virus (HSV)—and other, less common dermatologic manifestations.

HSV/VZV

Following the introduction of protease inhibitor-containing HAART, an increase in the incidence of HSV infection was noted, occurring in 14/193 of patients.[129] Of these, 12/14 (86%) cases occurred between 4 and 16 weeks. The incidence noted during entire study period was 6.2 episodes/100 patient-years, more than twice the incidence of 3.0 episodes/100 patient-years reported before the introduction of HAART.[129,130] This increased incidence, with a clustering of cases soon after HAART initiation, lent early support to these cases being IRIS. Subsequent IRIS case series estimate that between 5% and 12% of patients initiating HAART will develop VZV-IRIS.[17,18,20,27,129,131,132]

In addition to VZV-IRIS, herpes simplex virus (HSV) accounts for a significant burden of IRIS disease in patients initiating HAART. This is true in both adults and children (see the section on Pediatric IRIS, below). However, in adults HSV-IRIS manifests more commonly as orogenital disease, reflecting the higher prevalence of HSV type 2 disease in this population. In large case cohorts in developed settings, genital HSV disease accounted for 15% to 50% of all IRIS cases.[16,18] Genital HSV-IRIS disease appears to be common in Sub-Saharan cohorts as well, accounting for 9.7% of probable IRIS cases in a large cohort of 498 adult HIV-infected patients initiating HAART.[27]

Clinically, most patients experiencing VZV- or HSV-IRIS manifest presentations that are typical for the disease, such as dermatomal zoster distributions and vesicular genital eruptions.[16,18,129] However, severe cases can occur. In one such case, HAART initiation resulted in VZV-associated transverse myelitis and meningitis.[133] This case provides some of the only pathology in VZV-IRIS whereby CSF examination revealed most cells to be activated (CD38+ and CD69+) natural killer (NK) cells and CD8+ lymphocytes, suggesting a role for viral antigen-specific CD8+ lymphocytes in the pathogenesis of the disease. Treatment for such severe CNS or disseminated cases may require high-dose corticosteroids.[133] Otherwise, as in HIV-uninfected VZV patients, the use of oral acyclovir facilitates healing, shortens the duration of zoster-associated pain in HIV-infected patients, and may be used in combination with oral corticosteroids to shorten the duration of pain and improve quality of life.[134–136] No prospective trials involving the prophylactic use of antivirals for the prevention of HSV- or VZV-IRIS have been performed.

Other Dermatologic Manifestations

Common genital manifestations of importance are expansion of genital warts and molluscum contagiosum.[18,19,27] Common cutaneous manifestations include a generalized folliculitis, termed immune recovery folliculitis (see **Figure 17–4**),[137] which can be differentiated from HIV eosinophilic folliculitis, which is more chronic and lacks association with HAART initiation. Immune recovery folliculitis represented 39/144 (27.1%) of IRIS cases in a recent prospective South African cohort study.[27] Dermatologic IRIS manifestations are usually self-limited. Other dermatologic manifestations are less common and are listed in **Table 17–2**.

Cytomegalovirus (CMV)

Although cytomegalovirus (CMV) can present in unusual forms, such as CMV colitis[138] and encephalitis,[16] the most common infection manifestation is CMV retinitis. As with other opportunistic infections, the introduction of HAART changed the presentation of the disease. CMV-IRIS can present as either an unmasking or paradoxical form. Shortly after the introduction of HAART, the unmasking form of CMV-IRIS was described in five patients who developed CMV retinitis within 4 to 7 weeks of HAART initiation suggesting, a HAART-induced inflammatory immune response to subclinical CMV ocular infection through restored CMV-specific

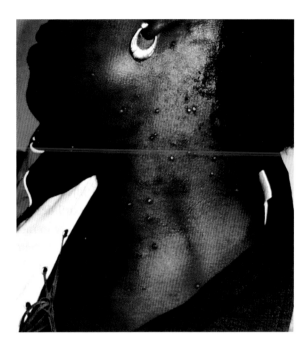

Figure 17–4. *Immune recovery folliculitis in a patient on antiretroviral therapy for 4 weeks.*

immunity.[139] Soon thereafter, a new presentation of CMV surfaced, exhibiting significant posterior segment ocular inflammation thought to be due to the presence of residual CMV antigens or proteins that serve as the antigenic stimulus for the syndrome. This paradoxical presentation, termed immune recovery vitritis (IRV) or immune recovery uveitis (IRU), occurs in patients with previously diagnosed and treated CMV retinitis.[140,141]

Estimates of CMV-IRIS are predominately derived from cohorts in resource-rich countries. One early, retrospective study reported the development of IRU in 19/30 (63%) of HAART responders with a CD4 cell count increase of ≥60 cells/mm^3 for ≥2 months and a pre-existing history of ocular CMV disease. In contrast, HAART non-responders exhibited no IRU. The median time to IRV was 43 weeks (95% confidence interval [CI]: 35–47).[142] Another estimate found that 5/33 (15.2%) of HAART responders exhibited symptoms of IRU.[143] A later prospective study involving 19 U.S. AIDS ophthalmology clinics reported that 31/176 (17.6%) of patients with a prior history of CMV retinitis developed IRU. Again, distinctions were made between HAART responders and nonresponders (CD4 count was ≥100 cells/mm^3 and also ≥50 cells/mm^3 higher than their observed nadir level at enrollment). Male gender, use of HAART, higher CD4 cell counts, and involvement of the posterior retinal pole were factors associated with a reduced risk for developing IRU, whereas prior use of intravitreous injections of cidofovir, large retinal lesions, and adequate immune recovery on HAART were associated with increased risk.[144]

Some progress has been made with a longitudinal cohort where 5/179 (2.8%) of patients were identified as having relapsing CMV retinitis at a median time 1.1 months from HAART initiation. All patients who suffered CMR retinitis IRIS were on anti-CMV therapy at the timing of the IRIS event. Compared to non-CMV IRIS patients, those experiencing CMV-IRIS exhibited significantly higher increases in CMV-specific IgG after HAART initiation and increased plasma levels of soluble CD30 (sCD30), a member of the tumor necrosis factor receptor (TNFR) super-family expressed on T cells, producing predominantly Th2 cytokines. Although CMV-IRIS patients exhibited a significant increase in CD4 cell counts, no difference was noted in CD8 cell counts.[141] In addition to these peripheral responses, histologic specimens of epiretinal mem-

causes, where most presentations occur within 3 months of HAART initiation and is a necessary, defining requirement for TB-IRIS.[26]

In addition to sarcoidosis, autoimmune thyroid disease is also common.[161] Detailed cases of autoimmune thyroid disease and Grave's disease provide some of the strongest support for pathologic rheumatologic IRIS manifestations, rather than simply incident rheumatologic disease. In one such case, a patient suffered from two episodes of autoimmune thyroid disease after two HAART initiation instances, supported by temporal dramatic increases in CD4 cell counts, suppression of thyroid stimulating hormone levels, and elevated free tetraiodothyronine and tri-iodothyronine levels. These episodes of Grave's disease were simultaneously accompanied by alopecia universalis, an autoimmune disease characterized by follicular cytotoxic CD8 T lymphocytes and CD4 lymphocytes.[162]

Other forms of autoimmune IRIS include systemic lupus erythematosus,[163] polymyositis,[164] Still's disease,[165,166] and rheumatoid arthritis.[167] Some rheumatologic diseases have decreased since HAART introduction, including reactive arthritis, psoriatic arthritis, and polyarthritis.[161] In their longitudinal cohort, the incidence of rheumatologic diseases did not significantly change between the pre-HAART and HAART eras. Rather, rheumatologic diseases with an inflammatory basis—such as reactive arthritis—decreased, and diseases such as diffuse infiltrative lymphocytosis syndrome persisted. This observation reinforces the fact that significant immune activation and elevated inflammation levels characterize HIV disease. For most patients, the introduction of HAART yields the beneficial responses of immune restoration and suppression of HIV RNA levels and their associated immune activation. Beneficial effects on the overall incidence of chronic inflammatory disease such as reactive arthritis are thus observed. However, in a subset of patients, this favorable balance is disrupted, culminating in IRIS through an as yet unknown immunologic mechanism.

Although treatment with corticosteroids is arguably beneficial in the setting of an infectious IRIS pathogen, their use in rheumatologic IRIS processes is perhaps more easily understandable, given their use in the management of these rheumatologic diseases outside of the context of IRIS, in association with their noninfectious pathogenesis. Most episodes of arthritis and inflammatory rheumatologic IRIS events respond to various steroid therapies.[161,167] However, adverse effects of steroid therapy on beneficial CD4 reconstitution have been observed, with increased difficulty in managing some patients' underlying HIV infection while on potent immunosuppressive medications.[166]

Other Noninfectious Manifestations of IRIS

Other uncommon noninfectious IRIS manifestations exhibit interesting insights. A case report highlighting the occurrence of IRIS in association with intradermal tattoo ink illustrates the common requirement of a precipitating antigen for occurrence of the syndrome, with overlying inflammation following the tattoo markings within 2 months of HAART initiation. Although a biopsy did not mention the specific infiltrative cell type, a granulomatous and eczematous reaction was described without the observation of any infectious organisms.[168] The occurrence of a granulomatous reaction in this case suggests a complex interplay between activated helper T lymphocytes, macrophages, and cytokine secretion such as tumor necrosis factor-α. In other manifestations of IRIS, such as HBV- and HCV-induced liver enzyme elevations, a hepatocytotoxic T cell and monocyte response within the liver as a result of elevated CXCL-10 levels and resulting IFN-γ is thought to be the primary mechanism.[156] Thus, from a common precipitating antigen, whether infectious or noninfectious, different immunologic mechanisms are thought to be responsible for the various clinical and immunohistologic manifestations of the syndrome.[169]

Other uncommon noninfectious IRIS occurrences are listed in **Table 17–2**.

Pediatric IRIS

By the end of 2007, the number of children receiving HAART in low- and middle-income countries rose to 200,000 up from 75,000 in 2005. This is still a minority of the estimated 780,000 children in need of HAART, with children constituting only 6% of the estimated 3 million HIV-infected people on HAART in low- and middle-income countries.[170] Mirroring the adult experience, this increasing access to pediatric HAART has also meant increasing reports of IRIS. Despite their young age, the underlying OI burden in this population is as at least as high, with up to 48% of children in highly endemic TB areas undergoing TB therapy at HAART initiation.[171]

As in adults, the diagnosis of IRIS in the pediatric population is based on clinical signs and symptoms. Although preliminary case definitions for pediatric IRIS have been presented,[172] the added difficulty of TB diagnosis in the infant and younger pediatric population make definitively fulfilling IRIS diagnostic criteria even more problematic than in adults. Nevertheless, easily recognized IRIS manifestations do occur, and numerous retrospective and prospective pediatric IRIS cohorts have been described in the literature.

Most early data on pediatric IRIS incidence is from retrospective studies conducted in Thailand, where 29/153 (19%) of patients experienced a total of 32 episodes of IRIS. The pattern is similar to that of adults. The majority of cases were due to mycobacterial organisms (14 episodes, 43%), and there were 3 episodes of *Cryptococcus neoformans* infection. Varicella-zoster virus and herpes simplex virus were frequent etiologies (7 episodes each).[173] This well-characterized cohort was followed by a prospective study in South Africa, where 34/162 (21%) of children developed IRIS. However, in contrast to the Thailand study, BCG-related complications were most frequent (24/34, 70.6%) in the South African study, with six demonstrating smear positive samples and three having concurrent *M. tuberculosis* complex cultures.[33]

Common Infectious Etiologies in the Pediatric Population

BCG Disease

One distinct difference in the presentation of IRIS in the pediatric population is the occurrence of IRIS after vaccination with Bacille Calmette-Guérin (BCG), a live attenuated *Mycobacterium bovis* vaccine. Irrespective of IRIS, disseminated BCG disease due to vaccination of HIV-infected children has been a concern and source of debate in the pediatric HIV vaccination literature. Following data that indicate HIV-infected children are at a substantially increased risk of developing disseminated BCG infection, which is associated with a mortality of 75% to 86%, [174,175] revisions to WHO guidelines included HIV infection as an absolute contraindication to BCG vaccination, even in areas of high rates of endemic TB.[176, 177]

The most well-characterized pediatric BCG cohort reported 21 BCG-related complications in 162 HIV-infected children following HAART initiation. In this series, complications occurred at a median of 34 days following HAART (interquartile range, 15–60 days). All 21 patients demonstrated ipsilateral regional disease and five demonstrated ulceration or abscess formation at the vaccination site.[33] Case reports of BCG-IRIS highlight the potential adverse effects of this vaccine in HIV-infected children. Clinical manifestations include limited lymphadenopathy and/or lymphadenitis, but can include more suppuration and abscess formation (**Figure 17–5**).[178,179] Abscess formation occurs within 4–10 weeks at the site of vaccination, although cases of BCG-IRIS have occurred as soon as one week postvaccination.[179, 180] Other presentations include disseminated BCG disease with bone and pulmonary involvement.[181]

TB and Other Mycobacteria

In addition to *M. bovis*, other tuberculous and nontuberculous mycobacteria have been implicated in pediatric IRIS. Cases of *M. tuberculosis* present most often with pulmonary manifestations, but extrapulmonary and disseminated cases do occur.[33,182,183] In general, TB-IRIS occurs soon after HAART initiation, and usually within the first 3 months. In a series of 11 HIV-infected children who experienced unmasking or paradoxical TB-IRIS, 7 experienced unmasking TB-IRIS after a median 25 days (range, 8–54 days) of starting HAART. Those experiencing the paradoxical form were on TB treatment at HAART initiation, with paradoxical reactions occurring between 6 and 105 days post-HAART initiation.[182] Unmasking and paradoxical pediatric pulmonary TB-IRIS cases can be as dramatic as those seen in adults, with worsening of pulmonary infiltrates or parenchymal disease in 90% and tracheal compression, with or without pleural effusions, in 45.5%.[181]

Herpes Simplex and Varicella Zoster Viruses

Although infrequently observed in one prospective pediatric IRIS study[33] and constituting all of observed IRIS cases in another,[184] other common etiologic agents involved in pediatric IRIS cohorts include varicella zoster virus (VZV) (21.9%–35.3% of IRIS events) and herpes simplex labialis (18.7%–35.3% of IRIS events).[173,183] These usually present in a typical fashion (for example, ulcerative cutaneous eruptions), are usually mild to moderate in severity, and are not associated with any increased risk of disseminated disease, with only one case of HSV encephalitis being reported in children.[173] Of 20 cases of VZV-IRIS reported in three large cohorts, eruptions were typical in appearance and presentation and none involved disseminated VZV or

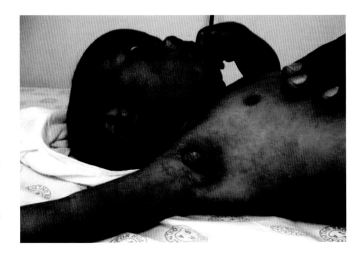

Figure 17–5. *BCG adenitis in a child following the initiation of antiretroviral therapy. Photo courtesy of the Harriet Shezi Clinic, Baragwanath Hospital, Johannesburg, South Africa.*

atypical lesions. Where reported, hospitalization occurred in only three patients and outcomes were favorable, with all patients responding to oral or intravenous acyclovir.[173,183,184]

Cryptococcus

Cryptococcal meningitis IRIS (CM-IRIS) is much less frequently observed in the pediatric population, mirroring the lower general incidence seen when compared with HIV infected adults, although underreporting may play a role. Of 83 episodes of pediatric IRIS reported across three continents, only three (3.6%) cases were due to CM-IRIS, all of which occurred in Thailand.[33,173,183] All three of these patients had CM diagnosed prior to HAART and were receiving fluconazole antifungal therapy at HAART initiation. All three suffered from headache and fever. One patient was noncompliant and demonstrated CSF cultures positive for *C. neoformans*, and the remaining two were diagnosed clinically and demonstrated positive serum cryptococcal antigen at the IRIS event. Due to the lack of cases in the pediatric population, specific recommendations for diagnosis and therapy for pediatric CM-IRIS cannot be made.

Other Etiologies

In addition to these infectious agents, additional rare IRIS presentations in children include Guillain-Barré syndrome,[173] pulmonary Kaposi's sarcoma,[181] and bacterial sepsis.[33] Although dermatologic IRIS has been reported in the form of severe seborrheic dermatitis,[33] pediatric dermatologic IRIS is underreported, possibly secondary to the occurrence of common dermatologic problems such as infant acne/folliculitis and contact dermatitis normally encountered in this population. In contrast to adults, noninfectious and rheumatologic IRIS manifestations are not reported, probably due to the lack of prevalence of such diseases in the pediatric population.

Predictive Factors and Immunopathogenesis of Pediatric IRIS

As with adults, predictive clinical factors for developing the syndrome are varied and often inconsistent across cohorts of pediatric patients. Furthermore, immunologic studies are often difficult to perform in the pediatric population secondary to limited blood sampling, access to well-characterized cohorts, and ethical considerations.

A number of epidemiologic studies have attempted to determine predictors of pediatric IRIS. As in adults, many of these efforts have focused immune assessment on the measurement of CD4 cell counts and HIV RNA levels. In all-cause IRIS, studies indicate that it is associated with a lower baseline CD4 percentage[33,173] and younger age (7 months versus 10 months, $p=0.007$).[33,178] Although these findings were not replicated in another study, children who experienced the syndrome had a higher baseline HIV RNA level[178,183] and at least one indicator of malnutrition.[183] The association of HIV-associated IRIS with malnutrition is provocative, given that IRIS and exuberant episodes of inflammation have been noted in malnourished children.[8] Such paradoxical reactions in severely malnourished children during therapeutic refeeding occurred in 29.1% of 4,382 famine victims, manifested as an exacerbation of a pre-existing infection or the emergence of a latent infection after 2 weeks of re-feeding. Contrary to expectation, those who experienced an incident infection exhibited higher mean weight gains than those who did not experience a paradoxical infection. Severe malnutrition results in several important host immunologic changes, particularly in immunologic mechanisms that are crucial

10. Crespo G, Cervera C, Michelena J, Marco F, Moreno A, Navasa M. Immune reconstitution syndrome after voriconazole treatment for cryptococcal meningitis in a liver transplant recipient. Liver Transpl 2008;14:1671–1674.

11. Egli A, Bergamin O, Mullhaupt B, Seebach JD, Mueller NJ, Hirsch HH. Cytomegalovirus-associated chorioretinitis after liver transplantation: case report and review of the literature. Transpl Infect Dis 2008;10:27–43.

12. Lortholary O, Fontanet A, Memain N, Martin A, Sitbon K, Dromer F. Incidence and risk factors of immune reconstitution inflammatory syndrome complicating HIV associated cryptococcosis in France. Aids 2005;19:1043–1049.

13. Singh N, Dromer F, Perfect JR, Lortholary O. Cryptococcosis in solid organ transplant recipients: current state of the science. Clin Infect Dis 2008;47:1321–1327.

14. Singh N, Perfect JR. Immune reconstitution syndrome and exacerbation of infections after pregnancy. Clin Infect Dis 2007;45:1192–1199.

15. French MA, Mallal SA, Dawkins RL. Zidovudine-induced restoration of cell-mediated immunity to mycobacteria in immunodeficient HIV-infected patients. Aids 1992;6:1293–1297.

16. French MA, Lenzo N, John M, et al. Immune restoration disease after the treatment of immunodeficient HIV-infected patients with highly active antiretroviral therapy. HIV Med 2000;1:107–115.

17. Jevtovic DJ, Salemovic D, Ranin J, Pesic I, Zerjav S, Djurkovic-Djakovic O. The prevalence and risk of immune restoration disease in HIV-infected patients treated with highly active antiretroviral therapy. HIV Med 2005;6:140–143.

18. Ratnam I, Chiu C, Kandala NB, Easterbrook PJ. Incidence and risk factors for immune reconstitution inflammatory syndrome in an ethnically diverse HIV type 1-infected cohort. Clin Infect Dis 2006;42:418–427.

19. Murdoch DM, Venter WD, Feldman C, Van Rie A. Incidence and risk factors for the immune reconstitution inflammatory syndrome in HIV patients in South Africa: a prospective study. AIDS 2008;22:601–610.

20. Huruy K, Mulu A, Mengistu G, et al. Immune reconstitution inflammatory syndrome among HIV/AIDS patients during highly active antiretroviral therapy in Addis Ababa, Ethiopia. Jpn J Infect Dis 2008;61:205–209.

21. Klotz SA, Aziz Mohammed A, Girmai Woldemichael M, Worku Mitku M, Handrich M. Immune reconstitution inflammatory syndrome in a resource-poor setting. J Int Assoc Physicians AIDS Care (Chic Ill) 2009;8:122–127.

22. French MA, Price P, Stone SF. Immune restoration disease after antiretroviral therapy. AIDS 2004;18:1615–1627.

23. Shelburne SA, Montes M, Hamill RJ. Immune reconstitution inflammatory syndrome: more answers, more questions. J Antimicrob Chemother 2006;57:167–170.

24. Castelnuovo B, Manabe YC, Kiragga A, Kamya M, Easterbrook P, Kambugu A. Cause-specific mortality and the contribution of immune reconstitution inflammatory syndrome in the first 3 years after antiretroviral therapy initiation in an urban African cohort. Clin Infect Dis 2009;49:965–972.

25. Colebunders R, John L, Huyst V, Kambugu A, Scano F, Lynen L. Tuberculosis immune reconstitution inflammatory syndrome in countries with limited resources. Int J Tuberc Lung Dis 2006;10:946–953.

26. Meintjes G, Lawn SD, Scano F, et al. Tuberculosis-associated immune reconstitution inflammatory syndrome: case definitions for use in resource-limited settings. Lancet Infect Dis 2008;8:516–523.

27. Haddow LJ, Easterbrook PJ, Mosam A, et al. Defining immune reconstitution inflammatory syndrome: evaluation of expert opinion versus 2 case definitions in a South African cohort. Clin Infect Dis 2009;49:1424–1432.

28. Robertson J, Meier M, Wall J, Ying J, Fichtenbaum CJ. Immune reconstitution syndrome in HIV: validating a case definition and identifying clinical predictors in persons initiating antiretroviral therapy. Clin Infect Dis 2006;42:1639-46.

29. International Network for the Study of HIV-Associated IRIS (INSHI). 2009. Accessed September 4, 2009, 2009, at http://www.inshi.umn.edu/.

30. Shelburne SA, 3rd, Darcourt J, White AC, Jr., et al. The role of immune reconstitution inflammatory syndrome in AIDS-related Cryptococcus neoformans disease in the era of highly active antiretroviral therapy. Clin Infect Dis 2005;40:1049–1052.

31. World Health Organization. Towards Universal Access: Scaling up priority HIV/AIDS interventions in the health sector. September 2009 Progress Report.

32. Manabe YC, Campbell JD, Sydnor E, Moore RD. Immune reconstitution inflammatory syndrome: risk factors and treatment implications. J Acquir Immune Defic Syndr 2007;46:456–462.

33. Smith K, Kuhn L, Coovadia A, et al. Immune reconstitution inflammatory syndrome among HIV-infected South African infants initiating antiretroviral therapy. AIDS 2009;23:1097–1107.

34. Pepper DJ, Marais S, Maartens G, et al. Neurologic manifestations of paradoxical tuberculosis-associated immune reconstitution inflammatory syndrome: a case series. Clin Infect Dis 2009;48:e96–107.

35. Bicanic T, Meintjes G, Rebe K, et al. Immune reconstitution inflammatory syndrome in HIV-associated cryptococcal meningitis: a prospective study. J Acquir Immune Defic Syndr 2009;51:130–134.

36. Kambugu A, Meya DB, Rhein J, et al. Outcomes of cryptococcal meningitis in Uganda before and after the availability of highly active antiretroviral therapy. Clin Infect Dis 2008;46:1694–1701.

37. Sungkanuparph S, Filler SG, Chetchotisakd P, et al. Cryptococcal immune reconstitution inflammatory syndrome after antiretroviral therapy in AIDS patients with cryptococcal meningitis: a prospective multicenter study. Clin Infect Dis 2009;49:931–934.

38. Sungkanuparph S, Jongwutiwes U, Kiertiburanakul S. Timing of cryptococcal immune reconstitution inflammatory syndrome after antiretroviral therapy in patients with AIDS and cryptococcal meningitis. J Acquir Immune Defic Syndr 2007;45:595–596.

39. Kaech SM, Hemby S, Kersh E, Ahmed R. Molecular and functional profiling of memory CD8 T cell differentiation. Cell 2002;111:837–851.

40. Davies MA, Meintjes G. Assessing the contribution of the immune reconstitution inflammatory syndrome to mortality in developing country antiretroviral therapy programs. Clin Infect Dis 2009;49:973–975.

41. Yiannoutsos CT, An MW, Frangakis CE, et al. Sampling-based approaches to improve estimation of mortality among patient dropouts: experience from a large PEPFAR-funded program in Western Kenya. PLoS One 2008;3:e3843.

42. Braitstein P, Brinkhof MW, Dabis F, et al. Mortality of HIV-1-infected patients in the first year of antiretroviral therapy: comparison between low-income and high-income countries. Lancet 2006;367:817–824.

43. Lawn SD, Harries AD, Anglaret X, Myer L, Wood R. Early mortality among adults accessing antiretroviral treatment programmes in sub-Saharan Africa. AIDS 2008;22:1897–1908.

44. Lawn SD, Bekker LG, Miller RF. Immune reconstitution disease associated with mycobacterial infections in HIV-infected individuals receiving antiretrovirals. Lancet Infect Dis 2005;5:361–373.

45. Breton G, Duval X, Estellat C, et al. Determinants of immune reconstitution inflammatory syndrome in HIV type 1-infected patients with tuberculosis after initiation of antiretroviral therapy. Clin Infect Dis 2004;39:1709–1712.

46. Burman W, Weis S, Vernon A, et al. Frequency, severity and duration of immune reconstitution events in HIV-related tuberculosis. Int J Tuberc Lung Dis 2007;11:1282–1289.

47. Kumarasamy N, Chaguturu S, Mayer KH, et al. Incidence of Immune Reconstitution Syndrome in HIV/Tuberculosis-Coinfected Patients After Initiation of Generic Antiretroviral Therapy in India. J Acquir Immune Defic Syndr 2004;37:1574–1576.

48. Lawn SD, Myer L, Bekker LG, Wood R. Tuberculosis-associated immune reconstitution disease: incidence, risk factors and impact in an antiretroviral treatment service in South Africa. AIDS 2007;21:335-41.

49. Manosuthi W, Chaovavanich A, Tansuphaswadikul S, et al. Incidence and risk factors of major opportunistic infections after initiation of antiretroviral therapy among advanced HIV-infected patients in a resource-limited setting. J Infect 2007;55:464–469.

50. Michailidis C, Pozniak AL, Mandalia S, Basnayake S, Nelson MR, Gazzard BG. Clinical characteristics of IRIS syndrome in patients with HIV and tuberculosis. Antivir Ther 2005;10:417–422.

51. Patel KK, Patel AK, Sarda P, Shah BA, Ranjan R. Immune reconstitution visceral leishmaniasis presented as hemophagocytic syndrome in a patient with AIDS from a nonendemic area: a case report. J Int Assoc Physicians AIDS Care (Chic Ill) 2009;8:217–220.

52. Serra FC, Hadad D, Orofino RL, et al. Immune reconstitution syndrome in patients treated for HIV and tuberculosis in Rio de Janeiro. Braz J Infect Dis 2007;11:462–465.

53. Shelburne SA, Visnegarwala F, Darcourt J, et al. Incidence and risk factors for immune reconstitution inflammatory syndrome during highly active antiretroviral therapy. Aids 2005;19:399–406.

54. Wendel KA, Alwood KS, Gachuhi R, Chaisson RE, Bishai WR, Sterling TR. Paradoxical worsening of tuberculosis in HIV-infected persons. Chest 2001;120:193–197.

55. Breen RA, Smith CJ, Bettinson H, et al. Paradoxical reactions during tuberculosis treatment in patients with and without HIV co-infection. Thorax 2004;59:704–707.

56. Manosuthi W, Kiertiburanakul S, Phoorisri T, Sungkanuparph S. Immune reconstitution inflammatory syndrome of tuberculosis among HIV-infected patients receiving antituberculous and antiretroviral therapy. J Infect 2006;53:357–363.

57. Navas E, Martin-Davila P, Moreno L, et al. Paradoxical reactions of tuberculosis in patients with the acquired immunodeficiency syndrome who are treated with highly active antiretroviral therapy. Arch Intern Med 2002;162:97–99.

58. Schiffer JT, Sterling TR. Timing of antiretroviral therapy initiation in tuberculosis patients with AIDS: a decision analysis. J Acquir Immune Defic Syndr 2007;44:229–234.

59. Abdool Karim SS, Naidoo K, Grobler A, et al. Timing of Initiation of Antiretroviral Drugs during Tuberculosis Therapy. N Engl J Med 2010;362:697–706.

60. Fishman JE, Saraf-Lavi E, Narita M, Hollender ES, Ramsinghani R, Ashkin D. Pulmonary tuberculosis in AIDS patients: transient chest radiographic worsening after initiation of antiretroviral therapy. AJR Am J Roentgenol 2000;174:43–49.

61. Buckingham SJ, Haddow LJ, Shaw PJ, Miller RF. Immune reconstitution inflammatory syndrome in HIV-infected patients with mycobacterial infections starting highly active anti-retroviral therapy. Clin Radiol 2004;59:505–513.

62. Schluger NW, Perez D, Liu YM. Reconstitution of immune responses to tuberculosis in patients with HIV infection who receive antiretroviral therapy. Chest 2002;122.597–3602.

63. Autran B, Carcelain G, Li TS, et al. Positive effects of combined antiretroviral therapy on CD4 T cell homeostasis and function in advanced HIV disease. Science 1997;277:112–116.

64. Bucy RP, Hockett RD, Derdeyn CA, et al. Initial increase in blood CD4(+) lymphocytes after HIV antiretroviral therapy reflects redistribution from lymphoid tissues. J Clin Invest 1999;103:1391–1398.

65. Murdoch DM, Venter WD, Van Rie A, Feldman C. Immune reconstitution inflammatory syndrome (IRIS): review of common infectious manifestations and treatment options. AIDS Res Ther 2007;4:9.

66. Bourgarit A, Carcelain G, Martinez V, et al. Explosion of tuberculin-specific Th1-responses induces immune restoration syndrome in tuberculosis and HIV co-infected patients. Aids 2006;20:F1–7.

67. Meintjes G, Wilkinson KA, Rangaka MX, et al. Type 1 helper T cells and FoxP3-positive T cells in HIV-tuberculosis-associated immune reconstitution inflammatory syndrome. Am J Respir Crit Care Med 2008;178:1083–1089.

68. Tan DB, Yong YK, Tan HY, et al. Immunological profiles of immune restoration disease presenting as mycobacterial lymphadenitis and cryptococcal meningitis. HIV Med 2008;9:307–316.

69. Seddiki N, Sasson SC, Santner-Nanan B, et al. Proliferation of weakly suppressive regulatory CD4+ T cells is associated with over-active CD4+ T-cell responses in HIV-positive patients with mycobacterial immune restoration disease. Eur J Immunol 2009;39:391–403.

70. Bourgarit A, Carcelain G, Samri A, et al. Tuberculosis-associated immune restoration syndrome in HIV-1-infected patients involves tuberculin-specific CD4 Th1 cells and KIR-negative gammadelta T cells. J Immunol 2009;183:3915–3923.

71. Murdoch DM, Suchard MS, Venter WD, et al. Polychromatic immunophenotypic characterization of T cell profiles among HIV-infected patients experiencing immune reconstitution inflammatory syndrome (IRIS). AIDS Res Ther 2009;6:16.

72. Meintjes G, Rangaka MX, Maartens G, et al. Novel relationship between tuberculosis immune reconstitution inflammatory syndrome and antitubercular drug resistance. Clin Infect Dis 2009;48:667–676.

73. Breen RA, Smith CJ, Cropley I, Johnson MA, Lipman MC. Does immune reconstitution syndrome promote active tuberculosis in patients receiving highly active antiretroviral therapy? Aids 2005;19:1201–1206.

74. Lawn SD, Badri M, Wood R. Tuberculosis among HIV-infected patients receiving HAART: long term incidence and risk factors in a South African cohort. AIDS 2005;19:2109–2116.

75. Bonnet MM, Pinoges LL, Varaine FF, et al. Tuberculosis after HAART initiation in HIV-positive patients from five countries with a high tuberculosis burden. AIDS 2006;20:1275–1279.

76. Girardi E, Sabin CA, d'Arminio Monforte A, et al. Incidence of Tuberculosis among HIV-infected patients receiving highly active antiretroviral therapy in Europe and North America. Clin Infect Dis 2005;41:1772–1782.

77. Zolopa A, Andersen J, Powderly W, et al. Early antiretroviral therapy reduces AIDS progression/death in individuals with acute opportunistic infections: a multicenter randomized strategy trial. PLoS One 2009;4:e5575.

78. Meintjes G, Wilkinson R, Morroni C, et al. Randomized Placebo-controlled Trial of Prednisone for the TB Immune Reconstitution Inflammatory Syndrome. In: 16th Conference on Retroviruses and Opportunistic Infections; 2009; Boston, MA; February 8–11; 2009.

79. Dooley DP, Carpenter JL, Rademacher S. Adjunctive corticosteroid therapy for tuberculosis: a critical reappraisal of the literature. Clin Infect Dis 1997;25:872–887.

80. Thwaites GE, Nguyen DB, Nguyen HD, et al. Dexamethasone for the treatment of tuberculous meningitis in adolescents and adults. N Engl J Med 2004;351:1741–1751.

81. Phillips P, Kwiatkowski MB, Copland M, Craib K, Montaner J. Mycobacterial lymphadenitis associated with the initiation of combination antiretroviral therapy. J Acquir Immune Defic Syndr Hum Retrovirol 1999;20:122–128.

82. Race EM, Adelson-Mitty J, Kriegel GR, et al. Focal mycobacterial lymphadenitis following initiation of protease-inhibitor therapy in patients with advanced HIV-1 disease. Lancet 1998;351:252–255.

83. Cabie A, Abel S, Brebion A, Desbois N, Sobesky G. Mycobacterial lymphadenitis after initiation of highly active antiretroviral therapy. Eur J Clin Microbiol Infect Dis 1998;17:812–813.

84. Behrens G, Knuth C, Schedel I, Mendila M, Schmidt RE. Highly active antiretroviral therapy. Lancet 1998;351:1057–1058; author reply 8–9.

85. Desimone JA, Jr., Babinchak TJ, Kaulback KR, Pomerantz RJ. Treatment of Mycobacterium avium complex immune reconstitution disease in HIV-1-infected individuals. AIDS Patient Care STDS 2003;17:617–622.

86. Dworkin MS, Fratkin MD. Mycobacterium avium complex lymph node abscess after use of highly active antiretroviral therapy in a patient with AIDS. Arch Intern Med 1998;158:1828.

87. del Giudice P, Durant J, Counillon E, et al. Mycobacterial cutaneous manifestations: a new sign of immune restoration syndrome in patients with acquired immunodeficiency syndrome. Arch Dermatol 1999;135:1129–1130.

88. Lawn SD, Bicanic TA, Macallan DC. Pyomyositis and cutaneous abscesses due to Mycobacterium avium: an immune reconstitution manifestation in a patient with AIDS. Clin Infect Dis 2004;36:461–463.

89. Aberg JA, Chin-Hong PV, McCutchan A, Koletar SL, Currier JS. Localized osteomyelitis due to Mycobacterium avium complex in patients with Human Immunodeficiency Virus receiving highly active antiretroviral therapy. Clin Infect Dis 2002;35:E8–E13.

90. Phillips P, Bonner S, Gataric N, et al. Nontuberculous mycobacterial immune reconstitution syndrome in HIV-infected patients: spectrum of disease and long-term follow-up. Clin Infect Dis 2005;41:1483–1497.

91. Cattelan AM, Trevenzoli M, Sasset L, Lanzafame M, Marchioro U, Meneghetti F. Multiple cerebral cryptococcomas associated with immune reconstitution in HIV-1 infection. AIDS 2004;18:349–351.

92. Trevenzoli M, Cattelan AM, Rea F, et al. Mediastinitis due to cryptococcal infection: a new clinical entity in the HAART era. J Infect 2002;45:173–179.

93. Haddow LJ, Sahid F, Moosa MY. Cryptococcal breast abscess in an HIV-positive patient: arguments for reviewing the definition of immune reconstitution inflammatory syndrome. J Infect 2008;57:82–84.

94. Jenny-Avital ER, Abadi M. Immune reconstitution cryptococcosis after initiation of successful highly active antiretroviral therapy. Clin Infect Dis 2002;35:e128–133.

95. Putignani L, Antonucci G, Paglia MG, et al. Cryptococcal lymphadenitis as a manifestation of immune reconstitution inflammatory syndrome in an HIV-positive patient: a case report and review of the literature. Int J Immunopathol Pharmacol 2008;21:751–756.

96. Bicanic T, Harrison T, Niepieklo A, Dyakopu N, Meintjes G. Symptomatic relapse of HIV-associated cryptococcal meningitis after initial fluconazole monotherapy: the role of fluconazole resistance and immune reconstitution. Clin Infect Dis 2006;43:1069–1073.

97. King MD, Perlino CA, Cinnamon J, Jernigan JA. Paradoxical recurrent meningitis following therapy of cryptococcal meningitis: an immune reconstitution syndrome after initiation of highly active antiretroviral therapy. Int J STD AIDS 2002;13:724–726.

98. Shelburne SA, 3rd, Hamill RJ, Rodriguez-Barradas MC, et al. Immune reconstitution inflammatory syndrome: emergence of a unique syndrome during highly active antiretroviral therapy. Medicine (Baltimore) 2002;81:213–227.

99. Boelaert JR, Goddeeris KH, Vanopdenbosch LJ, Casselman JW. Relapsing meningitis caused by persistent cryptococcal antigens and immune reconstitution after the initiation of highly active antiretroviral therapy. AIDS 2004;18:1223–1224.

100. Lawn SD, Bekker LG, Myer L, Orrell C, Wood R. Cryptococcocal immune reconstitution disease: a major cause of early mortality in a South African antiretroviral programme. AIDS 2005;19:2050–2052.

101. Woods ML, 2nd, MacGinley R, Eisen DP, Allworth AM. HIV combination therapy: partial immune restitution unmasking latent cryptococcal infection. Aids 1998;12:1491–1494.

102. Antinori S, Ridolfo A, Fasan M, et al. AIDS-associated cryptococcosis: a comparison of epidemiology, clinical features and outcome in the pre and post HAART eras. Experience of a single centre in Italy. HIV Med 2009;10:6–11.

103. Lortholary O, Poizat G, Zeller V, et al. Long-term outcome of AIDS-associated cryptococcosis in the era of combination antiretroviral therapy. AIDS 2006;20:2183–191.

104. Chang YC, Kwon-Chung KJ. Isolation of the third capsule-associated gene, CAP60, required for virulence in Cryptococcus neoformans. Infect Immun 1998;66:2230–2236.

105. Graybill JR, Sobel J, Saag M, et al. Diagnosis and management of increased intracranial pressure in patients with AIDS and cryptococcal meningitis. The NIAID Mycoses Study Group and AIDS Cooperative Treatment Groups. Clin Infect Dis 2000;30:47–54.

106. Saag MS, Graybill RJ, Larsen RA, et al. Practice guidelines for the management of cryptococcal disease. Infectious Diseases Society of America. Clin Infect Dis 2000;30:710–718.

107. Haubrich RH, Haghighat D, Bozzette SA, Tilles J, McCutchan JA. High-dose fluconazole for treatment of cryptococcal disease in patients with human immunodeficiency virus infection. The California Collaborative Treatment Group. J Infect Dis 1994;170:238–242.

108. Albrecht H, Hoffmann C, Degen O, et al. Highly active antiretroviral therapy significantly improves the prognosis of patients with HIV-associated progressive multifocal leukoencephalopathy. Aids 1998;12:1149–1154.

109. Clifford DB, Yiannoutsos C, Glicksman M, et al. HAART improves prognosis in HIV-associated progressive multifocal leukoencephalopathy. Neurology 1999;52:623–625.

110. Tassie JM, Gasnault J, Bentata M, et al. Survival improvement of AIDS-related progressive multifocal leukoencephalopathy in the era of protease inhibitors. Clinical Epidemiology Group. French Hospital Database on HIV. AIDS 1999;13:1881–1887.

111. Collazos J, Mayo J, Martinez E, Blanco MS. Contrast-enhancing progressive multifocal leukoencephalopathy as an immune reconstitution event in AIDS patients. Aids 1999;13:1426–1428.

112. Miralles P, Berenguer J, Lacruz C, et al. Inflammatory reactions in progressive multifocal leukoencephalopathy after highly active antiretroviral therapy. AIDS 2001;15:1900–1902.

113. Safdar A, Rubocki RJ, Horvath JA, Narayan KK, Waldron RL. Fatal immune restoration disease in human immunodeficiency virus type 1-infected patients with progressive multifocal leukoencephalopathy: impact of antiretroviral therapy-associated immune reconstitution. Clin Infect Dis 2002;35:1250–1257.

114. Vendrely A, Bienvenu B, Gasnault J, Thiebault JB, Salmon D, Gray F. Fulminant inflammatory leukoencephalopathy associated with HAART-induced immune restoration in AIDS-related progressive multifocal leukoencephalopathy. Acta Neuropathol 2005;109:449–455.

115. Gasnault J, Kahraman M, de Goer de Herve MG, Durali D, Delfraissy JF, Taoufik Y. Critical role of JC virus-specific CD4 T-cell responses in preventing progressive multifocal leukoencephalopathy. AIDS 2003;17:1443–1449.

116. Falco V, Olmo M, del Saz SV, et al. Influence of HAART on the clinical course of HIV-1-infected patients with progressive multifocal leukoencephalopathy: results of an observational multicenter study. J Acquir Immune Defic Syndr 2008;49:26–31.

117. Tan K, Roda R, Ostrow L, McArthur J, Nath A. PML-IRIS in patients with HIV infection: clinical manifestations and treatment with steroids. Neurology 2009;72:1458–1464.

118. Kotecha N, George MJ, Smith TW, Corvi F, Litofsky NS. Enhancing progressive multifocal leukoencephalopathy: an indicator of improved immune status? Am J Med 1998;105:541–543.

119. Holkova B, Takeshita K, Cheng DM, et al. Effect of highly active antiretroviral therapy on survival in patients with AIDS-associated pulmonary Kaposi's sarcoma treated with chemotherapy. J Clin Oncol 2001;19:3848–3851.

120. Martinelli C, Zazzi M, Ambu S, Bartolozzi D, Corsi P, Leoncini F. Complete regression of AIDS-related Kaposi's sarcoma-associated human herpesvirus-8 during therapy with indinavir. AIDS 1998;12:1717–1719.

121. Connick E, Kane MA, White IE, Ryder J, Campbell TB. Immune reconstitution inflammatory syndrome associated with Kaposi sarcoma during potent antiretroviral therapy. Clin Infect Dis 2004;39:1852–1855.

122. Leidner RS, Aboulafia DM. Recrudescent Kaposi's sarcoma after initiation of HAART: a manifestation of immune reconstitution syndrome. AIDS Patient Care STDS 2005;19:635–644.

123. Weir A, Wansbrough-Jones M. Mucosal Kaposi's sarcoma following protease inhibitor therapy in an HIV-infected patient. AIDS 1997;11:1895–1896.

124. Volkow PF, Cornejo P, Zinser JW, Ormsby CE, Reyes-Teran G. Life-threatening exacerbation of Kaposi's sarcoma after prednisone treatment for immune reconstitution inflammatory syndrome. AIDS 2008;22:663–665.

125. Godoy MC, Rouse H, Brown JA, Phillips P, Forrest DM, Muller NL. Imaging features of pulmonary Kaposi sarcoma-associated immune reconstitution syndrome. AJR Am J Roentgenol 2007;189:956–965.

126. Little RF, Wyvill KM, Pluda JM, et al. Activity of thalidomide in AIDS-related Kaposi's sarcoma. J Clin Oncol 2000;18:2593–2602.

127. Ueno T, Mitsuishi T, Kimura Y, et al. Immune reconstitution inflammatory syndrome associated with Kaposi's sarcoma: successful treatment with interferon-alpha. Eur J Dermatol 2007;17:539–540.

128. Bower M, Nelson M, Young AM, et al. Immune reconstitution inflammatory syndrome associated with Kaposi's sarcoma. J Clin Oncol 2005;23:5224–5228.

129. Martinez E, Gatell J, Moran Y, et al. High incidence of herpes zoster in patients with AIDS soon after therapy with protease inhibitors. Clin Infect Dis 1998;27:1510–1513.

130. Whitley RJ, Gnann JW, Jr. Herpes zoster in patients with human immunodeficiency virus infection--an ever-expanding spectrum of disease. Clin Infect Dis 1995;21:989–990.

131. Domingo P, Torres OH, Ris J, Vazquez G. Herpes zoster as an immune reconstitution disease after initiation of combination antiretroviral therapy in patients with human immunodeficiency virus type-1 infection. Am J Med 2001;110:605–609.

132. Dunic I, Djurkovic-Djakovic O, Vesic S, Zerjav S, Jevtovic D. Herpes zoster as an immune restoration disease in AIDS patients during therapy including protease inhibitors. Int J STD AIDS 2005;16:475–478.

133. Clark BM, Krueger RG, Price P, French MA. Compartmentalization of the immune response in varicella zoster virus immune restoration disease causing transverse myelitis. Aids 2004;18:1218–1221.

134. Gnann JW, Jr., Crumpacker CS, Lalezari JP, et al. Sorivudine versus acyclovir for treatment of dermatomal herpes zoster in human immunodeficiency virus-infected patients: results from a randomized, controlled clinical trial. Collaborative Antiviral Study Group/AIDS Clinical Trials Group, Herpes Zoster Study Group. Antimicrob Agents Chemother 1998;42:1139–1145.

135. Whitley RJ, Weiss H, Gnann JW, Jr., et al. Acyclovir with and without prednisone for the treatment of herpes zoster. A randomized, placebo-controlled trial. The National Institute of Allergy and Infectious Diseases Collaborative Antiviral Study Group. Ann Intern Med 1996;125:376–383.

136. Wood MJ, Johnson RW, McKendrick MW, Taylor J, Mandal BK, Crooks J. A randomized trial of acyclovir for 7 days or 21 days with and without prednisolone for treatment of acute herpes zoster. N Engl J Med 1994;330:896–900.

137. Bouscarat F, Maubec E, Matheron S, Descamps V. Immune recovery inflammatory folliculitis. AIDS 2000;14:617-618.

138. von Both U, Laffer R, Grube C, Bossart W, Gaspert A, Gunthard HF. Acute cytomegalovirus colitis presenting during primary HIV infection: an unusual case of an immune reconstitution inflammatory syndrome. Clin Infect Dis 2008;46:e38–40.

139. Jacobson MA, Zegans M, Pavan PR, et al. Cytomegalovirus retinitis after initiation of highly active antiretroviral therapy. Lancet 1997;349:1443–1445.

140. Karavellas MP, Lowder CY, Macdonald C, Avila CP, Jr., Freeman WR. Immune recovery vitritis associated with inactive cytomegalovirus retinitis: a new syndrome. Arch Ophthalmol 1998;116:169–175.

141. Schrier RD, Song MK, Smith IL, et al. Intraocular viral and immune pathogenesis of immune recovery uveitis in patients with healed cytomegalovirus retinitis. Retina 2006;26:165–169.

142. Karavellas MP, Plummer DJ, Macdonald JC, et al. Incidence of immune recovery vitritis in cytomegalovirus retinitis patients following institution of successful highly active antiretroviral therapy. J Infect Dis 1999;179:697–700.

143. Nguyen QD, Kempen JH, Bolton SG, Dunn JP, Jabs DA. Immune recovery uveitis in patients with AIDS and cytomegalovirus retinitis after highly active antiretroviral therapy. Am J Ophthalmol 2000;129:634–639.

144. Kempen JH, Min YI, Freeman WR, et al. Risk of immune recovery uveitis in patients with AIDS and cytomegalovirus retinitis. Ophthalmology 2006;113:684–694.

145. Karavellas MP, Azen SP, MacDonald JC, et al. Immune recovery vitritis and uveitis in AIDS: clinical predictors, sequelae, and treatment outcomes. Retina 2001;21:1–9.

146. Kosobucki BR, Goldberg DE, Bessho K, et al. Valganciclovir therapy for immune recovery uveitis complicated by macular edema. Am J Ophthalmol 2004;137:636–638.

147. Song MK, Azen SP, Buley A, et al. Effect of anti-cytomegalovirus therapy on the incidence of immune recovery uveitis in AIDS patients with healed cytomegalovirus retinitis. Am J Ophthalmol 2003;136:696–702.

148. Wohl DA, Kendall MA, Owens S, et al. The safety of discontinuation of maintenance therapy for cytomegalovirus (CMV) retinitis and incidence of immune recovery uveitis following potent antiretroviral therapy. HIV Clin Trials 2005;6:136–146.

149. Arevalo JF, Mendoza AJ, Ferretti Y. Immune recovery uveitis in AIDS patients with cytomegalovirus retinitis treated with highly active antiretroviral therapy in Venezuela. Retina 2003;23:495–502.

150. Henderson HW, Mitchell SM. Treatment of immune recovery vitritis with local steroids. Br J Ophthalmol 1999;83:540–545.

151. John M, Flexman J, French MA. Hepatitis C virus associated hepatitis following treatment of HIV-infected patients with HIV protease inhibitors: an immune restoration disease? Aids 1998;12:2289–2293.

152. Kim HN, Harrington RD, Shuhart MC, et al. Hepatitis C virus activation in HIV-infected patients initiating highly active antiretroviral therapy. AIDS Patient Care STDS 2007;21:718–723.

153. Filippini P, Coppola N, Pisapia R, et al. Impact of occult hepatitis B virus infection in HIV patients naive for antiretroviral therapy. AIDS 2006;20:1253–1260.

154. Pogany K, Zaaijer HL, Prins JM, Wit FW, Lange JM, Beld MG. Occult hepatitis B virus infection before and 1 year after start of HAART in HIV type 1-positive patients. AIDS Res Hum Retroviruses 2005;21:922–926.

155. Hoffmann CJ, Charalambous S, Martin DJ, et al. Hepatitis B virus infection and response to antiretroviral therapy (ART) in a South African ART program. Clin Infect Dis 2008;47:1479–1485.

156. Crane M, Oliver B, Matthews G, et al. Immunopathogenesis of hepatic flare in HIV/hepatitis B virus (HBV)-coinfected individuals after the initiation of HBV-active antiretroviral therapy. J Infect Dis 2009;199:974–981.

157. Turnbull EL, Lopes AR, Jones NA, et al. HIV-1 epitope-specific CD8+ T cell responses strongly associated with delayed disease progression cross-recognize epitope variants efficiently. J Immunol 2006;176:6130–6146.

158. Dunn C, Brunetto M, Reynolds G, et al. Cytokines induced during chronic hepatitis B virus infection promote a pathway for NK cell-mediated liver damage. J Exp Med 2007;204:667–680.

159. De Rosa FG, Audagnotto S, Bargiacchi O, et al. Resolution of HCV infection after highly active antiretroviral therapy in a HIV-HCV coinfected patient. J Infect 2006;53:e215–218.

160. Konopnicki D, Mocroft A, de Wit S, et al. Hepatitis B and HIV: prevalence, AIDS progression, response to highly active antiretroviral therapy and increased mortality in the EuroSIDA cohort. AIDS 2005;19:593–601.

161. Calabrese LH, Kirchner E, Shrestha R. Rheumatic complications of human immunodeficiency virus infection in the era of highly active antiretroviral therapy: emergence of a new syndrome of immune reconstitution and changing patterns of disease. Semin Arthritis Rheum 2005;35:166–174.

162. Sereti I, Sarlis NJ, Arioglu E, Turner ML, Mican JM. Alopecia universalis and Graves' disease in the setting of immune restoration after highly active antiretroviral therapy. Aids 2001;15:138-140.

163. Diri E, Lipsky PE, Berggren RE. Emergence of systemic lupus erythematosus after initiation of highly active antiretroviral therapy for human immunodeficiency virus infection. J Rheumatol 2000;27:2711-2714.

164. Calza L, Manfredi R, Colangeli V, Freo E, Chiodo F. Polymyositis associated with HIV infection during immune restoration induced by highly active anti-retroviral therapy. Clin Exp Rheumatol 2004;22:651-652.

165. DelVecchio S, Skidmore P. Adult-onset Still's disease presenting as fever of unknown origin in a patient with HIV infection. Clin Infect Dis 2008;46:e41–43.

166. Lawson E, Bond K, Churchill D, Walker-Bone K. A case of immune reconstitution syndrome: adult-onset Still's disease in a patient with HIV infection. Rheumatology (Oxford) 2009;48:446–447.

167. Bell C, Nelson M, Kaye S. A case of immune reconstitution rheumatoid arthritis. Int J STD AIDS 2002;13:580–581.

168. Silvestre JF, Albares MP, Ramon R, Botella R. Cutaneous intolerance to tattoos in a patient with human immunodeficiency virus: a manifestation of the immune restoration syndrome. Arch Dermatol 2001;137:669-670.

169. Price P, Murdoch DM, Agarwal U, Lewin SR, Elliott JH, French MA. Immune restoration diseases reflect diverse immunopathological mechanisms. Clin Microbiol Rev 2009;22:651–663.

170. World Health Organization. Towards Universal Access: Scaling up priority HIV/AIDS interventions in the health sector: Progress Report 2008.

171. Walters E, Cotton MF, Rabie H, Schaaf HS, Walters LO, Marais BJ. Clinical presentation and outcome of tuberculosis in human immunodeficiency virus infected children on anti-retroviral therapy. BMC Pediatr 2008;8:1.

172. Boulware DR, Callens S, Pahwa S. Pediatric HIV immune reconstitution inflammatory syndrome. Curr Opin HIV AIDS 2008;3:461–467.

173. Puthanakit T, Oberdorfer P, Akarathum N, Wannarit P, Sirisanthana T, Sirisanthana V. Immune reconstitution syndrome after highly active antiretroviral therapy in human immunodeficiency virus-infected thai children. Pediatr Infect Dis J 2006;25:53–58.

174. Fallo A, Torrado L, Sanchez A, Cerqueiro C, Schargrodsky L, Lopez E. Delayed complications of Bacillus Calmette-Guerin (BCG) vaccination in HIV-infected children. In: International AIDS Society Conference. Rio de Janeiro, Brazil; July 24–27, 2005.

175. Hesseling AC, Marais BJ, Gie RP, et al. The risk of disseminated Bacille Calmette-Guerin (BCG) disease in HIV-infected children. Vaccine 2007;25:14–18.

176. Cotton MF, Schaaf HS, Lottering G, Weber HL, Coetzee J, Nachman S. Tuberculosis exposure in HIV-exposed infants in a high-prevalence setting. Int J Tuberc Lung Dis 2008;12:225–227.

177. Mak TK, Hesseling AC, Hussey GD, Cotton MF. Making BCG vaccination programmes safer in the HIV era. Lancet 2008;372:786–787.

178. Nuttall JJ, Davies MA, Hussey GD, Eley BS. Bacillus Calmette-Guerin (BCG) vaccine-induced complications in children treated with highly active antiretroviral therapy. Int J Infect Dis 2008;12:e99–105.

179. Puthanakit T, Oberdorfer P, Punjaisee S, Wannarit P, Sirisanthana T, Sirisanthana V. Immune reconstitution syndrome due to bacillus Calmette-Guerin after initiation of antiretroviral therapy in children with HIV infection. Clin Infect Dis 2005;41:1049–1052.

180. Siberry GK, Tessema S. Immune reconstitution syndrome precipitated by bacille Calmette Guerin after initiation of antiretroviral therapy. Pediatr Infect Dis J 2006;25:648–649.

181. Kilborn T, Zampoli M. Immune reconstitution inflammatory syndrome after initiating highly active antiretroviral therapy in HIV-infected children. Pediatr Radiol 2009;39:569–574.

182. Zampoli M, Kilborn T, Eley B. Tuberculosis during early antiretroviral-induced immune reconstitution in HIV-infected children. Int J Tuberc Lung Dis 2007;11:417–423.

183. Wang ME, Castillo ME, Montano SM, Zunt JR. Immune reconstitution inflammatory syndrome in human immunodeficiency virus-infected children in Peru. Pediatr Infect Dis J 2009;28:900–903.

184. Tangsinmankong N, Kamchaisatian W, Lujan-Zilbermann J, Brown CL, Sleasman JW, Emmanuel PJ. Varicella zoster as a manifestation of immune restoration disease in HIV-infected children. J Allergy Clin Immunol 2004;113:742–746.

185. North RJ, Jung YJ. Immunity to tuberculosis. Annu Rev Immunol 2004;22:599–623.

186. Woodward B, Hillyer L, Hunt K. T cells with a quiescent phenotype (CD45RA+) are overabundant in the blood and involuted lymphoid tissues in wasting protein and energy deficiencies. Immunology 1999;96:246–253.

187. Najera O, Gonzalez C, Toledo G, et al. CD45RA and CD45RO isoforms in infected malnourished and infected well-nourished children. Clin Exp Immunol 2001;126:461–465.

188. Rodriguez L, Gonzalez C, Flores L, Jimenez-Zamudio L, Graniel J, Ortiz R. Assessment by flow cytometry of cytokine production in malnourished children. Clin Diagn Lab Immunol 2005;12:502–507.

189. World Health Organization. Improving the diagnosis and treatment of smear-negative pulmonary and extrapulmonary tuberculosis among adults and adolescents: recommendations for HIV-prevalent and resource-constrained settings. Geneva: Stop TB Department, Department of HIV/AIDS, World Health Organization; 2006.

190. Rapose A, Sarvat B, Sarria JC. Immune reconstitution inflammatory syndrome presenting as pericarditis and pericardial effusion. Cardiology 2008;110:142–144.

191. Pfeffer G, Prout A, Hooge J, Maguire J. Biopsy-proven immune reconstitution syndrome in a patient with AIDS and cerebral toxoplasmosis. Neurology 2009;73:321–322.

192. Tremont-Lukats IW, Garciarena P, Juarbe R, El-Abassi RN. The immune inflammatory reconstitution syndrome and central nervous system toxoplasmosis. Ann Intern Med 2009;150:656–657.

193. Crump JA, Tyrer MJ, Lloyd-Owen SJ, Han LY, Lipman MC, Johnson MA. Military tuberculosis with paradoxical expansion of intracranial tuberculomas complicating human immunodeficiency virus infection in a patient receiving highly active antiretroviral therapy. Clin Infect Dis 1998;26:1008–1009.

194. Lee CH, Lui CC, Liu JW. Immune reconstitution syndrome in a patient with AIDS with paradoxically deteriorating brain tuberculoma. AIDS Patient Care STDS 2007;21:234–239.

195. Maggi P, Volpe A, Bellacosa C, et al. The role of immune reconstitution in the onset of subclinical atheromasic lesions. J Acquir Immune Defic Syndr 2009;52:524–525.

196. Dautremer J, Pacanowski J, Girard PM, Lalande V, Sivignon F, Meynard JL. A new presentation of immune reconstitution inflammatory syndrome followed by a severe paradoxical reaction in an HIV-1-infected patient with tuberculous meningitis. AIDS 2007;21:381–382.

197. Nolan RC, Chidlow G, French MA. Parvovirus B19 encephalitis presenting as immune restoration disease after highly active antiretroviral therapy for human immunodeficiency virus infection. Clin Infect Dis 2003;36:1191–1194.

198. Sinclair J, Sissons P. Latency and reactivation of human cytomegalovirus. J Gen Virol 2006;87:1763–1779.

199. Archuleta S. Neurologic complications of varicella-zoster virus reactivation in a person with HIV/AIDS. AIDS Read 2007;17:58, 64–66.

200. Patel AK, Patel KK, Shah SD, Desai J. Immune reconstitution syndrome presenting with cerebral varicella zoster vasculitis in HIV-1-infected patient: a case report. J Int Assoc Physicians AIDS Care (Chic Ill) 2006;5:157–160.

201. Furrer H, Malinverni R. Systemic inflammatory reaction after starting highly active antiretroviral therapy in AIDS patients treated for extrapulmonary tuberculosis. Am J Med 1999;106:371–372.

202. Goldsack NR, Allen S, Lipman MC. Adult respiratory distress syndrome as a severe immune reconstitution disease following the commencement of highly active antiretroviral therapy. Sex Transm Infect 2003;79:337–338.

203. Richardson D, Rubinstein L, Ross E, et al. Cystic lung lesions as an immune reconstitution inflammatory syndrome (IRIS) in HIV-TB co-infection? Thorax 2005;60:884.

204. Bell HC, Heath CH, French MA. Pulmonary Mycobacterium celatum immune restoration disease: immunopathology and response to corticosteroid therapy. AIDS 2005;19:2047–2049.

205. Lawn SD. Acute respiratory failure due to Mycobacterium kansasii infection: immune reconstitution disease in a patient with AIDS. J Infect 2005;51:339–340.

206. Manfredi R, Nanetti A, Tadolini M, et al. Role of Mycobacterium xenopi disease in patients with HIV infection at the time of highly active antiretroviral therapy (HAART). Comparison with the pre-Haart period. Tuberculosis (Edinb) 2003;83:319–328.

207. Cailhol J, Pizzocolo C, Brauner M, Bouchaud O, Abgrall S. A delayed immune reconstitution inflammatory syndrome. AIDS 2007;21:115–116.

208. Hasse B, Strebel B, Thurnheer R, Uhlmann F, Krause M. Chronic necrotizing pulmonary aspergillosis after tuberculosis in an HIV-positive woman: an unusual immune reconstitution phenomenon? AIDS 2005;19:2179–2181.

209. Scott C, Staughton RC, Bunker CJ, Asboe D. Acne vulgaris and acne rosacea as part of immune reconstitution disease in HIV-1 infected patients starting antiretroviral therapy. Int J STD AIDS 2008;19:493–495.

210. Phillips P, Lee JK, Wang C, Yoshida E, Lima VD, Montaner J. Chylous ascites: a late complication of intra-abdominal Mycobacterium avium complex immune reconstitution syndrome in HIV-infected patients. Int J STD AIDS 2009;20:285–287.

211. Batista MD, Porro AM, Maeda SM, et al. Leprosy reversal reaction as immune reconstitution inflammatory syndrome in patients with AIDS. Clin Infect Dis 2008;46:e56–60.

212. Chow D, Okinaka L, Souza S, Shikuma C, Tice A. Hansen's disease with HIV: a case of immune reconstitution disease. Hawaii Med J 2009;68:27–29.

213. Couppie P, Abel S, Voinchet H, et al. Immune reconstitution inflammatory syndrome associated with HIV and leprosy. Arch Dermatol 2004;140:997–1000.

214. Couppie P, Domergue V, Clyti E, et al. Increased incidence of leprosy following HAART initiation: a manifestation of the immune reconstitution disease. AIDS 2009,23:1599–1600.

215. Menezes VM, Sales AM, Illarramendi X, et al. Leprosy reaction as a manifestation of immune reconstitution inflammatory syndrome: a case series of a Brazilian cohort. AIDS 2009;23:641–643.

216. Wittram C, Fogg J, Farber H. Immune restoration syndrome manifested by pulmonary sarcoidosis. AJR Am J Roentgenol 2001;177:1427.

217. Viani RM. Sarcoidosis and interstitial nephritis in a child with acquired immunodeficiency syndrome: implications of immune reconstitution syndrome with an indinavir-based regimen. Pediatr Infect Dis J 2002;21:435–438.

218. Ingiliz P, Appenrodt B, Gruenhage F, et al. Lymphoid pneumonitis as an immune reconstitution inflammatory syndrome in a patient with CD4 cell recovery after HAART initiation. HIV Med 2006;7:411–414.

219. Schaller J, Carlson JA. Erythema nodosum-like lesions in treated Whipple's disease: signs of immune reconstitution inflammatory syndrome. J Am Acad Dermatol 2009;60:277–288.

220. Intalapaporn P, Poovorawan Y, Suankratay C. Immune reconstitution syndrome associated with parvovirus B19-induced pure red cell aplasia during highly active antiretroviral therapy. J Infect 2007;55(1):90–91.

221. Weber E, Gunthard HF, Schertler T, Seebach JD. Spontaneous splenic rupture as manifestation of the immune reconstitution inflammatory syndrome in an HIV type 1 infected patient with tuberculosis. Infection 2009;37:163–165.

222. Cuttelod M, Pascual A, Baur Chaubert AS, et al. Hemophagocytic syndrome after highly active antiretroviral therapy initiation: a life-threatening event related to immune restoration inflammatory syndrome? AIDS 2008;22:549–551.

223. Kim AC, Lupatkin HC. Strongyloides stercoralis infection as a manifestation of immune restoration syndrome. Clin Infect Dis 2004;39:439–440.

224. Lanzafame M, Faggian F, Lattuada E, Antolini D, Vento S. Strongyloidiasis in an HIV-1-infected patient after highly active antiretroviral therapy-induced immune restoration. J Infect Dis 2005;191:1027.

225. Taylor CL, Subbarao V, Gayed S, Ustianowski AP. Immune reconstitution syndrome to Strongyloides stercoralis infection. Aids 2007;21:649–650.

226. Sriaroon C, Mayer CA, Chen L, Accurso C, Greene JN, Vincent AL. Diffuse intra-abdominal granulomatous seeding as a manifestation of immune reconstitution inflammatory syndrome associated with microsporidiosis in a patient with HIV. AIDS Patient Care STDS 2008;22:611–612.

227. Nacher M, Vantilcke V, Mahamat A, et al. Increased incidence of cutaneous mycoses after HAART initiation: a benign form of immune reconstitution disease? AIDS 2007;21:2248–2250.

228. Ramirez-Amador VA, Espinosa E, Gonzalez-Ramirez I, Anaya-Saavedra G, Ormsby CE, Reyes-Teran G. Identification of oral candidosis, hairy leukoplakia and recurrent oral ulcers as distinct cases of immune reconstitution inflammatory syndrome. Int J STD AIDS 2009;20:259–261.

229. Acosta RD, Itzkowitz SL. Immune reconstitution syndrome masquerading as ulcerative colitis in a patient with HIV. Gastrointest Endosc 2008;68:1197–1198; discussion 8.

230. O'Leary JG, Zachary K, Misdraji J, Chung RT. De novo autoimmune hepatitis during immune reconstitution in an HIV-infected patient receiving highly active antiretroviral therapy. Clin Infect Dis 2008;46:e12–14.

231. Knysz B, Bolanowski M, Klimczak M, Gladysz A, Zwolinska K. Graves' disease as an immune reconstitution syndrome in an HIV-1-positive patient commencing effective antiretroviral therapy: case report and literature review. Viral Immunol 2006;19:102–107.

232. Perez N, Del Bianco G, Murphy JR, Heresi GP. Graves' disease following successful HAART of a perinatally HIV-infected 11-year-old. AIDS 2009;23:645–646.

Part V

TREATMENT

Chapter 18   TREATMENT OF HIV

LAURA WATERS, ANDREW SCOURFIELD, AND
MARK NELSON

When a lot of remedies are suggested for a disease,
that means it can't be cured.

—ANTON CHEKHOV

Introduction

The rate of evolution of antiretroviral therapy (ART) has been phenomenal since the late 1980s, when the first agent, zidovudine, was introduced. Huge amounts of research and investment have resulted in more than 20 licensed drugs from five individual drug classes, with more agents and classes in various stages of development. Highly active antiretroviral therapy (HAART)—the combination of at least three drugs from two or more classes—became possible with the advent of a second ART class, protease inhibitors (PIs). Following the introduction of HAART in the mid- to late 1990s, dramatic reductions in both HIV- and "non-HIV–related" morbidity and mortality resulted.[1] Prior to this, in the pre-HAART era, treatment consisted of sequential monotherapy or dual therapy with nucleoside reverse transcriptase inhibitors (NRTIs), which yielded, at best, short-term immunologic and virologic responses and was associated with high rates of NRTI resistance.

Current consensus guidelines—as this book goes to press, from the European AIDS Clinical Society [EACS], 2009; the U.S. Department of Health and Human Services Panel [DHHS], 2009; the International AIDS Society [IAS], 2010; and the British HIV Association [BHIVA], 2008)—recommend two NRTIs with a boosted PI or non-nucleoside reverse transcriptase inhibitor (NNRTI) for initial therapy. The EACS, DHHS, and IAS guidelines also list the integrase inhibitor raltegravir as an alternative and preferred option, respectively.

Antiretroviral Targets

Most licensed antiretroviral drugs target a step in the replication cycle of HIV by blocking one of three viral enzymes:

- Reverse transcriptase: NRTIs (including tenofovir, abacavir, and lamivudine) and NNRTIs (including efavirenz, nevirapine, and etravirine)
- Protease: PI (including darunavir, atazanavir, and lopinavir)
- Integrase: integrase inhibitors (II; raltegravir).

A fourth class, entry inhibitors, can be divided into fusion inhibitors (for example, enfuvirtide) and coreceptor antagonists. HIV utilizes one of two coreceptors on the surface of host cells, CCR5 or CXCR4. Maraviroc is the only licensed CCR5 antagonist to date and demonstrates virologic efficacy only in subjects with CCR5-using HIV; CXCR4 blockers are in much earlier stages of development. The fact that coreceptor antagonists block a host rather than a viral target has created some concerns about long-term safety. Fortunately, nature has provided a model for CCR5 blockade that supports the safety of this approach. Some individuals carry CCR5 genes with a deletion of 32 base pairs (delta 32 mutations). The homozygous and heterozygous state occurs in approximately 1% and 15% of northern European Caucasians, respectively. Homozygosity results in an absence of functioning cell surface CCR5 receptor (and high-level resistance to HIV-1 acquisition), but relatively normal immune function.[2–4] Heterozygotes have lower expression of CCR5,[5] normal immune function,[3] and delayed HIV-1 progression.[6] In terms of other medical conditions, the homozygous state is associated with an increased risk for symptomatic West Nile virus (and other flavivirus infections), a possible predisposition to multiple sclerosis, and improved kidney transplant survival. Heterozygotes experience more severe sarcoidosis and systemic lupus erythematosus, but milder rheumatoid arthritis and multiple sclerosis.[7–9]

Antiretroviral classes in development include maturation inhibitors, Vpu inhibitors, RNase H inhibitors, and strategies based on RNA interference (RNAi). Maturation inhibitors interfere with the final stages of HIV processing, resulting in the release of noninfectious virions. Bevirimat was the first agent in this class and is furthest in development (phase 2). It works by disrupting the conversion of capsid protein (p25) to mature protein (p24). Other investigational maturation inhibitors include MPC-9055[10] and dolabella diterpene, an extract of Brazilian brown algae.[11] Vpu is an accessory HIV gene. BIT225, an agent that has completed phase Ib/IIa studies, inhibits the late phase of the viral life cycle and reduces HIV-1 release from macrophage reservoirs.[12] Ribonuclease H (RNase H) is part of reverse transcriptase and inhibition of this step results in potent HIV inhibition in vitro.[13] Short sequences of RNA can promote RNA degradation and, therefore, can inhibit viral replication; due to the high mutation rate of HIV, agents targeting multiple, conserved regions of the RNA genome are likely to be most effective.[14] Recent data on a new type of class that targets the interaction between the integrase enzyme and a critical cofactor (LEDGF, or p75) have been presented and clinical data are awaited.[15]

Nucleoside Reverse Transcriptase Inhibitors (NRTIs)

As reflected in treatment guidelines mentioned above, NRTIs remain the core of initial therapy and are also important in subsequent lines of treatment. To date, no NRTI-sparing strategy has out-performed NRTI-based regimens for initial therapy, although in ACTG5142, the NRTI-sparing arm (EFV+LPV/r) was virologically noninferior to EFV 2 NRTI.[16]

Modern NRTI drugs such as tenofovir show higher rates of efficacy and lower rates of toxicity than older NRTIs, particularly thymidine analogs (zidovudine [AZT] and stavudine [d4T]).[17] Mitochondrial toxicity, the underlying cause of many NRTI toxicities, is much less frequent with agents such as lamivudine, emtricitabine, tenofovir, and abacavir, supported by in vitro data showing low levels of mitochondrial toxicity.[18] The thymidine analogs AZT and d4T are no longer recommended in resource-rich settings due to their association with several mitochondrial toxicities, particularly lipoatrophy.[19] Didanosine remains an alternative NRTI option (with lamivudine or emtricitabine) in the British and European guidelines (BHIVA 2008 and EACS 2009) and is listed, in combination with emtricitabine and efavirenz, as an "acceptable" option in the DHHS recommendations (DHHS 2009). Issues with didanosine include mitochondrial toxicity, a possible association with myocardial infarction (MI),[20] and increasing evidence of an association with noncirrhotic portal hypertension.[21–23] Didanosine should not be coadministered with tenofovir due to high virologic failure rates when this backbone was used with an NNRTI[24] and an interaction between the two agents that resulted in an increased risk for toxicity and blunted CD4 rise.[25]

NRTI-related toxicities continue to be important and, not infrequently, treatment-limiting. Prior to the introduction of pharmacogenomic screening, hypersensitivity was the main treatment-limiting adverse event associated with abacavir use, leading to discontinuation in up to 8% of patients in clinical trials. Abacavir hypersensitivity is strongly correlated with the presence of the HLA-B*5701 allele, and the use of prospective HLA-B*5701 testing has led to marked reduction in the incidence of hypersensitivity in clinical cohorts.[26] In a prospective, randomized trial, HLA-B*5701 screening significantly reduced suspected hypersensitivity and eliminated immunologically confirmed (by skin patch testing) hypersensitivity.[27] It must be cautioned that, despite the value of genetic screening, clinical diagnosis remains the key and abacavir should be discontinued in any patient with suspected hypersensitivity, regardless of HLA-B*5701 status.[28]

A more recent concern related to abacavir is an apparent increased risk of cardiovascular events, specifically MI. The DAD study, a large European cohort study, analyzed the impact of individual NRTI on MI risk. Contrary to the initial hypothesis that the older NRTI would increase MI risk, it was abacavir actually fared worst in the analysis, with recent use increasing the risk of MI by 90%; and didanosine use increased the risk for MI by approximately 40%.[29] A more recent analysis confirmed a significantly increased risk of MI with recent abacavir exposure, and showed no increased risk with tenofovir use.[20] Since then, other analyses have supported or refuted the DAD results, and a recently presented 96-week trial comparing abacavir plus lamuvidine (Kivexa) with emtricitabine plus tenofovir (Truvada) and efavirenz with atazanavir/ritonavir in a four-arm, randomized design showed no excess of significant cardiovascular events in Kivexa recipients compared with those who received Truvada.[30] However, the balance of current evidence is that abacavir should, if possible, be avoided in patients with high cardiovascular risk as reflected in three consensus guidelines (BHIVA 2008, EACS 2009, and DHHS 2009). Biologic mechanisms that account for an association between abacavir and MI may include increased platelet reactivity[31,32] and endothelial dysfunction.[33]

Tenofovir may be associated with renal toxicity, although in clinical trials this is infrequent and a rare cause of treatment discontinuation.[17,34] Earlier studies focused on estimated glomerular filtration rate (eGFR), using creatinine-based formulae, and generally showed a small, nonprogressive decline in eGFR with tenofovir. More recent data has focused on markers of proximal tubular dysfunction (such as proteinuria, glycosuria, and elevated fractional phosphate excretion); although more frequent with tenofovir,[35–37] the clinical significance of mild tubular dysfunction remains uncertain. A small, longitudinal study showed more marked changes in markers of proximal tubular function in patients on tenofovir than in those on other NRTIs and immediate improvements among those who discontinued tenofovir.[38]

One study showed a clear correlation between intracellular tenofovir concentrations and tubular dysfunction,[39] which may explain the higher rates of tubular abnormalities, observed with tenofovir plus a PI in one large cohort study,[36] as PIs interact with renal tubular efflux pumps. A strong correlation between tenofovir tubular toxicity and variations of a particular transport protein allele was observed in one small study.[39] Larger studies in heterogeneous populations will be required in order to determine the future utility of pharmacogenomics in predicting this and other toxicities. In addition to its renal effects, tenofovir is associated with small, statistically significant reductions in bone mineral density (BMD) in clinical trials[17,30,34] and has

with rilpivirine failure is the E138K which causes cross-class NNRTI resistance; EFV failure most commonly produces the K103N mutation which does not impair susceptibility to ETR.

A fixed-dose, single-tablet combination of tenofovir/emtricitabine/rilpivirine is planned,[66] and rilpivirine is also being studied as an intramuscular injectable formulation.[67] Healthy volunteer studies investigating the safety of this formulation as pre-exposure prophylaxis are ongoing.[68]

Protease Inhibitors

It was the development of PIs in the mid-1990s that heralded the advent of HAART, and between 1995 and 1996 three PIs (saquinavir, ritonavir, and indinavir) were licensed in quick succession. By combining two NRTIs with a PI, patients could, for the first time, expect durable viral suppression; and this basic HAART formula has barely changed since then. However, despite their efficacy, early PIs were complex to take and were associated with high rates of treatment-limiting toxicities, particularly gastrointestinal. The development of NNRTIs a few years later offered a simpler, more tolerable option, but in 2000, the introduction of boosting— using low, subtherapeutic doses of ritonavir to pharmacologically slow hepatic metabolism of other PIs—enabled significant improvements in the class with lower, less frequent doses and even higher genetic barriers to resistance.

Boosted PIs are now considered standard, with a limited role for unboosted atazanavir in ritonavir-intolerant patients (BHIVA 2008 and DHHS 2009 guidelines). Full-dose ritonavir and indinavir are no longer recommended treatment options due to high rates of toxicity, and only the WHO guidelines still list nelfinavir as an option only if boosted PIs are unavailable. British, European, and American guidelines (IAS 2008, EACS 2009, and DHHS 2009) lists boosted atazanavir, lopinavir, darunavir, saquinavir (twice-daily preferred to once-daily administration) and fosamprenavir as preferred or alternative options for initial therapy.

There have been several head-to-head comparisons of boosted PIs for initial therapy. Once-daily darunavir demonstrated superior virologic efficacy to lopinavir at 48 weeks in the ARTE-MIS study,[69] although atazanavir, noninferior to lopinavir at week 48 in the CASTLE study, was statistically superior to lopinavir by week 96 (predominantly driven by adverse events).[70] Both darunavir and atazanavir exhibited lower rates of grade 2–4 diarrhea over 48 weeks than lopinavir at 4% and 2%, respectively, versus around 10% for the comparator. Atazanavir is also the only boosted PI to date to show comparable efficacy to efavirenz in ACTG 5202;[30] lopinavir with two NRTIs failed to show noninferiority to efavirenz in ACTG 5142.[16] Twice-daily fosamprenavir/ritonavir (700/100 mg) was noninferior to lopinavir/ritonavir at 48 weeks, with similar rates of gastrointestinal toxicity, each coadministered with Kivexa, in the KLEAN study.[71] In terms of later lines of therapy, atazanavir/ritonavir performed similarly to lopinavir/ritonavir (each with tenofovir plus one other NRTI) in treatment-experienced subjects, although in the subset with four or more PI mutations, lopinavir was associated with higher rates of viral suppression.[72] Darunavir/ritonavir twice daily was superior to lopinavir/ritonavir in treatment-experienced, lopinavir-naïve individuals.[73] In addition, virologic failure on darunavir was associated with fewer new resistance mutations than lopinavir.

Saquinavir is generally well-tolerated and demonstrated similar 48-week virologic efficacy first-line as lopinavir/ritonavir (both dosed twice daily with tenofovir/emtricitabine) in the GEMINI study.[74] Gastrointestinal events and triglyceride elevations were less common on saquinavir/ritonavir (1000/100 mg twice daily), but there were numerically more virologic failures (7% on saquinavir vs. 3% on lopinavir), and one patient on saquinavir developed treatment-emergent major PI mutations. Although pharmacokinetic studies support once-daily dosing of saquinavir, there is a lack of clinical data so only twice-daily dosing is approved.[75]

As a class, PIs tend to be associated with gastrointestinal toxicity, particularly nausea, diarrhea, and lipid elevations. As outlined previously, newer PIs have better gastrointestinal tolerability profiles. Atazanavir is associated with smaller lipid elevations than lopinavir; darunavir, although causing smaller increases in triglycerides than lopinavir, yields similar changes in total:high-density lipoprotein cholesterol ratio. Although many studies present statistically significant differences in lipids between different agents, the clinical significance of these may be less marked.

An as yet unresolved issue is the contribution of PIs to an elevated risk for cardiovascular disease. A 2006 analysis of the DAD cohort showed PIs as a class to be associated with a cumulative increased risk for myocardial infarction, independent of any lipid effect. An updated analysis quantified the contribution of four individual PIs: lopinavir, indinavir, nelfinavir, and saquinavir, and only the former two were associated with a significantly increased MI risk, suggesting this association may not be cross-class. Currently, there are insufficient patient years of exposure to atazanavir and darunavir to warrant individual analysis in DAD, but a Canadian cohort analysis of 125 patients with MI and 1,084 controls found no association between recent or cumulative atazanavir exposure and MI risk.[76]

Finally, although not recommended in current treatment guidelines, PI monotherapy is an increasingly popular option for patients with NRTI tolerability or toxicity issues, and many studies support the use of lopinavir/ritonavir as a single agent. On the whole, lopinavir/ritonavir performs better in an induction maintenance manner than as initial therapy. In addition, two recent studies yielded promising results for darunavir/ritonavir once[77] and twice[78] daily as a switch strategy in virologically suppressed individuals. Trials of atazanavir/ritonavir as monotherapy have been small and have yielded disappointing results.[79–81] In terms of cerebrospinal fluid (CSF) penetration, both lopinavir/ritonavir and darunavir/ritonavir achieve therapeutic concentrations, but on atazanavir/ritonavir, approximately 50% of patients will have CSF concentrations less than the IC50 for wild-type viruses. CNS efficacy is a possible concern with PI monotherapy. In MONOI, two patients developed neurologic symptoms on darunavir/ritonavir monotherapy, and both had detectable CSF viremia despite suppressed plasma HIV-1 RNA. A recent meta-analysis concluded that, overall, PI monotherapy is inferior to HAART, but acknowledged that results are better as a switch option for patients who have been undetectable on HAART for at last 6 months. In addition, the incidence of low-level viremia (between 50 and 500 copies/mL) is more common on PI monotherapy regimens.[82] Importantly, low level viraemia on PI monotherapy is rarely associated with resistance development and re-intensification will complete viral suppression; as a strategy, PI monotherapy could be cost-saving.

Integrase Inhibitors

The only integrase inhibitor approved to date is raltegravir, with elvitegravir in phase 3 trials. These and other agents in development act on the preintegration complex—composed of integrase bound to viral DNA—to inhibit strand transfer and block the incorporation of viral DNA into the host genome.

As previously outlined, raltegravir is now recommended by the DHHS 2009 and IAS 2010 guidelines and is an alternative first-line option in the EACS 2009 recommendations.

Raltegravir was initially studied in highly treatment-experienced individuals with triple-class resistance. Patients were randomized to optimize background therapy (OBT) with either placebo or raltegravir (400 mg twice daily). At week 96, 57% of raltegravir recipients and 26% of placebo recipients had a viral load less than 50 copies/mL ($p<0.001$), with corresponding CD4 cell increases of 123 and 49 cells/mm^3 ($p<0/001$), respectively.[83] Raltegravir performed well across different baseline CD4 and HIV-RNA strata. Patients with active OBT (genotypic sensitivity score) experienced numerically higher rates of viral suppression on raltegravir than on placebo, although this difference was not statistically significant. Of the 112 patients experiencing virologic failure on raltegravir with resistance test results available, 65% had integrase resistance mutations at one of three residues (Y143, Q148 or N155), usually with at least one other mutation. Adverse events were similar in both study arms; creatine kinase elevations were numerically more common on raltegravir, although not clinically significant and, after initial concerns, malignancy rates were near identical in both treatment arms (3.0 and 2.6 cases per 100 person-years in the raltegravir and placebo groups, respectively).

Raltegravir was compared to efavirenz (each with tenofovir/lamivudine) in treatment-naïve patients in the 004 Study, a phase 2 dose-finding double-blind trial. Patients were randomized to receive efavirenz or one of four raltegravir doses, and after week 48, all raltegravir recipients were continued on the 400 mg twice-daily dosage. Raltegravir produced faster viral suppression than efavirenz, but by week 24, suppression rates were similar; at week 48, 83% to 88% of patients on raltegravir and 87% of those on efavirenz had a viral load less than 50 copies/mL.[84] Raltegravir was well tolerated with fewer adverse events, particularly CNS effects, and exerted a minimal effect on lipids. These results were maintained out to 192 weeks, with 74% of patients on raltegravir and efavirenz maintaining viral suppression.[85] Similar results were achieved in the phase 3 STARTMRK study, comparing raltegravir to efavirenz, each with a Truvada backbone.[86] The primary endpoint (proportion with HIV-RNA <50 copies/mL at 48 weeks, noncompleter = failure) was met by 86.1% of the raltegravir group and 81.9% on efavirenz; efficacy was similar across different baseline CD4 and HIV-RNA strata. Again, patients on raltegravir experienced significantly faster viral suppression, significantly fewer drug-related clinical adverse events, and significantly smaller increases in total cholesterol, low-density lipoprotein cholesterol and triglycerides.

Although pharmacokinetic data supports once daily use of raltegravir,[87] a recent press release confirmed that, in a large trial, once daily RAL failed to meet non-inferiority against the twice daily RAL dose (each with Truvada) for 1st line therapy; the trial has been discontinued by the Data Safety and Monitoring Board.[88]

However, all switches are not equal, and a randomized, blinded trial was conducted in which patients on lopinavir/ritonavir plus at least two NRTIs were randomly assigned to continue that regime or switch the PI component to raltegravir. Despite significant improvements in lipids (the primary endpoint), there were more virologic failures in the raltegravir arm, so noninferiority criteria were not met.[89]

Entry Inhibitors

The injectable fusion inhibitor, enfuvirtide, has been largely superseded by newer oral agents. Despite this, enfuvirtide previously played a very important role in patients with limited treatment options and may continue to do so in selected patients. Although the addition of enfuvirtide in patients on suppressive HAART yielded no impact on residual viremia or resting CD4 infection,[90] addition of the agent to initial HAART may be associated with more rapid viral decay.[91,92] For women presenting in pregnancy, short-term addition of enfuvirtide to HAART could be beneficial in terms of achieving viral suppression prior to delivery, especially as recent data have suggested we should be starting HAART earlier in pregnancy—particularly among women with high presenting HIV-RNA—in order to reach an undetectable viral load before birth.[93] Enfuvirtide, like most antiretroviral drugs, is not approved for use in pregnancy, but no teratogenicity has been shown in animal studies and the drug does not appear to cross the placenta.[94]

Data regarding the immunologic impact of adding enfuvirtide to initial HAART are conflicting. A small study of first-line therapy randomized patients with an initial CD4 count <50 cells/mm^3 to lopinavir/ritonavir and two NRTIs alone or with enfuvirtide (for at least 6 months or until viral suppression) and showed immune benefits in the enfuvirtide arm, including faster time to CD4 >200 cells/mm^3 (18 vs. 48 weeks; p=0.01) and higher CD4 percentage at all time points up to 48 weeks.[95] No CD4 cell count differences were observed over 48 weeks in a randomized study of HAART with and without enfuvirtide in treatment-experienced individuals, but median baseline CD4 cell counts were over 380 cells/mm^3 in both arms.[96]

The mechanism of action of coreceptor antagonists was outlined in the introduction, and further discussion will be limited to CCR5 blockers. Maraviroc is, to date, the only approved CCR5 antagonist; this agent has demonstrated efficacy in treatment-naïve[96] and highly treatment-experienced subjects.[97] Of note, maraviroc initially failed to demonstrate noninferiority to efavirenz in the original analysis of the MERIT study (which used the "standard" phenotypic tropism assay, Trofile), but was noninferior in a retrospective analysis using a more sensitive version of the same assay (Trofile ES), which made 15% of the initial study population ineligible due to previously undetected CXCR4-using virus. Despite the enhanced sensitivity of the new Trofile assay, tropism testing by this method is limited by cost and availability and there are now numerous algorithms to estimate tropism based on genotypic sequencing (predominantly the V3 loop). Several studies have compared genotypic and phenotypic methods and, on the whole, correlation is high. A post hoc analysis of the MOTIVATE studies (maraviroc vs. placebo, each with optimized background regimen, in highly treatment-experienced patients) found that geno2pheno, a genotypic algorithm that combines V3 sequencing with clinical data such as CD4 and clade, predicted virologic response as well as Trofile.[98] In a German cohort of 92 patients, geno2pheno and Trofile also performed similarly in predicting 12-week virologic response to a maraviroc-containing regimen.[99] By genotypic tropism sequencing, the MVC once and twice daily arms of MERIT yielded similar virological responses to EFV.[100] Available data suggest that tropism switch while on suppressive HAART is uncommon,[101] therefore a switch to CCR5 antagonists in patients with suppressed plasma HIV-RNA could be guided by pretreatment tropism results or by genotypic analysis of a current PBMC DNA sample.

There has long been debate regarding whether or not maraviroc provides immunologic benefits over and above those achieved secondary to viral suppression, triggered by data from MOTIVATE showing that even subjects with non-R5 HIV-RNA experienced a better CD4 rise if they received maraviroc (compared with placebo).[102] An analysis of MERIT showed that some markers of immune activation normalized more rapidly in the maraviroc than in the efavirenz arm,[103] but there is no evidence yet that this is associated with clinical benefits in the longer term. In addition, maraviroc has been studied as an "add-in" in patients stable on suppressive HAART. In one small study, adding maraviroc failed to improve CD4 cell counts in a group of patients with discordant response to HAART (undetectable HIV-RNA but suboptimal CD4 rise).[104] A larger pilot study (n=34) added maraviroc to stable HAART in patients who had experienced viral suppression for at least 48 weeks but whose CD4 counts remained below 250 cells/mm^3. Although there was a marginal improvement in CD4 slope, there was no significant increase in CD4 count after 24 weeks.[105] However, there was reduction in the levels of CD4 and CD8 activation and in markers of apoptosis, but, again, the clinical significance of this is unclear.

Vicriviroc is a once-daily CCR5 antagonist which, like PIs, requires ritonavir boosting. The recently presented findings of VICTOR-E3 and VICTOR-E4, two phase 3, double-blind studies comparing vicriviroc with placebo (each with optimized background therapy) in treatment-experienced subjects resulted in cessation of further development of vicriviroc in this patient group. All patients received optimized background containing at least two active drugs (including a boosted PI), but 60% received three or more active drugs. At week 48, the proportion of patients with an undetectable (less than 50 copies/mL) viral load were similar in each arm (62% on placebo and 64% on vicriviroc).[106] However, among participants receiving two or fewer active background drugs, 70% on vicriviroc achieved viral suppression compared with 55% on placebo (p=0.02). The success rates seen in the placebo arm were markedly better than in the placebo arms of earlier studies in similarly experienced patients, which undoubtedly is due to the wider availability of active drugs for patients with extensive drug resistance. It could be argued that no agent could have beaten placebo in the same study, which raises important questions for trial design in the future.

An earlier study of vicriviroc with two NRTIs for initial therapy was terminated early due to an excess of early virologic failures, but a study using vicriviroc as part of an NRTI-sparing strategy (with atazanavir/ritonavir) is ongoing.

Ultimately, CCR5 antagonists have yet to feature in first-line treatment guidelines, but if genotypic testing proves useful, this well-tolerated, lipid-friendly class may play a greater role in the future.

Conclusions

Most HIV-infected individuals with access to antiretroviral therapy can now expect an excellent prognosis and, as adequate immune restoration is achieved, a near-normal life expectancy. This has been driven by not only better understanding and management of HIV-related morbidities, but—probably most importantly—due to marked improvements in antiretroviral therapy. However, there remain limitations with current antiretrovirals, particularly regarding long-term toxicities. New antiretroviral treatment classes and strategies, including NRTI-sparing regimens and new methods to predict and monitor drug-related toxicities, will play increasingly important roles in optimizing and individualizing therapy for the long term.

References

1. van Sighem A, Gras L, Reiss P, Brinkman K, de Wolf F; on behalf of the ATHENA national observational cohort study. Life expectancy of recently diagnosed asymptomatic HIV-infected patients approaches that of uninfected individuals. AIDS 2010; Epub ahead of print.
2. McNicholl JM, Smith DK, Qari SH, Hodge T. Host genes and HIV: the role of the chemokine receptor gene CCR5 and its allele. Emerg Infect Dis 1997;3(3):261–271.
3. Liu R, Paxton WA, Choe S. Homozygous defect in HIV-1 coreceptor accounts for resistance of some multiply-exposed individuals to HIV-1 infection. Cell 1996;86(3):367–377.
4. Samson M, Libert F, Doranz BJ et al. Resistance to HIV-1 infection in caucasian individuals bearing mutant alleles of the CCR-5 chemokine receptor gene. Nature 1996;382(6593):722–725.

5. Wu L, Paxton WA, Kassam N et al. CCR5 levels and expression pattern correlate with infectability by macrophage-tropic HIV-1, in vitro. J Exp Med 1997;185(9):1681–1691.

6. de Roda Husman AM, Koot M, Cornelissen M et al. Association between CCR5 genotype and the clinical course of HIV-1 infection. Ann Intern Med 1997;127(10):882–890.

7. Ahlenstiel G, Woitas RP, Rockstroh J, Spengler U. CC-chemokine receptor 5 (CCR5) in hepatitis C--at the crossroads of the antiviral immune response? J Antimicrob Chemother 2004;53(6):895–898.

8. Glass WG, McDermott DH, Lim JK et al. CCR5 deficiency increases risk of symptomatic West Nile virus infection. J Exp Med 2006;203(1):35–40.

9. Klein RS. A Moving Target: The Multiple Roles of CCR5 in Infectious Diseases. J Infecti Dis 2008;197:183–186.

10. Beelen A, Otto J, Fidler M, et al. Phase 1, Single Ascending Oral Dose Study of the Safety, Tolerability, and Pharmacokinetics of a Novel HIV-1 Maturation Inhibitor in HIV- Healthy Volunteers. 16th Conference on Retroviruses and Opportunistic Infections Montreal, Canada; February 8–11, 2009. Abstract 570.

11. Abreu C, Da Costa L, Ferreira W et al. New HIV-1 Maturation Inhibitor Extracted from Brazilian Brown Algae Dictyota pfaffii. 16th Conference on Retroviruses and Opportunistic Infections Montreal, Canada; February 8–11, 2009. Abstract 562.

12. Khoury G, Ewart G, Luscombe C, Miller M, Wilkinson J. The Antiviral Efficacy of the Novel Compound BIT225 Against HIV-1 Release from Human Macrophages. Antimicrob Agents Chemother 2010;54(2):835–845.

13. Williams P, Staas D, Venkatraman S et al. Inhibitors of the RNase H Activity of Reverse Transcriptase as an Approach to New HIV-1 Antiretroviral Agents. 16th Conference on Retroviruses and Opportunistic Infections Montreal, Canada; February 8–11, 2009. Abstract 559.

14. Choi S, Ban H, Son J et al. Effective and Sustained Suppression of HIV-1 Infection in Humanized Mice by Combinatorial RNA Interference. 16th Conference on Retroviruses and Opportunistic Infections Montreal, Canada; February 8–11, 2009. Abstract 564.

15. Christ F, Voet A, Marchand A et al. First-in-class Inhibitors of LEDGF/p75-integrase Interaction and HIV replication. 17th Conference on Retroviruses & Opportunistic Infections. San Francisco. February 16–19, 2010. Abstract 49.

16. Riddler SA, Haubrich R, DiRienzo AG et al; AIDS Clinical Trials Group Study A5142 Team. Class-sparing regimens for initial treatment of HIV-1 infection. N Engl J Med 2008;358(20):2095–2106.

17. Arribas JR, Pozniak AL, Gallant JE et al. Tenofovir disoproxil fumarate, emtricitabine, and efavirenz compared with zidovudine/lamivudine and efavirenz in treatment-naive patients: 144-week analysis. J Acquir Immune Defic Syndr 2008;47(1):74–78.

18. Birkus G, Hitchcock MJ, Cihlar T. Assessment of mitochondrial toxicity in human cells treated with tenofovir: comparison with other nucleoside reverse transcriptase inhibitors. J Antimicrob Agents Chemother 2002;46(3):716–723.

19. Dubé MP, Komarow L, Mulligan K et al; Adult Clinical Trials Group 384. Long-term body fat outcomes in antiretroviral-naive participants randomized to nelfinavir or efavirenz or both plus dual nucleosides. Dual X-ray absorptiometry results from A5005s, a substudy of Adult Clinical Trials Group 384. J Acquir Immune Defic Syndr 2007;45(5):508–514.

20. Worm SW, Sabin C, Weber R et al. Risk of myocardial infarction in patients with HIV infection exposed to specific individual antiretroviral drugs from the 3 major drug classes: the data collection on adverse events of anti-HIV drugs (D:A:D) study. J Infect Dis 2010;201(3):318–330.

21. Maida I, Garcia-Gasco P, Sotgiu G et al. Antiretroviral associated portal hypertension: a new clinical condition? Prevalence, predictors and outcome. Antivir Ther 2008;13(1):103–107.

22. Kovari H, Ledergerber B, Peter U et al. Association of noncirrhotic portal hypertension in HIV-infected persons and antiretroviral therapy with didanosine: a nested case-control study. Clin Infect Dis 2009;49(4):626–635.

23. Scourfield AT, Waters LJ, Holmes P et al. Non-cirrhotic portal hypertension in HIV mono-infected individuals. HIV Med 2009 Apr 1–3; 10(Suppl 1):13 (abstract no. O28).

24. Maitland D, Moyle G, Hand J et al. Early virologic failure in HIV-1-infected subjects on didanosine/tenofovir/efavirenz: 12-week results from a randomized trial. AIDS 2005;19:1183–1188.

25. Waters L, Maitland D, Moyle GJ. Tenofovir and didanosine: a dangerous liaison. AIDS Read 2005 Aug;15(8):403–406, 413.

26. Waters LJ, Mandalia S, Gazzard B, Nelson M. Prospective HLA-B*5701 screening and abacavir hypersensitivity: a single centre experience. AIDS 2007;21(18):2533–2534.

27. Mallal S, Phillips E, Carosi G et al; PREDICT-1 Study Team. HLA-B*5701 screening for hypersensitivity to abacavir. N Engl J Med. 2008 Feb 7;358(6):568–579.

28. ViiV Healthcare UK Ltd. Ziagen Summary of Product Characteristics. 20th November 2009. Accessed 16 May 2010 at, www.medicines.org.uk.

29. Lundgren JD, Neuhaus J, Babiker A et al; Strategies for Management of Anti-Retroviral Therapy/INSIGHT; DAD Study Groups. Use of nucleoside reverse transcriptase inhibitors and risk of myocardial infarction in HIV-infected patients. AIDS 2008;22(14):F17–24.

30. Daar E, Tierney C, Fischl M et al. ACTG 5202: Final Results of ABC/3TC or TDF/FTC with either EFV or ATV/r in Treatment-naive HIV-infected Patients. 17th Conference on Retroviruses & Opportunistic Infections (CROI 2010). San Francisco. February 16–19, 2010. Abstract 59LB.

31. Satchell S, O'Connor E, Peace A et al. Platelet Hyper-Reactivity in HIV-1-infected Patients on Abacavir-containing ART. 16th Conference on Retrovirus and Opportunistic Infections, Montreal, Canada, February 2009. Abstract 151LB.

32. Tsoupras AB, Chini M, Tsogas N et al. Anti-Platelet-Activating Factor Effects of Highly Active Antiretroviral Therapy (HAART): A New Insight in the Drug Therapy of HIV Infection? AIDS Res Hum Retroviruses 2008;24(8):1079–1086.

33. Hsue PY, Hunt PW, Wu Y et al. Association of abacavir and impaired endothelial function in treated and suppressed HIV-infected patients. AIDS 2009;23(15):2021–2027.

34. Gallant JE, Staszewski S, Pozniak AL et al; 903 Study Group. Efficacy and safety of tenofovir DF vs stavudine in combination therapy in antiretroviral-naive patients: a 3-year randomized trial. JAMA 2004 Jul;292(2):191–201.

35. Smith KY, Patel P, Fine D et al; HEAT Study Team. Randomized, double-blind, placebo-matched, multicenter trial of abacavir/lamivudine or tenofovir/emtricitabine with lopinavir/ritonavir for initial HIV treatment. AIDS 2009;23(12):1547–1556.

36. Fux C, Opravil M, Cavassini M et al. Tenofovir and PI Use Are Associated with an Increased Prevalence of Proximal Renal Tubular Dysfunction in the Swiss HIV Cohort Study. 16th Conference on Retrovirus and Opportunistic Infections, Montreal, Canada, February 2009. Abstract 743.

37. HJ Stellbrink, G Moyle, C Orkin et al. Assessment of Safety and Efficacy of Abacavir/Lamivudine and tenofovir/Emtricitabine in Treatment-Naive HIV-1 Infected Subjects. ASSERT: 48-Week Result. 12th European AIDS Conference. Cologne, Germany. November 11–14, 2009.

38. Kinai E, Hanabusa H. Progressive renal tubular dysfunction associated with long-term use of tenofovir DF. AIDS Res Hum Retroviruses 2009;25(4):387–394.

39. Rodriguez Novoa S, Labarga P, Soriano V et al. Predictors of Kidney Tubulopathy in HIV Patients Treated with Tenofovir: A Pharmacogenetic Study. 16th Conference on Retrovirus and Opportunistic Infections, Montreal, Canada, February 2009. Abstract 37.

40. Woodward CL, Hall AM, Williams IG et al. Tenofovir-associated renal and bone toxicity. HIV Med 2009 Sep;10(8):482–487.

41. Calmy A, Fux CA, Norris R et al. Low bone mineral density, renal dysfunction, and fracture risk in HIV infection: a cross-sectional study. J Infect Dis 2009;200(11):1746–1154.

42. Bruera D, Luna N, David DO, et al. Decreased bone mineral density in HIV-infected patients is independent of antiretroviral therapy. AIDS 2003;17:1917–1923.

43. Fodale V, Mazzeo, A, Praticò C et al. Fatal exacerbation of peripheral neuropathy during lamivudine therapy: evidence for iatrogenic mitochondrial damage. Anaesthesia 2006;60(8):806–810.

44. Gilead Sciences Ltd. Emtriva Summary of Product Characteristics. 22nd September 2008. Accessed at www.medicines.org.uk on 16th May 2010.

45. Accessed 28 June 2010 at http://www.aidsmap.com/en/news/C9CB26F5-748A-43F1-9B29-8475FB8F0C73.asp.

46. Accessed 21 December 2009 at, http://www.koronispharma.com/news-2009-05-19.html.

47. Lanier R, Lampert B, Robertson A, Almond M & Painter G. Hexadecyloxypropyl Tenofovir Associates Directly with HIV and Subsequently Inhibits Viral Replication in Untreated Cells. 16th Conference on Retrovirus and Opportunistic Infections, Montreal, Canada, February 2009. Abstract 37. Abstract 556.

48. van Leth F, Phanuphak P, Ruxrungtham K et al. Comparison of first-line antiretroviral therapy with regimens including nevirapine, efavirenz, or both drugs, plus stavudine and lamivudine: a randomised open-label trial, the 2NN Study. Lancet 2004 Apr 17;363(9417):1253–1263.

49. Viramune Summary of Product Characteristics. Boehringer Ingelheim Limited; 10th January 2008. Accessed at www.medicines.org on 7th June 2010.

50. Sax PE. Report from the 5th IAS Conference on HIV Pathogenesis Treatment and Prevention. Nevirapine vs. boosted atazanavir - the ARTEN Study. AIDS Clin Care 2009 Oct;21(10):80.

51. Macías J, Castellano V, Merchante N et al. Effect of antiretroviral drugs on liver fibrosis in HIV-infected patients with chronic hepatitis C: harmful impact of nevirapine. AIDS 2004;18(5):767–774.

52. Berenguer J, Bellón JM, Miralles P et al. Association between exposure to nevirapine and reduced liver fibrosis progression in patients with HIV and hepatitis C virus coinfection. Clin Infect Dis 2008;46(1):137–143.

53. Torti C, Costarelli S, De Silvestri A et al. Analysis of severe hepatic events associated with nevirapine-containing regimens: CD4+ T-cell count and gender in hepatitis C seropositive and seronegative patients. Drug Saf 2007;30(12):1161–1169.

54. Labarga P, Soriano V, Vispo ME et al. Hepatotoxicity of antiretroviral drugs is reduced after successful treatment of chronic hepatitis C in HIV-infected patients. J Infect Dis 2007;196(5):670–676.

55. Muñoz-Moreno JA, Fumaz CR, Ferrer MJ et al. Neuropsychiatric symptoms associated with efavirenz: prevalence, correlates, and management. A neurobehavioral review. AIDS Rev 2009;11(2):103–109.

56. Boffito M, Jackson A, Lamorde M et al. Pharmacokinetics and safety of etravirine administered once or twice daily after 2 weeks treatment with efavirenz in healthy volunteers. J Acquir Immune Defic Syndr 2009;52(2):222–227.

57. Waters LJ, Fisher M, Winston A et al. A Phase IV, double-blind, multi centre, randomised, placebo-controlled, pilot study to assess the feasibility of switching individuals receiving efavirenz (EFV) with continuing central nervous system (CNS) adverse events (AE) to once daily etravirine (ETR) Second Joint Conference of the British HIV Association (BHIVA) with the British Association for Sexual Health and HIV (BASHH), 20–23 April 2010. Abstract O7.

58. Gutiérrez-Valencia A, Viciana P, Palacios R et al. Stepped-dose versus full-dose efavirenz for HIV infection and neuropsychiatric adverse events: a randomized trial. Ann Intern Med 2009;151(3):149–156.

59. Bangsberg D, Ragland K, Monk A & Deeks S. A One-pill, Once-daily Fixed-dose Combination of Efavirenz, Emcitrabine, and Tenofovir Disoproxil Fumarate Regimen Is Associated with Higher Unannounced Pill Count Adherence than Non-one-pill, Once-daily Regimens. 17th Conference on Retroviruses & Opportunistic Infections (CROI 2010). San Francisco. February 16–19, 2010. Abstract 510.

60. Intelence Summary of Product of Characteristics, Janssen-Cilag Ltd. 28th August 2009. Accessed 6 May 2010 at, www.medicines.org on .

61. Katlama C, Haubrich R, Lalezari J et al; DUET-1, DUET-2 study groups. Efficacy and safety of etravirine in treatment-experienced, HIV-1 patients: pooled 48 week analysis of two randomized, controlled trials. AIDS. 2009 Nov 13;23(17):2289–2300.

62. Yazdanpanah Y, Fagard C, Descamps D et al. High rate of virologic suppression with raltegravir plus etravirine and darunavir/ritonavir among treatment-experienced patients infected with multidrug-resistant HIV: results of the ANRS 139 TRIO trial. Clin Infect Dis 2009;49(9):1441–1449.

63. Ruxrungtham K, Pedro RJ, Latiff GH et al. Impact of reverse transcriptase resistance on the efficacy of TMC125 (etravirine) with two nucleoside reverse transcriptase inhibitors in protease inhibitor-naïve, nonnucleoside reverse transcriptase inhibitor-experienced patients: study TMC125-C227. HIV Med 2008;9(10):883–896.

64. Goebel F, Yakovlev A, Pozniak AL et al. Short-term antiviral activity of TMC278--a novel NNRTI--in treatment-naive HIV-1-infected subjects. AIDS 2006;20(13):1721–1726.

65a. Pozniak AL, Morales-Ramirez J, Katabira E et al; TMC278-C204 Study Group. Efficacy and safety of TMC278 in antiretroviral-naive HIV-1 patients: week 96 results of a phase IIb randomized trial. AIDS 2010;24(1):55–65.

65b. Cohen C, Molina J, Cahn P, et al. Pooled week 48 efficacy and safety results from ECHO and THRIVE, two double-blind, randomised, phase III trials comparing TMC278 versus efavirenz in treatment-naïve, HIV-1-infected patients. XVIII International AIDS Conference. Vienna, 2010.

65c. Cohen C, Molina J, Cahn P, Clotet B, Fourie J, Grinsztejn B, et al. Pooled week 48 safety and efficacy results from the ECHO and THRIVE phase III trials comparing TMC278 vs. EFV in treatment-naïve, HIV-1-infected patients. Tenth International Congress on Drug Therapy in HIV Infection. Glasgow, 2010.

66. Accessed 6 May 2010 at, http://www.reuters.com/article/idUSTRE56F6ZA20090716.

67. van't Klooster G, Verloes R, Baert L et al. Long-acting TMC278, a Parenteral Depot Formulation Delivering Therapeutic NNRTI Concentrations in Preclinical and Clinical Settings. 15th Conference on Retroviruses and Opportunistic Infections (CROI 2008). Boston, MA. February 3–6, 2008. Abstract 134.

68. TMC278-TiDP15-C158—A Study to Examine the Safety, Tolerability and Pharmacokinetics of a Single Dose or Three Successive Doses of Intramuscularly (IM) Injected Long Acting Formulation of TMC278. Accessed 6 May 2010 at, http://clinicaltrials.gov on.

69. Ortiz R, Dejesus E, Khanlou H et al. Efficacy and safety of once-daily darunavir/ritonavir versus lopinavir/ritonavir in treatment-naive HIV-1-infected patients at week 48. AIDS 2008;22(12):1389–1397.

70. Molina JM, Andrade-Villanueva J, Echevarria J et al. Once-daily atazanavir/ritonavir compared with twice-daily lopinavir/ritonavir, each in combination with tenofovir and emtricitabine, for management of antiretroviral-naive HIV-1-infected patients: 96-week efficacy and safety results of the CASTLE study. J Acquir Immune Defic Syndr 20101;53(3):323–332.

71. Eron J Jr, Yeni P, Gathe J Jr et al. The KLEAN study of fosamprenavir-ritonavir versus lopinavir-ritonavir, each in combination with abacavir-lamivudine, for initial treatment of HIV infection over 48 weeks: a randomised non-inferiority trial. Lancet 2006;368(9534):476–482.

72. Johnson M, Grinsztejn B, Rodriguez C et al. 96-week comparison of once-daily atazanavir/ritonavir and twice-daily lopinavir/ritonavir in patients with multiple virologic failures. AIDS 2006 Mar 21;20(5):711–718.

73. Madruga JV, Berger D, McMurchie M et al. Efficacy and safety of darunavir-ritonavir compared with that of lopinavir-ritonavir at 48 weeks in treatment-experienced, HIV-infected patients in TITAN: a randomised controlled phase III trial. Lancet 2007;370(9581):49–58.

74. Walmsley S, Avihingsanon A, Slim J et al. Gemini: a noninferiority study of saquinavir/ritonavir versus lopinavir/ritonavir as initial HIV-1 therapy in adults. J Acquir Immune Defic Syndr 2009;50(4):367–374.

75. Invirase Summary of Product Characteristics, Roche Products Limited. 4th October 2006. Accessed 6 May 2010 at, www.medicines.org.

76. Durand M, Sheehy O, Baril J-G et al. Relation between use of nucleoside reverse transcriptase inhibitors and risk of acute myocardial infarction (AMI): a nested case control study using Quebec's Public Health Insurance Database (RAMQ). Abstracts of the Fifth International AIDS Society Conference on HIV Pathogenesis, Treatment and Prevention, Cape Town, South Africa, 2009. Abstract TUPEB175.

77. Arribas JR, Horban A, Gerstoft J et al. The MONET trial: darunavir/ritonavir with or without nucleoside analogues, for patients with HIV RNA below 50 copies/ml. AIDS 2010,24(2):223–230.

78. Katlama C, Valentin MA, Algarte-Genin M et al. Efficacy of darunavir/ritonavir as single-drug maintenance therapy in patients with HIV-1 viral suppression: a randomized open-label non-inferiority trial, MONOI-ANRS 136 C. 5th IAS Conference on HIV Pathogenesis, Treatment and Prevention. July 19–22, 2009. Cape Town. Abstract WELBB102.

79. Swindells S, DiRienzo AG, Wilkin T et al. Regimen simplification to atazanavir-ritonavir alone as maintenance antiretroviral therapy after sustained virologic suppression. JAMA 2006; 296:806–814.

80. Karlstrom O, Josephson F, So nnerborg A. Early virologic rebound in a pilot trial of ritonavir-boosted atazanavir as maintenance monotherapy. J Acquir Immune Defic Syndr 2007; 44:417–422.

81. Vernazza P, Daneel S, Schiffer V et al. The role of compartment penetration in PI-monotherapy: the Atazanavir-Ritonavir Monomaintenance (ATARITMO) Trial. AIDS 2007; 21:1309–1315.

82. Bierman WF, van Agtmael MA, Nijhuis M, Danner SA, Boucher CA. HIV monotherapy with ritonavir-boosted protease inhibitors: a systematic review. AIDS 2009;23(3):279–291.

83. Steigbigel RT, Cooper DA, Teppler H et al. Long-term efficacy and safety of Raltegravir combined with optimized background therapy in treatment-experienced patients with drug-resistant HIV infection: week 96 results of the BENCHMRK 1 and 2 phase iii trials. Clin Infect Dis 2010; 50(4):605–612.

84. Markowitz M, Nguyen B-Y, Gotuzzo E et al. Rapid and Durable Antiretroviral Effect of the HIV-1 Integrase Inhibitor Raltegravir as Part of Combination Therapy in Treatment-Naive Patients With HIV-1 Infection: Results of a 48-Week Controlled Study. J Acquir Immune Defici Syndr 2007;46(2):125–133.

85. Gotuzzo E, Nguyen B-Y, Markowitz M et al. Sustained antiretroviral efficacy of raltegravir after 192 weeks of combination ART in treatment-naïve HIV-1 infected patients. 17th Conference on Retrovirusesand Opportunistic Infections. February 16–19, 2010; San Francisco, CA. Abstract #K-127; Poster #514.

86. Lennox JL, DeJesus E, Lazzarin A et al. Safety and efficacy of raltegravir-based versus efavirenz-based combination therapy in treatment-naïve patients with HIV-1 infection: a multicentre, double-blind randomised controlled trial. Lancet 2009;374: 96806.

87. Molto J, Valle M, Back D, Cedeno S, Watson V, Liptrott N, et al. Plasma and intracellular (PBMCs) pharmacokinetics of once-daily raltegravir (800mg) in HIV-infected patients. Antimicrob Agents Chemother . E-publication, ahead of print.

88. Merck Reports Initial Results of Phase III Study of ISENTRESS® (raltegravir) Investigational Once-Daily Dosing in Treatment-Naïve Adult Patients Infected with HIV-1, 2010

89. Eron JJ, Young B, Cooper DA et al. Switch to a raltegravir-based regimen versus continuation of a lopinavir-ritonavir-based regimen in stable HIV-infected patients with suppressed viraemia (SWITCHMRK 1 and 2): two multicentre, double-blind, randomised controlled trials. Lancet 2010;375(9712):396–407.

90. Archin NM, Cheema M, Parker D et al. Antiretroviral intensification and valproic acid lack sustained effect on residual HIV-1 viremia or resting CD4+ cell infection. PLoS One. 2010 Feb 23;5(2):e9390.

91. Joly V, Fagard C, Descamps D et al. Intensification of HAART through the Addition of Enfuvirtide in Naive HIV-infected Patients with Severe Immunosuppression Does Not Improve Immunological Response: Results of a Prospective Randomized Multicenter Trial (APOLLO - ANRS 130). 17th Conference on Retroviruses & Opportunistic Infections. San Francisco. February 16–19, 2010. Abstract 282.

92. Clotet B, Capetti A, Soto-Ramirez LE, Gatell JM, Rowell L, Salgo M, Schapiro JM. A randomized, controlled study evaluating an induction treatment strategy in which enfuvirtide was added to an oral, highly active antiretroviral therapy regimen in treatment-experienced patients: the INTENSE study. J Antimicrob Chemother. 2008 Dec;62(6):1374–1378.

93. Read P, Khan P, Mandalia S et al. When Should HAART Be Initiated in Pregnancy to Achieve an Undetectable Viral Load? 17th Conference on Retroviruses & Opportunistic Infections. San Francisco. February 16–19, 2010. Abstract 896.

94. Ceccaldi PF, Ferreira C, Gavard L, et al. Placental transfer of enfuvirtide in the ex vivo human placenta perfusion model. Am J Obstet Gynecol 2008; 198:433 e1–433 e2.

95. S Bonora, A Calcagno, C Cometto, et al. A Long-Term Immunological Advantage Associated with a Short-Term Additional Therapy with Enfuvirtide in the Treatment of HIV Very Late Presenters. 49th Interscience Conference on Antimicrobial Agents and Chemotherapy (ICAAC 2009). San Francisco. September 12–15, 2009. Abstract H-924.

96. Cooper DA, Heera J, Goodrich J et al. Maraviroc versus efavirenz, both in combination with zidovudine-lamivudine, for the treatment of antiretroviral-naive subjects with CCR5-tropic HIV-1 infection. J Infect Dis 2010 Mar 15;201(6):803–813.

97. Gulick RM, Lalezari J, Goodrich J et al; MOTIVATE Study Teams. Maraviroc for previously treated patients with R5 HIV-1 infection. N Engl J Med 2008;359(14):1429–1441.

98. Harrigan PR, McGovern R, Dong W et al. Screening for HIV tropism using population-based V3 genotypic analysis: a retrospective virologic outcome analysis using stored plasma screening samples from the MOTIVATE studies of maraviroc in treatment-experienced patients. Fifth International AIDS Society Conference on HIV Pathogenesis, Treatment and Prevention, Cape Town, abstract WeLBA101, 2009.

99. Obermeier M, Carganico A, Berg T, et al. The Berlin maraviroc cohort: influence of genotypic tropism testing results on therapeutic outcome. 7th European HIV Drug Resistance Workshop, March 25–27, 2009, Stockholm. Abstract 79.

100. McGovern R, Dong W, Zhong X, Knapp D, Thielen A, Chapman D, et al. Population-based Sequencing of the V3-loop Is Comparable to the Enhanced Sensitivity Trofile Assay in Predicting Virologic Response to Maraviroc of Treatment-naïve Patients in the MERIT Trial. 17th Conference on Retroviruses and Opportunistic Infections. San Francisco, CA, 2010

101. Seclén E, Del Mar González M, De Mendoza C, Soriano V, Poveda E. Dynamics of HIV tropism under suppressive antiretroviral therapy: implications for tropism testing in subjects with undetectable viraemia. J Antimicrob Chemother 2010;65(7):1493–1496.

102. Saag M, Ive P, Heera J et al. A multicenter, randomized, double-blind, comparative trial of a novel CCR5 antagonist, maraviroc vs efavirenz, both in combination with combivir (zidovudine/lamivudine), for the treatment of antiretroviral naive patients infected with R5 HIV-1: week 48 results of the MERIT study [abstract #WESS104]. In: 4th IAS Conference on HIV pathogenesis, treatment and prevention; July 2007; Sydney, Australia, 2007.

103. Funderburg N, Kalinowska M, Eason J et al. Differential effects of maraviroc (MVC) and efavirenz (EFV) on markers of immune activation (IA) and inflammation and their association with CD4 cell rises: a subanalysis of the MERIT study. In: Program and abstracts of the 49th Interscience Conference on Antimicrobial Agents and Chemotherapy; September 12–15, 2009; San Francisco, Calif. Abstract H-1582.

104. Stepanyuk O, Chiang TS; Dever LL et al. Impact of adding maraviroc to antiretroviral regimens in patients with full viral suppression but impaired CD4 recovery. AIDS 2009;23(14):1911–1913.

105. Wilkin T, Lalama C, Tenoria A et al. Maraviroc intensification for suboptimal CD4+ cell response despite sustained virologic suppression: ACTG 5256. Program and abstracts of the 17th Conference on Retroviruses and Opportunistic Infections; February 16–19, 2010; San Francisco, California. Abstract 285.

106. Gathe J, Diaz R, Fatkenheuer G et al. Phase 3 trials of vicriviroc in treatment-experienced subjects demonstrate safety but not significantly greater superiority over potent background regimens alone. Seventeenth Conference on Retroviruses and Opportunistic Infections, abstract 54LB, San Francisco, 2010.

Chapter 19 Treatment of Viral Infections

C. BEAU WILLISON, L. KATIE MORRISON, NATALIA MENDOZA, AND STEPHEN K. TYRING

Scientific principles and laws do not lie on the surface of nature. They are hidden, and must be wrested from nature by an active and elaborate technique of inquiry.

—JOHN DEWEY, *Reconstruction in Philosophy, 1920*

Introduction

Manifestations of viral infection may herald infection with the human immunodeficiency virus (HIV) or a change in an HIV-positive patient's immune function, and are a principal cause of morbidity in HIV-infected patients. Therefore, a thorough understanding of the potential viral pathogens that can affect HIV patients including the ability to recognize the associated signs and symptoms and initiate a proper treatment regimen is essential.

Herpes Simplex Virus

Background

Herpes simplex virus (HSV) is a double-stranded, encapsulated DNA virus belonging to the Herpesviridae family. Herpes simplex virus type 1 (HSV-1) and type 2 (HSV-2) are very common causes of disease in the general population as well as in HIV-infected patients. In the United States, 50% to 70% of the general population is infected with HSV-1 and 15% to 33% with HSV-2, with an even higher prevalence in the HIV-positive population. HSV-2 has a seroprevalence of 60% to 90% in HIV-infected persons.[1–3] HSV-1 is more commonly associated with orolabial herpes or herpes above the waistline and HSV-2 most commonly associated with genital herpes; however, HSV-1 is responsible for >70% of orolabial herpes, whereas ~70% of genital herpes is caused by HSV-2. Primary HSV infection occurs through contact with the skin or mucous membranes, where local viral replication occurs. Viral transmission can occur during periods of symptomatic and asymptomatic latent infection, and asymptomatic shedding of HSV-2 has been shown to be increased in HIV-positive patients compared to those unaffected by the disease.[4,5] HIV-infected patients with HSV-2 who underwent daily anogenital swabs demonstrated HSV-2 viral shedding in 29% of swabs while taking placebo compared to 4% while using daily suppressive oral valacyclovir (500 mg bid).[6,7] Some studies have also demonstrated that HSV-2 infection may increase the risk for HIV transmission, even above levels that might be expected to result from epidermal breach with HSV lesions.[8–13]

Characteristic of herpes viruses, the virus then spreads via sensory nerves to dorsal root ganglia, where latent infection is established; reactivation causes the virus to again travel distally along the sensory nerve, resulting in mucocutaneous vesicular eruptions.

Presentation/Diagnosis

Patients with symptomatic HSV infection usually present with grouped vesicles or ulcerative lesions (**Figures 19–1, 19–2, 19–3**). Primary orolabial infection in children lasts approximately 2 to 3 weeks and is characterized by fever and involvement of the buccal and gingival mucosa. In adults, primary orolabial HSV infection is characterized by pharyngitis and a mononucleosis syndrome.[14,15] Primary genital HSV infection is characterized by macules and papules followed by vesicles, which eventually ulcerate, with a total duration of around 3 weeks. Fever is often seen in primary infection. The recurrent outbreak of orolabial and genital herpes is often preceded by prodromal symptoms of tingling, burning, or pain, followed by erythema and a papular eruption that evolves into vesicles; these vesicles ulcerate, crust, and finally heal. HSV-1 infection is typically associated with a milder course than HSV-2. HIV-positive patients with

Figure 19–1. *Erosive herpes simplex in an AIDS patient in the intergluteal area. It is atypical in duration (months) and configuration (no grouped vesicles but an ulcerative plaque).*

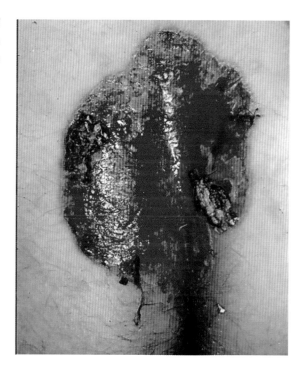

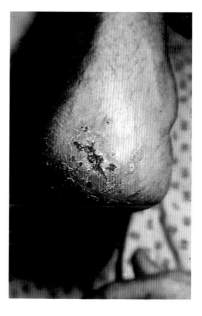

Figure 19–2. *Elbow in an AIDS patient showing positve culture for herpes simplex with erosions and eczematous dermatitis on the elbow.*

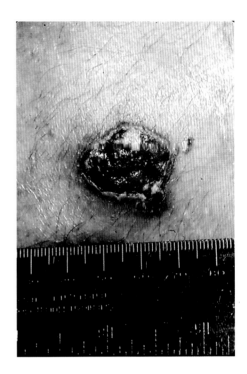

Figure 19–3. *Extremely painful herpes simplex virus infection in a AIDS patient on the knee present for over 6 months and very recalcitrant to therapy.*

advanced disease appear to have longer courses of symptomatic infection, with increased severity and more frequent recurrence rates compared to immunocompetent individuals.[16–20] Patients may also present with proctitis, characterized by fever, pruritus, severe rectal pain, and tenesmus. This primarily occurs in male patients and is the most common cause of nongonococcal proctitis in men who have sex with men (MSM).[21–23] Another AIDS-defining illness that patients may present with is HSV esophagitis, which is characterized by odynophagia and/or retrosternal pain. This typically is seen in patients with CD4 counts <50 cells/mm^3.[24–27] Patients may also present with encephalitis, which is typically caused by HSV-1 involvement in the temporal lobe. However, in HIV-positive patients, HSV encephalitis can involve many areas of the brain and brain stem outside of the limbic system. This can be very difficult to differentiate clinically from other causes of encephalitis, including cytomegalovirus (CMV) infection and toxoplasmosis.[28] HSV, like VZV, can also cause a rapidly progressive retinal necrosis known as acute retinal necrosis syndrome or progressive outer retinal necrosis (PORN). It is associated with pain, keratitis, and iritis, and must be recognized as quickly as possible to initiate intravenous antiviral treatment and thereby minimize possible vision loss.[29]

Treatment

Acyclovir, valacyclovir, and famciclovir have all been shown to lessen the severity of symptomatic HSV infection and to decrease the time to healing and shedding of virus. Primary mucocutaneous HSV infection is initially treated with the same therapy used for immunocompetent patients—either acyclovir (200–400 mg po 5 times daily × 10–14 days), valacyclovir (1,000 mg po bid × 7–10 days), or famciclovir (500 mg po bid × 7–10 days). Recurrent infection is treated with the same antivirals, but at different dosing and duration of therapy—acyclovir (200–400 mg po 5 times daily × 5–10 days), valacyclovir (500 mg po bid × 5–10 days), or famciclovir (500 mg po bid × 7–10 days). Patients with particularly severe or complicated cases or in those who cannot tolerate oral treatment, IV acyclovir (5mg/kg q8h × 7–10 days) can be used. Duration of antiviral therapy should be extended, when necessary, until lesions are completely crusted over.[1,14,30–36] For patients with frequent or severe recurrences (that is, 3 outbreaks in 6 months) continuous suppressive therapy may be considered. Suppressive therapy options include acyclovir (400–800 mg po 2–3 × day), famciclovir (250 mg po bid), valacyclovir (500 mg po bid or 1,000 mg po 1 × day).[37,38] Side effects from acyclovir and valacyclovir are rarely encountered at the recommended doses, but may include reversible nephrotoxicity and neurotoxicity. Famciclovir has not been found to produce any serious side effects. Patients with impaired renal function (creatinine clearance of <10mL/min for po acyclovir, <50mL/min for IV acyclovir and po valacyclovir, and <40mL/min for famciclovir) should receive appropriately reduced doses.[1] Although some studies have shown that daily HSV-2 antiviral therapy reduced plasma HIV-1 levels, a randomized, double-blind, placebo-controlled trial of twice-daily suppressive acyclovir treatment demonstrated no decrease in risk of HIV transmission.[6,7,39–42]

Acyclovir-resistant strains of HSV have been described in patients with HIV infection, particularly those with CD4+ T-lymphocyte counts of <50 cells/mm^3.[43–49] Acyclovir-resistant HSV infection should be suspected in patients who remain unresponsive to standard treatment for 14 days. These patients should have repeat viral cultures performed for antiviral susceptibility. As not all recalcitrant HSV infections are acyclovir-resistant, initially increasing the dose (acyclovir 800 mg po q4h 5 × day) or switching to an alternative therapy with either valacyclovir or famciclovir is a prudent first step. If this regimen continues to fail or susceptibility testing indicates acyclovir resistance, the treatment of choice is foscarnet, 40mg/kg IV tid, until lesions have completely re-epithelialized.[14,50–55] Some reports have suggested IV cidofovir as a possible alternative in resistant HSV infections; however, a significant side-effect profile and lack of sufficient data warrant further studies to determine its role as a suitable agent.[56–61] Alternatively, some topical antiviral treatments may be effective in acyclovir-resistant HSV infection. One option that is suggested by the U.S. Centers for Disease Control and Prevention (CDC) is cidofovir gel 1%, applied once daily for 5 consecutive days. Other options include trifluridine ophthalmic solution, applied tid, and foscarnet cream 1%, applied 5 times daily. Side effects of these topical treatments are most commonly associated with local irritation.[1,62–66]

Patients with HSV esophagitis or proctitis should be treated for 10 to 14 days with either acyclovir (400 mg po 5 × day), acyclovir (5 mg/kg q8h), or valacyclovir (500 mg po bid). Visceral or central nervous system (CNS) HSV infections are treated with IV acyclovir 10–15mg/kg q8h for 14–21 days. However, even with appropriate IV antiviral treatment, HSV encephalitis is associated with very high morbidity and mortality. In one study, IV acyclovir given at 10 mg/kg every 8 hours for 10 to 14 days was shown to decrease mortality at 3 months to 19% compared to 50% in patients treated with vidarabine therapy.[1,14,21,22,27,30,31,67–70]

Proper administration of highly-active antiretroviral therapy (HAART) in an effort to maintain immune function is also a crucial step in decreasing the severity and frequency of HSV infection in HIV-infected patients.

Varicella Zoster Virus

Background

Varicella zoster virus (VZV) is a double-stranded, encapsulated DNA virus belonging to the Herpesviridae family. Only one serotype of VZV exists, and seven genotypes have been identified.[71] It is the cause of two separate clinical diseases, varicella (chickenpox) and herpes zoster (shingles). Primary infection occurs via airborne virus exposure or through contact with non-crusted varicella or zoster vesicles in susceptible individuals. Primary varicella is contagious from around 2 days prior to rash onset to 4 to 5 days after. Since 1995, children have been routinely vaccinated against VZV.[72] Studies have shown that 95% of the U.S. population has serologic evidence of VZV infection by age 20, and 99.6% of people 40 to 49 years of age demonstrated VZV seropositivity.[73,74] Herpes zoster occurs with the reactivation of dormant VZV, which resides in sensory dorsal or cranial root ganglia, as is found in HSV infection. Clinical VZV disease has been shown to occur with increased frequency in HIV-infected patients and is associated with a more severe clinical course, with an increased rate of complications and a relapse rate of around 20%.[29,75,76] Shingles can occur in patients with any CD4+ count, but the incidence has been found to be higher in patients with lowered immune function, and can be one of the first signals of immunodeficiency. The incidence of herpes zoster is thought to be around 15-fold higher in HIV-positive patients compared to age-matched, seronegative controls.[77–84]

Presentation

Primary varicella or chickenpox has an incubation of ~15 days and classically presents as a rash that starts with macules, quickly evolves into papules, and then to vesicles surrounded by erythema, which eventually pustulate and scab over (**Figure 19–4**). The rash begins on the head and spreads to the trunk and extremities. Lesions are classically found concurrently in all stages of development—that is, the simultaneous appearance of papules, vesicles, and crusted lesions. The rash can be preceded by prodromal symptoms of fever, malaise, anorexia, or headache.

Herpes zoster presents classically as a painful cutaneous eruption of vesicles in a unilateral and dermatomal distribution, which can be preceded by prodromal symptoms of tingling, burning, or pain. Adjacent dermatomal involvement may be seen in ~20% of cases.[85] The lesions gradually pustulate, crust, and heal. The chronic pain syndrome that is one of the most common and feared complications of herpes zoster is called postherpetic neuralgia (PHN). Although still a rare occurrence, HIV-positive patients are more frequently found to have adjacent and, even very rarely, nonadjacent dermatomal involvement.[29,86] Herpes zoster involving the first branch of the trigeminal nerve (V1) has been called herpes zoster ophthalmicus (HZO). HZO can be associated with devastating ocular complications, including permanent loss of vision, and warrants early, aggressive antiviral treatment. Acute retinal necrosis (ARN), varicella-zoster virus retinitis (VZVR), PORN, or rapidly progressive herpetic retinal necrosis (RPHRN) have all been described in HIV-positive patients. These syndromes are associated with pain, keratitis, and iritis

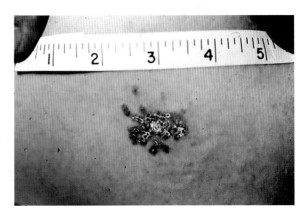

Figure 19–4. *Varicella virus on the lower back of an AIDS patient. Similar smaller grouped crusts and vesicles ocurred for many months widely scattered over the trunk and occasionally the extremities.*

and can be complicated by bilateral involvement and retinal detachment. These can occur after or during HZO, or even with herpes zoster involving remote dermatomes. Fundoscopic examination is part of a proper workup; findings include granular, yellow or pale gray, nonhemorrhagic peripheral lesions. HSV can also cause an identical condition. Rapid recognition and initiation of intravenous antiviral treatment for this condition is crucial to minimize complications. Complete loss of vision is reported to occur in 75% to 85% of involved eyes.[87–94] Atypical herpes zoster lesions—such as disseminated disease, verrucous or hyperkeratotic lesions, ecthymatous lesions, and pinpoint papules—are also found in HIV-infected patients.[94,95] Visceral involvement has rarely been reported in HIV-infected patients.[96] CNS involvement may occur in HIV-positive patients, even without a history of cutaneous zoster-like eruptions.[79,97–103]

Treatment

Varicella: Primary varicella may be treated with oral acyclovir (20 mg/kg, to a maximum dose of 800 mg, 5 × day) until the lesions are healed. This treatment has been well studied in immunocompetent children, adolescents, and adults and has been shown to speed up the time to cessation of new lesion formation, decrease the overall number of lesions formed, and decrease constitutional symptoms such as fever. Unfortunately, no controlled, prospective trials have evaluated the effect of antiviral therapy on HIV-positive patients with primary varicella, so treatment guidelines must be extrapolated from existing studies on immunocompetent individuals. Intravenous antiviral treatment (IV acyclovir 10 mg/kg q8h) is usually reserved for particularly severe or complicated cases. Other antivirals such as valacyclovir and famciclovir have not been as thoroughly evaluated for the treatment of chickenpox, and these are not available in suspension; however, their antiviral properties suggest that they may be as effective as acyclovir.[104–106] Prevention of chickenpox with the live-attenuated varicella vaccine has been approved and recommended for healthy children in the U.S. since 1995. It is also currently recommended that HIV-infected children who are asymptomatic and not significantly immunosuppressed receive the vaccine.[107–110]

Herpes Zoster: When initiated within 72 hours of onset of herpes zoster in immunocompetent hosts, acyclovir, valacyclovir (1.0 g po tid), and famciclovir (500 mg po tid) have all been shown to effectively decrease the duration of viral shedding, decrease new lesion formation, hasten lesion healing, and decrease the duration of zoster-related pain. However, valacyclovir and famciclovir are considered superior therapeutic options due to their pharmacokinetic properties. In HIV-infected individuals, in contrast to the standard duration of therapy of 7 to 10 days, treatment should continue until complete lesion resolution has occurred.[111–114] As with chickenpox, severe, atypical, and/or complicated cases of herpes zoster (for example, visceral or CNS involvement, pneumonitis, retinitis, etc.) may be treated with IV antiviral therapy. VZV-induced retinal necrosis is particularly difficult to treat, and some suggest combination therapy with IV foscarnet, IV ganciclovir ± intravitreal foscarnet and/or ganciclovir.[87,116–122] Zoster-related pain can be very debilitating, and adequate pain management is usually warranted, with judicious use of analgesics such as nonsteroidal anti-inflammatory drugs (NSAIDs), opioids, and/or GABA analogs. The initiation of HAART may paradoxically increase the incidence of herpes zoster in HIV-positive patients via immune reconstitution; mechanisms by which this occurs are poorly understood at this time.[123–128]

Acyclovir-resistant VZV: Acyclovir-resistant strains of VZV have been demonstrated multiple times in HIV-infected patients, especially in those with very low CD4+ T lymphocyte

use and requires fluids with high-dose probenecid to prevent proximal renal tubular cell uptake of the drug.[175–177] Antiviral therapy for CMV-associated disease is often given as an initial "induction" regimen and then as a chronic "maintenance" regimen when needed.

Treatment of CMV esophagitis or colitis begins with a 3- to 6-week induction course of ganciclovir (5 mg/kg bid × 14–21 days), valganciclovir (900 mg po bid × 14–21 days), or foscarnet (90 mg/kg bid or 60 mg/kg q9h × 14–21 days). If symptomatic disease resolves after this course, therapy may be stopped. If the symptoms persist, switching antiviral regimens or adding another antiviral agent to the treatment regimen is recommended for an additional 3 to 6 weeks. If the symptoms persist or recur after initial resolution, repeat esophagogastroduodenoscopy (EGD) or colonoscopy should be performed for visualization and biopsy of suspicious lesions.[178–182]

Treatment of CMV retinitis in patients with AIDS begins with induction IV ganciclovir, at 5 mg/kg bid, or valganciclovir, 900 mg po bid for 14 to 21 days, followed by daily oral maintenance therapy of ganciclovir, 5 mg/kg, or valganciclovir, 900 mg, continued indefinitely. The oral maintenance regimen is not recommended if the patient has a disease that potentially may threaten central visual acuity. If the patient experiences progression of retinitis during the maintenance phase, retreatment with the twice-daily regimen should be given. Eighty percent to 90% of patients treated with this regimen experience improvement or stabilization of disease. Foscarnet may also be used, with an induction dose of 90 mg/kg IV q12h for 2 to 3 weeks, followed by 90 mg/kg IV daily maintenance therapy. Combination therapy with ganciclovir and foscarnet has demonstrated synergistic activity against CMV in vitro, and in clinical studies has been shown to prolong the progression of disease when compared to monotherapy; however, this synergism was not demonstrated in vivo and was associated with a decrease in quality of life in patients due to the burden of two intravenous infusions daily.[29,135,183–185] Intravenous use of cidofovir is another alternative, but has associated treatment-limiting nephrotoxicity, iritis, and hypotony in some studies.[135,186–190] Patients who are unable or unwilling to undergo systemic antiviral treatment may also be considered for intravitreal treatment. Ganciclovir may be given by intravitreal injection, at 400 μg per week for 2 to 3 weeks of induction, followed by weekly maintenance injections. Foscarnet may also be given by intravitreal injection, at 2,400 μg twice weekly for 2 to 3 weeks followed by weekly maintenance injections. Intravitreal injection of cidofovir has been used, but is generally avoided due to increased risk for iritis, uveitis, and hypotony with possible significant visual loss.[29,191] A ganciclovir intraocular implant was also approved in 1996, which must be surgically replaced every 5 to 8 months.[192–195] Another intravitreal treatment option that can be used in patients who cannot tolerate or who are resistant to other therapies is fomivirsen, an oligonucleotide antisense agent. Fomivirsen is administered by intravitreal injection, 0.05 mL (330 μg) 2 weeks apart, for a total of 2 doses.[196–197] The major problem with intraocular therapy alone is lack of systemic antiviral activity, which potentiates the development of CMV-associated disease (contralateral eye, viscera, etc.) elsewhere.[135,181,198–209]

CMV pneumonitis is treated in fashion similar to what is used for CMV esophagitis or colitis. Patients who are found to have evidence of CMV pneumonitis or who fail 1 to 2 weeks of treatment for other presumed pathogens are treated with a 3- to 6-week course of ganciclovir or foscarnet. If symptomatic disease resolves, therapy may be discontinued. If symptoms continue or recur, repeat evaluation with bronchoscopy should be performed. If a different pathogen is found, the proper treatment should be initiated. If evidence of CMV pneumonitis is found, re-induction with ganciclovir, foscarnet, or both should be given, followed by chronic maintenance therapy.[153]

CMV-associated encephalitis, polyradiculopathy, and/or myelitis are treated with combination foscarnet and ganciclovir, at induction dosing until maximum clinical improvement/

stabilization occurs, followed by a daily maintenance regimen, as tolerated by the patient, to prevent relapse. Rapid initiation of treatment is critical to obtaining an optimal clinical improvement.[29,135,210]

Epstein-Barr Virus

Background

Epstein-Barr virus (EBV) is a double-stranded, encapsulated DNA virus belonging to the Herpesviridae family and the Gammaherpesvirinae subfamily. All Gammaherpesvirinae viruses are capable of replication in lymphoid cells in vitro, and some are able to undergo lytic replication in epithelial cells and fibroblasts.[215] EBV is commonly known to cause infectious mononucleosis and is involved in the AIDS-defining illnesses of oral hairy leukoplakia (OHL), non-Hodgkin's lymphoma (NHL), and diffuse large B cell lymphoma (DLBCL). CNS lymphoma is virtually 100% EBV-positive, and around two-thirds of DLBCL outside the CNS is EBV-positive.[29,216,217] Like all viruses in the Herpesviridae family, EBV is known to cause active as well as latent infections. Transmission of EBV is through exposure of virus-containing oropharyngeal secretions of infected persons to susceptible individuals. Oral shedding of EBV virus has been shown to be increased in frequency in HIV-seropositive individuals.[218–220] Serologic studies have demonstrated that more than 95% of adults have been infected with EBV. Primary infection with EBV almost always precedes HIV infection, except in cases of vertical transmission of both viruses.

Presentation

Primary infection in children is largely asymptomatic, except for occasional reports of hepatosplenomegaly.[216] In adults and adolescents, primary infection is characterized by the classic acute infectious mononucleosis (AIM) symptoms, including fever, cervical lymphadenopathy, malaise, headache, and pharyngitis.[215,221] Heterophile antibodies, which react to antigens found on sheep, horse, and bovine erythrocytes, are found in 90% of primary EBV infections and are the basis for the Monospot test used in diagnosis.[222] When EBV infection is mistakenly treated with ampicillin or certain other penicillins, many patients will develop a characteristic morbiliform rash on the trunk and extremities that lasts for ~1 week and is followed by desquamation.[223,224] Patients with EBV-induced OHL present with corrugated "hairy" white plaques on the lateral surface of the tongue caused by epithelial hyperplasia; these plaques cannot be removed with gentle scraping, a feature which distinguishes OHL from oral candidiasis). About 20% of asymptomatic HIV-positive patients develop OHL, and the incidence increases with advanced HIV disease. OHL is rarely seen without some form of immunocompromise, and its presence warrants HIV testing.[225–228]

Treatment

The most effective method of managing EBV-associated disease in HIV-infected patients is optimization of their immune function with proper use of HAART.[216,229]

Patients with persistent OHL despite adequate HAART may be treated with systemic antiherpesvirus agents, including acyclovir, valganciclovir, foscarnet, and ganciclovir. Although these agents have been shown to produce clinical regression of OHL, cessation of therapy results in a high rate of recurrence.[29,230–237] Topical therapy with 25% podophyllin resin, an agent which binds tubulin and inhibits microtubule polymerization, has also been shown to be effective in treatment of OHL. Side effects are minimal and include mild burning/pain/discomfort and transient dysgeusia.[238–240]

Treatment of EBV-associated NHL requires systemic chemotherapy (see Chapter 24, which covers this and other HIV-related malignancies). Additionally, rituximab, an anti-CD20 monoclonal antibody, has been shown to be effective against NHL in HIV-negative patients, but has failed to demonstrate efficacy in HIV-infected individuals.[241–243] The role of systemic antiviral therapy with agents such as acyclovir, foscarnet, and ganciclovir remains unclear, and further investigation will be required before well-defined guidelines regarding their use in treatment or prevention of NHL are made.[244–252] AIDS-related DLBCL generally carries a very poor prognosis, but improvement has been seen with the advent of HAART.[216,253–256]

Kaposi's Sarcoma

Background

Kaposi's sarcoma (KS) is caused by human herpesvirus 8 (HHV-8, previously called Kaposi's sarcoma-associated herpesvirus, or KSHV). HHV-8 is a double-stranded DNA virus belonging to the Herpesviridae family, the Gamma-herpesvirinae subfamily, and the Rhadinovirus genus. Like all herpesviruses, HHV-8 produces both latent and lytic infections, which are presumed to be lifelong. KS is a spindle cell tumor generated from lymphatic endothelium which was first described in 1872 by Moris Kaposi, an Austrian dermatologist and dermatopathologist.[257,258] An infectious etiology has been suspected since the 1950s; this was reinforced by the prominent development of KS in AIDS, and KS was one of the first described HIV-associated opportunistic infections.[259–261] In the early period of the AIDS epidemic, KS was a very frequent presenting sign of HIV infection, occurring in ~79% of HIV-positive patients in 1981. This gradually decreased to ~25% in 1989, 9% in 1992, and <1% in 1997.[29] KS gained more exposure in the general public as an HIV-related manifestation with the 1993 Academy Award winning film *Philadelphia*, starring Tom Hanks as a homosexual man who was wrongly terminated from his job at a prestigious law firm after colleagues noticed KS lesions (which eventually lead to the discovery of his HIV status and sexual orientation). HHV-8 seropositivity is relatively rare in North American and northern European populations, occurring in only ~1% to 5% of the population.[216,257,262–265] The incidence appears to be higher in Italian and other Mediterranean peoples (~10%–20%) and highest in African populations (30%–80%).[266–275] Men who have sex with men appear to be 20 times more likely to present with KS when compared to similar immuno-compromised hemophiliac men.[276,277] A substantial decrease in the incidence of KS was reported in the mid-1980s with the advent of HAART, but recent studies have shown a resurgence of KS in patients with low HIV loads and high CD4+ T lymphocyte counts.[278–288] The exact mechanisms of viral transmission are not entirely clear, although horizontal transmission appears to be the predominant form of infection, and both sexual and nonsexual means of transmission are thought to play a role. Infection rates seem to be highest in bisexual and homosexual males; however, viral shedding has not been appreciably detected in semen of healthy donors but has been found in the semen of HIV-infected persons.[289] Both symptomatic and asymptomatic shedding in oropharyngeal secretions does occur, and blood-borne transmission during transfusion has been reported, although with low efficiency (~4% per infected transfusion).[290–292]

Presentation

Classic KS was first described in 1872 as an indolent tumor that occurred in elderly Mediterranean men. Since that time KS has been found in endemic areas of eastern Africa, often presenting in children with fatal lymphadenopathy. KS lesions were later noticed in immunocompromised organ transplant recipients, and then at an unexpectedly high rate in the MSM population during the early years of the HIV epidemic.[216] Cutaneous KS typically presents first as macular patches (similar to bruising), and gradually progresses to red or violaceous papules or plaques on the skin or mucous membranes in an at-risk patient. These lesions can eventually progress to ulceration in advanced disease. The cutaneous lesions may also resemble the lesions of bacillary angiomatosis, which is caused by *Bartonella henselae*, but in contrast to KS, bacillary angiomatosis lesions are typically painful, blanch with pressure, and are accompanied by systemic symptoms. Patients with gastrointestinal KS are frequently asymptomatic, but may present with pain, occult or gross fecal blood, dysphagia, or obstruction. Pulmonary KS may present with dyspnea, cough, or hemoptysis. Radiographically, pulmonary KS may demonstrate intrathoracic adenopathy involving the pleural surface, parenchyma, bronchial tree, hilar nodes, mediastinal nodes, pleural effusions, and diffuse or alveolar infiltrates. For all lesions, direct imaging via endoscopy or bronchoscopy is appropriate in order to obtain biopsy tissue, when possible, for histologic diagnosis. Diagnostic confirmation can be obtained with tissue immunostaining for LANA1 protein.[29,257,260,293–295]

Treatment

The first step in treatment of HIV-related KS is optimization of HAART, which is sometimes associated with a regression in KS lesions. However, KS lesions may occasionally worsen after the initiation of HAART, which is believed to be part of the immune reconstitution inflammatory syndrome (IRIS).[29,296–302]

For limited cutaneous lesions that are not life-threatening, treatment should consist of therapies that do not further compromise a patient's immune function. Local therapies such as a 9-cis-retinoic acid gel, cryotherapy with liquid nitrogen, and intralesional injections of vinblastine are viable options for treatment of such lesions.[303–306] Local treatment has not been shown to inhibit development of KS lesions elsewhere and is often associated with local side effects, such as discomfort/pain, hyper- or hypopigmentation, and eschar formation. Other local therapies with agents such as recombinant interferon-alpha (IFN-α), recombinant granulocyte/macrophage colony-stimulating factor (GM-CSF), recombinant platelet factor 4, and human chorionic gonadotropin have been examined in small clinical trials, but these have failed to demonstrate advantages over the previously mentioned local therapies.[307–310] Radiation therapy has also been shown to be an effective tool in the treatment of HIV-related KS. Radiation therapy is more commonly applied in cases of cutaneous and oral KS and less commonly used in cases of visceral disease. Adverse side effects of radiation therapy may be local irritation, dry desquamation, local alopecia, hyperpigmentation, radiation-induced edema, subcutaneous fibrosis, and, with oral radiation, altered gustatory sensation. HIV-infected persons also appear to be more sensitive to the adverse effects of radiation treatment, especially radiation-induced mucositis, than are noninfected populations.[311–316]

Systemic therapy, usually with either chemotherapy or IFN-α, is used to treat patients with severe disease (multiple lesions, severe symptoms, or visceral involvement). IFN-α therapy has been found to be especially effective in patients with higher CD4+T-lymphocyte counts (~80% responsive in patients with CD4+ T cell >600/μL and a response rate of <10% in patients with

CD4+ T cell <150/µL). IFN-α has the additional benefit of having antiretroviral activity.[317–319] Combination IFN-α and chemotherapy regimens have been studied but have not demonstrated clinical advantage to this point.[320–322] Some regimens of IFN-α therapy, particularly when used in combination with antiretrovirals such as zidovudine, have shown a dose-limiting effect of neutropenia, which may be prevented or counteracted with GM-CSF.[323–328] IFN-α alone may not be a suitable monotherapy for patients with rapidly progressive or symptomatic visceral disease due to a relatively long course of treatment (~6 months) before maximal clinical response is seen.[260]

Advanced cases of KS, which may be severely symptomatic or rapidly progressive, are generally treated with chemotherapy. Having a very low CD4+T lymphocyte count should not preclude a patient from receiving the necessary chemotherapy when indicated, and many of the studies that have examined these chemotherapeutic agents in HIV-positive patients have included severely immunocompromised subjects. Three chemotherapeutic agents—liposomal daunorubicin, liposomal doxorubicin, and paclitaxel—have been approved by the FDA specifically for treatment of KS. These are now considered first-line (doxorubicin) and second-line (paclitaxel and daunorubicin) agents for the treatment of advanced HIV-associated KS. However, many other agents have been shown to be clinically effective against KS, including etoposide, vinblastine, vincristine, bleomycin, doxorubicin, teniposide, vinorelbine, and epirubicine.[329–336] Liposomal doxorubicin is generally the first-line chemotherapeutic agent, administered at a dosage of 20mg/m^2 by slow intravenous infusion (over 30–60 min) every 3 weeks. It has been shown to have a response rate of ~59% with response duration of ~2.3 months.[337–339] Liposomal daunorubicin is given at a dosage of 40 mg/m^2 every 2 weeks and may be increased to 60 mg/m^2 if patients are unresponsive to the lower dose or in those who relapse. Liposomal daunorubicin has been shown to have a response rate of ~25%–59% with some experts asserting that the actual response rate is closer to ~25%. A 2002 prospective, randomized, double-blind trial of liposomal doxorubicin compared with daunorubicin in symptomatic cases of AIDS-related KS showed relief of KS-associated symptoms in 80% of those treated with liposomal doxorubicin compared with 63% of those treated with liposomal daunorubicin. The objective tumor response rates for liposomal doxorubicin and daunorubicin were 55% and 32%, respectively.[260,340] Liposomal doxorubicin alone, compared to combination with bleomycin and vincristine, has also been shown to be equally effective, with significantly lower rates of toxicity.[341] Paclitaxel functions as a mitotic spindle poison that causes mitotic arrest. Patients with advanced KS treated with paclitaxel, at doses of 135 mg/m^2 every 3 weeks or 100 mg/m^2 every 2 weeks intravenously over 3 hours, experienced an objective response rate of 69% and 59% respectively, which lasted for 7–10 months.[342–347] As with many chemotherapeutic agents, the use of these agents is often limited by potentially severe toxicities. Common toxicities seen with specific agents include neutropenia (with doxorubicin, etoposide, and vinblastine); cardiac toxicity (with high dose doxorubicin); alopecia and mucositis (with doxorubicin and etoposide); peripheral neuropathy (with vincristine); and fever and pulmonary fibrosis (with bleomycin). Some adverse effects, such as nausea, vomiting, and alopecia, can be minimized with the use of the liposomal version of the anthracycline agents rather than the free drug.[260,348–350]

Molluscum Contagiosum

Background

Molluscum contagiosum (MC) virus is a large enveloped double-stranded linear DNA virus belonging to the *Poxviridae* family and the *Molluscipoxvirus* genus. MCV is the most prevalent poxvirus infection and is spread by direct skin-to-skin contact, including via autoinoculation, and is also spread via fomites. MCV is commonly seen in healthy children <8 years of age and as a sexually transmitted disease in adults. The prevalence of clinical MC infection in healthy children in the U.S. is <5%. MCV is found with an increased frequency in immunocompromised populations; among HIV-infected patients, it has a prevalence of 5%–18%. This prevalence has notably decreased since the introduction of HAART.[351–356] Development of MC may also be an excellent indicator for the degree of immunocompromise.[357–358]

Presentation

MC presents as 3- to 6-mm, flesh colored papules with characteristic central umbilication. In healthy children, it usually presents with widespread papules on the trunk and face, and in adults it usually produces genital lesions. In immunocompromised persons, including those with HIV, MC can produce thousands of lesions, with increased incidence of facial involvement, bacterial superinfection, and treatment resistance.[351,353]

Treatment

MC is generally considered a self-limited disease, although complete resolution may not be seen for 6 months to 5 years, or even longer in immunocompromised patients. As a result, treatment is frequently initiated for aesthetic improvement, reduced risk of transmission, and reduced patient discomfort. Topical treatment options include trichloroacetic acid, podophyllin, retinoic acid, cantharidin, and imiquimod cream. Lesions may also be surgically removed via local excision, electrocautery and curettage, or with cryotherapy. Cryotherapy must commonly be repeated every 2 to 4 weeks for adequate control. Imiquimod 5% cream applied nightly is a treatment that can be used by patients at home.[359,360] Cidofovir, topical or IV, may also be an effective treatment.[361–363] Photodynamic therapy after 5-aminolevulinic acid topical application has also been reported with some success.[364,365] Recurrence with all treatment modalities is common in immunocompromised patients.[352,353] The most effective treatment and prophylaxis for MC infection in HIV-infected patients is initiation of HAART, which frequently will cause MC lesions to regress or completely resolve.[29,366]

JC Virus

Background

JC virus (JCV) is an unenveloped, double-stranded DNA virus belonging to the Polyomaviridae family. It is significant as the causative agent in progressive multifocal leukoencephalopathy (PML), a fatal demyelinating disease. JCV was first isolated by Padgett and colleagues in 1971 by inoculation of PML-affected brain tissue into primary cultures of human fetal glial cells. It was named JC after the initials of the infected patient.[367–369] JCV infection has been found to be ubiquitous in humans, with antibodies to JCV found in 10% of children 5 years of age and 76% of older adults. This prevalence has not been found to be different in immunocompromised populations, including HIV-infected patients.[370–373] However, symptomatic infection with development of PML is seen almost exclusively in immunocompromised patients—about 4% of patients with AIDS and in up to 8% of immunocompromised patients at autopsy.[29,367,369,374–377] The mode of JCV transmission is not well established, but is suspected to be through respiratory secretions.[369,378]

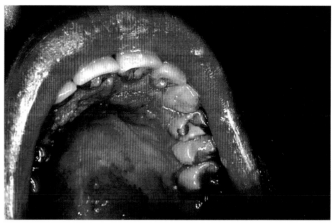

Figure 19–7. *This HIV-positive patient was exhibiting signs of a secondary condyloma acuminata infection, i.e., venereal warts. This intraoral eruption of condyloma acuminata, or venereal warts was caused by the human papilloma virus. (Courtesy of the Public Health Image Library for the Centers for Disease Control and Prevention.)*

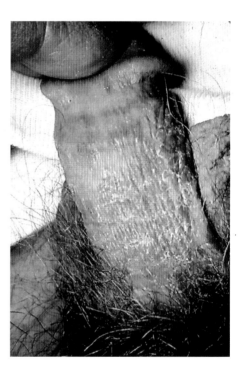

Figure 19–8. *Human papilloma virus on the genitalia in an AIDS patient which on biopsy showed squamous cell carcinoma in situ.*

topically applied 3%–5% acetic acid, which can make HPV lesions stand out as white patches or papules; however, this is not a very specific diagnostic test. The diagnosis of most lesions can be made based on clinical appearance (**Figure 19–8**), but when in doubt, a biopsy may be appropriate. A Papanicolaou smear and Dacron swab of mucous membranes for cytology and virology is a useful screening tool for detecting HPV disease.[29,433]

Treatment

Unlike many other opportunistic infections associated with HIV, the use of HAART does not appear to show a clear clinical benefit with respect to HPV disease. Studies have shown everything from no effect to possible improvement of genital condyloma, vulvar neoplasia, and CIN. Oral and anal HPV disease has typically been shown to be at best unresponsive to HAART and at times even worsened.[434-441]

Treatments available for HPV infection are aimed at symptomatic disease rather than eliminating infection. Many treatment options are available, ranging from topical to surgical, but all have limitations.[433]

Podophyllin, or its purified and standardized toxin, podofilox, are topical treatments that have been shown to be effective against warts and work by binding tubulin and inhibiting microtubule polymerization, and possibly also directly damaging HPV DNA.[442,443] Podophyllin is applied topically, once a week, for a total of up to 6 applications. Podofilox is applied topically, twice a day for 3 consecutive days per week, and may be used for up to 4 total cycles. Podofilox may also be used to suppress HPV lesions by once-daily application for 3 consecutive days per week, for up to 8 cycles. Podofilox has the added benefit of being more predictably effective and less toxic than podophyllin, and can be applied by the patient rather than by the provider. Side effects are mostly related to cutaneous irritation—discomfort, pain, itching, and ulceration/scarring; however, high doses may result in systemic toxicity, producing nausea, vomiting, neuropathy, seizure, coma, and even death. It is also potentially damaging to the kidneys, lungs, and bone marrow, and is contraindicated during pregnancy.[442,444] Complete response to podophyllin is typically found in 35% to 50% of cases, and recurrence occurs in 40% to 70%. Complete response to podofilox generally occurs in 60% to 70% of cases, with recurrence in 30% to 50%.[442,444,445]

Imiquimod is an immunomodulator that induces IFN-α and other cytokines. It has shown impressive results as a topical therapy for condyloma acuminatum and has been approved by the FDA for that purpose (5% imiquimod cream, Aldara). The recommended FDA topical dose of imiquimod is three times per week, and it can be applied by the patient. Complete response has been shown to occur in ~11%–62% of patients with recurrence rates of ~13%–29%.[446–450] Imiquimod has also been shown to be an effective adjuvant therapy in reducing recurrence rates after other treatments, such as surgical excision and electrocautery.[451–461] Adverse effects of topical imiquimod include local irritation, pain, erythema, ulceration, and swelling.

Bichloroacetic acid (BCA) and trichloroacetic acid (TCA) also have been found to be effective topical treatment for HPV. BCA and TCA work by acid hydrolysis and direct HPV DNA damage. They are both applied topically once per week for up to 6 total applications. Common adverse effects are similar to those seen with other topical treatments, including cutaneous irritation, itching, pain, ulceration, and scarring. Complete response to TCA is found in ~65%–80% of cases, with recurrence in ~50%. Unlike podophyllin and podofilox, these treatments are safe for use in pregnant females.[462–464]

5-fluorouracil (5-FU) is a structural analog of thymidine and a pyrimidine antagonist that disrupts DNA and RNA synthesis, making it particularly effective in rapidly dividing cells. Topically, it has been used for a wide variety of dermatologic conditions, including treatment and prophylaxis against HPV-associated condyloma acuminatum and intraepithelial neoplasia.[465–475] 5-FU may be applied topically as often as twice daily to external cutaneous tissue or internal vaginal mucosa (using an applicator) and has been used for durations of up to 10 weeks. However, application two times per week is associated with fewer side effects and appears to be clinically equivalent to more frequent dosing. Adverse effects are similar to those seen with other topical treatments and include application-site irritation, pain, itching, burns/ulceration, allergic dermatitis, and scarring.[476–479] 5-FU is not recommended for use in pregnant patients, although it has not been linked to congenital malformations.[480]

Cidofovir is a nucleoside analog that has been shown to be effective in the treatment of HPV-associated disease. This can be administered by intralesional injection, but has also shown modest results when applied as a topical gel formulation alone; even better results have been reported with the use of this drug in combination with electrocautery.[481–493]

Cryotherapy is one of the most common treatment modalities for cutaneous HPV disease and has been examined in multiple trials.[462,463,494–503] The most common cryotherapy agent is liquid nitrogen, but solid carbon dioxide (carbonic ice) and nitrous oxide may also be used. Cryotherapy may be delivered by direct contact, via cotton-tipped applicators and cryoprobes or by spray, which has the added benefit of reducing viral transmission.[504] Cryotherapy functions by producing local tissue necrosis at the site of application, but does little in the way of HPV DNA damage. The cryotherapy agent is usually applied until a small (1- 2-mm) ice halo forms around the lesion, some practitioners advocate allowing a complete thaw and refreeze of the lesion. Patients often experience brief discomfort and a stinging sensation, numbness, eventual blistering, and sometimes skin discoloration.[443,505–509] Complete response is achieved in ~65% to 85% of patients, but the recurrence rate is typically in the range of 20% to 40%. Cryotherapy can be a relatively safe method of treatment for virtually all patients and may even be used on cervical lesions during pregnancy.[510]

Cold-blade surgical excision using local anesthetic, with or without epinephrine for hemostatic control, and a scalpel or iridectomy scissors is a very simple and effective method of HPV treatment. Cold-blade excision is often combined with electrocautery. This treatment is generally well tolerated by patients, with some experiencing mild discomfort, bleeding, and scarring, and a few experiencing frank pain. Complete response is achieved in 46% to 92% of patients, and recurrence is seen in ~4% to 50% of cases.[511–519] Cold-blade excision of cervical lesions, or conization, has largely been replaced by newer techniques, such as electrosurgery, laser surgery, and cryotherapy.[520]

Electrosurgery techniques such as electrodesiccation, electrocautery, and electrocoagulation, are frequently used in the treatment of HPV disease, but still lack much needed well designed clinical evaluation. One randomized controlled trial demonstrated superiority of electrodesiccation over podophyllin and cryotherapy, with a complete response rate of 94% and recurrence rate of ~20% at 3 to 5 months of follow-up. Cryotherapy achieved a complete response of 79% with a recurrence rate of ~20%, and podophyllin achieved a complete response in 41% of patients and a recurrence rate of ~40%.[502] Electrosurgery may also be effective when combined with other treatments, such as cold-blade excision and interferon injections.[403] As previously mentioned, electrosurgical techniques such as loop electrosurgical excision procedure (LEEP) and large loop excision of transitional zone (LLETZ) have been shown to be very effective treatments for CIN, as they are well tolerated with no apparent subsequent adverse effect on fertility. However, electrosurgery is not recommended on the gravid cervix.[521–523] Providers using electrosurgical techniques as well as laser treatments for HPV should, in addition to donning standard surgical attire, utilize a smoke evacuation system to avoid possibly acquiring HPV infection due to HPV DNA that has been found to be present in the resultant smoke.[524–528]

Laser surgery is yet another effective option for treatment of HPV disease. Although many medical lasers, such as argon, KTP, and pulse dye lasers, have been shown to be effective against HPV lesions, the carbon dioxide (CO_2) laser is the best option when treating anogenital HPV lesions. Laser surgery has demonstrated a complete response in 90% to 100% of patients, but a relatively high relapse rate of 50% to 65%.[519,529–535] The possible role of adjuvant therapy with systemic interferon in an attempt to lower relapse rates remains unclear.[536–539] Laser surgery has also been used effectively in the treatment of CIN and oral HPV.[147–153] Adverse side effects of laser treatment include pain, bleeding, discharge, local tissue swelling, dysuria, meatal stenosis, and scarring.[513,529,547–550] As previously mentioned, smoke evacuation systems should be utilized due to potential infectious risk of smoke inhalation and contact. Laser therapy is not contraindicated in pregnant patients. Thermal ablation with infrared coagulation, another method of

HPV treatment, does not produce smoke and has been shown to be similar in clinical efficacy when compared with electrocautery.[551–553]

HPV treatment with interferon has been widely studied and has demonstrated clear antitumor and antiviral properties. Intralesional interferon treatment has been shown to be effective against HPV-associated disease, but, unfortunately, has demonstrated marginal results in HIV-infected patients.[536,538,554–567] Treatments with topical interferon preparations have not been clearly shown to be of benefit and are not currently available in the U.S.[568–572] Systemic treatment with interferon has also not shown a clear clinical advantage over existing therapies, nor has it been shown to be particularly useful as an adjuvant treatment when combined with existing therapies.[508,509,554,573–577] However, although further evaluation is needed, some promising results have been shown utilizing systemic pegylated IFN2b (PEG-IFN) in HIV-positive patients with condyloma acuminatum.[578] Known adverse side effects of interferon treatment are usually dose-dependent, reversible on cessation of treatment, and usually decrease with longitudinal exposure to the drug. The most common side effects are fever, chills, headache, malaise, fatigue, and myalgias. More serious adverse effects may include confusion, mood alteration, weight loss, nausea, vomiting, alopecia, peripheral neuropathy, neutropenia, thrombocytopenia, elevated hepatic transaminases, anemia, and hypertriglyceridemia. Some of the more common side-effects may be diminished with concomitant use of acetaminophen or NSAIDS.

Prevention of HPV-associated disease can be improved through patient education, the use of condoms, and regular health screening, including Papanicolaou smears. Recently approved HPV vaccines such as the quadrivalent vaccine against HPV types 6, 11, 16, and 18 (Gardasil) and the bivalent vaccine against HPV types 16 and 18 (Cervarix) are a great advance in the prevention of HPV-associated disease, especially those HPV types responsible for cervical malignancies.[579–584] However, their use in HIV-infected populations currently remains unclear.[585–587] Novel vaccines for use in HIV-positive populations are currently being investigated.[403,588–598]

Parvovirus B19

Background

Parvovirus B19 is a small, nonenveloped, single-stranded DNA virus belonging to the Parvoviridae family and the Erythrovirus genus. Parvovirus B19 was initially discovered by chance in 1975 evaluations of hepatitis B viral antigen tests.[599,600] It is most commonly associated with erythema infectiosum (fifth disease) in childhood, but is also associated with transient aplastic crisis, chronic anemia in immunocompromised patients, and hydrops fetalis.[601] Up to 80% of adults have been shown to have antibodies to parvovirus B19, but infection is usually controlled by an intact humoral immune system. Transmission is thought to be mostly through respiratory secretions from close contacts, droplets, and/or fomites. However, virus has also been found in urine and blood specimens, and vertical transmission to infants of mothers infected during pregnancy has also been shown.[602–606,609]

Presentation

In HIV-infected patients parvovirus B19 infection may present as chronic intractable anemia. Symptoms of this may include weakness/fatigue, dyspnea, palpitations, and/or pallor.

77. Tyndall MW, Nasio J, Agoki E, et al. Herpes zoster as the initial presentation of human immunodeficiency virus type 1 infection in Kenya. Clin Infect Dis 1995 Oct;21(4):1035–1037.

78. Holmberg SD, Buchbinder SP, Conley LJ, et al. The spectrum of medical conditions and symptoms before acquired immunodeficiency syndrome in homosexual and bisexual men infected with the human immunodeficiency virus. Am J Epidemiol 1995 Mar 1;141(5):395–404

79. Glesby MJ, Moore RD, Chaisson RE. Clinical spectrum of herpes zoster in adults infected with human immunodeficiency virus. Clin Infect Dis 1995 Aug;21(2):370–375.

80. Veenstra J, Krol A, van Praag RM, et al. Herpes zoster, immunological deterioration and disease progression in HIV-1 infection. AIDS 1995 Oct;9(10):1153–1158.

81. Engels EA, Rosenberg PS, Biggar RJ. Zoster incidence in human immunodeficiency virus-infected hemophiliacs and homosexual men, 1984–1997. District of Columbia Gay Cohort Study. Multicenter Hemophilia Cohort Study. J Infect Dis 1999 Dec;180(6):1784–1789.

82. Morgan D, Mahe C, Malamba S, et al. Herpes zoster and HIV-1 infection in a rural Ugandan cohort. AIDS 2001 Jan 26;15(2):223–229

83. Buchbinder SP, Katz MH, Hessol NA, et al. Herpes zoster and human immunodeficiency virus infection. J Infect Dis 1992 Nov;166(5):1153–1156.

84. Gnann JW Jr, Whitley RJ. Clinical practice. Herpes zoster. N Engl J Med 2002 Aug 1;347(5):340–346.

85. Veenstra J, van Praag RM, Krol A, et al. Complications of varicella zoster virus reactivation in HIV-infected homosexual men. AIDS 1996 Apr;10(4):393–399.

86. Ormerod LD, Larkin JA, Margo CA, et al. Rapidly progressive herpetic retinal necrosis: a blinding disease characteristic of advanced AIDS. Clin Infect Dis 1998 Jan;26(1):34–45.

87. Moorthy RS, Weinberg DV, Teich SA, et al. Management of varicella zoster virus retinitis in AIDS. Br J Ophthalmol 1997 Mar;81(3):189–194.

88. Batisse D, Eliaszewicz M, Zazoun L, et al. Acute retinal necrosis in the course of AIDS: study of 26 cases. AIDS 1996 Jan;10(1):55–60.

89. Miller RF, Brink NS, Cartledge J, et al. Necrotising herpetic retinopathy in patients with advance HIV disease. Genitourin Med 1997 Dec;73(6):462–466.

90. Purdy KW, Heckenlively JR, Church JA, et al. Progressive outer retinal necrosis caused by varicella-zoster virus in children with acquired immunodeficiency syndrome. Pediatr Infect Dis J 2003 Apr;22(4):384–386.

91. Garweg J, Böhnke M. Varicella-zoster virus is strongly associated with atypical necrotizing herpetic retinopathies. Clin Infect Dis 1997 Apr;24(4):603–608.

92. Short GA, Margolis TP, Kuppermann BD, et al. A polymerase chain reaction-based assay for diagnosing varicella-zoster virus retinitis in patients with acquired immunodeficiency syndrome. Am J Ophthalmol 1997 Feb;123(2):157–164.

93. Kashiwase M, Sata T, Yamauchi Y, et al. Progressive outer retinal necrosis caused by herpes simplex virus type 1 in a patient with acquired immunodeficiency syndrome. Ophthalmology 2000 Apr;107(4):790–794.

94. Kimya-Asadi A, Tausk FA, Nousari HC. Verrucous varicella zoster virus lesions associated with acquired immunodeficiency syndrome. Int J Dermatol 2000 Jan;39(1):77–78.

95. Castanet J, Rodot S, Lacour JP, et al. Chronic varicella presenting as disseminated pinpoint-sized papules in a man infected with the human immunodeficiency virus. Dermatology 1996;192(1):84–86.

96. Harrison RA, Soong S, Weiss HL, et al. A mixed model for factors predictive of pain in AIDS patients with herpes zoster. J Pain Symptom Manage 1999 Jun;17(6):410–417.

97. Iten A, Chatelard P, Vuadens P, et al. Impact of cerebrospinal fluid PCR on the management of HIV-infected patients with varicella-zoster virus infection of the central nervous system. J Neurovirol 1999 Apr;5(2):172–180.

98. Brown M, Scarborough M, Brink N, et al R. Varicella zoster virus-associated neurological disease in HIV-infected patients. Int J STD AIDS 2001 Feb;12(2):79–83.

99. Manian FA, Kindred M, Fulling KH. Chronic varicella-zoster virus myelitis without cutaneous eruption in a patient with AIDS: report of a fatal case. Clin Infect Dis 1995 Oct;21(4):986–988.

100. Kenyon LC, Dulaney E, Montone KT, et al. Varicella-zoster ventriculo-encephalitis and spinal cord infarction in a patient with AIDS. Acta Neuropathol 1996 Aug;92(2):202–205.

101. Liu JZ, Brown P, Tselis A. Unilateral retrobulbar optic neuritis due to varicella zoster virus in a patient with AIDS: a case report and review of the literature. J Neurol Sci 2005 Oct 15;237(1-2):97–101.

102. Franco-Paredes C, Bellehemeur T, Merchant A, et al. Aseptic meningitis and optic neuritis preceding varicella-zoster progressive outer retinal necrosis in a patient with AIDS. AIDS 2002 May 3;16(7):1045–1049.

103. Moulignier A, Pialoux G, Dega H, et al. Brain stem encephalitis due to varicella-zoster virus in a patient with AIDS. Clin Infect Dis 1995 May;20(5):1378–1380.

104. Gershon AA, Mervish N, LaRussa P, et al. Varicella-zoster virus infection in children with underlying human immunodeficiency virus infection. J Infect Dis 1997 Dec;176(6):1496–500.

105. von Seidlein L, Gillette SG, Bryson Y, et al. Frequent recurrence and persistence of varicella-zoster virus infections in children infected with human immunodeficiency virus type 1. J Pediatr 1996 Jan;128(1):52–57.

106. Arvin AM. Antiviral therapy for varicella and herpes zoster. Semin Pediatr Infect Dis 2002 Jan;13(1):12–21.

107. American Academy of Pediatrics. Committee on Infectious Diseases. Varicella vaccine update. Pediatrics 2000 Jan;105(1 Pt 1):136–141.

108. Levin MJ, Gershon AA, Weinberg A, et al. Immunization of HIV-infected children with varicella vaccine. J Pediatr 2001 Aug;139(2):305–310.

109. Prevention of varicella. Update recommendations of the Advisory Committee on Immunization Practices (ACIP). MMWR Recomm Rep 1999 May 28;48(RR-6):1–5.

110. Kaplan JE, Benson C, Holmes KH, et al. Guidelines for prevention and treatment of opportunistic infections in HIV-infected adults and adolescents: recommendations from CDC, the National Institutes of Health, and the HIV Medicine Association of the Infectious Diseases Society of America. MMWR Recomm Rep 2009 Apr 10;58(RR-4):1–207

111. Wood MJ, Kay R, Dworkin RH, et al. Oral acyclovir therapy accelerates pain resolution in patients with herpes zoster: a meta-analysis of placebo-controlled trials. Clin Infect Dis 1996 Feb;22(2):341–347.

112. Beutner KR, Friedman DJ, Forszpaniak C, et al. Valaciclovir compared with acyclovir for improved therapy for herpes zoster in immunocompetent adults. Antimicrob Agents Chemother 1995 Jul;39(7):1546–1553.

113. Tyring S, Barbarash RA, Nahlik JE, et al. Famciclovir for the treatment of acute herpes zoster: effects on acute disease and postherpetic neuralgia. A randomized, double-blind, placebo-controlled trial. Collaborative Famciclovir Herpes Zoster Study Group. Ann Intern Med 1995 Jul 15;123(2):89–96.

114. Tyring SK, Beutner KR, Tucker BA, et al. Antiviral therapy for herpes zoster: randomized, controlled clinical trial of valacyclovir and famciclovir therapy in immunocompetent patients 50 years and older. Arch Fam Med 2000 Sep-Oct;9(9):863–869.

115. Benson CA, Kaplan JE, Masur H, et al. Treating opportunistic infections among HIV-infected adults and adolescents: recommendations from CDC, the National Institutes of Health, and the HIV Medicine Association/Infectious Diseases Society of America. MMWR Recomm Rep 2004 Dec 17;53(RR-15):1–112.

116. Johnston WH, Holland GN, Engstrom RE Jr, et al. Recurrence of presumed varicella-zoster virus retinopathy in patients with acquired immunodeficiency syndrome. Am J Ophthalmol 1993 Jul 15;116(1):42–50.

117. Scott IU, Luu KM, Davis JL. Intravitreal antivirals in the management of patients with acquired immunodeficiency syndrome with progressive outer retinal necrosis. Arch Ophthalmol 2002 Sep;120(9):1219–1222.

118. Galindez OA, Sabates NR, Whitacre MM, et al. Rapidly progressive outer retinal necrosis caused by varicella zoster virus in a patient infected with human immunodeficiency virus. Clin Infect Dis 1996 Jan;22(1):149–151.

119. Pérez-Blázquez E, Traspas R, Méndez Marín I, et al. Intravitreal ganciclovir treatment in progressive outer retinal necrosis. Am J Ophthalmol 1997 Sep;124(3):418–421.

120. Ciulla TA, Rutledge BK, Morley MG, et al. The progressive outer retinal necrosis syndrome: successful treatment with combination antiviral therapy. Ophthalmic Surg Lasers 1998 Mar;29(3):198–206.

121. Spaide RF, Martin DF, Teich SA, et al. Successful treatment of progressive outer retinal necrosis syndrome. Retina 1996;16(6):479–487.

122. Meffert SA, Kertes PJ, Lim PL, et al. Successful treatment of progressive outer retinal necrosis using high-dose intravitreal ganciclovir. Retina 1997;17(6):560–562.

123. Vanhems P, Voisin L, Gayet-Ageron A, et al. The incidence of herpes zoster is less likely than other opportunistic infections to be reduced by highly active antiretroviral therapy. J Acquir Immune Defic Syndr 2005 Jan 1;38(1):111–113.

124. Martínez E, Gatell J, Morán Y, et al. High incidence of herpes zoster in patients with AIDS soon after therapy with protease inhibitors. Clin Infect Dis 1998 Dec;27(6):1510–1513.

125. Aldeen T, Hay P, Davidson F, et al. Herpes zoster infection in HIV-seropositive patients associated with highly active antiretroviral therapy. AIDS 1998 Sep 10;12(13):1719–1720.

126. Domingo P, Torres OH, Ris J, et al. Herpes zoster as an immune reconstitution disease after initiation of combination antiretroviral therapy in patients with human immunodeficiency virus type-1 infection. Am J Med 2001 Jun 1;110(8):605–609.

127. Tangsinmankong N, Kamchaisatian W, Lujan-Zilbermann J, et al. Varicella zoster as a manifestation of immune restoration disease in HIV-infected children. J Allergy Clin Immunol 2004 Apr;113(4):742–746.

128. French MA, Price P, Stone SF. Immune restoration disease after antiretroviral therapy. AIDS 2004 Aug 20;18(12):1615–1627.

129. Pahwa S, Biron K, Lim W, et al. Continuous varicella-zoster infection associated with acyclovir resistance in a child with AIDS. JAMA 1988 Nov 18;260(19):2879–882.

130. Jacobson MA, Berger TG, Fikrig S, et al. Acyclovir-resistant varicella zoster virus infection after chronic oral acyclovir therapy in patients with the acquired immunodeficiency syndrome (AIDS). Ann Intern Med 1990 Feb 1;112(3):187–191.

131. Bernhard P, Obel N. Chronic ulcerating acyclovir-resistant varicella zoster lesions in an AIDS patient. Scand J Infect Dis 1995;27(6):623–625.

132. Breton G, Fillet AM, Katlama C, et al. Acyclovir-resistant herpes zoster in human immunodeficiency virus-infected patients: results of foscarnet therapy. Clin Infect Dis 1998 Dec;27(6):1525–1527.

133. Collier AC, Meyers JD, Corey L, et al. Cytomegalovirus infection in homosexual men. Relationship to sexual practices, antibody to human immunodeficiency virus, and cell-mediated immunity. Am J Med 1987; 82:593–601.

134. Guinan ME, Thomas PA, Pinsky PF et al. Heterosexual and homosexual patients with the acquired immunodeficiency syndrome. A comparison of surveillance, interview, and laboratory data. Ann Intern Med 1984;100: 213–218.

135. Griffiths PD, Polis MA. Cytomegalovirus Disease. In: Dolin R, Masur H, Saag M AIDS Therapy. 3rd ed. New York: Elsevier 2008;p855–883.

136. Jacobson MA, Mills J. Serious cytomegalovirus disease in the acquired immunodeficiency syndrome (AIDS). Clinical findings, diagnosis, and treatment. Ann Intern Med 11988;08:585.

137. Kestelyn PG, Cunningham ET. HIV AIDS and blindness. Bull WHO 2001;79:208–213.

138. Hoover DR, Saah AJ, Bacellar H, et al. Clinical manifestations of AIDS in the era of Pneumocystis prophylaxis. Multicenter AIDS Cohort Study. N Engl J Med 1993;329:1922.

139. Bloom JN, Palestine AG. The diagnosis of cytomegalovirus retinitis. Ann Intern Med 1988;109:963.

140. Drew WL. Cytomegalovirus infection in patients with AIDS. Clin Infect Dis 1992;14:608.

141. Crowe SM, Carlin JB, Stewart KI, et al. Predictive value of CD4 lymphocyte numbers for the development of opportunistic infections and malignancies in HIV-infected persons. J Acquir Immune Dific Syndr1992; 5:1069.

142. Cope AV, Sabin C, Burroughs A, et al. Interrelationships among quantity of human cytomegalovirus (HCMV) DNA in blood, donor-recipient serostatus, and administration of methylprednisolone and antithymocyte globulin (ATG). J Med Virol 1999;58:182.

143. Gor D, Sabin C, Prentice HG, et al. Longitudinal fluctuations in cytomegalovirus load in bone marrow transplant patients: relationship between peak virus load, donor/recipient serostatus, acute GVHD and CMV disease. Bone Marrow Transplant 1998;21:597.

144. Pérez CL, Villarroel BJ, Reyes JA, et al. Eritrodermia exfoliativa y dermatitis infecciosa em um lactante infectado por El vírus linfotrópico humano-I (HTLV-I). Rev Chil Infectol 2007; 24:142–148.

145. Dodt KK, Jacobsen PH, Hofmann B, et al. Development of cytomegalovirus (CMV) disease may be predicted in HIV-infected patients by CMV polymerase chain reaction and the antigenemia test. AIDS 1997;11:F21.

146. Shinakai M, Bozzette SA, Powderly W, et al. Utility of urine and leukocyte cultures and plasma DNA polymerase chain reaction for identification of AIDS patients at risk for developing human cytomegalovirus disease. J Infect Dis 1997;175:302.

147. Bowen EF, Sabin CA, Wilson P, et al. Cytomegalovirus (CMV) viraemia detected by polymerase chain reaction identifies a group of HIV-positive patients at high risk of CMV disease. AIDS 1997;11:889.

148. Dieterich DT, Wilcox CM, Diagnosis and treatment of esophageal diseases associated with HIV infection. Practice Parameters Committee of the American College of Gastroenterology. Am J Gastroenterol 1996;91:2265.

149. Gallant JE, Moore RD, Richman DD, et al. Incidence and natural history of cytomegalovirus disease in patients with advanced human immunodeficiency virus disease treated with zidovudine. The Zidovudine Epidemiology Study Group. J Infect Dis 1992;166:1223.

150. Dieterich DT, Rahmin M, Cytomegalovirus colitis in AIDS: presentation in 44 patients and a review of the literature. J Acquir Immune Defic syndr 1991;4:S29.

151. Wallace JM, Hannah J. Cytomegalovirus pneumonitis in patients with AIDS. Findings in an autopsy series. Chest 1987;92:198.

152. Jacobsen MA, Mills J, Rush J, et al. Morbidity and mortality of patients with AIDS and first-episode Pneumocystis carinii pneumonia unaffected by concomitant pulmonary cytomegalovirus infection. Am rev Respir Dis 11991;44:6.

153. Rodriguez-Barradas MC, Stool E, Musher DM, et al. Diagnosing and treating cytomegalovirus pneumonia in patients with AIDS. Clin Infect Dis 1996;23:76.

154. Petito CK, Cho ES, Lemann W, et al. Neuropathology of acquired immunodeficiency syndrome (AIDS): an autopsy review. J Neuropathol Exp Neurol 1986;45;635.

155. Arribas JR, Clifford DB, Fichtenbaum CJ, et al. Level of cytomegalovirus (CMV) DNA in cerebrospinal fluid of subjects with AIDS and CMV infection of the central nervous system. J Infect Dis 1995;172:527.

156. Arribas JR, Storch GA, Clifford DB, et al. Cytomegalovirus encephalitis. Ann Intern Med 1996;125:577.

157. Holland NR, Power C, Mathews VP, et al. Cytomegalovirus encephalitis in acquired immunodeficiency syndrome (AIDS). Neurology 1994;44:507.

158. Kalayjian RC, Cohen ML, Bonomo RA, et al. Cytomegalovirus ventriculoencephalitis in AIDS: A suyndrome with distinct clinical and pathologic features. Medicine (Baltimore) 1993;72:67.

159. Morgello S, Cho ES, Nielsen S, et al. Cytomegalovirus encephalitis in patients with acquired immunodeficiency syndrome: an autopsy study of 30 cases and a review of the literature. Hum Pathol 1987;18:289

160. Wolf DG, Spector SA. Diagnosis of human cytomegalovirus central nervous system disease in AIDS patients by DNA amplification from cerebrospinal fluid. J Infect Dis 1992;166:1412.

161. Bchar R, Wilcy C, McCutchan JA. Cytomegalovirus polyradiculoneuropathy in acquired immune deficiency syndrome. Neurology 1987;37:557.

162. McCutchan JA. Cytomegalovirus infections of the nervous system in patients with AIDS. Clin Infect Dis 1995;20:747.

163. Miller RF, Fox JD, Thomas P, et al. Acute lumbosacral polyradiculopathy due to cytomegalovirus in advanced HIV disease: CSF findings in 17 patients. J Neurol Neurosurg Psychiatry1996;61:456.

164. So YT, Olney RK. Acute lumbosacral polyradiculopathy in acquired immunodeficiency syndrome: experience in 23 patients. Ann Neurol 1994;35:53

165. Kaplan JE, Hanson D, Dworkin MS, et al. Epidemiology of human immunodeficiency vuris-associated opportunistic infections in the United States in the era of highly active antiretroviral therapy. Clin Infect Dis 2000;30:S5.

166. Steininger C, Puchhammer-Stöckl E, Popow-Kraupp T. Cytomegalovirus disease in the era of highly active antiretroviral therapy (HAART). J Clin Virol 2006;37(1):1–9.

167. Jabs DA, Van Natta ML, Thorne JE, et al. Course of cytomegalovirus retinitis in the era of highly active antiretroviral therapy: 2. Second eye involvement and retinal detachment. Ophthalmology 2004;111:2232.

168. Cheng Y, Huang ES, Lin JC, et al. Unique spectrum of activity of 9-{1,3-dihydroxy-2-propoxy)methyl]-guanine against herpesviruses in vitro and its mode of action against herpes simplex virus type 1. Proc Natl Acad Sci USA 1983;80:2767–2770.

169. Drew WL. Cytomegalovirus infection in patients with AIDS. Clin Infect Dis 1992;14:608.

170. 170.CMV-38. Ericksson B, Oberg B, Wahren B. Pyrophosphate analogues as inhibitors of DNA polymerases of cytomegalovirus, herpes simplex virus and cellular origin. Biochim Biophys Acta 1982;696:115.

171. Ostrander M, Cheng YC. Properties of herpes simplex virus type 1 and type 2 DNA polymerase. Biochim Biophys Acta 1980;609:232.

172. Sandstrom EG, Kaplan JC, Byington RE, et al. Inhibition of human T-cell lymphotropic virus type III in vitro by phosphonoformate. Lancet 1985;1:1480.

173. Deray G, Martinez F, Katlama C, et al. Foscarnet nephrotoxicity: mechanism, incidence and prevention. Am J Nephrol 1989;9:316.

174. Yin MT, Brust JCM, Van Tieu H, et al. (2009). Antiherpesvirus, Anti-Hepatitis Virus, and Anti-Respiratory Virus Agents. In: Richman DD, Whitley RJ, Hayden FG Clincal Virology. 3rd ed. Washington, DC: ASM Press 2009,p217–264.

175. Lalezari JP, Drew WL, Glutzer E, et al. (S)-1-[3-hydroxy-2-(phosphonylmethoxy)propyl]cytosine (cidofovir): results of a phase I/II study of a novel antiviral nucleoside analogue. J Infect Dis 1995;171:788.

176. Polis MA, Spooner KM, Baird BF, et al. Anticytomegaloviral activity and safety of cidofovir in patients with human immunodeficiency virus infection and cytomegalovirus viruria. Antimicrob Agents Chemother 1995;39:882.

177. Cihlar T, Lin DC, Pritchard JB, et al. The antiviral nucleoside analogs cidofovir and adefovir are novel substrates for human and rat renal organic anion transporter 1. Mol Pharmacol 1999;56:570.

178. Dieterich DT, Kotler DP, Busch DF, et al. Ganciclovir treatment of cytomegalovirus colitis in AIDS: a randomized, double-blind, placebo-controlled multicenter study. J Infect Dis 1993;167:278.

179. Blanshard C, Benhamou Y, Dohin E, et al. Treatment of AIDS-associated gastrointestinal cytomegalovirus infection with foscarnet and ganciclovir: a randomized comparison. J Infect Dis 1995;172:622.

180. Blanshard C, Treatment of HIV-related cytomegalovirus disease of the gastrointestinal tract with foscarnet. J Acquir Immune Dific Syndr 1992;5:S25.

181. Buhles WC Jr, Mastre BJ, Tinker AJ, et al. Ganciclovir treatment of life- or sight-threatening cytomegalovirus infection: experience in 314 immunocompromised patients. Rev Infect Dis 1988;10:S495.

182. Nelson MR, Connolly GM, Hawkins DA, et al. Foscarnet in the treatment of cytomegalovirus infection of the esophagus and colon in patients with the acquired immune deficiency syndrome. Am J Gastroenterol 1991;86:876.

183. Studies of Ocular Complications of AIDS Research Group ACTG. Combinatino foscarnet and ganciclovir therapy vs monotherapy for the treatment of relapsed cytomegalovirus retinitis in patients with AIDS: the Cytomegalovirus Retretment Trial. Arch Ophthalmol 1996;23.

184. Henderly DE, Freeman WR, Causey DM, et al. Cytomegalovirus retinitis and response to therapy with ganciclovir. Ophthalmology 1987;94:425.

185. Mattes FM, Hainsworth EG, Geretti AM, et al. A randomized, controlled trial comparing ganciclovir to ganoiolovir plus fooonrnet (onoh at half dooo) for preemptive therapy of cytomegalovirus infection in transplant recipients. J Infect Dis 2004;189:1355.

186. Gowdey G, Lee RK, Carpenter WM. Treatment of HIV-related hairy leukoplakia with podophyllum resin 25% solution. Oral Surg Oral Med Oral Pathol Oral Radiol Endod 1995;79:64–67.

187. Goedert JJ, Cote TR, Virgo P, et al. Spectrum of AIDS associated malignant disorders. Lancet 1998;351:1833–1839.

188. Cote TR, Biggar RJ, Rosenberg PS, et al. Non-Hodgkin's lymphoma among people with AIDS: incidence, presentation and public health burden. AIDS/Cancer Study Group, Int J Cancer 1997;73:645–650.

189. Lennette ET, Blackbourn DJ, Levy JA. Antibodies to human herpesvirus type 8 in the general population and in Kaposi's sarcoma patients. Lancet 1996;348:858–861.

190. Howard MR, Whitby D, Bahadur G, et al. Detection of human herpesvirus 8 DNA in semen from HIV-infected individuals but not healthy semen donors. AIDS 1997;11:F15–19.

191. Viera J, Huang ML, Koelle DM, Corey L. Transmissible Kaposi's sarcoma-associated herpesvirus (human herpesvirus 8) in saliva of men with a history of Kaposi's sarcoma. J Virol 1997;71:7083–7087.

192. Engstrom RE Jr, Holland GN. Local therapy for cytomegalovirus retinopathy. Am J Ophthalmol 1995;120:376–385.

193. Martin DF, Parks DJ, Mellow SD, et al. Treatment of cytomegalovirus retinitis with an intraocular sustained-release ganciclovir implant. A randomized controlled clinical trial. Arch Ophthalmol 1994;112:1531–1539.

194. Musch DC, Martin DF, Gordon JF, et al, Ganciclovir Implant Study Group. Treatment of cytomegalovirus retinitis with a sustained-release ganciclovir implant. N Engl J Med 1997; 337:83–90.

195. Kappel PJ, Charonis AC, Holland GN, Narayanan R, Kulkarni AD, Yu F, Boyer DS, Engstrom RE Jr, Kuppermann BD; Southern California HIV/Eye Consortium. Outcomes associated with ganciclovir implants in patients with AIDS-related cytomegalovirus retinitis. Ophthalmology 2006 Apr;113(4):683.e1–8.

196. Cesarman E, Chang Y, Moore PS, et al. Kaposi's sarcoma-associated herpesvirus-like DNA sequences in AIDS-related body-cavity based lymphomas. N Engl J Med 1995;332:1186–1191.

197. Nador RG, Cesarman E, Chadburn A, et al. Primary effusion lymphoma: a distinct clinicopathologic entity associated with the Kaposi's sarcoma-associated herpes virus. Blood 1996;88:645–656.

198. Cantrill HL, Henry K, Melroe NH, et al. Treatment of cytomegalovirus retinitis with intravitreal ganciclovir. Long-term results. Ophthalmology 1989;96:367.

199. Henry K, Cantrill H, Fletcher C, et al. use of intravitreal ganciclovir (dihydroxy propoxymethyl guanine) for cytomegalovirus retinitis in a patient with AIDS. Am J Ophthalmol 1987;103:17.

200. Schulman J, Peyman GA, Horton MB, et al. Intraocular 9-([2-hydroxy-1-(hydroxymethyl) ethoxyl] methyl) guanine levels after intravitreal and subconjunctival administration. Ophthalmic Surg 1986;178:429.

201. Young S, McCluskey P, Minassian DC, et al. Retinal detachment in cytomegalovirus retinitis: intravenous versus intravitreal therapy. Clin Experiment Ophthalmol 2003;31:96.

202. Martin DV, Parks DJ, Mellow SD, et al. Treatment of cytomegalovirus retinitis with an intraocular sustained-release ganciclovir implant. A randomized controlled clinical trial. Arch Ophthalmol 1994;112:1531.

203. Jabs DA, Enger C, Haller J, et al. Retinal detachments in patients with cytomegalovirus retinitis. Arch Ophthalmol 1991;109:794.

204. Kempen JH, Jabs DA, Dunn JP, et al. Retinal detachment risk in cytomegalovirus retinitis related to the acquired immunodeficiency syndrome. Arch Ophthalmol 2001;119:33.

205. Musch DC, Martin DF, Gordon JF, et al. Treatment of cytomegalovirus retinitis with a sustained-release ganciclovir implant. The Ganciclovir Implant Study Group. N Engl J Med 1997;337:83.

206. Anonymous. Valganciclovir, a more potent oral therapy for CMV retinitis in AIDS, approved by FDA. Clin Infect Dis 2001;32.

207. Brown F, Banken L, Saywell K, et al. Pharmacokinetics of valganciclovir and ganciclovir following multiple oral dosages of valganciclovir in HIV- and CMV-seropositive volunteers. Clin Pharmacokinet 1999;37:167.

208. Martin DF, Sierra-Madero J, Walmsley S, et al. A controlled trial of valganciclovir as induction therapy for cytomegalovirus retinitis. N Engl J Med 2002;346:1119.

209. Diaz-Llopis M, Espana E, Munos G, et al. High dose intravitreal foscarnet in the treatment of cytomegalovirus retinitis in AIDS. Br J Ophthalmol 1994;78:120.

210. Anduze-Faris BM, Fillet AM, Gozlan J, et al. Induction and maintenance therapy of cytomegalovirus central nervous system infection in HIV-infected patients. AIDS 2000;14:517.

211. Whitley RJ, Jacobson MA, Friedberg DN, et al. Guidelines for the treatment of cytomegalovirus diseases in patients with AIDS in the era of potent antiretroviral therapy: recommendations of an international panel. International AIDS Society-USA. Arch Intern Med 1998;158:957.

212. Gallant JE, Moore RD, Richman DD, et al. Incidence and natural history of cytomegalovirus disease in patients with advanced immunodeficiency virus disease treated with zidovudine. The Zidovudine Epidemiology Study Group. J Infect Dis 1992;166:1223.

213. Yust I, Fox Z, Burke M et al. Retinal and extraocular cytomegalovirus end-organ disease in HIV infected patients in Europe: a EuroSIDA study, 1994–2001. Eur J Clin Microbiol Infect Dis 2004; 23: 550–559.

214. Steininger C. Clinical relevance of cytomegalovirus infection in patients with disorders of the immune system. Clin Microbiol Infect 2007;13:953–963.

215. Luzuriaga K, Sullivan JL. Epstein-Barr Virus. In: Richman DD, Whitley RJ, Hayden FG Clinical Virology. 3rd ed. Washington DC: ASM Press 2009;P521–536.

216. Johannsen E. Epstein-Barr Virus and Kaposi Sarcoma-Associated Herpesvirus. In: Dolin R, Masur H, Saag M AIDS Therapy. 3rd ed. New York: Elsevier 2008;P885–897.

217. Hamilton-Dutoit SJ, Raphael M, Audouin J, et al. In situ demonstration of Epstein-Barr virus small RNAs (EBER 1) in acquired immunodeficiency syndrome-related lymphomas: correlation with tumor morphology and primary site. Blood 81993;2:619–624.

218. Jenson H, McIntosh K, Pitt J, et al. Natural history of primary Epstein-Barr virus infection in children of mothers infected with human immunodeficiency virus type 1. J Infect Dis 1999;179:1395–404.

219. Luxton JC, Williams I, Weller I, Crawford DH. Epstein-Barr virus infection of HIV-seropositive individuals is transiently suppressed by high-dose acyclovir treatment. AIDS 1993;7:1337–1343.

220. Ferbas J, Rahman MA, Kingsley LA, et al. Frequent oropharyngeal shedding of Epstein-Barr virus in homosexual men during early HIV infection. AIDS 1992;6:1273–11278.

221. Cooper NR, Moore MD, Nemerow GR. Immunobiology of CR2, the B lymphocyte receptor for Epstein-Barr virus and the C3d complement fragment. Annu Rev Immunol 1988;6:85–113.

222. Evans AS, Niederman JC, Cenabre LC, et al. A prospective evaluation of heterophile and Epstein-Barr virus-specific IgM antibody tests in clinical and subclinical infectious mononucleosis: Specificity and sensitivity of the tests and persistence of antibody. J Infect Dis 1975132:546–554,.

223. Bartlett BL, Tyring SK. Viral Infections of the Skin. In: Richman DD, Whitley RJ, Hayden FG Clinical Virology. 3rd ed. Washington DC: ASM Press.2009; P109–131.

224. Patel BM. Skin rash with infectious mononucleosis and ampicillin. Pediatrics 1967;40:910–911.

225. Feigal DW, Katz MH, Greenspan JS, et al. The prevalence of oral lesions in HIV-infected homosexual and bisexual men: three San Francisco epidemiological cohorts. AIDS 1992;6:95–100.

226. Epstein JB, Sherlock CH, Greenspan JS. Hairy leukoplakia-like lesions following bone-marrow transplantation. AIDS 1991;5:101–102.

227. Greenspan D, Greenspan JS, de Souza Y, et al. Oral hairy leukoplakia in an HIV-negative renal transplant recipient. J Oral Pathol Med 1989;18:32–34.

228. Wurapa AK, Luque AE, Menegus MA. Oral hairy leukoplakia: a manifestation of primary infection with Epstein-Barr virus? Scand J Infect Dis 1999;31:505–506.

229. Patton LL, McKaig R, Strauss R, et al. Changing prevalence of oral manifestations of human immune-deficiency virus in the era of protease inhibitor therapy. Oral Surg Oral Med Oral Pathol Oral Radiol Endod 2004;89:299–304.

230. Resnick L, Herbst JS, Ablashi DV, et al. Regression of oral hairy leukoplakia after orally administered acyclovir therapy. JAMA 1988;259:384–388.

231. Glick M, Pliskin ME. Regression of oral hairy leukoplakia after oral administration of acyclovir. Gen Dent 1990;38:374–375.

232. Laskaris G, Laskaris M, Theodoridou M. Oral hairy leukoplakia in a child with AIDS. Oral Surg Oral Med Oral Pathol Oral Radiol Endod 1995;79:570–571.

233. Naher H, Helfrich S, Hartmann M, et al. EBV replication and therapy of oral hairy leukoplakia using acyclovir. Hautarzt 1990;41:680–682.

234. Greenspan D, De Souza YG, Conant MA, et al. Efficacy of desciclovir in the treatment of Epstein-Barr virus infection in oral hairy leukoplakia. J Acquir Immune Defic Syndr 1990;3:571–578.

235. Newman C, Polk BV. Resolution of oral hairy leukoplakia during therapy with 9-(1,3-dihydroxy-2-propoxymethyl)guanine (DHPG). Ann Intern Med 1987;107:348–350.

489. Husak R, Zouboulis CC, Sander-Bähr C, Hummel M, Orfanos CE. Refractory human papillomavirus-associated oral warts treated topically with 1-3% cidofovir solutions in human immunodeficiency virus type 1-infected patients. Br J Dermatol 2005 Mar;152(3):590–591.

490. Coremans G, Margaritis V, Snoeck R, Wyndaele J, De Clercq E, Geboes K. Topical cidofovir (HPMPC) is an effective adjuvant to surgical treatment of anogenital condylomata acuminata. Dis Colon Rectum 2003 Aug;46(8):1103-8; discussion 1108–1109.

491. Matteelli A, Beltrame A, Graifemberghi S, et al. Efficacy and tolerability of topical 1% cidofovir cream for the treatment of external anogenital warts in HIV-infected persons. Sex Transm Dis 2001 Jun;28(6):343–346.

492. Orlando G, Fasolo MM, Beretta R, et al. Combined surgery and cidofovir is an effective treatment for genital warts in HIV-infected patients. AIDS 2002 Feb 15;16(3):447–450.

493. Snoeck R, Noel JC, Muller C, et al. Cidofovir, a new approach for the treatment of cervix intraepithelial neoplasia grade III (CIN III). J Med Virol 2000 Feb;60(2):205–209.

494. Ghosh AK. Cryosurgery of genital warts in cases in which podophyllin treatment failed or was contraindicated. Br J Vener Dis 1977 Feb;53(1):49–53.

495. Balsdon MJ. Cryosurgery of genital warts. Br J Vener Dis 1978 Oct;54(5):352–353.

496. Simmons PD, Langlet F, Thin RN. Cryotherapy versus electrocautery in the treatment of genital warts. Br J Vener Dis 1981 Aug;57(4):273–274.

497. Dodi G, Infantino A, Moretti R, Scalco G, Lise M. Cryotherapy of anorectal warts and condylomata. Cryobiology 1982 Jun;19(3):287–288.

498. Bergman A, Bhatia NN, Broen EM. Cryotherapy for treatment of genital condylomata during pregnancy. J Reprod Med 1984 Jul;29(7):432–435.

499. Bashi SA. Cryotherapy versus podophyllin in the treatment of genital warts. Int J Dermatol 1985 Oct;24(8):535–536.

500. Sand PK, Shen W, Bowen LW, Ostergard DR. Cryotherapy for the treatment of proximal urethral condyloma acuminatum. J Urol 1987 May;137(5):874–876.

501. Matsunaga J, Bergman A, Bhatia NN. Genital condylomata acuminata in pregnancy: effectiveness, safety and pregnancy outcome following cryotherapy. Br J Obstet Gynaecol 1987 Feb;94(2):168–172.

502. Stone KM, Becker TM, Hadgu A, Kraus SJ. Treatment of external genital warts: a randomised clinical trial comparing podophyllin, cryotherapy, and electrodesiccation. Genitourin Med 1990 Feb;66(1):16–19.

503. Damstra RJ, van Vloten WA. Cryotherapy in the treatment of condylomata acuminata: a controlled study of 64 patients. J Dermatol Surg Oncol 1991 Mar;17(3):273–276.

504. Jones SK, Darville JM. Transmission of virus particles by cryotherapy and multi-use caustic pencils: a problem to dermatologists? Br J Dermatol 1989 Oct;121(4):481–486.

505. Dachow-Siwiec E. Technique of cryotherapy. Clin Dermatol 1985 Oct-Dec;3(4):185–188.

506. Hatch KD. Cryotherapy. Baillieres Clin Obstet Gynaecol 1995 Mar;9(1):133–143.

507. Grimmett RH. Liquid nitrogen therapy. Histologic observations. Arch Dermatol 1961 Apr;83:563–567.

508. Bonnez W, Oakes D, Bailey-Farchione A, et al. A randomized, double-blind, placebo-controlled trial of systemically administered interferon-alpha, -beta, or -gamma in combination with cryotherapy for the treatment of condyloma acuminatum. J Infect Dis 1995 May;171(5):1081–1089.

509. Bonnez W, Oakes D, Bailey-Farchione A, et al. A randomized, double-blind trial of parenteral low dose versus high dose interferon-beta in combination with cryotherapy for treatment of condyloma acuminatum. Antiviral Res 1997 Jun;35(1):41–52.

510. Bergman A, Matsunaga J, Bhatia NN. Cervical cryotherapy for condylomata acuminata during pregnancy. Obstet Gynecol 1987 Jan;69(1):47–50.

511. Thomson JP, Grace RH. The treatment of perianal and anal condylomata acuminata: a new operative technique. J R Soc Med 1978 Mar;71(3):180–185.

512. Jensen SL. Comparison of podophyllin application with simple surgical excision in clearance and recurrence of perianal condylomata acuminata. Lancet 1985 Nov 23;2(8465):1146–1148.

513. Duus BR, Philipsen T, Christensen JD, Lundvall F, Søndergaard J. Refractory condylomata acuminata: a controlled clinical trial of carbon dioxide laser versus conventional surgical treatment. Genitourin Med 1985 Feb;61(1):59–61.

514. Gollock JM, Slatford K, Hunter JM. Scissor excision of anogenital warts. Br J Vener Dis 1982 Dec;58(6):400–401.

515. Khawaja HT. Treatment of condyloma acuminatum. Lancet 1986 Jan 25;1(8474):208–209.

516. Simmons PD, Thomson JP. Scissor excision of penile warts: case report. Genitourin Med 1986 Aug;62(4):277–278.

517. McMillan A, Scott GR. Outpatient treatment of perianal warts by scissor excision. Genitourin Med 1987 Apr;63(2):114–115.

518. Bonnez W, Oakes D, Choi A, et al. Therapeutic efficacy and complications of excisional biopsy of condyloma acuminatum. Sex Transm Dis 1996 Jul-Aug;23(4):273–276.

519. Kreuter A, Brockmeyer NH, Altmeyer P, Wieland U: Anal intraepithelial neoplasia in HIV infection. J Dtsch Dermatol Ges 2008;6:925–934.

520. Jones HW 3rd. Cone biopsy in the management of cervical intraepithelial neoplasia. Clin Obstet Gynecol 1983 Dec;26(4):968–979.

521. Wright TC Jr, Gagnon S, Richart RM, Ferenczy A. Treatment of cervical intraepithelial neoplasia using the loop electrosurgical excision procedure. Obstet Gynecol 1992 Feb;79(2):173–178.

522. Prendiville W. Large loop excision of the transformation zone. Clin Obstet Gynecol 1995 Sep;38(3):622–639.

523. Bigrigg A, Haffenden DK, Sheehan AL, Codling BW, Read MD. Efficacy and safety of large-loop excision of the transformation zone. Lancet 1994 Jan 1;343(8888):32–34.

524. Sawchuk WS, Weber PJ, Lowy DR, et al. Infectious papillomavirus in the vapor of warts treated with carbon dioxide laser or electrocoagulation: detection and protection. J Am Acad Dermatol 1989 Jul;21(1):41–49.

525. Bergbrant IM, Samuelsson L, Olofsson S, et al. Polymerase chain reaction for monitoring human papillomavirus contamination of medical personnel during treatment of genital warts with CO2 laser and electrocoagulation. Acta Derm Venereol 1994 Sep;74(5):393–395.

526. Garden JM, O'Banion MK, Shelnitz LS, et al. Papillomavirus in the vapor of carbon dioxide laser-treated verrucae. JAMA 1988 Feb 26;259(8):1199–202.

527. Kashima HK, Kessis T, Mounts P, et al. Polymerase chain reaction identification of human papillomavirus DNA in CO2 laser plume from recurrent respiratory papillomatosis. Otolaryngol Head Neck Surg 1991 Feb;104(2):191–195.

528. Gloster HM Jr, Roenigk RK. Risk of acquiring human papillomavirus from the plume produced by the carbon dioxide laser in the treatment of warts. J Am Acad Dermatol 1995 Mar;32(3):436–441.

529. Reid R. The management of genital condylomas, intraepithelial neoplasia, and vulvodynia. Obstet Gynecol Clin North Am 1996 Dec;23(4):917–991.

530. Herd RM, Dover JS, Arndt KA. Basic laser principles. Dermatol Clin 1997 Jul;15(3):355–372.

531. Hruza GJ. Laser treatment of warts and other epidermal and dermal lesions. Dermatol Clin 1997 Jul;15(3):487–506.

532. Reid R. Laser surgery of the vulva. Obstet Gynecol Clin North Am 1991 Sep;18(3):491–510.

533. Ferenczy A. Laser treatment of genital human papillomavirus infections in the male patient. Obstet Gynecol Clin North Am 1991 Sep;18(3):525–535.

534. Bhatta KM. Lasers in urology. Lasers Surg Med 1995;16(4):312–330.

535. Dorsey JH. Laser surgery for cervical intraepithelial neoplasia. Obstet Gynecol Clin North Am 1991 Sep;18(3):475–489.

536. Reid R, Greenberg MD, Pizzuti DJ, et al. Superficial laser vulvectomy. V. Surgical debulking is enhanced by adjuvant systemic interferon. Am J Obstet Gynecol 1992 Mar;166(3):815–820.

537. Hoyme UB, Hagedorn M, Schindler AE, et al. Effect of adjuvant imiquimod 5% cream on sustained clearance of anogenital warts following laser treatment. Infect Dis Obstet Gynecol 2002;10(2):79–88.

538. Randomized placebo-controlled double-blind combined therapy with laser surgery and systemic interferon-alpha 2a in the treatment of anogenital condylomata acuminatum. The Condylomata International Collaborative Study Group. J Infect Dis 1993 Apr;167(4):824–829.

539. Nieminen P, Aho M, Lehtinen M, et al. Treatment of genital HPV infection with carbon dioxide laser and systemic interferon alpha-2b. Sex Transm Dis 1994 Mar-Apr;21(2):65–69.

540. Cox JT. Management of cervical intraepithelial neoplasia. Lancet 1999 Mar 13;353(9156):857–859.

541. Martin-Hirsch PL, Paraskevaidis E, Kitchener H. Surgery for cervical intraepithelial neoplasia. Cochrane Database Syst Rev 2000;(2):CD001318.

542. Wetchler SJ. Treatment of cervical intraepithelial neoplasia with the CO2 laser: laser versus cryotherapy. A review of effectiveness and cost. Obstet Gynecol Surv 1984 Aug;39(8):469–473.

543. Morris M, Tortolero-Luna G, Malpica A, et al. Cervical intraepithelial neoplasia and cervical cancer. Obstet Gynecol Clin North Am 1996 Jun;23(2):347–410.

544. Townsend DE, Richart RM. Cryotherapy and carbon dioxide laser management of cervical intraepithelial neoplasia: a controlled comparison. Obstet Gynecol 1983 Jan;61(1):75–78.

545. Mathevet P, Dargent D, Roy M, Beau G. A randomized prospective study comparing three techniques of conization: cold knife, laser, and LEEP. Gynecol Oncol 1994 Aug;54(2):175–179.

546. Convissar RA. Laser palliation of oral manifestations of human immunodeficiency virus infection. J Am Dent Assoc 2002 May;133(5):591-8; quiz 624–625.

547. Bellina JH. The use of the carbon dioxide laser in the management of condyloma acuminatum with eight-year follow-up. Am J Obstet Gynecol 1983 Oct 15;147(4):375–378.

548. Calkins JW, Masterson BJ, Magrina JF, et al. Management of condylomata acuminata with the carbon dioxide laser. Obstet Gynecol 1982 Jan;59(1):105–108.

549. Krogh J, Beuke HP, Miskowiak J, et al. Long-term results of carbon dioxide laser treatment of meatal condylomata acuminata. Br J Urol 1990 Jun;65(6):621–623.

550. Bar-Am A, Shilon M, Peyser MR, Ophir J, Brenner S. Treatment of male genital condylomatous lesions by carbon dioxide laser after failure of previous nonlaser methods. J Am Acad Dermatol 1991 Jan;24(1):87–89.

551. Bekassy Z, Weström L. Infrared coagulation in the treatment of condyloma acuminata in the female genital tract. Sex Transm Dis 1987 Oct Dec;14(4):209–212.

552. Goldstone SE, Kawalek AZ, Huyett JW. Infrared coagulator: a useful tool for treating anal squamous intraepithelial lesions. Dis Colon Rectum 2005 May;48(5):1042–1054.

553. Stier EA, Goldstone SE, Berry JM, et al. Infrared coagulator treatment of high-grade anal dysplasia in HIV-infected individuals: an AIDS malignancy consortium pilot study. J Acquir Immune Defic Syndr 2008 Jan 1;47(1):56–61.

554. Rockley PF, Tyring SK. Interferons alpha, beta and gamma therapy of anogenital human papillomavirus infections. Pharmacol Ther 1995 Feb;65(2):265–287.

555. Friedman-Kien AE, Eron LJ, Conant M, et al. Natural interferon alfa for treatment of condylomata acuminata. JAMA 1988 Jan 22-29;259(4):533–538.

556. Vance JC, Bart BJ, Hansen RC, et al. Intralesional recombinant alpha-2 interferon for the treatment of patients with condyloma acuminatum or verruca plantaris. Arch Dermatol 1986 Mar;122(3):272–277.

557. Eron LJ, Judson F, Tucker S, et al. Interferon therapy for condylomata acuminata. N Engl J Med 1986 Oct 23;315(17):1059–1064.

558. Reichman RC, Oakes D, Bonnez W, et al. Treatment of condyloma acuminatum with three different interferons administered intralesionally. A double-blind, placebo-controlled trial. Ann Intern Med 1988 May;108(5):675–679.

559. Welander CE, Homesley HD, Smiles KA, et al. Intralesional interferon alfa-2b for the treatment of genital warts. Am J Obstet Gynecol 1990 Feb;162(2):348–354.

560. Douglas JM Jr, Eron LJ, Judson FN, et al. A randomized trial of combination therapy with intralesional interferon alpha 2b and podophyllin versus podophyllin alone for the therapy of anogenital warts. J Infect Dis 1990 Jul;162(1):52–59.

561. Handley JM, Horner T, Maw RD, et al. Subcutaneous interferon alpha 2a combined with cryotherapy vs cryotherapy alone in the treatment of primary anogenital warts: a randomised observer blind placebo controlled study. Genitourin Med 1991 Aug;67(4):297–302.

562. Bornstein J, Pascal B, Zarfati D, et al. Recombinant human interferon-beta for condylomata acuminata: a randomized, double-blind, placebo-controlled study of intralesional therapy. Int J STD AIDS 1997 Oct;8(10):614–621.

563. Dinsmore W, Jordan J, O'Mahony C, et al. Recombinant human interferon-beta in the treatment of condylomata acuminata. Int J STD AIDS 1997 Oct;8(10):622–628.

564. Trizna Z, Evans T, Bruce S, et al. A randomized phase II study comparing four different interferon therapies in patients with recalcitrant condylomata acuminata. Sex Transm Dis 1998 Aug;25(7):361–365.

565. Gaspari AA, Zalka A. Interferon gamma immunotherapy for generalized verrucosis in the setting of chronic immunodeficiency. J Am Acad Dermatol 1998 Feb;38:286–287.

566. Beutner KR, Reitano MV, Richwald GA, Wiley DJ. External genital warts: report of the American Medical Association Consensus Conference. AMA Expert Panel on External Genital Warts. Clin Infect Dis 1998 Oct;27(4):796–806.

567. Douglas JM Jr, Rogers M, Judson FN. The effect of asymptomatic infection with HTLV-III on the response of anogenital warts to intralesional treatment with recombinant alpha 2 interferon. J Infect Dis 1986 Aug;154(2):331–334.

568. Vesterinen E, Meyer B, Cantell K, et al. Topical treatment of flat vaginal condyloma with human leukocyte interferon. Obstet Gynecol 1984 Oct;64(4):535–538.

569. Keay S, Teng N, Eisenberg M, et al. Topical interferon for treating condyloma acuminata in women. J Infect Dis 1988 Nov;158(5):934–939.

570. Syed TA, Cheema KM, Khayyami M, et al. Human leukocyte interferon-alpha versus podophyllotoxin in cream for the treatment of genital warts in males. A placebo-controlled, double-blind, comparative study. Dermatology 1995;191(2):129–132.

571. Syed TA, Khayyami M, Kriz D, et al. Management of genital warts in women with human leukocyte interferon alpha vs. podophyllotoxin in cream: a placebo-controlled, double-blind, comparative study. J Mol Med 1995 May;73(5):255–258.

572. Syed TA, Ahmadpour OA. Human leukocyte derived interferon-alpha in a hydrophilic gel for the treatment of intravaginal warts in women: a placebo-controlled, double-blind study. Int J STD AIDS 1998 Dec;9(12):769–772.

573. Armstrong DK, Maw RD, Dinsmore WW, et al. A randomised, double-blind, parallel group study to compare subcutaneous interferon alpha-2a plus podophyllin with placebo plus podophyllin in the treatment of primary condylomata acuminata. Genitourin Med 1994 Dec;70(6):389–393.

574. Yliskoski M, Cantell K, Syrjänen K, et al. Topical treatment with human leukocyte interferon of HPV 16 infections associated with cervical and vaginal intraepithelial neoplasias. Gynecol Oncol 1990 Mar;36(3):353–357.

575. Bornstein J, Ben David Y, Atad J, Pascal B, Revel M, Abramovici H. Treatment of cervical intraepithelial neoplasia and invasive squamous cell carcinoma by interferon. Obstet Gynecol Surv 1993 Apr;48(4):251–260.

576. Rotola A, Costa S, Di Luca D, et al. Beta-interferon treatment of cervical intraepithelial neoplasia: a multicenter clinical trial. Intervirology 1995;38(6):325–331.

577. Gonzalez-Sanchez JL, Martinez-Chequer JC, Hernandez-Celaya ME, et al. Randomized placebo-controlled evaluation of intramuscular interferon beta treatment of recurrent human papillomavirus. Obstet Gynecol 2001 Apr;97(4):621–624.

578. Brockmeyer NH, Poffhoff A, Bader A, et al. Treatment of condylomata acuminata with pegylated interferon alfa-2b in HIV-infected patients. Eur J Med Res 2006 Jan 31;11(1):27–32.

579. Barr E, Sings HL. Prophylactic HPV vaccines: new interventions for cancer control. Vaccine 2008 Nov 18;26(49):6244–6257.

580. Shefer A, Markowitz L, Deeks S, et al. Early experience with human Papillomavirus vaccine introduction in the United States, Canada and Australia. Vaccine 2008;26(Suppl 10):K68–K75.

581. Harper DM, Franco EL, Wheeler CM, et al. Sustained efficacy up to 4–5 years of a bivalent L1 virus-like particle vaccine against human papillomavirus types 16 and 18: follow-up from a randomized control trial. Lancet 2006;367:1247–1255.

582. Garland SM, Hernandez-Avila M, Wheeler CM, et al. Quadrivalent vaccine against human papillomavirus to prevent anogenital diseases. N Engl J Med 2007;356:1928–1943.

583. The FUTURE II Study Group. Quadrivalent vaccine against human Papillomavirus to prevent high-grade cervical lesions. N Engl J Med 2007;356:1915–1927.

584. Paavonen J, Jenkins D, Bosch FX, et al. Efficacy of a prophylactic adjuvanted bivalent L1 virus-like-particle vaccine against infection with human Papillomavirus types 16 and 18 in young women: an interim analysis of a phase III double-blind, randomised controlled trial. Lancet 2007;369:2161–2170.

585. Palefsky JM, Gillison ML, Strickler HD: Chapter 16: HPV vaccines in immunocompromised women and men. Vaccine 2006;24(Suppl 3):S3/140–S3/146.

586. De Vuyst H, Franceschi S: Human papillomavirus vaccines in HIV-positive men and women. Curr Opin Oncol 2007, 19:470–475.

587. Schiller JT, Castellsague X, Villa LL, Hildesheim A: An update of prophylactic human papillomavirus L1 viruslike particle vaccine clinical trial results. Vaccine 2008, 26(Suppl 10):K53–K61.

588. Koutsky LA, Ault KA, Wheeler CM, et al. A controlled trial of a human papillomavirus type 16 vaccine. N Engl J Med 2002 Nov 21;347(21):1645–1651.

589. Villa LL, Costa RL, Petta CA, et al. Prophylactic quadrivalent human papillomavirus (types 6, 11, 16, and 18) L1 virus-like particle vaccine in young women: a randomised double-blind placebo-controlled multicentre phase II efficacy trial. Lancet Oncol 2005 May;6(5):271–278.

590. Garland SM, Hernandez-Avila M, Wheeler CM, et al. Quadrivalent vaccine against human papillomavirus to prevent anogenital diseases. N Engl J Med 2007 May 10;356(19):1928–1943.

591. Ault KA; Future II Study Group. Effect of prophylactic human papillomavirus L1 virus like-particle vaccine on risk of cervical intraepithelial neoplasia grade 2, grade 3, and adenocarcinoma in situ: a combined analysis of four randomized clinical trials. Lancet 2007 Jun 2;369(9576):1861–1868.

592. Joura EA, Leodolter S, Hernandez-Avila M, et al. Efficacy of a quadrivalent prophylactic human papillomavirus (types 6, 11, 16, and 18) L1 virus-like-particle vaccine against high-grade vulval and vaginal lesions: a combined analysis of three randomised clinical trials. Lancet 2007 May 19;369(9574):1693–1702.

593. Harper DM, Franco EL, Wheeler C, et al. Efficacy of a bivalent L1 virus-like particle vaccine in prevention of infection with human papillomavirus types 16 and 18 in young women: a randomised controlled trial. Lancet 2004 Nov 13–19;364(9447):1757–1765.

594. Harper DM, Franco EL, Wheeler CM, et al. Sustained efficacy up to 4.5 years of a bivalent L1 virus-like particle vaccine against human papillomavirus types 16 and 18: follow-up from a randomized control trial. Lancet 2006 Apr 15;367(9518):1247–1255.

595. Muñoz N, Bosch FX, Castellsagué X, et al. Against which human papillomavirus types shall we vaccinate and screen? The international perspective. Int J Cancer 2004 Aug 20;111(2):278–285.

596. Anderson JS, Hoy J, Hillman R, et al. A randomized, placebo-controlled, dose-escalation study to determine the safety, tolerability, and immunogenicity of an HPV-16 therapeutic vaccine in HIV-positive

participants with oncogenic HPV infection of the anus. J Acquir Immune Defic Syndr 2009 Nov 1;52(3):371–381.

597. Steinbrook R. The potential of human papillomavirus vaccines. N Engl J Med 2006 Mar 16;354:1109–1112. Erratum in N Engl J Med 2006;355:745.

598. Palefsky JM, Berry JM, Jay N, et al. A trial of SGN-00101 (HspE7) to treat high-grade anal intraepithelial neoplasia in HIV-positive individuals. AIDS 2006;20:1151–1155.

599. Anderson LJ, Erdman DD. Human Parvoviruses. In: Richman DD, Whitley RJ, Hayden FG Clinical Virology. 3rd ed. Washington DC: ASM Press 2009;P645–661.

600. Cossart YE, Field AM, Cant B, Widdown D. Parvovirus-like particles in human sera. Lancet 1975 Jan 11;1(7898):72–73.

601. Young NS, Brown KE. Parvovirus B19. N Engl J Med 2004 Feb 5;350(6):586–597.

602. Anderson MJ, Higgins PG, Davis LR, et al. Experimental parvoviral infection in humans. J Infect Dis 1985 Aug;152(2):257–265.

603. Heegaard ED, Brown KE. Human parvovirus B19. Clin Microbiol Rev 2002 Jul;15(3):485–505.

604. Plummer FA, Hammond GW, Forward K, et al. An erythema infectiosum-like illness caused by human parvovirus infection. N Engl J Med 1985 Jul 11;313(2):74–79.

605. Koch WC, Adler SP. Human parvovirus B19 infections in women of childbearing age and within families. Pediatr Infect Dis J 1989 Feb;8(2):83–87.

606. Prospective study of human parvovirus (B19) infection in pregnancy. Public Health Laboratory Service Working Party on Fifth Disease. BMJ 1990 May 5;300(6733):1166–1170.

607. Koduri PR, Kumapley R, Valladares J, et al. Chronic pure red cell aplasia caused by parvovirus B19 in AIDS: use of intravenous immunoglobulin- a report of eight patients. Am J Hematol 1999 May;61(1):16–20.

608. Kurtzman G, Frickhofen N, Kimball J, et al. Pure red-cell aplasia of 10 years' duration due to persistent parvovirus B19 infection and its cure with immunoglobulin therapy. N Engl J Med 1989 Aug 24;321(8):519–523.

609. Moore RD. Hematologic Disease. In: Dolin R, Masur H, Saag M AIDS Therapy. 3rd ed. New York: Elsevier 2008;P1187–1205.

610. Blattner WA, Charurat ME. Human Lymphotropic viruses: HTLV-1 and HTLV-2. In: Richman DD, Whitley RJ, Hayden FG Clinical Virology. 3rd ed. Washington DC: ASM Press 2009;P709–736.

611. Poiesz BJ, Ruscetti FW, Gazdar AF, et al. Detection and isolation of type C retrovirus particles from fresh and cultured lymphocytes of a patient with cutaneous T-cell lymphoma. Proc Natl Acad Sci U S A 1980 Dec;77(12):7415–7419.

612. Barré-Sinoussi F, Chermann JC, Rey F, et al. Isolation of a T-lymphotropic retrovirus from a patient at risk for acquired immune deficiency syndrome (AIDS). Science 1983 May 20;220(4599):868–871.

613. Gallo RC, Salahuddin SZ, Popovic M, et al. Frequent detection and isolation of cytopathic retroviruses (HTLV-III) from patients with AIDS and at risk for AIDS. Science 1984 May 4;224(4648):500–503.

614. Sarngadharan MG, DeVico AL, Bruch L, et al. HTLV-III: the etiologic agent of AIDS. Princess Takamatsu Symp 1984;15:301–308.

615. Biggar RJ, Ng J, Kim N, et al. Human leukocyte antigen concordance and the transmission risk via breast-feeding of human T cell lymphotropic virus type I. J Infect Dis 2006 Jan 15;193(2):277–282.

616. Biggar RJ, Miley WJ, et al. Provirus load in breast milk and risk of mother-to-child transmission of human T lymphotropic virus type I. J Infect Dis 2004 Oct 1;190(7):1275–1278.

617. Larsen O, Andersson S, da Silva Z, et al. Prevalences of HTLV-1 infection and associated risk determinants in an urban population in Guinea-Bissau, West Africa. J Acquir Immune Defic Syndr 2000 Oct 1;25(2):157–163.

618. Wiktor SZ, Pate EJ, Rosenberg PS, et al. Mother-to-child transmission of human T-cell lymphotropic virus type I associated with prolonged breast-feeding. J Hum Viro 1997 Nov–Dec;1(1):37–44.

619. Manns A, Wilks RJ, Murphy EL, et al. A prospective study of transmission by transfusion of HTLV-I and risk factors associated with seroconversion. Int J Cancer 1992 Jul 30;51(6):886–891.

620. Miyamura F, Kako S, Yamagami H, et al. Successful treatment of young-onset adult T cell leukemia/lymphoma and preceding chronic refractory eczema and corneal injury by allogeneic hematopoietic stem cell transplantation. Int J Hematol 2009 Oct;90(3):397–401.

621. Hanchard B, LaGrenade L, Carberry C, et al. Childhood infective dermatitis evolving into adult T-cell leukaemia after 17 years. Lance 1991;338:1593–1594.

622. Tsukasaki K, Yamada Y, Ikeda S, et al. Infective dermatitis among patients with ATL in Japan. Int J Cancer 1994;57:293.

623. Manns A, Hisada M, La Grenade L. Human T-lymphotropic virus type I infection. Lancet 1999;353:1951–1958.

624. Oliveira MF, Bittencourt AL, Brites C, et al. HTLV-I associated myelopathy/tropical spastic paraparesis in a 7-year-old boy associated with infective dermatitis. J Neurol Sci 2004; 222: 35–38.

625. Gonçalves DU, Guedes AC, Carneiro-Proietti ABF, et al. HTLV-I associated infective dermatitis may be an indolent HTLV-I associated lymphoma. Braz J Infect Dis 2000; 4: 100–102.

626. Spudich SS, Price RW. (2008). Neurological Disease. In: Dolin R, Masur H, Saag M AIDS Therapy. 3rd ed. New York: Elsevier. P1075-1101.

627. Nakagawa M, Izumo S, Ijichi S, et al. HTLV-I-associated myelopathy: analysis of 213 patients based on clinical features and laboratory findings. J Neurovirol 1995 Mar,1(1).50-61.

628. Nakagawa M, Nakahara K, Maruyama Y, et al. Therapeutic trials in 200 patients with HTLV-I-associated myelopathy/ tropical spastic paraparesis. J Neurovirol 1996 Oct;2(5):345–355.

629. Kitze B, Puccioni-Sohler M, Schäffner J, et al. Specificity of intrathecal IgG synthesis for HTLV-1 core and envelope proteins in HAM/TSP. Acta Neurol Scand 1995 Sep;92(3):213–217.

630. Kitze B, Brady JN. Human T cell lymphotropic retroviruses: association with diseases of the nervous system. Intervirology 1997;40(2-3):132–142.

631. Izumo S, Umehara F, Kashio N, et al. Neuropathology of HTLV-1-associated myelopathy (HAM/TSP). Leukemia 1997 Apr;11 Suppl 3:82–84.

632. Murphy EL, Fridey J, Smith JW, et al. HTLV-associated myelopathy in a cohort of HTLV-I and HTLV-II-infected blood donors. The REDS investigators. Neurology 1997 Feb;48(2):315–320.

633. Lehky TJ, Flerlage N, Katz D, et al. Human T-cell lymphotropic virus type II-associated myelopathy: clinical and immunologic profiles. Ann Neurol 1996 Nov;40(5):714–723.

634. Gessain A, Barin F, Vernant JC, et al. Antibodies to human T-lymphotropic virus type-I in patients with tropical spastic paraparesis. Lancet 1985;2(8452):407–410.

635. Osame M, Usuku K, Izumo S, et al. HTLV-I associated myelopathy, a new clinical entity. Lancet 1986;1(8488):1031–1032.

636. Oh U, Jacobson S. Treatment of HTLV-I-associated myelopathy/tropical spastic paraparesis: toward rational targeted therapy. Neurol Clin 2008 Aug;26(3):781–797, ix-x.

637. Saavedra-Lauzon A, Johnson RA. Dermatologic Disease. In: Dolin R, Masur H, Saag M AIDS Therapy. 3rd ed. New York: Elsevier 2008;P1121–1155.

638. Oliveira Mde F, Brites C, Ferraz N, et al. Infective dermatitis associated with the human T cell lymphotropic virus type I in Salvador, Bahia, Brazil. Clin Infect Dis 2005 Jun 1;40(11):e90–96.

639. Maragno L, Casseb J, Fukumori LM, et al. Human T-cell lymphotropic virus type 1 infective dermatitis emerging in adulthood. Int J Dermatol 2009 Jul;48(7):723–730.

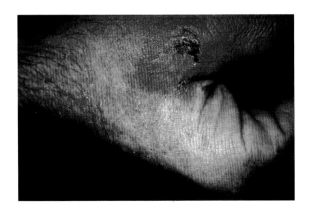

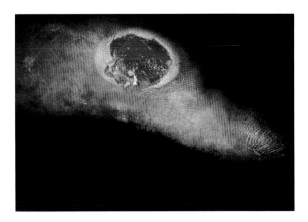

Figure 20–2. *Hemmorrhagic crust in the center of an erythemtous vesicular plaque on an AIDS patient dorsal hand near the thumb. Cellulitis and ulceration from a staphylococcal infection such as this can arise rapidly in immunosuppressed patients. (Courtesy of the Public Health Image Library of the Centers for Disease Control and Prevention.)*

Figure 20–3. *Mal perforans ulcer secondar to a staph infection on a red erosive base in an AIDS patient mimicking a diabetic pressure ulcer. In this case the ulceration is an acute staphylococcus ulcer arising on the foot and penetrating faster and more deeply than would be expect in a patient with a normal immune system. (Courtesy of the Public Health Image Library of the Centers for Disease Control and Prevention.)*

obvious, fluid can usually be expressed easily with slight pressure. If abscess formation is present, incision and drainage with lavage is crucial for successful treatment. A variety of individuals are known to be at risk for CA-MRSA SSTIs, presumably related to crowded conditions and/or frequent skin-to-skin contact: children, individuals with a prior history of MRSA infection, men who have sex with men, military personnel, athletes (especially those involved in contact sports), incarcerated persons, Native Americans, Pacific Islanders, injection drug users, and household contacts or day care center contacts of those with MRSA.[27–41] HIV-infected individuals are also at a higher risk for recurrent SSTIs.[40]

Musculoskeletal infections are the most common invasive CA-MRSA infections in children.[26,38,42–44] The most common sites of osteomyelitis in children are the long bones, such as the tibia and femur.[46] It has been demonstrated that the presence of PVL has been associated with greater complications, prolonged course of illness, and increased frequency of subperiosteal abscesses.[47–48] Adjacent venous thrombophlebitis with subsequent septic pulmonary emboli has also been linked to CA-MRSA containing PVL.[46] In adults, the vertebrae are the most common sites of hematogenous osteomyelitis.[49] Myositis and pyomyositis often occur with concomitant osteomyelitis, and they often are preceded by an injury to the involved region. Necrotizing fasciitis is typically associated with either current or previous injection drug use. The most common areas affected are the buttocks, legs, arms, and shoulders. Extensive debridement is often required for successful treatment.

Pneumonia due to *S. aureus* is a common occurrence throughout the world, often associated with a preceding influenza infection. A survey of 59 hospitals in the United States identified MRSA as a potential pathogen in 8.9% of community-acquired pneumonia, 26.5% of healthcare-associated pneumonia, 22.9% of hospital-acquired pneumonia, and 14.6% of ventilator-associated pneumonia cases.[50] HIV-infected individuals have approximately a 10-fold increased risk for bacterial pneumonia compared to HIV-uninfected individuals.[51] The risk increases with declining CD4 counts. Necrotizing pneumonia is closely associated with MRSA strains that produce PVL. The clinical presentation typically includes fever, cough productive of purulent sputum, dyspnea, chest pain, and rapid deterioration to include hemoptysis, pleural effusions, cavitation, and empyema. Leukopenia is surprisingly common.[52] Chest radiographs often demonstrate multilobar involvement, with or without pleural effusions. Cavitation on a chest radiograph of a younger patient with high fever and significant dyspnea should raise the suspicion for MRSA.[53–59] The fatality rate associated with CA-MRSA necrotizing pneumonia can be as high as 60%.[52]

Both CA-MRSA and HCA-MRSA are culprits in bacteremia. CA-MRSA has been a major cause of infective endocarditis in injection drug users, whereas HCA-MRSA endocarditis tends to occur in patients with diabetes and/or those receiving hemodialysis.[46] It is a very common cause of both native and prosthetic valve endocarditis.[60–63] Symptoms classically consist of fever, tachycardia, hypotension, and a new murmur. Nonspecific signs, such as arthralgias, myalgias, and chest pain, are variable. Specific cutaneous signs include Janeway lesions and Osler's nodes. In a study of *S. aureus* septicemia, 44% of HIV-positive patients had nasopharyngeal colonization compared to 31% of HIV-negative patients and 23% of healthy hospital staff.[64] Complications include mycotic aneurysms, stroke, multiple emboli, heart failure, and intracardiac abscesses. A high mortality rate—up to 30%—is associated with bacteremia.[65–68] Approximately one-third of patients with bacteremia have metastatic complications, especially if prosthetic material is present.[69]

Other possible clinical syndromes in HIV-infected individuals include meningitis, liver abscess,[70] retropharyngeal abscess with mediastinal extension and jugular vein thrombosis similar to Lemierre's syndrome,[71] and orbital infections.[72–73]

CA-MRSA isolates tend to be susceptible to clindamycin, and they less often exhibit resistance to multiple non-β-lactam drugs.[74] Clindamycin susceptibility testing may be misleading, as the organism may demonstrate inducible resistance. This requires subsequent testing, called the D-test, to determine the potential for successful treatment with clindamycin. Nearly all isolates are susceptible to TMP-SMX, rifampin, linezolid, and the tetracyclines. Rifampin is not acceptable for monotherapy in any situation due to the high frequency of mutations resulting in resistance;[75] however, it may be used as adjunct therapy with TMP-SMX or doxycycline. Linezolid tends to be cost-prohibitive in many instances, and resistance has been seen in some cases.[76] For parenteral treatment, vancomycin is considered the drug of choice, with clindamycin, daptomycin, tigecycline, and quinupristin-dalfopristin as potential other options, as there has been a slowly increasing number of cases of vancomycin intermediately-sensitive and vancomycin resistant strains of MRSA.[77] Intravenous linezolid has only been shown to be efficacious in the treatment of MRSA pneumonia.[78] Intravenous TMP-SMX has not been well studied, but it has been used with variable success in the U.S. Ceftobiprole, a member of a new class of cephalosporins, has promising potential in treating complicated SSTIs and pneumonias, but it has not yet been approved by the U.S. Food and Drug Administration (FDA) at the time of this publication.

Streptococcus pneumoniae

Streptococcus pneumoniae (also referred to as pneumococcus) is a gram-positive coccus with a lancet-shaped appearance (**Figure 20–4**). In addition to the pneumococcal cell wall, nearly all clinical isolates also have a polysaccharide capsule, which consists of mainly teichoic acid and

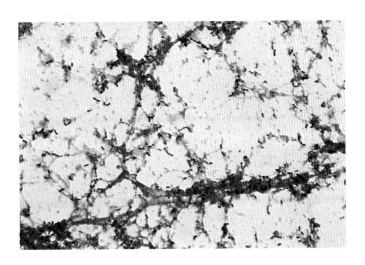

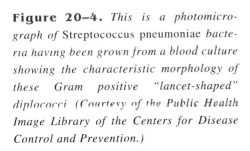

Figure 20–4. *This is a photomicrograph of* Streptococcus pneumoniae *bacteria having been grown from a blood culture showing the characteristic morphology of these Gram positive "lancet-shaped" diplococci (Courtesy of the Public Health Image Library of the Centers for Disease Control and Prevention.)*

peptidoglycan. The capsule provides protection from ingestion and killing by host phagocytic cells; however, anticapsular antibody is protective against pneumococcal infection, and this is the premise for vaccination. Pneumococci commonly colonize the nasopharynx of humans. These organisms are easily transmitted from one individual to another as a result of close contact, but infection is generally not regarded as contagious because so many factors intervene between acquisition of the organism and development of disease.[79] Outbreaks can occur, most commonly associated with crowding and close contact, such as in military camps, prisons, and nursing homes.[80–82]

S. pneumoniae has been long recognized as a major cause of pneumonia, meningitis, sinusitis, and otitis media; however, it has also been found to cause endocarditis, septic arthritis, and peritonitis. The most frequent symptoms of pneumococcal pneumonia include cough, fever, chills, shortness of breath, and fatigue. Patients typically have a grayish, anxious appearance that is distinct from that of individuals with viral or *Mycoplasma* pneumonia. Chest radiography typically demonstrates a lobar pneumonia. The most common complication of pneumococcal pneumonia is empyema. The occurrence of pneumococcal otitis media or bacteremia is seasonal, perhaps because of the association with viral respiratory illnesses. A November-April clustering, with a clear peak in February, has been described for otitis media among schoolchildren.[83] In contrast, invasive disease in adults clearly reaches a peak in the middle of winter, inversely related to ambient temperature and directly associated with the peak of viral respiratory disease.[84–85] Except during an epidemic of meningococcal infection, *S. pneumoniae* is the most common cause of bacterial meningitis in adults.[86] Meningitis may result from direct extension from the sinuses or middle ear or from bacteremia.[87–88] Soft tissue infections may occur in persons infected with HIV or those with connective tissue disorders.[89–90]

Mortality from bacterial pneumonia is higher in patients with HIV who have a CD4 cell count of less than 100 cells/mm^3, radiographic progression of disease on therapy, and shock. As with other opportunistic infections, use of potent antiretroviral combination therapy decreases the risk of bacterial pneumonia, but not to the rate of individuals who were HIV-negative even when the CD4 cell count normalizes.[91] The most commonly identified pathogen in HIV-related bacterial pneumonia is *S. pneumoniae*, followed closely by *H. influenzae* (see below).[92–93] Although both typically are seen with a relatively acute illness and focal consolidation on chest radiography, *Haemophilus influenzae* may rarely cause a more subacute illness with diffuse interstitial infiltrates, more suggestive of *Pneumocystis* pneumonia. The frequency of pneumococcal disease can be reduced by the administration of the 23-valent pneumococcal vaccine to patients whose CD4+ T-cell counts are above 200 cells/mm^3.[94]

Until recently, nearly all clinical isolates of *S. pneumoniae* have been sensitive to penicillin. In the past 20 years, the number of drug-resistant isolates has increased globally. The most common form of resistance is acquired by stepwise mutations of the bacterial genes which encode for penicillin-binding proteins (PBPs). These genes are considered "mosaic genes" in that the coding region includes segments of genetic material derived from other related streptococcal species. These mutations are chromosomally mediated and do not appear to alter the virulence of the organism, meaning that penicillin-resistant pneumococci are neither more nor less virulent than penicillin-sensitive pneumococci. The altered PBP genes appear to spread readily to other strains of pneumococci in a horizontal fashion, and these mutations appear to be stable. Resistance to other β-lactam antibiotics, such as the cephalosporins, is also mediated by altered PBPs. Resistance to other antibiotics can be acquired through conjugation with other related streptococci, such that there is a change in the antimicrobial target, as with the macrolides, fluoroquinolones, and trimethoprim. Several risk factors have been identified for the development of drug-resistant pneumococcus: age less than 6 years, advanced age, recent treatment with antibiotics, multiple comorbid diseases, attendance at day care centers, HIV infection and other immunocompromised states, recent hospitalization, and residence in a nursing home or prison. Treatment should be guided by susceptibility testing; however, empiric therapy should be instituted in the presence of obvious symptoms. If the prevalence of penicillin-resistant strains exceeds 15%, then wider-spectrum antibiotics, including amoxicillin-clavulanate, are preferred. Other non-penicillin–based potential therapeutic agents include third-generation cephalosporins, fluoroquinolones, TMP-SMX, and vancomycin. For pneumococcal meningitis, the recommended therapeutic regimen includes ceftriaxone and vancomycin, pending susceptibility testing. If the organism is found to be penicillin-sensitive, the preferred treatment is high-dose intravenous penicillin.[87]

Two major vaccines against pneumococcal infections are: a 23-polyvalent vaccine and a heptavalent vaccine. The heptavalent vaccine is recommended for all children between 2 and 23 months of age; the 23-valent vaccine is recommended for anyone older than 2 years of age who is at substantially increased risk for developing pneumococcal infection and/or a serious complication of such an infection.[95] Included in this classification are individuals who: (1) are older than 65 years of age, (2) have anatomic or functional asplenia, cerebrospinal fluid leak, diabetes mellitus, alcoholism, cirrhosis, chronic renal insufficiency, chronic pulmonary disease, or advanced cardiovascular disease, (3) have compromised immunity, such as multiple myeloma, lymphoma, Hodgkin's disease, HIV infection, organ transplantation, or chronic use of glucocorticoids, (4) are in genetic risk groups, including Native Americans and Alaskans, and (5) are residents in potential outbreak zones, including nursing homes.[92] Due to waning immunity, repeat vaccination is recommended every 5 years. The problem with vaccination is that those who need it most—such as HIV-infected individuals—are least likely to respond appropriately to the vaccination due to the diminished ability to make IgG to polysaccharide antigens.

Salmonella spp.

Salmonella are gram-negative, non-spore–forming bacilli in the family Enterobacteriaceae. They are effective pathogens that cause a spectrum of disease in humans and animals, including domesticated and wild mammals, reptiles, birds, and insects. More than 2,000 separate serotypes have been identified. Some serotypes, such as *S. typhi*, *S. paratyphi*, and *S. sendai*, are highly adapted to humans and have no other known natural hosts, whereas others, such as *S. typhimurium*, have a broad host range. Transmission is via ingestion of contaminated materials, particularly raw fruits and vegetables, oysters and other shellfish, and contaminated water. Eggs, poultry, and other dairy products are some of the more well-recognized sources. Outbreaks have been described in the summer months where children consume contaminated egg salad. The incubation period is about 1 to 3 weeks, and it is considered communicable until all *Salmonella* organisms have been eradicated from the stool or urine. Host factors are important and disease is more likely in immunocompromised individuals, sickle cell disease, and achlorhydria. Although typhoid fever represents a classic example of invasive and systemic human infection, there is no increase in susceptibility of severity in individuals with immunosuppression. Nontyphoidal *Salmonella* infections, on the other hand, have a dramatically more severe and invasive presentation in HIV-infected persons.[96] Nontyphoidal *Salmonella* infections are the leading cause of community-acquired bacteremia in HIV-infected individuals worldwide.[97, 98]

A range of clinical syndromes are associated with *Salmonella* infections, including diarrheal disease, typhoid fever, osteomyelitis, arthritis, abscesses, and bacteremia. Typhoid fever is caused by *S. typhi* or *S. paratyphi* serotypes A, B, and C. The symptoms initially are quite non-specific: low-grade fever, abdominal cramping, and diarrhea. Over the next week, the fever rises to high levels, hypotension develops, relative bradycardia may occur, and the infected individual appears very ill. About one-third will exhibit rose spots, a faint salmon-colored, maculopapular rash on the trunk (**Figure 20–5**).[99] Complications include gastrointestinal bleeding and intestinal perforation, both of which are life-threatening. The disease entity is unique in that the infection occurs twice within its life cycle. The ileum is the site of both initial invasion as well as secondary infection in typhoid. The organism gains access to the mesenteric lymph nodes and undergoes replication in the reticuloendothelial system, including the spleen, liver, and gallbladder. The release of new organisms occurs into two main compartments: the intestinal tract and the bloodstream. Once in the bloodstream, the bacteria can seed any other location, notably the bone, joints, and urinary tract. After re-entering the intestinal tract, the organisms reinfect the ileum and cause significant invasion and secondary bacteremia and resultant bleeding at the site of invasion. This cycle continues until interrupted by antibiotics, sufficient host immune control, or death. The potential exists for chronically infected asymptomatic human carriers, where the organism typically colonizes the gallbladder. These chronic carriers are at an increased risk for carcinoma of the gallbladder.[100]

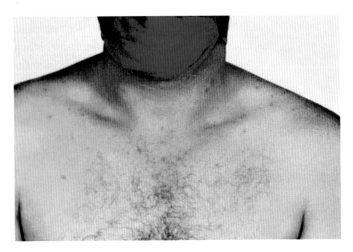

Figure 20–5. *Rose spots on the chest of a patient with typhoid fever due to the bacterium* Salmonella typhi. *(Courtesy of the Public Health Image Library of the Centers for Disease Control and Prevention.)*

Gastroenteritis caused by nontyphoidal *Salmonella* typically occurs within 6 to 48 hours after ingestion of contaminated food or water. Symptomatically, it is indistinguishable from other forms of gastroenteritis, with nausea, vomiting, and diarrhea of loose, nonbloody stool. Fever, abdominal cramping, chills, headache, and myalgias may also occur. Rarely, a syndrome of "pseudoappendicitis" may develop.[101] After resolution of symptoms, the mean duration of carriage in nontyphoidal *Salmonella* in the stool is 4 to 5 weeks and varies by serotype. Antimicrobial therapy may increase the duration of carriage.[102] Hospitalization may occur secondary to dehydration, and death is a rare complication. However, a disproportionate number of deaths occur among the elderly, especially those residing in long-term care facilities, and among immunocompromised patients, including those with HIV, flares of lupus, or those with rheumatologic disease currently being treated with antitumor necrosis factor antibody therapy.[103–107]

Bacteremia with nontyphoidal *Salmonella* in HIV-positive patients is a nonspecific febrile illness. Typically, this occurs with severe immunosuppression, with CD4+ T-cell counts <200 cells/mm^3. Hepatosplenomegaly may occur in about half of cases.[108] Metastatic seeding may occur in a variety of locations, causing cavitary lung lesions, endocarditis with or without mycotic aortic aneurysm, splenic abscesses, spontaneous peritonitis, pyomyositis, brain abscess, cerebral empyema, septic arthritis, and acalculous cholecystitis.[109–114]

Early diagnosis and the prompt administration of appropriate antibiotics will prevent severe complications and decrease mortality from typhoid fever. Fluoroquinolones are the most effective class of agents for treating drug-susceptible *Salmonella*. For quinolone-resistant strains, which have been increasing in incidence in Asia, the drug of choice is azithromycin, 1 gram daily for 7 days. In cases of severe typhoid fever, requiring parenteral treatment and hospitalization, quinolones are still the drug of choice; in cases of quinolone resistance, treatment with third-generation cephalosporins is preferred.[115] *Salmonella* bacteremia should be treated with both a third-generation cephalosporin and quinolone until susceptibilities return. Recurrent or high-grade bacteremia should prompt an investigation for endovascular abnormalities.[116,117] Bacteremia in severely immunosuppressed patients requires at least 4 to 6 weeks of therapy with a fluoroquinolone, TMP-SMX, or ceftriaxone to attempt eradication of the organism and to decrease the risk for recurrent bacteremia. If relapse occurs, then long-term suppressive oral therapy should be instituted.[118]

Two typhoid vaccines currently are available: (1) Ty21a, an oral, live attenuated *S. typhi* vaccine, and (2) a parenteral Vi capsular polysaccharide vaccine. The oral vaccine is contraindicated in pregnancy, those taking antimicrobial therapy, and immunocompromised hosts.

Pseudomonas spp.

Pseudomonas aeruginosa is the major pathogenic species in the family Pseudomonadaceae. It is an aerobic, Gram-negative bacillus, usually with a single flagellum. Strains that produce polysaccharide capsules (glycocalyx) are mucoid in colony appearance (**Figure 20–6**), with some strains producing pigment based on proteins produced (e.g., pyocyanin makes a blue pigment). In the 1800s, *P. aeruginosa* was found to be a cause of serious wound and surgical infections. In 1925, Osler thought it was more of a secondary or opportunistic invader of damaged tissues rather than a primary cause of infection in healthy tissue. It has been recognized as a major pathogen since the 1960s due to its ability to cause infections in the immunocompromised and burned hosts, in patients with cystic fibrosis, and because of its role as a nosocomial pathogen in healthcare facilities. Since it is commonly found in soil, water, and plants, it is an impor-

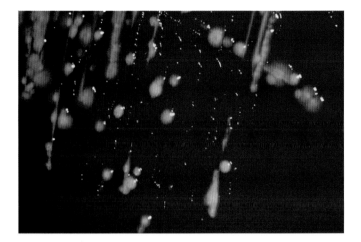

Figure 20-6. *This photograph depicts the mucoid colonial growth pattern displayed by* Pseudomonas aeruginosa *bacteria growing on a blood agar plate. (Courtesy of the Public Health Image Library of the Centers for Disease Control and Prevention.)*

tant cause of community-acquired infections. It has been associated with skin infections related to the use of hot tubs, whirlpools, and swimming pools.[119] It can cause ulcerative keratitis associated with contact lens solution[120,121] and is a frequent cause of otitis externa.[122] It is associated with puncture wound infections, classically when there are puncture wounds of the feet through tennis shoes. Pseudomonal endocarditis can occur with the use of injection drugs.[123]

P. aeruginosa is among the top five causes of nosocomial bacteremia, and severe infection often leads to sepsis. Mortality can be high, especially in immunosuppressed or neutropenic patients and burn victims.[124–126] The most frequently documented sources are the respiratory and urinary tracts. The clinical presentation is similar to any other sepsis-type syndrome; however, one distinctive clinical distinction is the appearance of ecthyma gangrenosa lesions, which occurs almost exclusively in markedly neutropenic patients. They are small, painful, reddish, maculopapular, well-circumscribed lesions that have a geographic margin and begin as pink, darken to purple, finally becoming black and necrotic. These lesions are teeming with bacteria. The mainstays of treatment of pseudomonal bacteremia include aggressive antimicrobial therapy, fluid resuscitation to reverse profound hypovolemia from distributive shock, supportive care, and removal of the most likely source of the organism if at all possible (for example, an indwelling catheter). There is no clear consensus as to the appropriate treatment for bacteremia: antipseudomonal β-lactam monotherapy or as a part of combination therapy with an aminoglycoside is commonly used.[127–131] The most accepted empiric treatment plan would include combination therapy until the results of susceptibility testing are available.

The respiratory tract remains the most frequent site of infection with *P. aeruginosa*. It is one of the most frequent causes of ventilator-associated pneumonia. It is also an important pathogen in community-acquired pneumonia, notably for HIV-infected individuals with low CD4+ T cell counts.[132] The clinical symptoms of acute pneumonia are very similar to those seen in pneumonia from nonpseudomonal causes: fever, cough, chills, copious sputum, and pleuritic chest pain. Necrotizing pneumonia is not uncommon. Treatment is similar to that of bacteremia. One additional potential therapeutic option is aerosolized aminoglycosides, as they have demonstrated the ability to reduce intrapulmonary densities of *P. aeruginosa*; however, there are no randomized controlled trials to date comparing aerosolized aminoglycosides to traditional parenteral antipseudomonal agents.[133,134]

Bone and joint infections can occurs as a result from bacteremia, direct inoculation into bone, or from spread from a contiguous infection. Bacteremia resulting from injection drug use has been associated with the development of vertebral osteomyelitis as well as sternoclavicular joint arthritis.[135,136] The clinical syndrome is quite indolent, with symptoms present for weeks to months prior to diagnosis. Fever is variably present. There may be localized erythema or tenderness to palpation. Leukocytosis is not always present, but the erythrocyte sedimentation rate is nearly always elevated. Osteomyelitis of the foot has been documented after puncture wounds as the organism has been found to reside between the layers of the rubber soles of sneakers.[137,138] This has been most well-documented in the field of pediatrics. Treatment for osteomyelitis, without concomitant endocarditis, can be accomplished with a single agent, such as ciprofloxacin or an aminoglycoside for a total of 4 to 6 weeks. If endocarditis is present, then therapy should be directed at treating the endocarditis, rather than the bone or joints involved.

Eye infections typically result from direct inoculation into the tissue related to trauma or surface injury caused by contact lenses. All eye infections with *Pseudomonas* have the potential to become extremely devastating, rapidly leading to loss of sight. Keratitis is the most frequent ocular manifestation in clinical practice. It is considered to be an ocular emergency due to the fact that it can rapidly progress. The typical treatment is topical antibiotics. Endophthalmitis is the most feared infection because nearly all cases result in some form of visual impairment.[139] It can be caused by penetrating injuries, surgery, perforation of a corneal ulcer, or seeding from bacteremia. The disease follows a fulminant course, with severe pain, chemosis, decreased visual acuity, anterior uveitis, vitreitis, and panophthalmitis occurring. The treatment of choice is parenteral and intravitreal antibiotics.

Ear infections with *P. aeruginosa* can be mild (swimmer's ear) to serious, life-threatening infections. Swimmer's ear is commonly seen as a result of underchlorinated swimming pools and macerated skin of the auditory canal. Purulent exudate may be visualized. Treatment is often antipseudomonal antibiotic ear drops. Malignant otitis externa is the dreaded form, which typically begins with infection of the external auditory canal with penetration into the surrounding cartilage and eventual extension to the middle ear, mastoid air cells, and temporal bone. This can be a devastating infection in diabetic patients, HIV-infected individuals, and elderly patients.[140–142] The most serious complication is extension into the venous sinuses of the brain and/or the carotid artery, causing thrombosis and subsequent infarction. Involvement of the fifth, sixth, and/or seventh cranial nerves may occur during the extension of the infection, and facial paralysis tends to be an early finding. Treatment consists of antipseudomonal antibiotics and debridement of necrotic tissue.

Urinary tract infections tend to occur as a complication of the presence of a foreign body such as a stone, stent, or catheter in the urinary tract. This provides a source of bacteremia via ascending infection. If a foreign body is present, removal is necessary for full recovery. Most treatment courses of antibiotics last 10 to 14 days, unless a renal abscess or bacteremia develops.

Endovascular infections, such as infective endocarditis, can occur from bacteremia and can involve both native and prosthetic valves. The right side of the heart tends to be affected more often than the left, and multivalvular disease is common. Fever is often the presenting symptom, and chest pain, with or without hemoptysis, may occur, indicating pulmonary involvement due to septic embolization to the lungs. Skin manifestations are rare, and ecthyma gangrenosum is not seen in endocarditis. Therapy often consists of synergistic combinations of antibiotics, such as an antipseudomonal β-lactam and an aminoglycoside. There have been cases of relapse, suggesting the need for adjunctive surgical therapy, which is a delicate matter given that prosthetic valve insertion has not been successful and cardiac decompensation may occur.

P. aeruginosa infections in HIV-infected patients were rather common prior to the advent of highly-active antiretroviral therapy (HAART). The infections were both nosocomial and community-acquired, but they have been mostly community-acquired since the era of HAART. It was thought that the infections would occur primarily as a result of neutropenia, with a low CD4+ T-cell count often associated with disseminated infection. The clinical presentation tends to be underwhelming and similar to that seen in HIV-uninfected individuals. Subsequently, it can be thought of as disproportionate to the potential severity of the disease, as the infection can be fatal. The most common form of infection is pneumonia, with or without bacteremia. Symptoms are similar to those experienced by HIV-uninfected patients; however, there is a greater prevalence of cavitary lesions in HIV-infected patients.[143–145] Another distinctive feature of pseudomonal disease associated with HIV infection is a higher incidence of relapses, especially with pulmonary disease, sinusitis, and bacteremia. However, treatment regimens are identical for HIV-infected and -uninfected patients.

Bartonella spp.

Bartonella species are small, pleomorphic fastidious gram-negative bacilli that can cause clinical illness in both immunocompetent and immunocompromised individuals. Humans are incidental hosts in most cases, with transmission via arthropod vectors or direct inoculation. Four species of *Bartonella* have been associated with human disease: *B. henselae, B. quintana, B. bacilliformis,* and *B. elizabethae* (**Table 20–1**). *B. henselae*, the causative agent of cat scratch disease, uses the cat flea as its major vector for cat-to-cat transmission. Its transmission to humans is not well-defined, but it has been linked to interaction with cats, including being licked, scratched, and bitten by them. More importantly, the highest risk of developing bacillary angiomatosis (BA) in HIV-infected individuals is associated with kittens or cats under 1 year of age.[146]

Bacillary angiomatosis is characterized by neovascular proliferation involving skin and regional lymph nodes, typically appearing late in HIV infection due to severe immunosuppression.[147–152] It can appear in a variety of internal organs, including the liver, spleen, bone, brain, lung, heart valves, bowel, and uterine cervix.[151–162] Dermatologic manifestations mimic Kaposi's sarcoma, which may be differentiated by skin biopsy, with specific staining of tissue to demonstrate clumps of bacilli. In the absence of dermatologic features, diagnosis is often delayed due to the nonspecific nature of the clinical presentation, typically consisting of fever, lymphadenopathy, hepatosplenomegaly, and anemia.[160] Bacillary peliosis refers to the hepatic involvement with *B. henselae* in immunocompromised hosts.

Cat-scratch disease is almost exclusively caused by *B. henselae*. It is the most commonly recognized manifestation of human infection with *Bartonella*. In the United States, an estimated 25,000 cases occur annually.[163] The "typical" presentation begins with a cutaneous papule or

TABLE 20–1	**Infections Due to *Bartonella* spp. in Humans**			
	Disease			
	B. henselae	**B. quintana**	**B. bacilliformis**	**B. elizabethae**
	Cat-scratch disease[a] Endocarditis[a,b] Bacillary angiomatosis[b] Relapsing bacteremia with fever[b]	Trench fever[a] Endocarditis[a,b] Bacillary angiomatosis[b] Relapsing bacteremia with fever[b]	Bartonellosis[a]	Endocarditis[a]

[a]Immunocompetent hosts. [b]Immunocompromised hosts.
Source: Adapted from Regnery et al.[152]

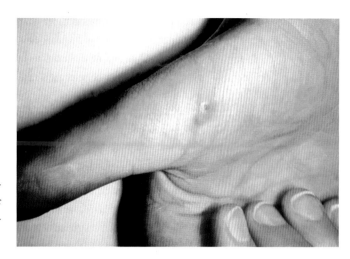

Figure 20–7. *Pustule of cat-scratch disease, skin of thumb. (Courtesy of the Public Health Image Library of the Centers for Disease Control and Prevention.)*

pustule (**Figure 20–7**) approximately 3 to 10 days after animal contact and inoculation, lasting up to 3 weeks.[164–166] Regional lymphadenopathy develops 1 to 7 weeks later, and is the most prominent and common manifestation. Low-grade fever tends to be present, with malaise or fatigue being less commonly reported. Lymph node enlargement and suppuration may persist for months. Direct needle aspiration can be useful for diagnostic purposes as well as for symptomatic relief. Hypercalcemia may complicate lymphadenopathy as a result of endogenous overproduction of active vitamin D associated with granuloma formation.[167] Other, less common, clinical features include myalgia, arthropathy, tendonitis, neuralgia, and osteomyelitis. The most common atypical presentation of cat-scratch disease is Parinaud's oculoglandular syndrome, characterized by a self-limited granulomatous conjunctivitis with ipsilateral preauricular lymphadenitis.[168,169] Other atypical manifestations include hepatitis, splenitis, pneumonitis, osteitis, encephalopathy, and neuroretinitis.[170,171] Both *B. henselae* and *B. quintana* have been implicated in a few cases of HIV-associated brain lesions, meningoencephalitis, encephalopathy, intracerebral BA, and neuropsychiatric disease.[157, 172–176]

Historically, the diagnosis required at least three of the following four criteria: (1) history of animal contact, with the presence of a scratch or primary skin or eye lesion; (2) aspiration of "sterile" pus from the lymph node, or culture and other laboratory testing that excluded other etiologic possibilities; (3) a positive cat-scratch disease skin test; and (4) a lymph node biopsy revealing pathology consistent with cat scratch disease. The skin test antigen was originally prepared from "sterile" pus derived from cat-scratch disease lymphadenitis from other patients. The test antigen was never standardized or manufactured commercially. Given the potential risk of transmitting other pathogens, the skin test is no longer used as a diagnostic criterion. Serology has primarily replaced skin testing in diagnosing *Bartonella* infections. Culturing may be difficult to attain due to the fact that typical concentrations of sodium polyanethol sulfate found in blood culture media inhibit *B. henselae* growth. Culturing also requires cell-free media, optimally on freshly prepared rabbit-heart infusion agar plates, but traditional fresh blood or chocolate agar plates may suffice in sustaining growth of the organisms.[177] Staining with silver impregnation techniques (for example, Warthin-Starry stain) is necessary for identifying organisms in tissue biopsies.

Successful treatment of *Bartonella* infections has been reported with several antimicrobial agents, including erythromycin, doxycycline, chloramphenicol, azithromycin, TMP-SMX, ciprofloxacin, gentamicin, and rifampin. The optimal length of treatment has not been well studied, but the general recommendation is treatment for at least 2 to 3 months for cutaneous bacillary angiomatosis and 3 to 4 months for severe disease, such as osteomyelitis or bacillary peliosis. Case reports of neuroretinitis treated with two effective antimicrobial agents for at least 6 weeks have demonstrated an accelerated rate of resolution.[172,174,178]

Treponema pallidum

Treponema pallidum, the causative agent of syphilis, is a thin, gram-negative, tightly-coiled spirochete. It can be visualized only with dark-field (rather than traditional light) microscopy. No culture systems for *T. pallidum* are clinically available. Syphilis occurs exclusively in humans and is most commonly spread by sexual contact. Other possible modes of transmission include transplacentally to the newborn and via blood transfusion. A person is considered most infectious early in the disease course, and gradually becomes less infectious as the disease progresses untreated. The number of reported new cases of syphilis in the United States has waxed and waned since its discovery. It reached a peak incidence during World War II; after the discovery of penicillin and aggressive public health intervention, the nadir was in the mid-1980s. A dramatic resurgence occurred in the late 1980s and early 1990s, only to fall again in the late 1990s. Subsequently, there has been another rise in incidence, mainly in the subpopulation of men who have sex with men, both HIV-infected and HIV-non-infected. (**Figure 20–8**) Syphilis remains a global epidemic, however, with an annual incidence of more than 12 million cases.[179–181]

Within hours to days after *T. pallidum* penetrates the intact mucous membrane or gains access through broken skin, it enters the lymphatics and bloodstream and disseminates throughout the body. The average dividing time is roughly 30 to 33 hours. Clinical lesions typically appear once the infectious burden reaches 10^7 organisms/mg of tissue. In untreated individuals, the disease progresses through a set series of stages: primary, secondary, latent, and tertiary. The primary stage is heralded by a chancre, a nontender ulcerative lesion representing the site of inoculation. The incubation period ranges from 3 to 90 days, with a median of 3 weeks. The chancre is often unrecognized, as it is both painless and typically inconspicuous, often lasting only 24 to 48 hours, but may be present up to 8 weeks, especially in immunocompromised hosts. The chancre shows indurated borders and a clean nonpurulent base (**Figure 20–9**); however, it is teeming with spirochetes and is therefore highly infectious. Most often, the chancre is solitary;

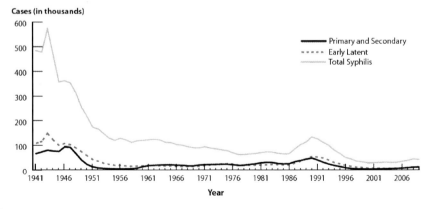

Figure 20–8. *Syphilis—Reported Cases by Stage of Infection: United States, 1941–2009. Source: U.S. Centers for Disease Control and Prevention. (http://www.cdc.gov/std/stats09/figures/33.htm; last accessed 01/27/11.)*

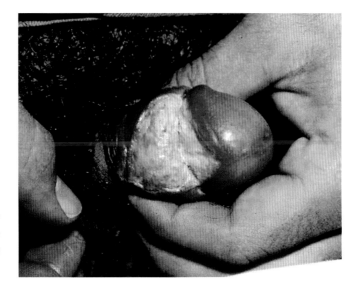

Figure 20–9. *Large and atypical chancre on the penile shaft indicative of syphilis infection. The patient was later found to be positive also for HIV. (Courtesy of Ted Rosen, MD.)*

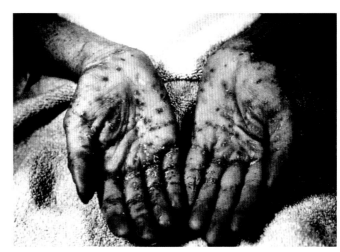

Figure 20–10. *This photograph shows keratotic lesions on the palms of this patient's hands due to a secondary syphilitic infection. (Courtesy of the Public Health Image Library of the Centers for Disease Control and Prevention.)*

however, in HIV-infected individuals, there may be multiple chancres.[182] The secondary stage represents dissemination of the organism, typically occurring 2 to 12 weeks after inoculation. The characteristic hallmark in this stage is a rash, notably involving the palms and soles (**Figure 20–10**). The rash can appear as macular, papular, maculopapular, pustular, papulosquamous, or urticarial forms.[183] Other unique features include follicular syphilides, patches of alopecia (**Figure 20–11**), hepatitis (with transaminases reaching up to 10 times the upper limit of normal and a disproportionately elevated alkaline phosphatase),[184] and condylomata lata [large, fleshy, flat papular lesions in the genital region (**Figure 20–12**)]. Constitutional symptoms, including fever, myalgias, and weight loss, are common. It is not uncommon to find secondary-stage symptoms while the chancre is still present in those infected with HIV. After the secondary stage subsides, the infected individual enters into the latent phase, during which diagnosis can only be made with serologic testing. The latent phase can be further subdivided into an "early" stage, during which relapses are common, and a "late" stage, in which relapses are unlikely. A clinical diagnostic distinction is that the "early latent" stage is when there has been a negative serologic test within the past year, and the "late latent" stage is when there is either no history of a serologic test or a negative serologic test more than one year prior to the current positive serologic test. Tertiary syphilis refers to disseminated disease that notably affects blood vessels, such as the vaso vasorum of the aorta and the small arteries of the central nervous system. The

positive despite adequate successful treatment. In HIV-infected individuals, the RPR may remain persistently elevated, despite adequate treatment. This is mainly due to B-cell dysfunction, resulting in polyclonal antibody stimulation. This phenomenon is called the "serofast" state. Despite this, successful treatment should still result in a four-fold decrease in the RPR titer. A definitive diagnosis of neurosyphilis is made by cerebrospinal fluid analysis using the VDRL test (as the RPR is an insensitive test)[185,189,199,200] or a positive real-time PCR DNA test specific for *T. pallidum*. The diagnosis of congenital syphilis is typically made either by testing the mother at the time of birth or by identifying characteristic clinical features in the neonate through physical examination, radiographic, and ultrasonographic studies.

The genome consists of a single circular chromosome that lacks apparent transposable elements, suggesting that it is extremely conserved and stable. This is the most likely reason as to why the organism has remained exquisitely sensitive to penicillin for more than 70 years. Therapy is based on the stage of syphilis at the time of diagnosis (**Table 20–3**). If individuals have a documented anaphylaxis to penicillin, doxycycline may be an option in primary, secondary, and latent syphilis. In penicillin-allergic patients with tertiary or neurosyphilis, many experts recommend penicillin desensitization. Ocular syphilis, presenting with either anterior and/or panuveitis, is a frequent complication of acute and chronic neurosyphilis, and thus should be treated with antibiotic regimens appropriate for neurosyphilis. Ocular syphilis appears to be seen with increasing frequency in individuals infected with HIV.[201] Treatment in any stage, but especially important in earlier stages due to the high organismal burden, has the potential to elicit the Jarisch-Herxheimer reaction. This is a systemic response to the massive release of heat-stable protein from the dead organisms. Symptoms typically appear 1 to 2 hours after the initial treatment, last 12 to 24 hours, and they consist of fever, chills, myalgias, headache, tachycardia, hyperventilation, vasodilation with flushing, and mild hypotension.[202] The reaction is self-lim-

TABLE 20–3	Recommended Treatments Based on Stage of Syphilis		
Stage	**Adult, Recommended**	**Adult, Alternative**	**Children**
Primary, secondary, early latent	Benzathine penicillin G, 2.4 million units IM × 1	Doxycycline 100 mg po BID × 2 weeks Tetracycline 500 mg po BID × 2 weeks Ceftriaxone 1gram IM/IV daily × 7–10 days	Benzathine penicillin G 50,000 units/kg × 1 (max: 2.4 million units)
Late latent, tertiary	Benzathine penicillin G, 2.4 million units IM weekly × 3	Doxycycline 100mg po BID × 4 weeks Tetracycline 500 mg po BID × 4 weeks	Benzathine penicillin G, 50,000units/kg weekly × 3 (max: 2.4 million units/dose)
Neurosyphilis	Aqueous penicillin G, 3–4 million units IV q4 hours × 10–14 days	Procaine penicillin 2–4 million units IM daily with probenecid 500 mg q6 hours × 10–14 days Ceftriaxone 2 g IM/IV daily × 10–14 days	

ited and often responds to the concomitant routine administration of nonsteroidal anti-inflammatory drugs and fluid hydration. Corticosteroids can also abort the reaction.

Unfortunately, humoral antibodies to the *Treponema* are only partially protective, and they only become more absolute the longer the infection remains untreated. This explains why an individual has the potential to become reinfected with *T. pallidum* and may exhibit the same degree of symptoms as in the previous/initial infection.[203] Untreated HIV-infected individuals have a propensity to develop more severe disease, and have an increased risk for manifesting a more protracted and malignant course, complicated by more constitutional symptoms, greater organ involvement, atypical rashes, and symptomatic neurosyphilis.[203–210] After treatment, aggressive serologic follow-up is recommended at intervals of 1, 2, 3, 6, 9, 12, and 24 months.[210–213]

Haemophilus influenzae

Haemophilus influenzae is a small, Gram-negative bacterium whose only host is humans. It is nearly exclusively found in the upper airway, with the genital tract being the only other potential location. One of the most pathogenic strains is the B strain; however, with the advent of childhood immunization in the United States, natural infection with *H. influenzae* type B is rare. As a result, nontypeable strains are the typical pathogenic bacteria that cause sinopulmonary disease. A unique feature of *Haemophilus* species, which renders them difficult to treat and responsible for recurrent infections, is the ability to create a biofilm that is relatively resistant to host defense mechanisms and penetration of antibiotics.

In individuals with chronic obstructive pulmonary disease or with immunodeficiency, nontypeable *H. influenzae* is an important cause of pneumonia.[214,215] The clinical presentation is quite similar to that of pneumonia caused by other bacteria (including *Streptococcus pneumoniae*): fever, cough productive of purulent sputum, and dyspnea. Chest radiography may demonstrate patchy or lobar infiltrates. *H. influenzae* can also cause bacteremia, which carries significant mortality in those who have underlying conditions such as HIV infection, cancer, and alcoholism.[216] There are cases of epididymo-orchitis in prepubertal boys due to *H. influenzae* type B, and there has been documentation of disease in an adult with HIV infection. The presentation is similar regardless of age, with symptoms of acute scrotal pain and fever. Complications include torsion and scrotal abscess.[217]

Treatment for most sinopulmonary infections often is successful with oral antibiotics alone. About 30% of nontypeable strains are β-lactamase producers, and therefore treatment with β-lactams requires the addition of a β-lactamase inhibitor. More severe infections, including bacteremia, require parenteral antibiotics, such as extended-spectrum cephalosporins, ampicillin-sulbactam, or fluoroquinolones.

Actinomyces israelii

Actinomyces are gram-positive, "higher order" bacteria that are related to the *Nocardia* species. The most common *Actinomyces* species causing pathologic disease is *Actinomyces israelii*, accounting for nearly 75% of all cases. These organisms are members of the normal oropharyngeal flora, with 100% colonization by the age of 2 years.[218] These bacteria are also natural inhabitants of the colon and female genital tract. They typically exhibit low virulence, but when

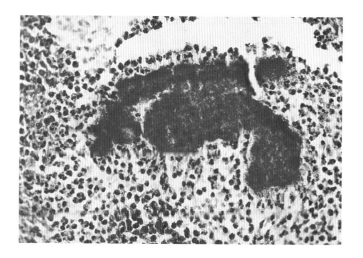

Figure 20–14. *This micrograph depicts histopathologic changes due to the gram-positive organism, Actinomyces israelii. Using a modified Fite-Faraco stain, a "sulfur granule" is shown in the middle of the image. These granules actually represent colonies of A. israelii, a gram-positive, anaerobic filamentous bacteria. (Courtesy of the Public Health Image Library of the Centers for Disease Control and Prevention.)*

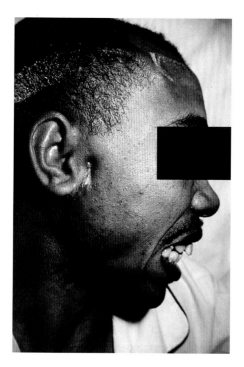

Figure 20–15. *A patient with Actinomycosis on the left side of the face. Actinomyces spp, bacteria, are normally found in the oral cavity is an opportunistic pathogen usually seen only in immunosuppressed patients. Lesions involve long standing swelling, suppuration and the formation of an abscess or granuloma. (Courtesy of the Public Health Image Library of the Centers for Disease Control and Prevention.).*

they invade tissue, they form tiny, visible clumps commonly referred to as "sulfur granules," based on their yellow color (**Figure 20–14**). There have been no documented cases of person-to-person transmission.[219] Penetration of the mucosal membrane is integral to the pathogenesis of these bacteria. Oral-cervicofacial infections are frequently associated with dental procedures, trauma, radiation, or oncologic surgical procedures.[220] Pulmonary infections often arise in the setting of aspiration. Gastrointestinal and intra-abdominal infections typically occur in the settings of intestinal surgery, diverticulitis, appendicitis, or foreign bodies such as fish bones or intrauterine devices.[221,222]

The most classically recognized clinical presentation is oral-cervicofacial disease, accounting for the majority of cases of infection. Typically, there is a painless soft tissue swelling at the angle of the mandible or high in the cervical neck (**Figure 20–15**). Other presentations include abscess, mass lesion, or rarely an ulcerative lesion.[223] The bacteria may spread to adjacent areas with complete disregard for anatomical architecture, potentially invading the carotid artery, the orbital cavity, cranium, cervical spine, or trachea.[222, 224–226] Pulmonary disease typically occurs following an aspiration event or as a complication of cervicofacial disease. Symptoms range from indolent cough without fever to cavitary lesions, resembling tuberculosis. One distinct feature characteristic of *Actinomyces* is its ability to create sinus tracts, such as from the lung to the chest wall.[219] There have been few cases of esophageal actinomycosis in HIV-positive patients, typically associated with recurrent oral or esophageal ulcers.[227,228] Pelvic actinomycosis is often seen as a complication of intrauterine devices (IUDs). Disease rarely develops within the first year of implantation, and the risk of infection increases with the length of time the IUD is in place.[229] Infection can also occur within months after the removal of the IUD. The most common presentation is an indolent course of fever, weight loss, abdominal pain, and abnormal vaginal bleeding, and/or discharge.[230] Hematogenous dissemination of infection is rare.

Intravenous penicillin G and surgical debridement are the mainstays of effective treatment for actinomycosis. Antibiotic treatment tends to be long-term, with the switch to an oral regimen after 2 to 4 weeks of intravenous therapy. For those with documented hypersensitivity to the β-lactams, other effective antibiotics include erythromycin, tetracycline, and clindamycin.

Rhodococcus equi and *Nocardia* spp.

Nocardia and *Rhodococcus* belong to the same family, Nocardiaceae (nocardioform organisms), and therefore will be discussed together. *Rhodococcus equi* is the major pathogen causing clinical disease in humans, notably in immunocompromised hosts with defective cell-mediated immunity.[231–233] More than 85% of cases in the literature have occurred in immunocompromised hosts, with HIV infection accounting for about two-thirds of them.[234] The "equi" designation refers to the fact that the organism was first isolated from infected horses. Approximately 20% to 30% of infected humans report contact with horses. The bacterium is an inhabitant of soil, and infection typically occurs via inhalation, although direct inoculation and ingestion are also potential means of acquisition.[235, 236] The primary clinical syndrome is pulmonary disease, occurring in about 80% of all cases,[234] with the most characteristic radiographic finding being cavitary upper lobe pneumonia.[237] The onset of pulmonary disease is insidious and it progresses rather slowly, with cough, pleuritic chest pain, and fever. Weight loss occurs over time. Given these symptoms, in conjunction with a cavitary upper lobe lesion and a partial acid-fast staining, cases are often misdiagnosed as pulmonary tuberculosis.[238,239] Bacteremia and dissemination may result, allowing for extrapulmonary involvement in about 20% of cases. Complications of pulmonary infection include lung abscesses, pleural effusion, empyema, pneumothorax, endobronchial lesions, pericarditis, cardiac tamponade, and mediastinitis.[240–243] Extrapulmonary infection occurs in approximately 25% of those who have no evidence of pulmonary infection, with the brain and the skin being the two most common locations.[240,244,245] Typical dermatologic manifestations include cellulitis, subcutaneous nodules, wound infection, and abscess. *R. equi* has also been identified as a cause of lymphocytic meningitis in immunocompetent hosts.[246] Another group of cases was associated with direct inoculation, such as a penetrating ocular injury or wound infection.

Due to the frequency of relapses, prolonged combination therapy is strongly recommended. Therapeutic options include erythromycin, vancomycin, fluoroquinolones, glycopeptides, carbapenems, aminoglycosides, and linezolid.[234,240,247–249] The severity of the illness and/or immunosuppression dictate the number of therapeutic agents; localized, non-CNS infections

133. Palmer LB, Smaldone GC, Simon SR, et al: Aerosolized antibiotics in mechanically ventilated patients: delivery and response. Critical Care Med 1998;26:31–39.

134. Parker AF, Couch L, Fiel SB, et al: Tobramycin solution for inhalation reduces sputum *Pseudomonas aeruginosa* density in bronchiectasis. Am J Respir Crit Care Med 2000;162:481–485.

135. Sapico FL, Montgomerie JZ: Vertebral osteomyelitis in intravenous drug abusers: report of three cases and review of the literature. Rev Infect Dis 1980;2:196–206.

136. . Bayer AS, Chow AW, Louie JS, et al: Sternoarticular pyoarthrosis due to gram-negative bacilli: report of eight cases. Arch Intern Med 1977;137;1036–1040.

137. Lang AG, Peterson HA: Osteomyelitis following puncture wounds of the foot in children. J Trauma 1976;16:993–999.

138. Fisher MC, Goldsmith JF, Gilligan PH: Sneakers as a source of *Pseudomonas aeruginosa* in children with osteomyelitis following puncture wounds. J Ped 1985;106:607–609

139. Eifrig CW, Scott IU, Flynn Jr HW, et al: Endophthalmitis caused by *Pseudomonas aeruginosa*. Ophthalmology 2003,110.1714–1717

140. Chandler JR: Malignant external otitis. Laryngoscope 1968;78:1257–1294.

141. Hern JD, Almeyda J, Thomas DM, et al: Malignant otitis externa in HIV and AIDS. J Laryngol Otol 1996;110:770–775.

142. Ress BD, Luntz M, Telischi FF, et al: Necrotizing external otitis in patients with AIDS. Laryngoscope 1997;107:456–460

143. Manfredi R, Nanetti A, Ferri M, et al: *Pseudomonas* spp. complications in patients with HIV disease: an eight-year clinical and microbiological survey. Eur J Epid 2000;16:111–118.

144. Dropulic LK, Leslie JM, Eldred LJ, et al: Clinical manifestations and risk factors of *Pseudomonas aeruginosa* infection in patients with AIDS. J Infect Dis 1995;171:930–937.

145. Gallant JE, Ko AH: Cavitary pulmonary lesions in patients infected with human immunodeficiency virus. Clin Infect Dis 1996;22:671–682

146. Tappero JW, Mohle-Boetani J, Koehler JE, et al. The epidemiology of bacillary angiomatosis and bacillary peliosis. JAMA 1993;269:770–775.

147. Stoler MH, Bonfiglio TA, Steigbigel RT, et al: An atypical subcutaneous infection associated with acquired immune deficiency syndrome. Am J Clin Path 1983;80:714–718.

148. Cockerell CJ, Webster GF, Whitlow MA, et al: Epithelioid angiomatosis: a distinct vascular disorder in patients with the acquired immunodeficiency syndrome or AIDS-related complex. Lancet 1987;2:6544–6546.

149. LeBoit PE, Egbert BM, Stoler MH, et al: Epithelioid haemangioma-like vascular proliferation in AIDS: manifestation of cat scratch disease bacillus infection? Lancet 1988;l:960–963.

150. Spach DH, Callis KP, Paauw DS, et al. Endocarditis caused by *Rochalimaea Quintana* in a patient infected with human immunodeficiency virus. J Clin Microbiol 1993;31:692–694.

151. Hadfield RL, Warren R, Kass M, Brun E, Levy C. Endocarditis caused by *Rochalimaea henselae*. Human Pathol 1993;24:1140–1141.

152. Regnery RL, Childs JE, Koehler JE. Infections associated with *Bartonella* species in persons infected with human immunodeficiency virus. Clin Infect Dis 1995;21(Suppl 1):S94–S98.

153. Slater LN, Welch DF, Min K-W: *Rochalimaea henselae* causes bacillary angiomatosis and peliosis hepatis. Arch Intern Med 1992;152:602–606

154. Koehler JE, LeBoit PE, Egbert BM, et al: Cutaneous vascular lesions and disseminated cat-scratch disease in patients with the acquired immunodeficiency syndrome (AIDS) and AIDS-related complex. Ann Intern Med 1988;109:449–455.

155. Milam MW, Balerdi MJ, Toney JF, et al: Epithelioid angiomatosis secondary to disseminated cat scratch disease involving the bone marrow and skin in a patient with acquired immune deficiency syndrome: a case report. Amer J Med 1990;88:180–183.

156. Kemper CA, Lombard CM, Deresinski SC, et al: Visceral bacillary epithelioid angiomatosis: possible manifestations of disseminated cat scratch disease in the immunocompromised host: a report of two cases. Amer J Med 1990;89:216–222.

157. Spach DH, Panther LA, Thorning DR, et al: Intracerebral bacillary angiomatosis in a patient infected with the human immunodeficiency virus. Ann Intern Med 1992;116:740–742.

158. Koehler JE, Cederberg L: Intraabdominal mass associated with gastrointestinal hemorrhage: a new manifestation of bacillary angiomatosis. Gastroenterology 1995;109:2011–2014.

159. Coche E, Beigelman C, Lucidarme O, et al: Thoracic bacillary angiomatosis in a patient with AIDS. AJR: Am J Roentgenology 1995;165:56–58.

160. Mohle-Boetani JC, Koehler JE, Berger TG, et al: Bacillary angiomatosis and bacillary peliosis in patients infected with the human immunodeficiency virus: clinical characteristics in a case control study. Clin Infect Dis 1996;22:794–800.

161. Huh YB, Rose S, Schoen RE, et al: Colonic bacillary angiomatosis. Ann Intern Med 1996;124:735–737.

162. Long SR, Whitfield MJ, Eades C, et al: Bacillary angiomatosis of the cervix and vulva in a patient with AIDS. Obstet Gynecol 1996;881:709–711.

163. Jackson LA, Perkins BA, Wenger JD: Cat scratch disease in the United States: an analysis of three national databases. Am J Public Health 1993;83:1707–1711.

164. Carithers HA: Cat-scratch disease: an overview based on a study of 1,200 patients. Am J Dis Child 1985;139:1124–1133.

165. Moriarty R, Margileth A: Cat scratch disease. Infect Dis Clin North Amer 1987,1.575–590.

166. Margileth AM: Cat scratch disease. Adv Ped Infect Dis 1993;8:1–21.

167. Bosch X: Hypercalcemia due to endogenous overproduction of active vitamin D in identical twins with cat-scratch disease. JAMA 1998;279:532–534.

168. Parinaud H: Conjonctivite infectieuse par les animaux. Annales d'Oculistique 1889;101:252–253.

169. Cassady JV, Culbertson CS: Cat-scratch disease and Parinaud's oculoglandular syndrome. Arch Ophthalmol 1953;50:68–74.

170. Abbasi S, Chesney PJ: Pulmonary manifestations of cat scratch disease: a case report and review of the literature. Ped Infect Dis J 1995;14:547–548.

171. Muszynski M, Eppes J, Riley H: Granulomatous osteolytic lesion of the skull associated with cat scratch disease. Ped Infect Dis J 1987;6:199–201.

172. Wong MT, Dolan MJ, Lattuada Jr CP, et al: Neuroretinitis, aseptic meningitis, and lymphadenitis associated with *Bartonella* (*Rochalimaea*) *henselae* infection in immunocompetent patients and patients infected with human immunodeficiency virus type 1. Clin Infect Dis 1995;21:352–360

173. Schwartzman WA, Patnaik M, Barka NE, et al: *Rochalimaea* antibodies in HIV-associated neurologic disease. Neurology 1994;44:1312–1316.

174. Baker J, Ruiz-Rodriguez R, Whitfield M, et al: Bacillary angiomatosis: a treatable cause of acute psychiatric symptoms in human immunodeficiency virus infection. J Clin Psych 1995;56:161–166.

175. Patnaik M, Schwartzman WA, Peter JB: *Bartonella henselae*: detection in brain tissue of patients with AIDS-associated neurological disease [abstract]. J Invest Med 1995;43(Suppl 2):368A.

176. Schwartzman WA, Patnaik M, Angulo FJ, et al: *Bartonella* (*Rochalimaea*) antibodies, dementia, and cat ownership in human immunodeficiency virus-infected men. Clin Infect Dis 1995;21:954–959.

177. Welch DF, Hensel DM, Pickett DA, et al: Bacteremia due to *Rochalimaea henselae* in a child: practical identification of isolates in the clinical laboratory. J Clin Microbiol 1993;31:2381–2386.

178. Reed JB, Scales JK, Wong MT, et al: *Bartonella henselae* neuroretinitis in cat scratch disease. Ophthalmol 1998;105:459–466.

179. Zetola NM, Klausner JD: Syphilis and HIV infection: An update. Clin Infect Dis 2007;44:1222–1228.

180. Buchacz K, Klausner JD, Kerndt PR, et al: HIV incidence among men with early syphilis in Atlanta, San Francisco, and Los Angeles, 2004 to 2005. J Acquir Immune Defici Syndr 2008;47:234–240.

181. Fenton KA, Breban R, Vardavas JT, et al: Infectious syphilis in high-income settings in the 21st century. Lancet Infect Dis 2008;8:244–253.

182. Rompalo AM, Lawlor J, Seaman P, et al: Modification of syphilitic genital ulcer manifestations by coexistent HIV infection. Sex Transm Dis 2001;28:448–454.

183. Chapel TA: The signs and symptoms of secondary syphilis. Sexually Transmitted Diseases 1980;7:161–167.

184. Mullick CJ, Liappis AP, Benator DA, et al: Syphilitic hepatitis in HIV-infected patients: A report of 7 cases and review of the literature. Clin Infect Dis 2004;39:100–105.

185. Lugar A, Schmidt BL, Steyer K, et al: Diagnosis of neurosyphilis by examination of the cerebrospinal fluid. Br J Venereal Dis 1981;57:232–237.

186. Marra CM, Maxwell CL, Smith SL, et al: Cerebrospinal fluid abnormalities in patients with syphilis: Association with clinical and laboratory features. J Infect Dis 2004;189:369–376

187. Lukehart S, Hook EW, Baker-Zander SH, et al: Invasion of the central nervous system by *Treponema pallidum*: Implications for diagnosis and therapy. Ann Intern Med 1988;109:855–862.

188. Tramont EC: Neurosyphilis in patients with human immunodeficiency virus infection. N Engl J Med 1994;332:1169–1170

189. Gurvinder PT, Kaur S, Gupta R, et al: Syphilitic panuveitis and asymptomatic neurosyphilis: A marker of HIV infection. International Journal of STDs and AIDS 2001;12:754–756.

190. Aldave AJ, King JA, Cunningham ET: Ocular syphilis. Current Opinions in Ophthalmology 2001;12:433–441.

191. Ormerod LD, Pukin JE, Sobel JD: Syphilitic posterior uveitis: Correlative findings and significance. Clin Infect Dis 2001;32:1661–1673.

192. Parc CE, Chahed S, Patel SV, et al: Manifestations and treatment of ocular syphilis during an epidemic in France. Sex Transm Dis 2007;34:553–33647.

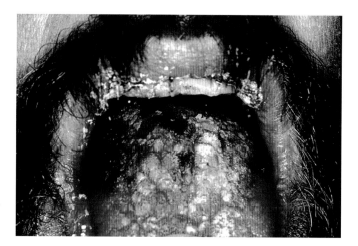

Figure 21–1. *This HIV/AIDS patient presented with a chronic secondary opportunistic oral candidiasis infection. (Courtesy of the Public Health Image Library of the Centers for Disease Control and Prevention.)*

Oral thrush becomes increasingly common as the CD4 cell count falls. At CD4 counts <50/mm^3, esophageal thrush also becomes common. In people with HIV infection, resistance to azole antifungals is associated with severe immunosuppression (<50 CD4 cells/mm^3), more episodes treated with antifungal drugs, and longer median duration of systemic azole treatment.[49]

Esophageal candidiasis is an AIDS-defining illness, according to the 1993 CDC classification system and usually occurs in patients with CD4 counts <100/mm^3. Concomitant oral candidiasis is often present. Esophagitis may also lead to septicemia and disseminated candidiasis. Symptoms include burning pain in the substernal area, dysphagia, nausea, and vomiting. The clinical diagnosis relies on radiologic and endoscopic findings, which usually shows white mucosal plaques with erythema, resembling those seen in oral candidiasis.

Candida pneumonia is very rare. Pulmonary candidiasis can be acquired by either hematogenous dissemination causing a diffuse pneumonia or by bronchial extension in patients with oropharyngeal candidiasis. It tends to be a late or terminal manifestation of HIV infection, usually occurring as a part of disseminated candidiasis, which may include candidal endocarditis, meningitis, or hepatosplenic candidiasis.

Invasive candidiasis is not common in patients with AIDS, and it usually occurs when there is drug-induced neutropenia or use of indwelling catheters.[8] Hematogenous dissemination may then occur to one or more other organ systems, with the formation of numerous microabscesses. Hematogenous dissemination can lead to brain abscess or chronic meningitis. There is an increasing incidence of candidemia by species other than *C. albicans*.

Laboratory Diagnosis

Direct Microscopy. Skin and nail scrapings, urine, sputum, bronchial washings, oral/throat swabs, cerebrospinal fluid (CSF), pleural fluid, blood, and tissue biopsies from various visceral organs and indwelling catheter tips are the common samples taken in suspected cases of candidiasis[30] and are examined under the microscope using either 10% potassium hydroxide (KOH) and/or gram-stained smears. Tissue sections are stained using periodic acid Schiff (PAS), Grocott's methenamine silver (GMS), or Gram's stain. Specimens are examined for the presence of small, round to oval, thin-walled, clusters of budding yeast cells (blastoconidia) and branching pseudohyphae (**Figures 21–2** and **21–3**).

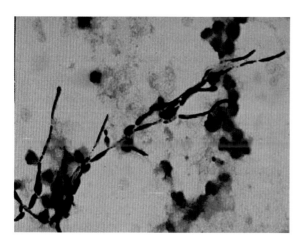

Figure 21–2. *Photomicrograph of budding yeasts with pseudohyphae in oral swab smear due to* Candida *spp. (Gram's stain; magnification 1,000×).*

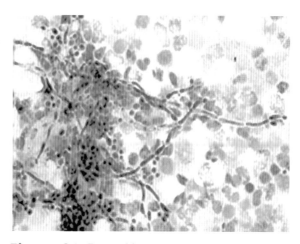

Figure 21–3. *Budding yeast cells with pseudohyphae in a smear of sputum due to* Candida *spp. (PAS stain; magnification 1,000×).*

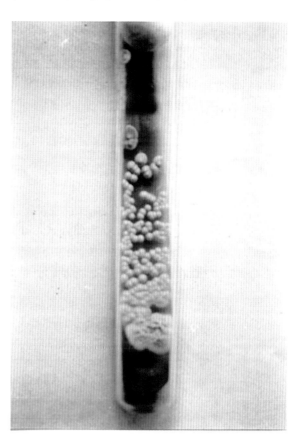

Figure 21–4. *Macroscopic appearance of* Candida spp. *(5-day-old culture, on Sabouraud dextrose agar).*

Culture. Plaques can be cultured, although cultures rarely are indicated. Colonies are typically white to cream colored with a smooth, glabrous to waxy surface (**Figure 21–4**). The genus *Candida* is characterized by globose to elongate yeast-like cells or blastoconidia that reproduce by multilateral budding. Most *Candida* species are also characterized by the presence of well-developed pseudohyphae, but this feature may be absent in *C. glabrata.* Arthroconidia and colony pigmentation are always absent. Within the genus *Candida*, fermentation, nitrate assimilation and carbohydrate assimilation, germ tube formation, and morphology on corn meal agar are used for identification of different species. [30, 50]

A positive culture from blood or other sterile body fluid or tissue biopsy is considered significant. Lysis centrifugation is currently the most sensitive method for the isolation of *Candida* from blood. Blood cultures often remain negative, even in patients who are dying from proven disseminated candidiasis.[30] However, positive culture from nonsterile specimens, such as sputum, bronchial lavage, esophageal brushings, urine, stool, and surgical drains, are of little diagnostic value.[30]

Pulmonary candidiasis is difficult to diagnose due to nonspecific radiologic and culture findings and most patients, especially those with granulocytopenia, present at autopsy. The presence of yeasts in alveolar lavage or sputum specimens is not specific and blood cultures may also be negative.[30]

Serology. Various serologic procedures have been devised to detect the presence of *Candida* antibodies, ranging from immunodiffusion to more sensitive tests, such as counter immunoelectrophoresis (CIE), enzyme-linked immunosorbent assay (ELISA), and radioimmunoassay (RIA). However, these are often negative in the immunocompromised patient, especially at the beginning of an infection.[30] The detection of antigen by immunologic methods such as ELISA or RIA, and polymerase chain reaction (PCR) testing have been used, but the latex agglutination (cand-tec)[48] test for glycoprotein antigen has proved to be the most useful and feasible.[30,50]

Diagnostic challenges still remain in the management of candidiasis, as there is no gold-standard approach; bloodstream culture is positive in only 50% of patients. Various nonculture methods like enolase and antibodies to enolase, mannoproteins, β-glucan metabolic product D-arabinitol, and DNA detection by PCR are still under development.

Treatment

Oral Candidiasis. Initial episodes of oropharyngeal candidiasis can be adequately treated with topical therapy, including clotrimazole troches (10 mg 5 × day until the lesions resolve, usually 7–14 days); nystatin suspension (500,000 units, gargled 4–5 times per day) or pastilles; or once-daily miconazole mucoadhesive tablets.[51]

Oral fluconazole (100–150 mg/day for 7–14 days) is as effective and, in certain studies, superior to topical therapy for oropharyngeal candidiasis. In addition, it is more convenient and typically is better tolerated. Therefore, oral fluconazole is considered the drug of choice.[52] Itraconazole oral solution for 7 to 14 days is as effective as oral fluconazole, but is less well tolerated. Posaconazole oral solution is also as effective as fluconazole and is generally better tolerated than itraconazole.[53] Alternatives to oral fluconazole are available, although few situations require that these drugs would be used in preference to fluconazole solely to treat mucosal candidiasis. In a multicenter, randomized study, posaconazole was proven more effective than fluconazole in sustaining clinical success after antifungal therapy was discontinued.[53] Ketoconazole and itraconazole capsules are less effective than fluconazole because of their more variable absorption. Using these agents to treat mucosal candidiasis is not reasonable if the other options are available.

For severe, recurrent, and refractory cases, itraconazole, 100–200 mg/day maintenance therapy may be indicated.

Esophageal Candidiasis. Oral fluconazole (100–400 mg/day) or itraconazole (200 mg/day) for 14 to 21 days is the preferred treatment.

Systemic antifungals are required for effective treatment of esophageal candidiasis. A 14- to 21-day course of either fluconazole (oral or IV) or oral itraconazole solution is highly effective. As with oropharyngeal candidiasis, oral ketoconazole or itraconazole capsules are less effective than fluconazole because of variable absorption. Although IV caspofungin or IV voriconazole are effective in treating esophageal candidiasis among HIV-infected patients, oral or IV fluconazole remain the preferred therapies. Voriconazole, now licensed and available in IV and PO forms, has been seen to clearly work for esophageal candidiasis in a study comparing voriconazole with fluconazole, with a success rate of 98% for voriconazole compared to 95% for fluconazole.[54]

In addition to caspofungin, two additional parenteral echinocandins, micafungin and anidulafungin, also are approved for the treatment of esophageal candidiasis. Although the three echinocandins are as effective as fluconazole in the treatment of esophageal candidiasis, they all appear to be associated with a greater relapse rate compared to fluconazole.[55,56]

Vulvovaginal candidiasis in HIV-infected women is usually uncomplicated (90% of cases) and responds readily to short-course oral or topical treatment with any of several therapies: oral fluconazole, topical azoles (clotrimazole, butaconazole, miconazole, ticonazole, or terconazole), and itraconazole oral solution. Severe or recurrent episodes of vaginitis require oral fluconazole or topical antifungal therapy for ≥7 days.[44]

The majority of studies clearly indicate that acute disseminated candidiasis is often rapidly fatal if not treated appropriately. Patients with a blood culture yielding *Candida* must receive antifungal therapy. Time of initiation of effective therapy for candidemia matters, as shown by studies by Morrell[57] (one hospital) and Garey[58] (four hospitals) with similar results of mortality: 15% if therapy begins on the day positive blood culture taken, 25% ~24 h later, 35% ~48 h later, and 40% ~72 h later.

Amphotericin B, 0.7 mg/kg/day, given alone and occasionally in combination with flucytosine, is the standard therapy, particularly for clinically unstable patients. Up to 70% of patients, including those infected with *C. krusei* and *C. glabrata,* will respond favorably.

Lipid formulations of amphotericin B, 3 to 5 mg/kg/day, are used frequently in patients likely to develop nephrotoxicity. Few clinical trials have compared efficacy for treatment of candidiasis in neutropenic and bone marrow transplant patients. The majority of reports are from the compassionate use of the lipid formulations in patients intolerant of or refractory to conventional amphotericin B.

Caspofungin, an echinocandin antifungal, is approved for treating candidemia and invasive candidiasis. Caspofungin was shown to be as effective as amphotericin B in a randomized, double-blind trial that included mostly nonneutropenic patients.

Dosages for Invasive Candidiasis (IC) and Esophageal Candidiasis (EC)

- Caspofungin: 70 mg load, then 50 mg/day
- Anidulafungin: 200 mg load, then 100 mg/day for IC; 100/50 for EC
- Micafungin: 50 mg/day for EC; not approved yet for IC, but dosage will likely be 100 mg/day

---

All three related compounds are IV only. They are mostly similar in safety, are very clean with nonrenal clearance (no adjustment required in renal failure), but caution is needed in hepatic failure. Echinocandins have no cross-resistance.

The Azoles—Dosages for Invasive Candidiasis (IC) and Esophageal Candidiasis (EC)

- Fluconazole: Load with 2 × daily doses; then 100–200 mg/day for EC; 400 mg/day for IC
- Voriconazole: Load with 6 mg/kg q12 h × 2 doses; then, 3–4 mg/kg/day for IC. Oral is 200 mg q12 h × 2 doses then 200 mg/day (IC & EC)

Patients with an invasive infection caused by a susceptible *C. albicans* isolate can be treated with fluconazole. Fluconazole therapy for candidiasis has been found to be equivalent to amphotericin B in nonneutropenic patients. Fluconazole may be considered in patients with susceptible isolates and in those not receiving prophylaxis.

Fluconazole, IV and PO forms are interchangeable. Renal clearance is needed (dose per creatinine level). Voriconazole is cleared by hepatic clearance (dose is decreased by 50% with mild to moderate failure, no data in severe failure), while IV modulation uses a cyclodextrin carrier that is cleared by the kidneys. It should be avoided in patients with failure.

As far as safety is concerned, both are quite good. Hepatic injury is the main risk. Both have typical range of P450/cytochrome azole problems; voriconazole is more prone to drug interactions.

The current practice in cases of candidemia is to continue therapy for at least 2 weeks after the last negative blood culture and until granulocytopenia and fever have resolved. Treatment until all signs and symptoms of the infection have been eradicated is required for patients with extensive visceral involvement. Follow-up treatment with oral fluconazole provides the opportunity to manage these cases on an outpatient basis.

Whenever required, removing central venous catheters is important to clear fungemia and to decrease the complications of candidiasis.

Management of Treatment Failure or Refractory Mucosal Candidiasis

Refractory oral or esophageal candidiasis is still reported in approximately 4%–5% of HIV-infected persons, typically in those patients with CD4 counts <50 cells/mm^3 who have received multiple courses of azole antifungals.[44] For severe, recurrent, and refractory cases, itraconazole 100–200 mg/day maintenance therapy may be indicated.

Treatment failure is typically defined as signs and symptoms of oropharyngeal or esophageal candidiasis that persist after more than 7–14 days of appropriate therapy. Cases of refractory oral thrush due to yeasts other than *Candida* spp., such as *Rhodotorula muciloginosa* and *Saccharomyces cerevisiae*, have been reported.[59,60] Endoscopy to confirm diagnosis and biopsy with fungal cultures is recommended and useful. Oral itraconazole solution is effective, at least transiently, in approximately two-thirds of persons with fluconazole-refractory mucosal candidiasis. Posaconazole immediate-release oral suspension (400 mg bid for 28 days) is effective in 75% of patients with azole-refractory oropharyngeal and/or esophageal candidiasis.[61]

Intravenous amphotericin B is usually effective and can be used in patients with refractory disease. Both conventional amphotericin B and lipid complex and liposomal amphotericin B have been used. Amphotericin B oral suspension (1 mL 4 × day of the 100 mg/mL suspension) is sometimes effective among patients with oropharyngeal candidiasis who do not respond to itraconazole. However, this product is not available in the U.S. Azole-refractory esophageal candidiasis also can be treated with posaconazole, anidulafungin, caspofungin, micafungin, or voriconazole.[44]

Voriconazole is effective for refractory candidiasis and treatment of fluconazole-resistant serious invasive *Candida* infections (including *C. krusei).* A series of patients have been collected from several different studies, with candidemia showing a 48% overall response, other invasive cases showing 41% overall response, and esophageal candidiasis showing a 61% overall response. Salvage data suggest activity across various species and with higher MICs.[62]

Preventing Recurrence

No primary or secondary prophylaxis (chronic maintenance therapy) for recurrent oropharyngeal or vulvovaginal candidiasis is recommended, as the therapy for acute disease is quite effective. In addition, factors such as the low mortality associated with mucosal candidiasis, the potential for resistant *Candida* organisms to develop, the possibility of drug interactions, and the cost of prophylaxis further argue against prophylaxis. However, the decision to use secondary prophylaxis should take into account the effect of recurrences on a patient's well-being and quality of life, the need for prophylaxis for other fungal infections, cost, toxicities, and most importantly, drug interactions.[63]

If recurrences are frequent or severe, oral fluconazole can be used for either oropharyngeal or vulvovaginal candidiasis.[64–66] A recent randomized clinical trial[67] has documented that the number of episodes of oropharyngeal candidiasis and other invasive fungal infections was statistically significantly lower in HIV patients with CD4 count <150 cells/mm^3 when receiving continuous (three times a week) fluconazole versus episodic treatment of recurrences. This clinical trial also proved that the development of clinically significant resistance was not higher in the group of continuous prophylaxis than in the group with episodic administration of fluconazole, provided that patients received ART.[67]

For recurrent esophageal candidiasis, daily fluconazole can be used. Oral posaconazole, twice daily, is also effective. However, potential azole resistance should be taken into account when long-term azoles are being considered.[44]

Secondary prophylaxis should be instituted in those patients with fluconazole-refractory oropharyngeal or esophageal candidiasis who have responded to echinocandins, voriconazole, or posaconazole therapy because of high relapse rate until ART produces immune reconstitution.[44]

Preventing Disease and Exposure

Candida organisms are common commensals on mucosal surfaces in healthy persons. No measures are available to reduce exposure to these fungi. Data from prospective controlled trials indicate that fluconazole can reduce the risk for mucosal (e.g., oropharyngeal, esophageal, and vaginal) candidiasis among patients with advanced HIV disease.[64–67] However, routine primary prophylaxis is not recommended because mucosal disease is associated with very low attributable mortality and acute therapy is highly effective. ART does reduce the likelihood of mucosal candidiasis.[44]

As far as drug activity and *Candida* species are concerned, amphotericin B (in all forms) is reliable for all species, with the occasional exceptions of *C. lusitaniae, C. guilliermondii, C. inconspicua, C. sake, C. kefyr,* and *C. rugosa* species. Fluconazole and itraconazole are not useful for *C. krusei* but may be useful for *C. glabrata.* Voriconazole and posaconazole may be used for *C. krusei* and often for *C. glabrata* (MICs rise, but respond). Resistance in *C. albicans* in the setting of HIV and OPC is a special case. Development of resistance during therapy is difficult to detect. MIC testing is as yet only meaningful for *Candida* spp. against fluconazole and perhaps voriconazole.

Resistance is very rare in amphotericin B, whereas it is common and of concern in azoles. *C. krusei* is often resistant; *C. glabrata* readily becomes resistant, whereas others only rarely become resistant. In the case of echinocandins, resistance definitely occurs but is rare as yet. High echinocandin MICs by current methods do not reliably predict failure. Only caspofungin has had wide use to date and, thus, all reports focus on this candin. *C. parapsilosis* seems most problematic. Although echinocandins are reliable for almost all Candida infections, resistance issues are slowly emerging.

Cryptococcosis

Cryptococcosis is a chronic, subacute to acute pulmonary, systemic or meningeal disease, initiated by the inhalation of basidiospores and/or desiccated yeast cells of *Cryptococcus neoformans*.

Currently, cryptococcosis is considered an AIDS-defining illness, and HIV testing is imperative whenever *C. neoformans* is recovered from clinical specimens.[68] It is the leading infectious cause of meningitis in patients with AIDS, and it is the initial AIDS-defining illness in approximately 2% of patients, generally occurring in patients with CD4 counts <100/mm^3. Before the advent of potent HAART, approximately 5% to 8% of HIV-infected patients in developed countries acquired disseminated cryptococcosis.[69] The majority of cases are observed in patients who have CD4 T lymphocyte counts of <50 cells/mm^3. The incidence has declined substantially since then.[70]

Before the AIDS era, cryptococcosis was a well-recognized but rare disease. Primary pulmonary infections are associated with no diagnostic symptoms and are usually subclinical. In dissemination, the fungus usually shows a predilection for the central nervous system (CNS), but skin, bones, and visceral organs may also become involved.

Clinical Manifestations

In humans, *C. neoformans* predominantly affects immunocompromised hosts and is the most common cause of fungal meningitis. Worldwide, 7% to 10% of patients with AIDS are affected. The spontaneous onset of CNS cryptococcosis is an AIDS-defining illness.[68] Meningitis is the predominant clinical presentation. Secondary cutaneous infections occur in up to 15% of patients with disseminated cryptococcosis, and their appearance often indicates a poor prognosis.[30]

Pulmonary cryptococcosis is the consequence of the inhalation of *C. neoformans* from various environmental sources. It is commonly accepted that the acquisition of the infection occurs early in life and that the disease is mostly related to a reactivation from a pulmonary site in immunocompromised hosts, such as patients infected with HIV.[30] Invasive pulmonary cryptococcosis may occur when primary infections do not resolve. In some patients, this leads to a more chronic pneumonia, progressing slowly over several years.[30] Pulmonary infections due to *C. neoformans* may be transitory and mild, and the diagnosis may be missed in the absence of symptoms and radiologic shadows.[71]

Dissemination to the brain and meninges is the most common clinical manifestation of cryptococcosis (75% to 90% of cases), and includes meningitis, meningoencephalitis, or expanding cryptococcoma.[72] Symptoms usually develop slowly, over several months, and, in 30% to 40% of cases initially include headache, followed by drowsiness, dizziness, irritability, confusion, nausea, and vomiting; neck stiffness and focal neurologic defects, such as ataxia, are not seen commonly.[72] Diminishing visual acuity and coma may also occur in later stages of the infection. In some cases, onset is acute, especially in patients with widespread disease; these patients may deteriorate rapidly and die in a matter of weeks.[72]

Infection of the brain and meninges is the most common clinical manifestation of cryptococcosis and also the most common cause of death from this disease. It generally occurs in patients with CD4 T cell counts $<200/mm^3$.[72,73] Cryptococcal infection should be suspected in all cases of meningitis in HIV-infected persons. Early diagnosis and treatment may alter the prognosis for these patients; hence, examination of the CSF should be considered in all HIV infected persons with symptoms of meningitis.[74]

In patients with AIDS, skin manifestations represent the second most common site of disseminated cryptococcosis. Lesions often occur on the head and neck and may present as papules, nodules, plaques, ulcers, abscesses, cutaneous ulcerated plaques, herpetiform lesions, or lesions simulating both molluscum contagiosum and Kaposi's sarcoma. Anal ulceration may also occur.[30]

Laboratory Diagnosis

Direct Microscopy. CSF, biopsy tissue, sputum, bronchial washings, pus, blood, and urine can all be collected, depending on the site of infection or the organ system involved. Lumbar puncture is the single most useful diagnostic test. In patients without AIDS, levels of glucose in the CSF are reduced in half of all cases. Protein levels are usually increased and lymphocytic pleocytosis is usually found. CSF abnormalities are less pronounced in patients with AIDS, although India ink smear is more often positive.[2,30]

Abnormalities on brain imaging—computed tomography (CT) or magnetic resonance imaging (MRI)—are seen in up to 20% of patients. Focal neurologic signs or seizures are unusual and occur in only about 10% of patients. CT abnormalities attributable to cryptococcus include meningeal enhancement and, rarely, ring-enhancing lesions from cryptococcomas. However, anatomic abnormalities in the brain parenchyma are usually attributable to other HIV-associated problems.[75]

An India ink preparation can be made for exudates and body fluids to demonstrate encapsulated yeast cells under the microscope. Sputum and pus may need to be digested with 10% KOH prior to India ink/Gram's staining (**Figures 21–5 and 21–6**). For tissue sections, PAS, GMS, hematoxylin and eosin (H&E), and mucicarmine stains are useful to demonstrate the polysaccharide capsule.[30,50] An India ink smear of centrifuged CSF sediment reveals encapsulated yeast in approximately 75% of patients with AIDS and 50% of non-AIDS cases.[30]

Culture is the gold standard for the diagnosis of cryptococcal infections. The primary isolation media used are Sabouraud's dextrose agar, with or without antibiotics. Translucent, smooth, gelatinous colonies, which later become very mucoid and creamy in color, are characteristic. Identification of the organism is based on gross and microscopic appearance, biochemical test results, and growth at 37°C. The results of nucleic acid hybridization or the formation of brown pigment on Niger seed agar can also be used for identification (**Figure 21–7**).

The fungus has four capsular serotypes, designated A, B, C, and D. Organisms are designated *C. neoformans* var. *neoformans* for serotypes A and D, and *C. neoformans* var. *gattii* for serotypes B and C.[2]

Pulmonary cryptococcosis mimics malignancy with regard to radiographic findings and symptoms. Sputum culture is positive in only 10% of cases. Occasionally, *C. neoformans* appears in one or more sputum specimens as an endobronchial saprophyte. Biopsy is usually required for diagnosis.[2,30] A positive culture of CSF is definitive. However, positive culture of

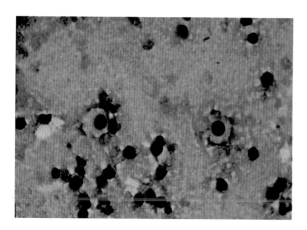

Figure 21–5. *Gram-positive budding yeast cells in a cerebrospinal fluid smear due to* Cryptococcus neoformans *(Gram's stain; magnification 1,000×).*

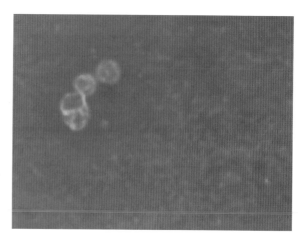

Figure 21–6. *Photomicrograph of an India ink preparation of a cerebrospinal fluid sample showing encapsulated budding spherical yeast cells of* Cryptococcus neoformans *(magnification 600×).*

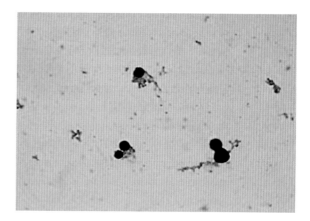

Figure 21–7. *Microscopic morphology of* Cryptococcus neoformans *(5-day-old culture on Sabouraud dextrose agar, Gram's stain; magnification 1,000×).*

respiratory secretions, especially in patients without clinical symptoms, should be interpreted with some caution until additional supporting evidence is available.[30]

Serology. The detection of cryptococcal capsular polysaccharide antigen in spinal fluid is the most rapid method for diagnosing patients with cryptococcal meningitis. In AIDS patients, cryptococcal antigen can be detected in the serum in nearly 100% of cases, whereas serum antigen tests are positive in only one-third of cases of pulmonary cryptococcosis.[30] Latex agglutination has a sensitivity and specificity of 91% and 92%, respectively.[76] Cryptococcal antigen in CSF and serum is very helpful in diagnosing cryptococcal meningitis, but its role as an indicator in monitoring the response to treatment is questionable; in a study in Thailand, 83.3% of a patient's CSF was still positive for cryptococcal antigen even when the culture was sterile after 10 weeks of therapy.[77]

Preventing Exposure/Disease

It is difficult to avoid exposure to *C. neoformans*, although it may help to avoid specific activities (such as those that include exposure to bird droppings) that can lead to an increased risk for infection.[44]

Routine testing of asymptomatic persons for serum cryptococcal antigen is not recommended, as the incidence of cryptococcal disease is low. Prospective, controlled trials indicate that fluconazole and itraconazole can reduce the frequency of primary cryptococcal disease among patients who have CD4 counts <50 cells/mm^3.[64,78]

However, routine antifungal prophylaxis to prevent cryptococcosis is not recommended because of the relative infrequency of cryptococcal disease, lack of survival benefits associated with prophylaxis, possibility of drug interactions, potential antifungal drug resistance, and cost.[44]

Treatment. For the induction phase, the recommended treatment is: amphotericin B, 0.7 mg/kg/day intravenously + 5 flucytosine, 100 mg/kg/day orally for 14 days. This should be followed by a consolidation phase: fluconazole, 400 mg/day for 8 weeks or until the culture is sterile. The maintenance/suppressive phase of treatment is: fluconazole, 200 mg/day lifelong, or continued until the CD 4 count is >200 cells/mm^3 for 3–6 months in patients on HAART.

Alternative regimens. Amphotericin B 0.7–1.0 mg/kg/day IV for 14 days (without 5 flucytosine), followed by fluconazole, 400–800 mg/day for 8–10 weeks, followed by itraconazole, 200 mg twice a day orally in the consolidation phase. Lipid amphotericin B formulations are used in cases that are refractory or intolerant to conventional amphotericin B.

Flucytosine plus various therapies have been tried in cryptococcal meningitis, and the results have been generally favorable, with increased success, increased rate in CSF sterilization with decreased amphotericin B dose and, thus, decreased nephrotoxicity and decreased relapse rates of HIV. Good results were obtained in a murine model of cryptococcosis treated with fluconazole + amphotericin B, but fluconazole given first was associated with a worse outcome.[79,80] A study of combination therapy for cryptococcal meningitis, testing serial quantitative CSF cultures, showed better results with amphotericin B + flucytosine, compared with amphotericin B + fluconazole and amphotericin B alone at full therapeutic doses.[81]

The clinical implications for today in cryptococcal infections are that adding 5 flucytosine is generally good; adding fluconazole may be better; and the amphotericin B + azole combination is often found to be positive.

It has been demonstrated that IFN-γ, when given as adjuvant therapy for cryptococcal meningitis, produced CSF cultures were more often negative at 2 weeks and a lower serum cryptococcal antigen. However, candins alone have minimal effects in cases of cryptococcosis; caspofungin + amphotericin B have yielded favorable results in vitro, but have no obvious in vivo advantage.

Management of Increased Intracranial Pressure. Raised intracranial pressure (ICP) accounts for more than 90% of deaths in the first 2 weeks of onset of cryptococcal meningitis; therefore, management of raised ICP is critical to the management of the disease. In patients with increased intracranial pressure, repeated daily lumbar punctures may be required until the opening CSF pressure is <200 mm H$_2$O. A lumbar drain or V-P shunt may be indicated if repeated lumbar punctures are inadequate to control intracranial pressure.

Management of Treatment Failure

Treatment failure is defined as either the lack of clinical improvement after 2 weeks of appropriate therapy (including management of increased ICP) or relapse after an initial clinical response, defined as either a positive CSF culture and/or a rising CSF cryptococcal antigen titer with an associated compatible clinical picture. Although fluconazole resistance has been reported with *C. neoformans,* it is rare in the U.S.[82] At this time, routine susceptibility testing is not recommended.[44]

The optimal therapy for patients with treatment failure has not been established. For those initially treated with fluconazole, therapy should be changed to amphotericin B, with or without flucytosine, and continued until a clinical response occurs. Liposomal amphotericin B (4–6 mg/kg/day) might yield improved efficacy over the deoxycholate formulation[83, 84] and should be considered in treatment failures. Higher doses of fluconazole in combination with flucytosine also might be useful. Caspofungin and other echinocandins have no in vitro activity against *Cryptococcus spp.* and, therefore, have no role in the clinical management of these patients. The newer triazoles—posaconazole and voriconazole—have activity against *Cryptococcus spp.* in vitro and may have a role in therapy. [44]

Preventing Recurrence

Patients who have completed the initial 10 weeks of therapy for acute cryptococcosis should be given fluconazole, 200 mg/day, as maintenance therapy, either lifelong or until immune reconstitution occurs as a consequence of HAART. Itraconazole is inferior to fluconazole for preventing the relapse of cryptococcal disease. [85, 86]

Pneumocystosis

Pneumocystosis is an opportunistic fungal infection of the respiratory system leading to interstitial plasma cell pneumonia, caused by a taxonomically unique fungus sharing biologic characteristics with protozoa. In contrast to the pre-AIDS era when *Pneumocystis* pneumonia (PCP) was uncommon, PCP is a major source of morbidity and mortality in immunocompromised patients. PCP is a result either of reactivation of latent infection or new exposure to the organism.

Study of the basic biology of the causative organism, *P. jiroveci,* has been severely hampered by the lack of a reliable in vitro cultivation system. Fortunately, advances in DNA analysis technology have allowed progress in the absence of a robust culture system. Major developmental stages of the organism include: the small (1–4 µm), pleomorphic trophozoite or trophic form; the 5- to 8-µm cyst, which has a thick cell wall and contains up to eight intracystic bodies; and the precyst, an intermediate stage. The life cycle of *P. jiroveci* probably involves asexual replication by the trophic form and sexual reproduction by the cyst, which ends in release of the intracystic bodies. An intracellular stage has not been identified.[2]

The hypothesized mechanism of transmission is via inhalation of airborne cysts that subsequently colonize the respiratory tract. In a major study at University of California, it was established that recurrent undiagnosed fevers, night sweats, oropharyngeal thrush, and unintentional weight loss were associated with risk for this infection among HIV-infected persons with CD4 counts above 200/mm^3. Subjects in whom CD4 counts declined to below 200/mm^3 and who were not receiving preventive therapy were nine times more likely to develop PCP within 6 months compared to subjects who received such therapy.[87] Analysis of AIDS surveillance data collected at the World Health Organization revealed that PCP was the most common AIDS-defining illness in Western Europe (17.8%).[88]

However, in developing countries, the prevalence of PCP has been much lower. In Africa, PCP occurs in only 9% of patients with new diagnoses of AIDS. The organism is ubiquitous worldwide. The low prevalence is thought to be due to lack of disease progression or lack of diagnosis. Another hypothesis is that other, more virulent organisms—such as those associated with tuberculosis—might be leading to pulmonary disease before PCP can manifest itself.[89]

Before the widespread use of primary PCP prophylaxis and effective ART, PCP occurred in 70% to 80%of patients with AIDS. 90% of cases occurred among patients with CD4 T-lymphocyte count of <200 mm^3.[90]

Clinical Manifestations

Typically, the onset of symptoms of PCP is gradual. Fever, a mild and dry cough, shortness of breath, rapid breathing, bluish skin (cyanosis), pain at the end of inspiration, and joint pain are the most common symptoms with the following frequency: nonproductive cough (59%–91%), fever (79%–100%), dyspnea (29%–95%), chest pain (14%–23%), and sputum production (23%–30%).

In patients infected with HIV, the disease course tends to have a more subtle presentation, with a longer prodrome and milder symptoms than in patients not infected with HIV.[11] The median duration of symptoms in HIV-infected patients before diagnosis of PCP is 28 days, with a range of presentations varying from a fulminant to a chronic course.[91, 92] The most common manifestations of PCP among HIV-infected patients are progressive exertional dyspnea, fever, nonproductive cough, and chest discomfort.[90]

On chest examination crackles/crepitations, signs of focal lung consolidation, or acute bronchospasm may be present. Lung examination may be normal in many patients. Although the classic findings of diffuse central (perihilar) alveolar or interstitial infiltrates may be found in some cases, less common findings include patchy, asymmetric infiltrates, pneumatoceles, and pneumothorax. Upper lobe disease occurs only with inhaled pentamidine. Pleural effusions and intrathoracic adenopathy are rare.[30] A normal chest x-ray is found in 0%–39% of cases. The radiographic improvement of PCP with resolution of chest x-ray findings may lag behind clinical improvement, as some patients have persistent abnormalities months after treatment.[93]

Although *P. jiroveci* usually remains confined to the lungs, cases of disseminated infection have occurred in both HIV-infected and non-HIV-infected patients. One risk factor for extrapulmonary spread in patients with HIV is the administration of aerosolized pentamidine. The most common sites of extrapulmonary involvement are the lymph nodes, spleen, liver, and bone marrow. Clinical manifestations range from incidental findings at autopsy to specific organ involvement. Histopathology examination reveals the presence of *P. jiroveci* and the characteristic associated foamy material.[2]

Oral, intravenous, and inhaled medications are used in the treatment of PCP. Pentamidine, dapsone, and trimethoprim/sulfamethoxazole (TMP-SMX) are the most commonly used agents. Adverse reactions from the medications used to treat the infection include respiratory failure. PCP can be life-threatening, and death may occur due to respiratory failure. Early treatment reduces the fatality rate.[30]

Laboratory Diagnosis

Direct Microscopy. Samples such as induced sputum, bronchioalveolar lavage (BAL) fluid, and bronchial or lung biopsy can be collected. BAL fluids are considered better than induced sputum samples, but since the load is higher in HIV-infected patients, induced sputum samples give comparable results.[94]

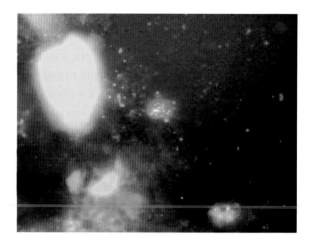

Figure 21–8. *Photomicrograph of* Pneumocystis carinii *cluster of cysts and trophozoites in characteristic apple-green honeycomb appearance with respiratory cells in induced sputum (direct immunofluorescence stain; magnification 400×).*

Induced sputum is sensitive and specific for diagnosing PCP in HIV-infected patients, depending on the laboratory method employed. They can be subjected to either direct microscopy or PCR, as this organism has not been successfully cultured on artificial media.[30]

Sputum induction for direct fluorescent antibody (DFA) test for pneumocystis can be done if PCP is strongly suspected. This is a very sensitive method for the detection of *P. jiroveci* (**Figure 21–8**).

Special stains such as Giemsa, GMS, and toluidine blue O staining can also be used. Different stains color various stages of the life cycle. GMS and toluidine blue stain the cyst stage, whereas Giemsa stain and its modifications are used for both the cyst and the trophozoite stages. Cysts of *P. jiroveci* are Gram-negative on smears of induced sputum or BAL fluids.[2,30]

In the diagnosis of PCP, PCR has been shown to increase the sensitivity of the diagnosis from induced sputum specimens. In a study in the U.S. in 1998 the sensitivity of PCR for the BAL specimens was as high as 100%, with a specificity of 98%; for induced sputum, the sensitivity and specificity of PCR were 94% and 90%, respectively.[95]

Treatment

Preferred Treatment Regimens. Trimethoprim, 15–20 mg/kg/day with sulfamethoxazole, 75–100 mg/kg per day, orally or intravenously in 3 or 4 divided doses, is given for 21 days. This is equivalent to cotrimoxazole double-strength tablets (160/800), two tablets three times a day.[96,97] The recommended duration of therapy for PCP is 21 days.[98] The probability and rate of response to therapy depend on the agent used, the number of previous PCP episodes, severity of illness, degree of immunodeficiency, and timing of initiation of therapy.[44]

Patients with moderate to severe disease should receive corticosteroids: prednisone, 40 mg orally twice a day for 5 days, tapering to 40 mg orally once a day for 5 days, and then 20 mg per day until completion of treatment.[99,100,101]

Alternate Regimens.

1. Trimethoprim (15 mg/kg/day) orally, along with dapsone, 100 mg/day orally, for 21 days.[97,102]

2. Clindamycin (600–900 mg intravenously every 6–8 hour, or 300–450 mg orally every 6 hours) with primaquine (15–30 mg/day base orally) for 21 days is recommended.[103–105]

3. Pentamidine (3–4 mg/kg/day intravenously for 21 days) is reserved for severe cases.[105–107]

Management of Treatment Failure

Clinical failure is defined as lack of improvement or worsening of respiratory function documented by arterial blood gas measurements after at least 4–8 days of anti-PCP treatment. Treatment failure attributed to treatment-limiting toxicities occurs in up to one-third of patients.[97] Switching to another regimen is the appropriate management for treatment-related toxicity. Failure attributed to lack of drug efficacy occurs in approximately 10% of those with mild to moderate disease. No convincing clinical trials exist on which to base recommendations for the management of treatment failure attributed to lack of drug efficacy. Clinicians should wait at least 4–8 days before switching therapy for lack of clinical improvement. In the absence of corticosteroid therapy, early and reversible deterioration within the first 3 to 5 days of therapy is typical, probably because of the inflammatory response caused by antibiotic-induced lysis of organisms in the lung. Other concomitant infections must be excluded as a cause for clinical failure; bronchoscopy with BAL should be strongly considered to evaluate for this possibility, even if this procedure was done prior to initiating therapy. [108, 109]

Primary prophylaxis. Primary prophylaxis is indicated in all HIV-infected patients with CD4 counts <200 cells/mm^3 or in the presence of any other AIDS-defining illness.[110–112]

One double-strength tablet of TMP-SMX once a day is recommended. This also confers cross-protection against toxoplasmosis[113] and selected common respiratory bacterial infections.[114,115]

Alternative prophylaxis regimens include:

1. Dapsone, 100 mg once daily or 50 mg twice daily.[115]
2. Aerosolized pentamidine, 300 mg/month, delivered by a special aerosol device.[116]
3. Dapsone, 200 mg/week, with pyrimethamine, 75 mg/week, with leucovorin 25 mg/week.[117–119]

Primary pneumocystis prophylaxis should be discontinued for adult and adolescent patients who have responded to ART with an increase in CD counts to >200 cells/mm^3 for at least 3 months.[44]

Discontinuing primary prophylaxis among these patients is recommended because prophylaxis adds limited disease prevention i.e., for PCP, toxoplasmosis, or bacterial infections[120,121] and because discontinuing drugs reduces pill burden, potential for drug toxicity, drug interactions, selection of drug-resistant pathogens, and cost. Prophylaxis should be reintroduced if the CD4 count decreases to <200 cells/mm^3.[44]

Secondary prophylaxis is recommended for all patients after an episode of *Pneumocystis* pneumonia and should be continued until the CD4 count is >200 cells/mm^3 on two occasions over 6 months. Discontinuing secondary prophylaxis for such patients is recommended because the drugs add limited disease prevention (i.e., for PCP, toxoplasmosis, or bacterial infections) and because discontinuing drugs reduces pill burden, potential for drug toxicity, drug interactions, selection of drug-resistant pathogens, and cost. Prophylaxis should be reintroduced if the CD4 count decreases to <200 cells/mm^3. If PCP recurs at a CD4 count of ≥200 cells/mm^3, lifelong prophylaxis should be administered.[44]

Aspergillosis

Aspergillosis may present as a well defined clinical syndrome involving a variety of sites and organ systems: pulmonary, disseminated, and cutaneous. *Aspergillus fumigatus*, found in >90%

of infections,[122] is the most common cause of aspergillosis, causing the most severe disease in humans. However, *A. flavus*, *A. niger*, and several other species can also cause disease.[30]

In HIV-infected patients, lungs and the CNS are the most frequent sites of disease. Patients usually present with fever and focal neurologic abnormalities. Invasion of lung tissue is confined almost entirely to immunosuppressed patients. Invasive aspergillosis occurs among patients with advanced HIV infection and was more common before the advent of HAART.[123,124]

The relative paucity of aspergillus infection in the setting of HIV disease is probably due to relatively intact phagocytic cell function that accompanies the T-cell dysfunction in these patients. Although AIDS, per se, is not considered a risk factor for invasive pulmonary aspergillosis, the underlying risk factors—including neutropenia, use of corticosteroids, and intravenous drug abuse puts these patients at substantial risk. In keeping with this hypothesis, more than half of patients with AIDS who develop invasive aspergillosis have either neutropenia, usually secondary to ganciclovir or corticosteroid treatment as additional risk factors.[125]

Data analyzed from the U.S. Adult and Adolescent Spectrum of HIV Disease (ASD) project in 2000 revealed 228 cases of aspergillosis among 35,252 HIV-infected persons, yielding an overall incidence of 3.5 cases/1,000 PY. The incidence of aspergillosis was significantly higher among people 35 years old, homosexual men, and in the setting of a white blood cell count <2,500 cells/mm^3, CD4 count <100 cells/mm^3, prior history of an opportunistic infection, and prescribed medications associated with neutropenia. The median survival in AIDS patients with invasive aspergillosis is 3 months, with only 26% surviving >1 year.[124]

Patients who have had HIV-associated aspergillosis typically had CD4 counts <100 cells/mm^3, a history of other AIDS-defining OIs, and were not receiving HAART.[126]

Clinical Manifestations

Pulmonary Aspergillosis. The clinical manifestations of pulmonary aspergillosis are many, ranging from harmless saprophytic colonization to acute invasive disease. Endobronchial saprophytic pulmonary aspergillosis presents as a chronic productive cough, often with hemoptysis, in a patient with prior chronic lung disease, such as TB, sarcoidosis, bronchiectasis, or histoplasmosis.

Invasive aspergillosis in the immunocompromised host presents as an acute, rapidly progressive, densely consolidated pulmonary infiltrate. Infection progresses by direct extension across tissue planes and by hematogenous dissemination to the lung, brain, and other organs. CT is particularly valuable in suggesting the diagnosis of invasive pulmonary aspergillosis.

Aspergillosis in HIV-infected patients most commonly involves the lung, presenting as fever, cough, and dyspnea. Typically, the CD4 cell count is below 50 cells/mm^3. Roughly half of these patients have neutropenia or have been recently treated with glucocorticoids. Bilateral diffuse or focal pulmonary infiltrates with a tendency to cavitate constitute the most common radiologic manifestations. Aspergillus infection may have an unusual presentation in the respiratory tract of patients with AIDS, where it gives the appearance of a pseudomembranous tracheobronchitis.[2]

Disseminated Aspergillosis. Hematogenous dissemination to other visceral organs may occur, especially in patients with severe immunosuppression or intravenous drug addiction. Abscesses may occur in the brain (cerebral aspergillosis), kidney (renal aspergillosis), heart, (endocarditis, myocarditis), bone (osteomyelitis), and gastrointestinal tract. Ocular lesions (mycotic keratitis, endophthalmitis, and orbital aspergilloma) may also occur, either as a result of dissemination or following local trauma or surgery.[48]

Cutaneous Aspergillosis. Cutaneous aspergillosis is a rare manifestation that is usually a result of dissemination from primary pulmonary infection in the immunosuppressed patient. However, cases of primary cutaneous aspergillosis also occur, usually as a result of trauma or colonization. Lesions manifest as erythematous papules or macules with progressive central necrosis.[48]

Laboratory Diagnosis

Direct Microscopy. Sputum, bronchial washings, and tracheal aspirates from patients with pulmonary disease are examined for direct microscopy in wet mounts in either 10% KOH mounts and/or Gram-stained smears.[68] Tissue sections or sputum smears are stained with H&E, GMS, and PAS and are examined for dichotomously branched, septate hyphae.

Interpretation. The presence of hyaline, branching septate hyphae, consistent with aspergillus in any specimen, from a patient with supporting clinical symptoms is considered significant. Biopsy and evidence of tissue invasion is of particular importance.[50]

Culture. Clinical specimens are inoculated onto primary isolation media, like Sabouraud's dextrose agar. Colonies are fast-growing and may be white, yellow, yellow-brown, brown-to-black, or green in color, depending on the species isolated.

Identification. Aspergillus colonies consist mostly of a dense felt of erect conidiophores. Conidiophores terminate in a vesicle covered with either a single palisadelike layer of phialides (uniseriate) or a layer of subtending cells (metulae), which bear small whorls of phialides (biseriate structure). The vesicle, phialides, metulae, and conidia form the conidial head[68] (**Figure 21–9**).

Interpretation. Aspergillus species are well recognized as common environmental airborne contaminants, so a positive culture from a nonsterile specimen, such as sputum, is not proof of infection. However, the detection of aspergillus (especially *A. fumigatus* and *A. flavus*) in sputum cultures from patients with appropriate predisposing conditions is likely to be of diagnostic importance and empiric antifungal therapy should be considered.[50] The repeated isolation

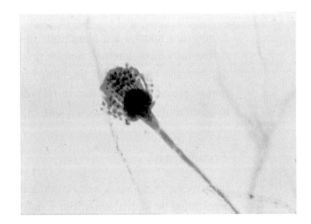

Figure 21–9. *Photomicrograph of an* Aspergillus fumigatus *fruiting structure (4-day-old culture on Sabouraud dextrose agar, lactophenol cotton blue preparation; magnification 400×).*

of aspergillus from sputum or the demonstration of hyphae in sputum or BAL fluid suggests endobronchial colonization or infection.[2]

In patients with advanced AIDS, fever, and cough, the isolation of aspergillus from respiratory secretions raises the possibility of aspergillosis and, thus, should prompt bronchoscopy. Fungus ball of the lung is usually detectable by chest x-ray. Biopsy is usually required for the diagnosis of invasive aspergillosis of the lung, nose, paranasal sinus, bronchi, or sites of dissemination. Blood cultures are rarely positive, even in patients with infected cardiac valves (native or prosthetic).[2]

Serology. Immunodiffusion tests for the detection of antibodies to *Aspergillus* species have proven to be of value in the diagnosis of allergic, aspergilloma, and invasive aspergillosis. However, they should be correlated with other clinical and diagnostic data.[127] Detection of galactomannan antigen in serum suggests the diagnosis, but false-positive results are frequent.[2]

The diagnosis of invasive aspergillosis is considered proven, highly probable, or probable depending on a battery of tests.[49] When hyphae are seen on direct microscopy and positive aspergillus culture is obtained from a biopsy and deep tissue specimen, it is proven invasive aspergillosis. Highly probable invasive aspergillosis should be the conclusion in the presence of any two of the following: hyphae in fibroscopic samples, positive aspergillus culture from BAL fluid or bronchial aspirate, or positive antigenemia by Pastorex aspergillus test. Probable invasive aspergillosis is defined by finding one of the following: positive culture from fibroscopic sample, seroconversion, or increase in specific aspergillus antibody concentration.[128]

Commercially available sandwich ELISA for the detection aspergillus detects circulating Galactomannan antigen with sensitivity limits of 1.0 ng/mL of serum. Aspergillus assay has been reported to have sensitivities of over 90% for patients with confirmed aspergillosis (histopathology and/or positive blood culture).[129] In a study of immunosuppressed patients from Japan, the sensitivity of latex agglutination was 44%, and specificity was 93%. Sensitivity tended to be lower in patients with invasive pulmonary aspergillosis localized to the lung than in those with disseminated invasive aspergillosis.[130]

Diagnostic challenges remain in the management of aspergillosis, as reliable techniques are not well established. Although cultures of sputum, BAL fluid, and tissue are fairly specific, sensitivity in proven cases is only 25% to 50%. Antibody detection is not useful in most patients. Galactomannan detection is potentially useful and PCR testing is under development.

Imaging. X-ray and CT scan can be very useful.

Preventing Exposure/Disease

Aspergillus species are ubiquitous in the environment, and exposure is unavoidable. Avoiding particularly dusty environments is prudent, especially in areas such as those created by construction because spore counts might be higher in these settings. No data are available on the prevention of primary aspergillosis in HIV-infected patients, although posaconzaole has been reported to be effective among patients with hematologic malignancy and neutropenia.[131]

Treatment

Invasive aspergillosis is a devastating infection for severely immunocompromised patients; treatment must be started early and a definitive diagnosis must be pursued to exclude other pathogens. Treatment of aspergillosis in the HIV-infected population has not been examined systematically. The recommended treatment for invasive aspergillosis in patients without HIV infection is voriconazole.[132] Voriconazole is the drug of choice, but should be used cautiously with HIV PIs and efavirenz.[44]

Preferred Regimen. For invasive disease, voriconazole (6 mg/kg IV twice a day for 2 days followed by 4 mg/kg twice a day for 1 week, and then 200 mg twice a day) is recommended. Voriconazole has shown superior results to conventional amphotericin B for treatment of invasive aspergillosis in an open, randomized trial consisting primarily of HSCT recipients and patients with hematologic malignancies. In a randomized trial comparing voriconazole with amphotericin B in 277 patients, voriconazole was associated with superior response (53% vs. 32% for amphotericin B), and superior survival (71% vs. 58%).[133]

Amphotericin B deoxycholate (1 mg/kg/day) or lipid-formulation amphotericin B (5 mg/kg/day) are alternatives, as is caspofungin (50 mg/day) and posaconazole. Other echinocandins, such as micafungin and anidulafungin, also are reasonable alternatives.[44.]

The length of therapy is not established and may be prolonged, and should continue at least until the peripheral blood CD4 count is >200 cells/mm^3 and there is evidence of clinical response.[44]

Management of Treatment Failure

The overall prognosis is poor among patients with advanced immunosuppression and in the absence of effective HAART. No data are available to guide recommendations for the management of treatment failure. If voriconazole was used initially, substitution with amphotericin B, posaconazole, or echinocandins might be considered. The amphotericin B or echinocandins would be a reasonable choice for those who began therapy with voriconazole or posaconazole.[44]

Lipid formulation of amphotericin B (usually, 5 mg/kg/day) should be used in cases that are refractory or intolerant to conventional amphotericin B. A multicenter, randomized trial comparing the lipid formulation with conventional amphotericin B in the treatment of neutropenic patients with either documented invasive mycosis or suspected invasive pulmonary aspergillosis reported superior efficacy and safety for the lipid formulation.[134]

Caspofungin has shown efficacy and safety in patients with documented invasive aspergillosis who did not respond to or were intolerant of prior antifungal therapy. Forty-one percent of patients receiving caspofungin responded favorably.[135] Oral itraconazole can be used as chronic therapy, but oral voriconazole is increasingly preferred. G-CSF and GM-CSF have been used adjunctively with antifungal agents to treat aspergillosis. No controlled trials have assessed the effectiveness of this adjunctive therapy.

Surgery is indicated if localization of the lesions poses a direct threat of invasion of a major vessel with the risk of fatal hemorrhage, or for excision of localized infection after a period of antifungal therapy. It is essential to see a clinical and radiologic response before therapy is discontinued. If therapy is needed on an outpatient basis after the patient has responded to initial therapy, oral itraconazole or voriconazole should be prescribed.

Preventing Recurrence. No data are available for the basis of a recommendation for or against chronic maintenance or suppressive therapy among patients who have successfully completed an initial course of treatment.[44]

Discontinuing Secondary Prophylaxis (Chronic Maintenance Therapy)

An AIDS Clinical Treatment Group (ACTG)-sponsored study reported that discontinuing itraconazole was safe for patients who have been treated for histoplasmosis and who have a good immunologic response to HAART.[169] Antifungal discontinuation in patients with AIDS appears to be safe for those who meet the following criteria: at least 1 year of itraconazole therapy, negative blood cultures, serum and urine antigen levels <2 ng/mL, CD4 T lymphocyte count >150 cells/mm³ while on HAART. Suppressive therapy should be resumed if the CD4 count decreases to <150 cells/mm³.[44]

Blastomycosis

Blastomycosis is a chronic granulomatous and suppurative disease having a primary pulmonary stage that is followed by dissemination to other body sites, chiefly the skin and bone. *Blastomyces dermatitidis* is a thermally dimorphic fungus, producing mycelia with 2- to 10-mm, round to oval or pear-shaped conidia at 25°C, and broad-based budding yeast cells with thick refractile walls varying in size from 8 mm to 15 mm, sometimes up to 30 mm in diameter, at 37°C.[170] It occurs characteristically in North America and is frequent in the southeastern U.S. Blastomycosis is of historic importance in that the microorganisms were later grown in culture from markedly scattered areas in Africa.[171] In recent years, cases have been diagnosed in Asia and Europe.[172,173] All available clinical and epidemiologic evidence indicates that humans and lower animals contract blastomycosis from some source in nature. However, the natural habitat of *B. dermatitidis* is not definitely known. The presence of decaying organic material appears to be required to support the sustained growth of *B. dermatitidis* in soil.[30]

Blastomycosis is not considered an AIDS-defining infection; nevertheless, in some practice settings, a distinct increase in incidence and severity of the disease occurring in immunocompromised hosts has been observed.[174] HIV-infected patients may experience reactivation of previously dormant foci of blastomycosis once T-cell-mediated immunity fails. Most cases of blastomycosis in patients with AIDS have occurred in those with CD4 counts below 200 cells/mm³.[170] The disease is particularly progressive in AIDS patients when the CD4 count drops below 200 cells/mm³.[175]

Blastomycosis is an uncommon disease, even in endemic areas. Blastomycosis-complicating AIDS is an extremely uncommon infection, with only a few series being reported, even from endemic areas.[170] Two patterns of disease are associated with HIV infection: localized pulmonary disease and disseminated extrapulmonary disease.

Clinical Manifestations

Pulmonary Blastomycosis. Blastomycosis is indolent in onset and patients present with chronic symptoms such as cough, fever, malaise, and weight loss. The lesions become more extensive, with continued suppuration and eventual necrosis and cavitation. Occasionally, patients present with an acute onset of infection, with development of high fever, chills, productive cough, myalgia, arthralgia, and pleuritic chest pain. Chest radiographic findings are variable and are not diagnostic.[170] In most individuals, pulmonary lesions are asymptomatic and are not detected until the infection has spread to other organs.[30]

Cutaneous Blastomycosis. Hematogenous spread gives rise to cutaneous lesions in more than 70% of patients. These tend to be painless and present either as raised verrucous lesions with irregular borders or as ulcers. The face, upper limbs, neck, and scalp are the most frequent sites involved.[30]

Osteoarticular Blastomycosis. Osteoarticular infection occurs in about 30% of patients, with the spine, pelvis, cranial bones, ribs, and long bones most commonly involved. Patients often remain asymptomatic until the infection spreads into contiguous joints or into adjacent soft tissue, causing subcutaneous abscesses. Radiologic findings are often nonspecific, and arthritis occurs in up to 10% of patients. Genitourinary blastomycosis is seen involving the prostate, epididymis, or testis, with hematogenous spread to the brain causing meningitis and spinal or brain abscess. Other organs may also be involved, and choroiditis and endophthalmitis have been reported.[30]

Patients with AIDS may develop fulminant blastomycosis, with widespread dissemination following endogenous reactivation of previous infection. Clinically, the disease in immunocompromised patients is potentially much more severe and is characterized by disseminated multiple organ involvement, including frequent involvement of the CNS.[176]

Laboratory Diagnosis

Direct Microscopy. Skin scrapings, sputum and bronchial washings, CSF, pleural fluid and blood, bone marrow, and urine are examined using 10% KOH and/or calcofluor white mounts. Tissue sections are stained using PAS, GMS, or Gram's stain, as for body fluids.

Histopathology is the most important method of diagnosis, with tissue sections showing large, broad-based, unipolar, budding, yeastlike cells, 8–15 μm in diameter. Positive direct microscopy demonstrating characteristic yeastlike cells from any specimen should be considered significant.

Culture. Clinical specimens are inoculated onto Sabouraud's dextrose agar and brain-heart infusion agar, with or without 5% sheep's blood. A positive culture from any of the above specimens should be considered significant. Cultures are positive in more than 90% of patients.[170]

Serology. Serologic tests are of limited value in the diagnosis of blastomycosis. Serologic tests for antibodies are typically negative and not useful for diagnosis of blastomycosis.[170] Antibody detection can be done using immunodiffusion.[11]

Treatment Per IDSA Endemic Mycoses Guidelines 2008

- Mild to moderate pulmonary disease: iltraconazole for 6–12 months
- Mild to moderate disseminated disease: itraconazole for 6–12 months
- Osteoarticular: itraconazole for 6–12 months
- Severe disease: lipid amphotericin B for 1–2 weeks, followed by itraconazole
- Immunosuppressed: lipid amphotericin B for 1–2 weeks, followed by oral azole therapy for at least 12 months
- CNS disease: lipid amphotericin B for 4–6 weeks followed by itraconazole, voriconazole, or high-dose itraconazole

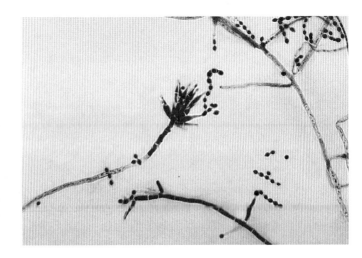

Figure 21–11. *This photomicrograph depicts a conidia-laden conidiophore of a* Penicillium marneffei *fungal organism.* Penicillium *spp. are known to cause penicilliosis which usually affects immunocompromised individuals such as those with AIDS or those undergoing chemotherapy.* P. marneffei *is normally acquired though inhalation of airborne spores. (Courtesy of the Public Health Image Library of the Centers for Disease Control and Prevention.)*

Treatment

There is an increased role for lipid formulations of amphotericin B and step-down therapy with amphotericin B followed by azoles. There is a possible increase in the role of voriconazole and posaconazole, along with therapeutic monitoring required. Clinical reports of success have been demonstrated with voriconazole, although there are as yet no reports regarding posaconazole. Ketocnazole and fluconazole have largely been removed from the list of therapeutic options for treating blastomycosis.

Therapeutic drug monitoring. Itraconazole levels should be obtained 2 weeks after starting therapy and should be between 1 and 0.1 µg/mL.

Penicilliosis

Penicillium marneffei is the causative agent of penicilliosis, an increasingly important mycosis associated with AIDS patients in Southeast Asia, including Manipur, and Assam in India.[177–181] It exhibits thermal dimorphism by growing in living tissue or in culture at 37°C as a yeastlike fungus or in culture at temperatures below 30°C as a mold (**Figure 21–11**). It has a propensity to cause disease in the normal host as well as in immunosuppressed patients, but significantly, it has now become a major opportunistic pathogen in HIV-positive patients in Indochina.[30]

In the areas of endemicity in Southeast Asia, India, and China, *P. marneffei* infection is regarded as an AIDS-defining illness, and the severity of the disease depends on the immunologic status of the infected individual. Most naturally occurring infections have been in residents of, or travelers to, Southeast Asia, especially northern Thailand, Vietnam, Hong Kong, Taiwan and southern China, and Eastern India. Imported cases of *P. marneffei* infections have been reported from Australia, France, Italy, Netherlands, the UK, and the U.S.[30,182–184]

Little is known about the ecology, epidemiology, or pathogenesis of *P. marneffei* infection. Bamboo rats are known to be asymptomatic carriers of the fungus, and it is unclear whether they are an important reservoir for human infection or act only as sentinel animals that are susceptible to infection from an environmental source.[185]

Clinical Manifestations

In patients with normal immunity, *P. marneffei* infection may either be focal or disseminated. Both clinical and histologic appearances strongly resemble those of TB—for example, suppurative lymphadenopathy. In HIV-infected patients, *P. marneffei* infection is usually disseminated at the time of diagnosis. Commonly, the skin, reticuloendothelial system, lung, and gut are infected. Fungemia is present in the majority of cases, and other organ systems—including kidney, bones, joints, and pericardium—may also be involved. Patients usually present with nonspecific symptoms of fever, anemia, and weight loss. Skin lesions are most commonly papules, often with a central necrotic umbilication, similar in appearance to those seen in molluscum contagiosum, usually located on the face, trunk and extremities.[30] The majority of cases of penicilliosis are observed in patients who have CD4 T lymphocyte counts of <100 cells/mm^3.[186] The infection is associated with a high mortality rate if timely treatment with appropriate antifungal drugs is not administered.[187]

Laboratory Diagnosis

Direct Microscopy. A Giemsa- or GMS-stained smear of a skin biopsy or bone marrow aspirate is a rapid and sensitive diagnostic method to demonstrate the presence of typical yeast-like cells with a central septa, either within histiocytes or scattered through the tissue. The yeast-cells are spherical to ellipsoidal, 2 to 6 μm in diameter, and divide by fission rather than budding, a characteristic visible on stained smears that distinguishes *P. marneffei* from *Histoplasma capsulatum.*[30] Tissue sections show small, oval to elliptical yeastlike cells, 3 μm in diameter, either packed within histiocytes or scattered through the tissue. Occasional, large, elongated sausage-shaped cells up to 8 μm long with distinctive septa may be present.[30]

Culture. Clinical specimens are inoculated onto Sabouraud's dextrose agar. Typical yellow-pink colonies with distinctive red diffusible pigment is characteristic of *P. marneffei.*[30]

Serology. Although a monoclonal antibody-based ELISA has been developed,[188] a direct immunofluorescence test is the test of choice for specific diagnosis. Serologic diagnosis by antigen detection does not have high sensitivity (immunodiffusion, 58.8%; latex agglutination, 76.5%) and antibody detection is not very helpful, especially in immunocompromised patients.[189]

Preventing Exposure/Disease

Available information does not support specific recommendations regarding exposure avoidance. However, patients with advanced HIV disease should avoid visiting the disease-endemic areas.[44]

Treatment

P. marneffei is highly susceptible to miconazole, itraconazole, ketoconazole, and 5-flucytosine. Amphotericin B has intermediate antifungal activity, whereas fluconazole is the least active.[187]

The recommended treatment is amphotericin B at a dosage of 0.6 mg/kg/day IV for 2 weeks, followed by oral itraconazole at a dosage of 400 mg/day for a subsequent duration of 10 weeks.[190] Consideration should be given to simultaneous administration of treatment for penicilliosis and initiation of HAART to improve outcome.[44]

Patients with mild disease can be initially treated with oral itraconazole, 400 mg/day for 8 weeks[191] followed by 200 mg/day for prevention of recurrence. Itraconazole capsules are better absorbed when taken with or immediately after a meal. Itraconazole oral solution could be taken on an empty stomach.

Management of Treatment Failure

Alternative treatment options for penicilliosis have not been established.

For those whose initial therapy has failed, the approach to treatment should consist of reinitiating parenteral amphotericin B followed by another course of oral itraconazole, coupled with optimizing HAART. It is important to address obstacles to adherence, avoid adverse drug interactions, and ensure that adequate absorption and serum concentrations of itraconazole are achieved.[44]

A small case series reported good outcomes with voriconazole.[192]

Preventing Recurrence

In Thailand, approximately 50% of patients have a reported relapse of *P. marneffei* infection within 6 months after discontinuation of antifungal therapy.[191] A that double-blind, placebo-controlled trial of oral itraconazole, conducted in Chiang Mai, Thailand, demonstrated that 200 mg/day, given for secondary prophylaxis in AIDS patients, reduced the relapse rate of *P. marneffei* from 57% to 0% ($p < 0.001$).[193]

All patients who successfully complete treatment for penicilliosis should be given secondary prophylaxis (chronic maintenance therapy) with oral itraconazole at a dosage of 200 mg/day.[44]

Discontinuing Secondary Prophylaxis (Chronic Maintenance Therapy)

No randomized controlled study exists that demonstrates the safety of discontinuing secondary prophylaxis for penicilliosis. However, an open-label, historical-controlled trial from Chiang Mai University Hospital (Chiang Mai, Thailand) indicated that no relapse of penicilliosis and invasive fungal infections occurred after discontinuation of itraconazole in patients receiving HAART and with CD4 T lymphocyte counts of >100 cells/mm^3.[194]

Discontinuing secondary prophylaxis for penicilliosis is recommended for AIDS patients who receive combination HAART and have CD4 counts >100 cells/mm^3 for ≥6 months. Secondary prophylaxis should be reintroduced if the CD4 count decreases to <100 cells/mm^3 or if penicilliosis recurs at a CD4 count of >100 cells/mm^3.[44]

Despite the availability of HAART, OIs continue to cause considerable morbidity and mortality, and appropriate identification and management is a must for effective management of HIV disease with HAART. Clinicians must be knowledgeable about optimal strategies for prevention and management of OIs to provide comprehensive high-quality care for these patients. Current strategies of management have been successful in various settings, but for effective management it is important to identify the "at-risk" patient.

Factors useful in identifying high-risk patients include: type of immunosuppression related to treatment, duration of neutropenia, degree of CD4 T-cell depletion, and underlying medical conditions/diseases.

Conclusion

Despite promising progress in antifungal therapy, many questions remain regarding comparative efficacy, pharmacodynamics, mechanism of action, basis of improved therapeutic index, long-term toxic effects, interactions with other drugs and cytokines, as well as role in first-line therapy, role in prophylactic therapy, initial and optimal doses, and pharmacoeconomics and cost-effectiveness.

Clinicians must be knowledgeable about optimal strategies for prevention and management of OIs to provide comprehensive, high-quality care for immunocompromised patients. The use of chemoprophylaxis, immunization, and better strategies for managing acute OIs are essential to improve quality of life and improve survival.[9]

In summary, important strategies to control infection include:

- Reducing exposure to pathogens
- Suppressing colonization
- Avoidance/limit of invasive procedures
- Enhancement of host defense
- Immunomodulation (cytokines—GCSF, IFN-γ) and white cell transfusions

Opportunistic infections remain a major complication of AIDS. Although HAART has led to a dramatic reduction in the frequency of opportunistic infection in the developed world, significant morbidity and mortality are still associated with the complications of HIV disease. Research regarding and access to newer antifungals and newer regimens is important for the acute management of opportunistic infections, as well as for counteracting the rising problems of resistance and intolerability. Restoration of the immune system with antiretrovial therapy will go a long way in the long-term management and prevention of future recurrences.

References

1. UNAIDS/WHO AIDS Epidemic Update: December 2005.
2. Fauci AS and Lane HC. Human Immunodeficiency Virus (HIV) Disease: AIDS and Related Disorders in Harrison's principles of internal medicine 14th ed. New York: The McGraw-Hill companies;1998.
3. Fahey JL, Taylor JMG, Detels R, Hofmann B, Melmed RBS, et al. The prognostic value of cellular and serologic markers in infection with human immunodeficiency virus type 1. N Engl J Med 1990;322:166–172.
4. Moss AR, Bacchetti P, Osmond D, Krampf W, Chaisson RE, et al. Seropositivity for HIV and the development of AIDS or AIDS related condition: three year follow up of the San Francisco General Hospital cohort. Br Med J 1988;296:745–750.
5. Eyster ME, Ballard JO, Gail MH, Drummond JE, Goedert JJ, et al. Predictive markers for the acquired immunodeficiency syndrome (AIDS) in hemophiliacs: persistence of p24 antigen and low T4 cell count. Ann Intern Med 1989;110:963–969.
6. George J, Hamida A, Das AK, Amarnath SK, Rao RS. Clinical and lab profiles of 60 patients with AIDS: a South Indian study. South East Asian J. Trop. Med Public Health 1996;27(4):686–690.
7. Sivaraman V, Gilbert F, Rao RS. HIV infection and pulmonary tuberculosis: Report of 6 cases. Ind J Tub 1992;39:35–43.
8. Aquina SR, Tarey SD, Ravinderan GD, Nagamani D, Ross C. Cryptococcal meningitis in AIDS-Need for early diagnosis. J Assoc. Physicians India 1996;44(3):178–180.
9. Walensky RP, Paltiel AD, Losina E, et al. The survival benefits of AIDS treatment in the United States. J Infect Dis 2006;194:11–19.
10. Palella FJ, Jr., Delaney KM, Moorman AC, et al. Declining morbidity and mortality among patients with advanced human immunodeficiency virus infection. HIV Outpatient Study Investigators. N Engl J Med 1998;338:853–860.
11. Detels R, Munoz A, McFarlane G, Kingsley LA, et al. Effectiveness of potent antiretroviral therapy on time to AIDS and death in men with known HIV infection duration: Multicenter AIDS Cohort Study Investigators. JAMA 1998;280:1497–1503.

63. Marty F, Mylonakis E. Antifungal use in HIV infection. Expert Opin Pharmacother 2002;3:91–102.

64. Powderly WG, Finkelstein D, Feinberg J, et al. A randomized trial comparing fluconazole with clotrimazole troches for the prevention of fungal infections in patients with advanced human immunodeficiency virus infection. N Engl J Med 1995;332:700–705.

65. Schuman P, Capps L, Peng G, et al. Weekly fluconazole for the prevention of mucosal candidiasis in women with HIV infection: a randomized, double-blind, placebo-controlled trial. Ann Intern Med 1997;126:689–696.

66. Havlir DV, Dube MP, McCutchan JA, et al. Prophylaxis with weekly versus daily fluconazole for fungal infections in patients with AIDS. Clin Infect Dis 1998;27:1369–1375.

67. Goldman M, Cloud GA, Wade KD, et al. A randomized study of the use of fluconazole in continuous versus episodic therapy in patients with advanced HIV infection and a history of oropharyngeal candidiasis. Clin Infect Dis 2005;41:1473–1480.

68. Koneman EW, Allen SD, Janda WM, Schreckenberger PC, Winn WC,Jr. Color atlas and textbook of diagnostic microbiology. 5th ed. Philadelphia. Lippincott Williams & Wilkins. 1997; 983–1057.

69. Aberg JA, Powderly WG. Cryptococcosis. In: Dolin R, Masur H, Saag MS, eds. AIDS Therapy. New York, NY: Churcill Livingstone 2002:498–510.

70. Mirza S, Phelan M, Rimland D, et al. The changing epidemiology of cryptococcosis: an update from population-based active surveillance in 2 large metropolitan areas, 1992-2000. Clin Infect Dis 2003;36:789–794.

71. Randhawa HS, Pal M. Occurrence and Significance of Cryptococcus Neoformans in the Respiratory Tract of Patients With Bronchopulmonary Disorders. J Clin Microbiol Jan. 1977:5–8.

72. Powdery WG. Cryptococcal Meningitis and AIDS. Clin Infect Dis 1993;17:837-842.

73. Wadhwa A, Kaur R, Bhalla P. Profile of central nervous system disease in HIV/AIDS patients with special reference to cryptococcal infections.Neurologist. 2008 Jul;14:247–251.

74. Manoharan G, Padmavathy BK, Vasanthi S, Gopalte R. Cryptococcal meningitis among HIV infected patients. Indian Journal of Medical Microbiology 2001;19:157–158.

75. Chuck SL, Sande MA. Infections with Cryptococcus neoformans in the acquired immunodeficiency syndrome. N Eng J Med 1989;321:794–799.

76. Stockman L and Roberts GD. Specificity of the latex test for cryptococcal antigen: a rapid, simple method for eliminating interference factors. J Clin Microbiol. 1983;17:945–947.

77. Sungkanuparph S, Vibhagool A, Kiatatchasai W. Cerebrospinal Fluid Cryptococcal Antigen Titer And Culture In Monitoring Treatment Response in AIDS—Associated Cryptococcal Meningitis. J Infect Dis Antimicrob Agents 2003;20:68–71.

78. McKinsey DS, Wheat LJ, Cloud GA, et al. Itraconazole prophylaxis for fungal infections in patients with advanced human immunodeficiency virus infection: randomized, placebo-controlled, double-blind study. Clin Infect Dis 1999;28:1049–1056.

79. Barchiesi F, Schimizzi AM, Caselli F, Novelli A, Fallani S, Giannini D, Arzeni D, Di Cesare S, Di Francesco LF, Fortuna M, Giacometti A, Carle F, Mazzei T, Scalise G. Interactions between triazoles and amphotericin B against Cryptococcus neoformans. Antimicrob Agents Chemother. 2000 Sep;44(9):2435–2441.

80. LeMonte AM, Washum KE, Smedema ML, Schnizlein-Bick C, Kohler SM, Wheat LJ.Amphotericin B combined with itraconazole or fluconazole for treatment of histoplasmosis.J Infect Dis. 2000 Aug;182(2):545–550.

81. Brouwer AE, Rajanuwong A, Chierakul W, Griffin GE, Larsen RA, White NJ, Harrison TS.Combination antifungal therapies for HIV-associated cryptococcal meningitis: a randomised trial.Lancet. 2004 May 29;363(9423):1764–1767.

82. Brandt ME, Pfaller M, Hajjeh R, et al. Trends in antifungal drug susceptibility of *Cryptococcus neoformans* isolates in the United States: 1992 to 1994 and 1996 to 1998. Antimicrob Agents Chemother 2001;45:3065–3069.

83. Chen SC. Cryptococcosis in Australasia and the treatment of cryptococcal and other fungal infections with liposomal amphotericin B. J Antimicrob Chemother 2002;49:57–61.

84. Leenders AC, Reiss P, Portegies P, et al. Liposomal amphotericin B (AmBisome) compared with amphotericin B both followed by oral fluconazole in the treatment of AIDS-associated cryptococcal meningitis. AIDS 1997;11:1463–1471.

85. Larsen RA. A comparison of itraconazole versus fluconazole as maintenance therapy for AIDS-associated cryptococcal meningitis. Clin Infect Dis 1999;28:297–298.

86. Powderly WG, Saag MS, Cloud GA, et al. A controlled trial of fluconazole or amphotericin B to prevent relapse of cryptococcal meningitis in patients with the acquired immunodeficiency syndrome. N Engl J Med 1992;326:793–798.

87. Stansell JD, Osmond DH, Charlebois E,et al. Predictors of Pneumocystis carinii pneumonia in HIV-infected persons. Pulmonary Complications of HIV Infection Study Group. Am J Respir Crit Care Med 1997;155:60–66.

88. Udwadia ZF, Doshi AV, Bhaduri AS. Pneumocystis carinii pneumonia in HIV infected patients from Mumbai. J Assoc Physicians India 2005;53:437–440.

89. Abouya YL, Beaumel A, Lucas S: Pneumocystis carinii pneumonia. An uncommon cause of death in African patients with acquired immunodeficiency syndrome. Am Rev Respir Dis 1992;145:617–620.

90. Schuman P, Capps L, Peng G, Vazquez J, el-Sadr W, Goldman AI, Alston B, Besch CL, Vaughn A, Thompson MA, Cobb MN, Kerkering T, Sobel JD. Weekly fluconazole for the prevention of mucosal candidiasis in women with HIV infection. A randomized, double-blind, placebo-controlled trial. Terry Beirn Community Programs for Clinical Research on AIDS. Ann Intern Med 1997,126:689–696.

91. Hoores DR, Soah AJ, Bacellar H et al. Clinical manifestations of AIDS in the era of Pneumocystis prophylaxis. NEJM 1993;329:1922–1926.

92. Murray JF, Garay SM, Hopewell PC, Mills J, Snider GL, Stover DE. Pulmonary complications of the acquired immunodeficiency syndrome: an update.Am Rev Respir Dis. 1987 Feb;135:504–509.

93. Datta D, Ali SA, Henken EM, Kellet H, Brown S, and Metersky ML. Pneumocystis carinii Pneumonia:The Time Course of Clinical and Radiographic Improvement. *Chest* 2003;124:1820-1823.

94. Bigby TD, Margolskee D, Curtis JL: The usefulness of induced sputum in the diagnosis of Pneumocystis carinii pneumonia in patients with the acquired immunodeficiency syndrome. Am Rev Respir Dis 1986 Apr;133: 515-8.

95. Caliendo AM, Hewitt PL, Allega JM, Keen A, Ruoff KL, Ferraro MJ. Performance of PCR assay for detection of Pneumocystis carinii from respiratory specimens. *J Clin Microb* 1998;36:979–982.

96. Hughes W, Leoung G, Kramer F, et al. Comparison of atovaquone (566C80) with trimethoprim-sulfamethoxazole to treat *Pneumocystis carinii* pneumonia in patients with AIDS. N Engl J Med 1993;328:1521–1527.

97. Safrin S, Finkelstein DM, Feinberg J, et al. Comparison of three regimens for treatment of mild to moderate *Pneumocystis carinii* pneumonia in patients with AIDS: a double-blind, randomized, trial of oral trimethoprim-sulfamethoxazole, dapsone-trimethoprim, and clindamycin-primaquine. Ann Intern Med 1996;124:792–802.

98. Kovacs JA, Hiemenz JW, Macher AM, et al. *Pneumocystis carinii* pneumonia: a comparison between patients with the acquired immunodeficiency syndrome and patients with other immunodeficiencies. Ann Intern Med 1984;100:663–671.

99. Nielsen TL, Eeftinck Schattenkerk JK, Jensen BN, et al. Adjunctive corticosteroid therapy for *Pneumocystis carinii* pneumonia in AIDS: a randomized European multicenter open label study. J Acquir Immune Defic Syndr 1992;5:726–731.

100. Bozzette SA, Sattler FR, Chiu J, et al. A controlled trial of early adjunctive treatment with corticosteroids for *Pneumocystis carinii* pneumonia in the acquired immunodeficiency syndrome. N Engl J Med 1990;323:1451–1457.

101. National Institutes of Health. Consensus statement on the use of corticosteroids as adjunctive therapy for *Pneumocystis* pneumonia in the acquired immunodeficiency syndrome. N Engl J Med 1990;323:1500–1504.

102. Medina I, Mills J, Leoung G, et al. Oral therapy for *Pneumocystis carinii* pneumonia in the acquired immunodeficiency syndrome: a controlled trial of trimethoprim–sulfamethoxazole versus trimethoprim-dapsone. N Engl J Med 1990;323:776–782.

103. Black JR, Feinberg J, Murphy RL, et al. Clindamycin and primaquine therapy for mild-to-moderate episodes of *Pneumocystis carinii* pneumonia in patients with AIDS. Clin Infect Dis 1994;18:905–913.

104. Toma E, Thorne A, Singer J, et al. Clindamycin with primaquine vs. Trimethoprim-sulfamethoxazole therapy for mild and moderately severe *Pneumocystis carinii* pneumonia in patients with AIDS: a multicenter, double-blind, randomized trial. Clin Infect Dis 1998;27:524–530.

105. Smego RA, Jr., Nagar S, Maloba B, Popara M. A meta-analysis of salvage therapy for *Pneumocystis carinii* pneumonia. Arch Intern Med 2001;161:1529–1533.

106. Conte JE, Jr., Chernoff D, Feigal DW, Jr., et al. Intravenous or inhaled pentamidine for treating *Pneumocystis carinii* pneumonia in AIDS: a randomized trial. Ann Intern Med 1990;113:203–209.

107. Wharton JM, Coleman DL, Wofsy CB, et al. Trimethoprim-sulfamethoxazole or pentamidine for *Pneumocystis carinii* pneumonia in the acquired immunodeficiency syndrome: a prospective randomized trial. Ann Intern Med 1986;105:37–44.

108. Baughman RP, Dohn MN, Frame PT. The continuing utility of bronchoalveolar lavage to diagnose opportunistic infection in AIDS patients. Am J Med 1994;97:515–522.

109. Stover DE, Zaman MB, Hajdu SI, et al. Bronchoalveolar lavage in the diagnosis of diffuse pulmonary infiltrates in the immunosuppressed host. Ann Intern Med 1984;101:1–7.

110. CDC. Guidelines for prophylaxis against Pneumocystis carinii pneumonia for persons infected with human immunodeficiency virus. MMWR 1989;38:1–9.

111. Phair J, Munoz A, Detels R, et al. The risk of *Pneumocystis carinii* pneumonia among men infected with human immunodeficiency virus type 1. Multicenter AIDS Cohort Study Group. N Engl J Med 1990;322:161–165.

112. Kaplan JE, Hanson DL, Navin TR, Jones JL. Risk factors for primary *Pneumocystis carinii* pneumonia in human immunodeficiency virus-infected adolescents and adults in the United States: reassessment of indications for chemoprophylaxis. J Infect Dis 1998;178:1126–1132.

113. Carr A, Tindall B, Brew BJ, et al. Low-dose trimethoprim-sulfamethoxazole prophylaxis for toxoplasmic encephalitis in patients with AIDS. Ann Intern Med 1992;117:106–111.

114. Hardy WD, Feinberg J, Finkelstein DM, et al. A controlled trial of trimethoprim- sulfamethoxazole or aerosolized pentamidine for secondary prophylaxis of *Pneumocystis carinii* pneumonia in patients with the acquired immunodeficiency syndrome. N Engl J Med 1992;327:1842–1848.

115. Bozzette SA, Finkelstein DM, Spector SA, et al. A randomized trial of three antipneumocystis agents in patients with advanced human immunodeficiency virus infection. N Engl J Med 1995;332:693–600.

116. Schneider MM, Hoepelman AI, Eeftinck Schattenkerk JK, et al. A controlled trial of aerosolized pentamidine or trimethoprim-sulfamethoxazole as primary prophylaxis against *Pneumocystis carinii* pneumonia in patients with human immunodeficiency virus infection. N Engl J Med 1992;327:1836–1841.

117. Podzamczer D, Salazar A, Jimenez J, et al. Intermittent trimethoprim- sulfamethoxazole compared with dapsone-pyrimethamine for the simultaneous primary prophylaxis of *Pneumocystis* pneumonia and toxoplasmosis in patients infected with HIV. Ann Intern Med 1995;122:75–761.

118. Opravil M, Hirschel B, Lazzarin A, et al. Once-weekly administration of dapsone/pyrimethamine vs. aerosolized pentamidine as combined prophylaxis for *Pneumocystis carinii* pneumonia and toxoplasmic encephalitis in human immunodeficiency virus-infected patients. Clin Infect Dis 1995;20:531–541.

119. Girard PM, Landman R, Gaudebout C, et al. Dapsone-pyrimethamine compared with aerosolized pentamidine as primary prophylaxis against *Pneumocystis carinii* pneumonia and toxoplasmosis in HIV infection. N Engl J Med 1993;328:1514–1520.

120. Mussini C, Pezzotti P, Govoni A, et al. Discontinuation of primary prophylaxis for *Pneumocystis carinii* pneumonia and toxoplasmic encephalitis in human immunodeficiency virus type I-infected patients: the changes in opportunistic prophylaxis study. J Infect Dis 2000;181:1635–1642.

121. Lopez Bernaldo de Quiros JC, Miro JM, et al. A randomized trial of the discontinuation of primary and secondary prophylaxis against *Pneumocystis carinii* pneumonia after highly active antiretroviral therapy in patients with HIV infection. N Engl J Med 2001;344:159–167.

122. Latgé JP. Aspergillus fumigatus and aspergillosis. Clin Microbiol Rev 1999;12:310–350.

123. Mylonakis E, Barlam TF, Flanigan T, Rich JD. Pulmonary aspergillosis and invasive disease in AIDS: review of 342 cases. Chest 1998;114:251–262.

124. Holding KJ, Dworkin MS, Wan PC, et al. Aspergillosis among people infected with human immunodeficiency virus: incidence and survival. Clin Infect Dis 2000;31:1253–1257.

125. Khoo SH, Denning DW. Invasive aspergillosis in patients with AIDS. Clin Infect Dis 1994;19 Suppl 1:S41–48.

126. Wallace JM, Lim R, Browdy BL, et al. Risk factors and outcomes associated with identification of *Aspergillus* in respiratory specimens from persons with HIV disease: Pulmonary Complications of HIV Infection Study Group. Chest 1998;114:131–137.

127. Eyer-Silva WA, Basílio-de-Oliveira CA, Morgado MG. HIV infection and AIDS in a small municipality in Southeast Brazil. Rev. Saúde Pública. 2005;39:6.

128. Hearn VM, Pinel C, Blachier S, Ambroise-Thomas P, Grillot R. Specific antibody detection in invasive aspergillosis by analytical isoelectrofocusing and immunoblotting methods. J Clin Microbiol 1995 Apr;33:982–986.

129. White PL, Archer AE, Barnes RA. Comparison of non-culture-based methods for detection of systemic fungal infections, with an emphasis on invasive Candida infections. J Clin Microbiol 2005 May;43: 2181–2187.

130. Kami M, Tanaka Y, Kanda Y,et al. Computed tomographic scan of the chest, latex agglutination test and plasma (1AE3)-beta-D-glucan assay in early diagnosis of invasive pulmonary aspergillosis: a prospective study of 215 patients. Haematologica 2000 Jul;85:745–752.

131. Cornely OA, Maertens J, Winston DJ, et al. Posaconazole vs. fluconazole or itraconazole prophylaxis in patients with neutropenia. N Engl J Med 2007;356:348–359.

132. Segal BH, Walsh TJ. Current approaches to diagnosis and treatment of invasive aspergillosis. Am J Respir Crit Care Med 2006;173:707–717.

133. Herbrecht R, Denning DW, Patterson TF et al. Voriconazole versus amphotericin B for primary therapy of invasive aspergillosis.N Engl J Med. 2002 Aug 8;347(6):408–415.

134. Leenders AC, Daenen S, Jansen RL et al. Liposomal amphotericin B compared with amphotericin B deoxycholate in the treatment of documented and suspected neutropenia-associated invasive fungal infections. Br J Haematol. 1998 Oct;103(1):205–212.

135. Maertens J, et al. *Proceedings of the 40th Interscience Conference on Antimicrobial Agents and Chemotherapy* [abstract 1103]. Toronto, 2000.

136. Nagy-Agren SE, Chu P, Smith GJ, Waskin HA, Altice FL. Zygomycosis (mucormycosis) and HIV infection: report of three cases and review. Acquir Immune Defic Syndr Hum Retrovirol 1995 Dec 1;10(4):441–449.

137. Guardia JA, Bourgoignie J, Diego J. Renal mucormycosis in the HIV patient. Am J Kidney Dis. 2000 May;35(5):E24.

138. Hejny C, Kerrison JB, Newman NJ, Stone CM. Rhino-orbital mucormycosis in a patient with acquired immunodeficiency syndrome (AIDS) and neutropenia. Am J Ophthalmol 2001;132(1):111–112.

139. Moraru RA, Grossman ME. Palatal necrosis in an AIDS patient: a case of mucormycosis. Cutis. 2000;66(1):15–18.

140. Connolly JE Jr, McAdams HP, Erasmus JJ, Rosado-de-Christenson ML.Opportunistic fungal pneumonia. J Thorac Imaging 1999;14(1):51–62.

141. Lagorce Pages C, Fabre A, Bruneel F, Zimmermann U, Henin D. Disseminated mucormycosis in AIDS. Ann Pathol 2000;20(4):343–345.

142. Fujii T, Takata N, Katsutani S, Kimura A. Disseminated mucormycosis in an acquired immunodeficiency syndrome (AIDS) patient. Intern Med 2003 Jan;42(1):129–130.

143. Samanta TK, Biswas J, Gopal L, Kumarasamy N, Solomon S. Panophthalmitis due to rhizopus in an AIDS patient: a clinicopathological study. Indian J Ophthalmol 2001 Mar;49 (1): 49–51.

144. Kaufman L, Mendoza L, and Standard PG. Immunodiffusion test for serodiagnosing subcutaneous zygomycosis. J Clin Microbiol 1990;28(9):1887–1890.

145. Center for Disease Control. Revision of the case definition of acquired immune deficiency syndrome for national reporting – United States. MMWR 1985;34: 373 –375.

146. Sarosi GA, Johnson PC. Disseminated Histoplasmosis in patients infected with human immunodeficiency virus. Clin Infect Dis1992;14:Suppl 1: S60–S67.

147. Wheat LJ. Histoplasmosis in Acquired immunodeficiency syndrome. Curr TopMed Mycol 1996;7:7–18.

148. McKinsey DS, Spiegel RA, Hutwagner L, et al. Prospective study of histoplasmosis in patients infected with human immunodeficiency virus: incidence, risk factors, and pathophysiology. Clin Infect Dis 1997;24:1195– 203.

149. Marshall BC, Cox JK, Jr., Carroll KC, and Morrison RE. Case report: Histoplasmosis as a cause of pleural effusion in the acquired immunodeficiency syndrome. Am J Med Sci 1990;300:98–101.

150. Wheat LJ, Connolly-Stringfield PA, Baker RL, Curfman MF, Eads ME, Israel,KS, Norris SA, Webb DH and Zeckel ML. Disseminated histoplasmosis in the acquired immune deficiency syndrome: clinical findings, diagnosis and treatment, and review of the literature. Medicine (Baltimore) 1990;69:361–374.

151. Loh FC, Yeo JF, Tan WC, Kumarasinghe G. Histoplasmosis presenting as hyperplastic gingival lesion. J Oral Pathol Med 1989;18: 533–536.

152. Reddy P, Gorelick DF, Brasher CA, Larsh H. Progressive disseminated histoplasmosis as seen in adults. Am J Med 1970;48: 629–636.

153. Chinn H, Chernoff DN, Migliorati CA, Silverman S, Green TL. Oral histoplasmosis in HIV—infected patients: a report of two cases. Oral Surg Oral. Med Oral Pathol Oral Radiol Endod 1995;79:710–714.

154. Casariego Z, Kelly GR, Perez H, et al. Disseminated histoplasmosis with orofacial involvement in HIV-1-infected patients with AIDS: manifestations and treatment. Oral Dis 1997;3:184–187.

155. Hernandez SL, Lopez de Blanc SA, Sambuelli RH, Roland H , Cornelli C, Lattanzi V, Carnelli MA. Oral histoplasmosis associated with HIV infection: a comparative study. J Oral Pathol Med 2004;33:445–450.

156. Wheat LJ, Connolly-Stringfield PA, Williams B, etal. Diagnosis of Histoplasmosis in patients with Acquired Immunodeficiency syndrome by detection of Histoplasma capsulatum polysaccharide antigen in Bronchoalveolar lavage fluid. Am Rev Respir Dis 1992;145:1421–1424.

157. Anand A. Diagnosis of systemic histoplasmosis in AIDS patients. South Med J 1993;86:844–845.

158. Bille J, Stockman L, Roberts GD, Horstmeier CE, and Ilstrup DM. Evaluation of a lysis-centrifugation system for recovery of yeast and filamentous fungi from blood. J Clin Microbiol 1983;18:469–471.

159. Wheat LJ, Connolly-Stringfield PA, Williams B, Connolly K, Blair R, Bartlett M, and Durkin M. Diagnosis of Histoplasmosis in patients with the acquired immunodeficiency syndrome by detection of Histoplasma capsulatum polysaccharide antigen in bronchoalveolar lavage fluid. Am Rev Respir Dis 1992;145:1421–1424.

160. Wheat LJ, Kohler RB, Tewari RP, Garten M, and French MLV. Significance of Histoplasma antigen in the cerebrospinal fluid of patients with meningitis. Arch Intern Med 1989;149:302–304.

161. Wheat LJ, Kohler RB, and Tewari RP. Diagnosis of disseminated histoplasmosis by detection of Histoplasma capsulatum antigen in serum and urine specimens. N Engl J Med 1986;314:83–88.

162. LeMonte AM, Washum KE, Smedema ML, Schnizlein-Bick C, Kohler SM, Wheat LJ.Amphotericin B combined with itraconazole or fluconazole for treatment of histoplasmosis.J Infect Dis. 2000 Aug;182(2):545–550.

163. Wheat LJ, Musial CE, Jenny-Avital E. Diagnosis and management of central nervous system histoplasmosis. Clin Infect Dis 2005;40:844–852.

164. Restrepo A, Tobon A, Clark B, et al. Salvage treatment of histoplasmosis with posaconazole. J Infect 2007;54:319–327.

165. Al-Agha OM, Mooty M, Salarieh A. A 43-year-old woman with acquired immunodeficiency syndrome and fever of undetermined origin: disseminated histoplasmosis. Arch Pathol Lab Med 2006;130:120–123.

166. Freifeld AG, Iwen PC, Lesiak BL, et al. Histoplasmosis in solid organ transplant recipients at a large Midwestern university transplant center. Transpl Infect Dis 2005;7:109–115.

167. Wheat LJ, Connolly P, Smedema M, et al. Activity of newer triazoles against *Histoplasma capsulatum* from patients with AIDS who failed fluconazole. J Antimicrob Chemother 2006;57:1235–1239.

168. Hecht FM, Wheat J, Korzun AH, et al. Itraconazole maintenance treatment for histoplasmosis in AIDS: a prospective, multicenter trial. J Acquir Immune Defic Syndr Hum Retrovirol 1997;16.100–107.

169. Goldman M, Zackin R, Fichtenbaum CJ, et al. Safety of discontinuation of maintenance therapy for disseminated histoplasmosis after immunologic response to antiretroviral therapy. Clin Infect Dis 2004;38:1485–1489.

170. Pappas PG, Pottage JC, Powderly WG, et al: Blastomycosis in patients with the acquired immunodeficiency syndrome. Ann Intern Med 1992;116:847–853

171. Utz JP. The pulmonary mycosis in bronchopulmonary diseases and related disorders. Cranston W Wolman, Carl Muschenheim eds. Harper & Ron Publishers, Maryland, New York. 1st edition 1972;p 418.

172. Ray D, Jairaj PS, Date A. North American Blastomycosis in a South Indian Girl—Report of a Case. Ind J Tub.1995;42–43.

173. Jambhekar NA, Shrikhande SS, Advani SH, Rao RS. Disseminated blastomycosis—a case report. Indian J Pathol Microbiol 1988;31:330–333.

174. Wheat J. Endemic mycosis in AIDS: a clinical review. Clin Microbiol Rev 1995;8:146–159.

175. Pappas PG, Threlkeld MG, Bedsole GD et al. Blastomycosis in patients with acquired immunodeficiency syndrome. Medicine1993;72:322–325.

176. Pappas PG. Blastomycosis in the immunocompromised patient. Semin Respir Infect 1997 Sep;12(3):243–251.

177. Supparatpinyo K, Khamwan C, Baosoung V, Nelson KE, Sirisanthana T. Disseminated *Penicillium marneffei* infection in Southeast Asia. Lancet 1994;344:110–113.

178. Clezy K, Sirisanthana T, Sirisanthana V, Brew B, Cooper DA. Late manifestations of HIV in Asia and the Pacific. AIDS 1994;8 (Suppl 2):35–43.

179. Kantipong P, Panich V, Pongsurachet V, Watt G. Hepatic penicilliosis in patients without skin lesions. Clin Infect Dis 1998;26:1215–1217.

180. Singh PN, Ranjana K, Singh YI, et al. Indigenous disseminated *Penicillium marneffei* infection in the state of Manipur, India: report of four autochthonous cases. J Clin Microbiol 1999;37:2699–2702.

181. Ranjana KH, Priyokumar K, Singh TJ, et al. Disseminated *Penicillium marneffei* infection among HIV-infected patients in Manipur state, India. J Infect Dis 2002;45:268–71.

182. Drouhet E. Penicilliosis due to Penicillium marneffei: a new emerging mycosis in AIDS patients traveling to or living in South east Asia. Review of 44 cases reported in HIV infected patients during last 5 years compared to 44 cases in HIV -ve patients reported over 20 years. J Mycol Med 1993;3:195–122.

183. Chariyalertsak S, Sirisanthana T, Saengwonloey O, Nelson KE. Clinical presentation and risk behaviors of patients with acquired immunodeficiency syndrome in Thailand, 1994–1998: regional variation and temporal trends. Clin Infect Dis 2001;32:955–962.

184. Taborda A, Arechavala AI. Paracoccidioidomycosis, In Sarosi GA, Davies SF (Eds): Fungal Diseases of the Lung, 2nd edition. New York, NY, Raven Press 1993;85–94.

185. Randhawa HS. Respiratory and Systemic Mycoses : An Overview. Indian J Chest Dis Allied Sci 2000;42:207–219.

186. Chariyalertsak S, Supparatpinyo K, Sirisanthana T, Nelson KE. A controlled trial of itraconazole as primary prophylaxis for systemic fungal infections in patients with advanced human immunodeficiency virus infection in Thailand. Clin Infect Dis 2002;34:277–284.

187. Supparatpinyo K, Nelson KE, Merz WG, et al. Response to antifungal therapy by human immunodeficiency virus-infected patients with disseminated *Penicillium marneffei* infections and in vitro susceptibilities of isolates from clinical specimens. Antimicrob Agents Chemother 1993;37:2407–2411.

188. Chaiyaroj SC, Chawengkirttikul R, Sirisinha S, Watkins P, and Srinoulprasert Y. Antigen Detection Assay for Identification of *Penicillium marneffei* Infection. J Clin Microbiol 2003 January;41(1): 432–434.

189. WHO Regional office for South east Asia. July 23, 2003. Standard Operating Procedures for The Laboratory Diagnosis Of Common Fungal Opportunistic Infections In HIV/AIDS Patients.

190. Sirisanthana T, Supparatpinyo K, Perriens J, Nelson KE. Amphotericin B and itraconazole for treatment of disseminated *Penicillium marneffei* infection in human immunodeficiency virus-infected patients. Clin Infect Dis 1998;26:1107–1110.

191. Supparatpinyo K, Chiewchanvit S, Hirunsri P, et al. An efficacy study of itraconazole in the treatment of *Penicillium marneffei* infection. J Med Assoc Thai 1992;75:688–691.

192. Supparatpinyo K, Schlamm HT. Voriconazole as therapy for systemic *Penicillium marneffei* infections in AIDS patients. Am J Trop Med Hyg 2007;77:350–353.

193. Supparatpinyo K, Perriens J, Nelson KE, Sirisanthana T. A controlled trial of itraconazole to prevent relapse of *Penicillium marneffei* infection in patients infected with the human immunodeficiency virus. N Engl J Med 1998;339:1739–1743.

194. Chaiwarith R, Charoenyos N, Sirisanthana T, Supparatpinyo K. Discontinuation of secondary prophylaxis against penicilliosis marneffei in AIDS patients after HAART. AIDS 2007;21:365–367.

Chapter 22 HIV/AIDS AND TB COINFECTION: A POLITICAL CALL TO ACTION

CAROLE P McARTHUR, JÜRGEN NOESKE, AND NICOLE PARRISH

I am what I am both as a result of people who respected and helped me, and of those who did not respect me and treated me badly.

—NELSON MANDELA

Introduction

The beginning of what is now known as acquired immunodeficiency syndrome (AIDS) is well established: a description of five young homosexuals in whom *Pneumocystis carinii* pneumonia and other "opportunistic" infections had developed, appeared in 1981.[1] Other reports followed, describing an abnormal ratio of lymphocyte subgroups with opportunistic infections, including tuberculosis, first in homosexual men, IV-drug abusers, and Haitians and then in risk groups ranging from blood transfusion recipients, infants, female sexual contacts of infected men, prisoners, and Africans. Published evidence of transmission of the syndrome through sexual intercourse, blood and blood products, and, finally, the isolation from a patient with AIDS of a new virus—now called human immunodeficiency virus (HIV)—associated with the syndrome left no doubt as to the viral origin of HIV/AIDS. The viral epidemic spread rapidly, from Haiti and Africa to other parts of the world.

HIV/AIDS and TB: The Evolution of a Deadly Partnership

In 1991, 10 years later, more than 10.1 million persons worldwide were reported to be infected with HIV, and more than 10% of infected individuals died. The incidence of HIV continued to increase worldwide, reaching an estimated 33.4 million [31.1 million–35.8 million] in 2008.[2] The total number of HIV-infected individuals increased 20% between 2000 and 2008, a prevalence roughly three-fold higher than in 1990. This increased prevalence reflected increased infections, together with the benefits of more accessible antiretroviral treatment. Despite a growing number of HIV-infected persons worldwide, the pandemic seems to have peaked in 1996, when 3.5 million [3.2 million–3.8 million] new HIV infections occurred vs. 2.7 million [2.4 million–3.0 million] in 2008, approximately 30% lower than at the epidemic's peak. Most of the global HIV/AIDS burden of 22.4 million (67%) infected individuals, are living in sub-Saharan Africa.

In parallel with the emerging HIV epidemic, the world witnessed a recrudescence of tuberculosis (TB) in the late 1980s and the early 1990s. Notably, as in the case of the HIV/AIDS epidemic, the etiology and epidemiology of the TB epidemic were very different for wealthy countries such as the U.S. and Western Europe than in the developing world. In the former, the TB epidemic had reached its peak at the turn of the 19th century, long before HIV/AIDS was discovered. TB incidence decreased, slowly at first, and then rapidly due to various social, economic, and medical factors. These included: (1) the demographic transition and stabilization of population growth during the Industrial Revolution in the late 19th and early 20th centuries in North America and Europe; (2) an unprecedented rise in living standards for all social classes; (3) impressive advances in scientific knowledge about *Mycobacterium tuberculosis* and the diseases it produces in humans; (4) the discovery of drugs such as streptomycin in 1944 and rifampicin in 1956; and (5) a clear concept of efficient TB treatment and control based on sound science. In retrospect, the transient rising incidence of TB in highly industrialized countries toward the end of the 20th century was caused by prematurely dismantled TB services. By that time, TB was finally limited to socially marginalize high-risk groups such as IV drug users, migrants from developing countries, and, over the past 30 years, HIV-infected individuals. Excess TB morbidity during this period did not seriously disturb indigenous populations.

Over the past 30 years, HIV/AIDS and TB evolved from independent diseases traditionally addressed separately by the World Health Organization (WHO) to a highly pathogenic coinfection threatening global control of both diseases. This coinfection complicates the pathogenesis, clinical presentation, diagnosis, management, treatment, and societal and economic aspects of each disease. Coinfection increases the number of active TB cases and reactivates latent TB, increasing morbidity and mortality. Approximately 9 million new cases of active TB occur annually, and latent TB infection exists in 2 billion people, or one-third of the world's population.[3–5] As 34.3 million people are now living with HIV (71% in sub-Saharan Africa),[4] clearly, significant overlap of both diseases exists. In fact, approximately 1.4 million (15%) of all new active TB cases are coinfected with HIV.[6] When stratified by individual country, the coinfection rate is even more alarming. In Africa, more than 50% of HIV-positive patients have TB. This number exceeds 80% in some locations.[6] Active TB has been shown to increase viral load in HIV infected patients which accelerates progression of both diseases, and increases HIV genetic heterogeneity through compartmentalization.[7] As a result, co-infection with these two pathogens is the greatest cause of death in HIV/AIDS patients.[4]

Both HIV and TB are intricately connected to poverty. This connection is even more pronounced in developing countries such as India and those on the African continent where public health resources are scarce, capacitance is poor, and infrastructure is often in disrepair or nonexistent. Unfortunately, corruption also flourishes in these settings. HIV is a relatively "modern" disease for which no cure exists, whereas TB—although one of the oldest diseases known to man—is generally curable with appropriate antibiotic therapy. Therein lies a paradox associated with this deadly disease: treatment for drug-susceptible TB is effective and inexpensive, yet it remains the leading infectious cause of morbidity and mortality worldwide. In 1993, the WHO declared TB a global emergency. However, the reality is that available means of treatment and control have not been widely applied, especially in many endemic regions of the globe. This raises important questions: Have control strategies failed because they have been incorrectly implemented? Or are the control strategies inherently flawed?

> *The history of tuberculosis has been one of scientific, medical and political failure … immense forces are counteracting efforts to tackle the spread of TB. Political and demographic factors, the HIV/AIDS epidemic, poverty and social*

marginalization, mass displacements of people, and growth of drug resistance... .

—*ZUMLA AND GANDY*, 2003[8]

Even more alarming has been the emergence of MDR-TB and XDR-TB strains, which are rapidly becoming the next global health emergency and are the harbingers of an impending pandemic.[9–14]

> *There is a gathering storm of drug-resistant tuberculosis and the strategy of the WHO and of other national and international health agencies ... has failed to control the disease or prevent the emergence of more threatening strains that are extremely resistant to the antibiotics available today.*[5]

MDR-TB is defined as *M. tuberculosis* resistant to isoniazid and rifampin; XDR-TB is MDR plus resistance to any fluoroquinolone and at least one of the injectable second-line drugs, amikacin, kanamycin, or capreomycin.[16] More than 500,000 cases of MDR-TB occurred in 2007,[18] and XDR-TB has been detected in 55 countries.[17]

Much of the drug resistance worldwide is the result of a complex interplay of a variety of factors, ranging from inadequate to inappropriate therapy. Inadequate therapy is intricately linked to noncompliance, poor patient follow-up, inaccessibility to required drugs, or accessibility to substandard drugs, all of which strain local resources and hinder control efforts. Inappropriate therapy is often connected to diagnostic impediments related to identification of those with TB and, in those who have been diagnosed, the failure to detect drug resistance. In addition, in many high-burden countries of the developing world, TB case detection is based solely on clinical signs and symptoms combined with bio sensitivity of smear microscopy, while drug resistance is determined by response to therapy. This syndromic management of TB has been facilitated by poor or unattainable diagnostic tools and a lack of laboratory infrastructure and health care support services in endemic regions of the globe. In such settings, patients are often empirically treated with standard first-line drug regimens until treatment failure is evident, when the use of more expensive, more toxic, longer-term, alternative second-line drugs is indicated. Unfortunately, standard drug regimens can be a death sentence for individuals with MDR-TB or XDR-TB.[15,19–22]

Currently, in developing countries, TB incidence and prevalence evolves differently and diagnosis and treatment is generally implemented within a different paradigm. Colonization first and, later, independence, together with aid for development, led to declining death rates from TB without concomitant industrialization, education, substantial improvement in living conditions, or fall in birth rates that were central features of the demographic transition in America and Europe.[23] Globally, the incidence of TB increased from 6.6 million cases in 1990 to 9.22 million cases in 2008. Most of the cases in 2007 were in Asia (55%) and Africa (31%), with a small proportion in the Eastern Mediterranean region (6%), Europe (5%), and the Americas (3%).[24] The African region and Asia together accounted for 84% of all notified new and relapsed cases of TB and for similar proportions of new smear-positive cases. Hence, tuberculosis remains one of the world's major public health challenges, being the most frequent cause of death from a single agent among persons between 15 and 49 years of age, causing more than 2 million (mostly young) adult deaths per year. **Figure 22–1** shows global trends in estimated TB incidence for high-income countries, for Africa in areas with high HIV incidence.

In a significant number of countries in sub-Saharan Africa, the TB epidemic was drastically influenced by the spread of HIV. From an epidemiologic point of view, the risk of TB in persons

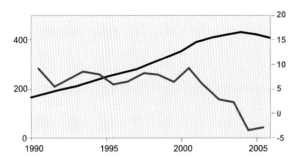

Figure 22–1a. *Africa: Countries with high HIV prevalence.*

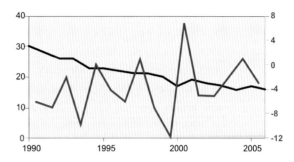

Figure 22–1b. *High-income countries.*

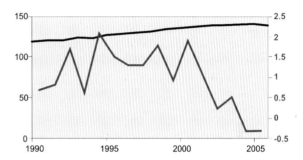

Figure 22–1c. *World.*

with HIV infection is modulated by several factors, the most important among them being the prevalence of latent infection in the population. A second factor, the likelihood of TB exposure, depends on the prevalence of active disease in the population.[25] In sub-Saharan Africa, about 33% of TB cases between 1985 and 1993 are estimated to have occurred because of the HIV epidemic.[2] Thus, as the latest WHO Global Tuberculosis Report shows in regard to the 2007 incidence figures, the number of notified cases rose similarly in Thailand, Vietnam, India, and Brazil, due to HIV coinfections:

> *Globally, the latest data suggest that there were 1.4 million new HIV-positive TB cases in 2007 (out of a total of 9.3 million incident cases of TB). This estimate is much higher than figures previously published by WHO in their annual reports. In this context, it is important to highlight that the estimated total number of incident TB cases (HIV-positive and HIV-negative combined) has changed only slightly. The reason for the much higher estimated number of HIV-positive TB cases is that the proportion of incident cases of TB who are estimated to be infected with HIV has been revised upwards, based on much more extensive data about HIV prevalence in TB patients. These data became available mostly in 2008 following the rapid expansion of routine HIV testing in TB patients since 2005–2006, notably in African countries. The African Region accounts for 79% of estimated HIV-positive TB cases; most of the remaining cases are in the South-East Asia Region.[6]*

These figures suggest that HIV-associated TB has increased almost four-fold from 4% in 1995[27] to 15% in 2007. Simply stated, the developing world harbors large numbers of cases of active TB.

Studies in the U.S. in the early 1990s, as well as in Europe and in central Africa, demonstrated the high risk of tuberculosis in persons with HIV infection.[28–30] The criteria for AIDS surveillance quickly included TB, in recognition of the close association of HIV infection with this disease. The 1987 criteria for AIDS in adults from the U.S. Centers for Disease Control and Prevention (CDC) included laboratory evidence of HIV infection together with opportunistic infections such as extrapulmonary TB. In 1993, pulmonary TB was added by the CDC to conditions defining AIDS. Numerous clinical, biologic, and epidemiologic studies confirmed the close interaction between TB and HIV-infection. The epidemiology of TB is altered by HIV in three major ways:[31] (1) reactivation of latent TB in HIV-infected individuals; (2) accelerated progression from infection with TB to disseminated TB; and (3) transmission and spreading of TB to the general population from those patients who develop disseminated disease. As one standard textbook for TB states: "…HIV infection may be the most potent risk factor for TB yet identified."[25] Conversely, there is much evidence for TB accelerating the course of HIV.

In 1988, the first World Aids Day was celebrated, recognizing the threat of a pandemic. In 1993, TB was recognized by WHO as global emergency. Responses to both epidemics developed separately, guided by international health politics until 2000, when a series of urgent meetings of the Global Working Group on TB/HIV of the World Health Organization (WHO) began.[33] A strategic framework to decrease the burden of TB/HIV was developed and guidelines were conceived and published.[31] In the UNAIDS Outcome Framework 2009–2011, tuberculosis ranked fifth among nine priority areas identified, and it was stated that "we can prevent people living with HIV from dying of tuberculosis."[34] Correspondingly, the Stop TB Strategic plan of 2006–2015 formulated its second priority to "address TB/HIV, MDR-TB, and other challenges" under the goal to "implement collaborative TB/HIV activities."[35]

More recently, the convergence of HIV/AIDS, drug-resistant TB, the current downturn in the global economy, and increasing poverty has been considered the "perfect storm"[36] to facilitate a global increase in the number of MDR- and XDR-TB cases. Of these new cases, ~95% in the HIV-negative population will develop latent TB, seeding the general population with future drug-resistant outbreaks, which may be difficult if not impossible to treat. Clearly, control of TB would result in a significant impact on HIV disease outcomes, and vice versa. However, TB research is at a critical juncture, and political and financial obstacles abound. Compounding the problem is the perception of TB as a relatively "common" disease, which has created markedly less media attention, attracted fewer activists, and generated a mere fraction of the necessary funding compared to the intricately related "modern" disease, HIV/AIDS. HIV/AIDS has attracted enormous media attention from the very beginning, arousing huge passions and leading to significant political activism. HIV/AIDS has become the disease of the 20th century, as illustrated by the advent of the upcoming XVIIIth annual World AIDS Conference to be held in Vienna (2010) and the dedication of December 1st as World AIDS Day. World Tuberculosis Day (March 24th), sponsored by the WHO and the International Union Against Tuberculosis and Lung Disease (IUATLD), is a much less celebrated or visible event, occurring each year since 1982. Yet international awareness of these deficits exist, as illustrated by the consensus reached by the Stop TB Partnership and the Treatment Action Group (TAG), which clearly stated that current funding was insufficient to meet benchmark goals for the control and treatment of TB.[37] Reversal of this 75% funding shortfall to meet the STOP TB/WHO strategic goals and the impending global health crisis will require enormous political leadership with an immediate response among policy makers, donors, researchers, and activists.

> *Global roadblocks in HIV/TB research and development must be removed promptly to continue and accelerate the progress seen during the past 5–10 years.[38]*

TB control in developing regions of the globe such as India, Africa, or China are clearly subject to a different paradigm in diagnosis, management, treatment, and control of both HIV and TB than in the developed, "Westernized" world of the U.S. or Europe. These differences are widely recognized by the scientific community, as is the global threat posed by the convergence of HIV/AIDS and TB. Thus, a massive paradigm shift on both sides is essential to extend and implement existing diagnostic tools and therapies from the developed to the developing world. We must accelerate the passage of diagnostic tools, new drugs, and vaccines through the appropriate pipelines and simultaneously look for innovative, local traditional therapies, which may be more readily accepted culturally.

The Current State of TB Diagnostic Development

Currently, identification and detection of resistance for the majority of the Mycobacteria species, including *M. tuberculosis*, require several weeks or months and multiple methodologies to complete. Existing methods range from simple smear microscopy for mycobacterial detection to labor- intensive and slow culture methods to advanced, costly, and, depending on the platform, technically demanding molecular assays used for speciation and detection of drug resistance. The sheer number and variety of tests required to progress from detection to identification and determination of drug resistance is often beyond the capacity of smaller clinical laboratories and, in the developing world, are completely out of reach. In all cases, including the most technically equipped laboratories, average turnaround times for reporting results are measured in weeks to months, not hours to days. More rapid and reliable methods for identification and detection of drug resistance in *M. tuberculosis* are urgently needed, as noted by an Institute of Medicine (IOM) report and the WHO/Global Plan to Stop TB, 2006–2015.[43] Rapid methods, many already in the pipeline (*www.finddiagnostics.org/programs/tb/pipeline.html*), would allow for earlier identification of patients with active TB and provide for more timely initiation of appropriate drug regimens for patients with resistant disease, including MDR- and XDR-TB. The major obstacle to these goals is lack of funding and, possibly, potential conflicts of interest, which may emerge amidst competing private and public agencies.

Current diagnostic development strategies center on the improvement of existing tests and the development of novel ones, with research being conducted in both the public and private sectors. These technologic advances and novel assays require critical, unbiased evaluation with practical considerations for implementation in high-burden settings. Toward this end, WHO established a process for evaluation and endorsement of new tools for TB control. In addition, the Global Plan to Stop TB 2006–2015 designed a framework to facilitate introduction and implementation of new diagnostics through its Retooling Task Force and monetary support from the Foundation for Innovative Diagnostics (FIND). **Table 22–1** shows several of the new or improved diagnostic tools already in use or in late-stage development; **Table 22–2** includes other diagnostics in early phases of development or those not currently endorsed by WHO.

A great disparity still exists between developed and developing countries in public health infrastructure and resources. Interestingly, however, the needs of developing countries, which carry the burden of HIV/TB, have begun to influence technology development globally. New technologies appropriate for the developing world are very much in the realm of point-of-care and rapid methods, which have been part of the U.S. and European armamentarium for many years. The concomitant rise in the standard of living, as well as the growth and competition from China and India, has stimulated western corporations to develop these technologies for sale and

TABLE 22–1	TB Diagnostic Technologies in Use or in Late Stage Development		
	Technology	**Description**	**Product**
	Liquid culture	Manual and commercial broth-based culture methods	BacT/ALERT 3D; MGIT
	Molecular line probe assay	Strip test for rapid identification of TB/INH and RIF resistance	Genotype® MTBDR and MTBDRplus; INNO LiPA Rif.TB
	Strip speciation	Detects TB-specific antigen from positive liquid or solid cultures	Capilia TB Rapid Diagnostic Test
	Automated detection and MDR screening	Automated sample processing/DNA amplification of TB and detection of RIF resistance	Cepheid GeneXpert device and MTB cartridge
	Colorimetric redox indicators	Detection of INH/RIF resistance using redox dyes in culture	Noncommercial method (Resazurin)
	Front-loaded smear microscopy	Same-day examination of patient specimens	N/A
	Interferon gamma release assay	Detection of cellular immune responses indicating TB infection	QuantiFERON®-TB Gold In Tube; T-SPOT.TB®
	LED fluorescence microscopy	Fluorescent microscopy based on light-emitting diodes (LEDs)	Fraen, LW Scientific, Zeiss
	Microscopic observation drug susceptibility (MODS)	Manual liquid culture technique, uses inverted light microscope for early growth detection	Noncommercial method
	New solid culture methods	Nitrate reductase assay, thin-layer agar culture	Noncommercial methods
	Sensititre MYCOTB Susceptibility Method	Microbroth dilution for susceptibility testing of MTB; 1st- and 2nd-line drugs; can be used to determine MICs	TREK Diagnostics

application in developing countries. However, the scale of the drug-sensitive and drug-resistant TB pandemic remains overwhelming. To eliminate TB as public health and development problem, the second Global Plan to Stop TB and the Stop TB Strategy clearly states the importance of bringing to the field new diagnostics, drugs, and vaccines. In the 2006–2015 Strategic Plan, the STOP TB New Diagnostic Working Group (NDWG) had aimed, by 2008, "to introduce an easy-to-use technology with accuracy similar to culture but capable of providing results in a few hours (or days) instead of weeks." This product would be "implementable at the first referral level (district laboratories) and to some extent also in peripheral labs (microscopy centers)." Such technology has not yet been introduced, although a variety of assays are in various stages of refinement.

Major progress has also been made in the development of molecular tools for active TB. However, cost is still an issue, and limitations remain for the application with smear-negative specimens or drug susceptibility testing. The need for rapid drug susceptibility testing is felt globally. National tuberculosis programs (NTPs) may find it bewildering to choose from among the variety of rapid tests. Correlation between phenotypic and genotypic DST remains problematic

TB I

TABLE 22–2	TB Diagnostic Technologies in Early Stage Development	
	Technology	**Developers**
	Breathalyser screening test	Rapid Biosensor Systems, Ltd.
	Loop-mediated isothermal amplification (LAMP)	Eiken Chemical Co.; FIND
	Lipoarabinomannan (LAM) detection in urine	Inverness Medical Innovations, Inc.
	Phage-based tests	BIOTEC Laboratories, Ltd.; Academic Laboratories
	Sodium hypochlorite microscopy	TDR
	Sputum filtration	Academic Laboratories
	TB patch test	Sequella
	Vital fluorescent staining of sputum smears	Academic Laboratories
	Rapid analysis of mycolic acids (RAM)	Academic Laboratories
	Paralens LED fluorescent microscopy	QBC Diagnostics
	CyScopeTB	Partec

The

due to our insufficient knowledge of the mutations underlying drug resistance.[39] The detection or management of monodrug-, polydrug- or multidrug-resistant TB requires access to sensitivity testing for several anti-TB drugs. This diagnostic capacity must be accessible quickly; indeed, the Stop TB Strategy specifies as one of its objectives "to achieve universal access to high-quality diagnosis and patient-centered treatment." Excellent microscopy remains crucial, but is challenging.

For molecular or other novel technologies to lead to a simple, reliable, inexpensive test to detect resistance to several antibiotics, important basic scientific challenges remain. Success has been achieved in the development of culture-based, rapid, simplified, and relatively inexpensive tool(s) for the detection of TB. The Capilia assay, which is being field-tested, is a fast, simple, lateral flow method that allows confirmation of MTB complex in culture in less than 15 minutes (**Figure 22–1**). Rapid molecular PCR-based screens have been developed for the detection of resistance to isoniazid and rifampicin. A first-generation LAMP-based assay (loop-mediated iso-thermal amplification technology platform), which does not require a thermocycler, may be able to be implemented at the microscopy level to detect MTB complex in 2011. Performance in the field has been confirmed for the MGIT TB and MGIT DST systems, and progress toward the detection of resistance to other drugs is ongoing and rapid. These technologies are FDA-registered and were approved by WHO in 2007, but are currently too expensive and sophisticated for most developing countries. Manual nucleic acid amplification tests (Hain and FIND), which allow the detection of resistance to rifampicin and isoniazid in 1 day, have also been developed, field-tested, and endorsed by WHO. There is a need to implement rapid nucleic acid amplification tests and point-of-care diagnostics with a flexible strategy in developing countries because, as stated by the STOP TB Partnership, "the wide array of products in the development pipeline …requires systems that can manage ongoing change and rapidly integrate the newly available tools…. A new tool may be superseded rapidly by an even newer tool within a short time-span

According to the WHO constitution, the major task of WHO is to combat disease, especially infectious diseases, and promote the general health of the people of the world. Over the past 5 to 10 years, the spread of HIV/TB has increasingly threatened public health in both developing and developed countries, giving rise to multiple international initiatives, working groups, and public awareness. The increase in public awareness has been fostered by a flurry of media reports, including several by U.S.-based media outlets, providing short-lived attention to individuals or cases. For example, in 2007, the U.S. Centers for Disease Control and Prevention (CDC) and WHO reported that a U.S. citizen with extensively drug-resistant TB had traveled internationally, sparking global outrage and concern.[32] Another example is former South African President Thabo Mbeki's vocal and somewhat controversial stance on HIV/AIDS, for which he received worldwide criticism.[41] In a speech given at the 13th International AIDS Conference in July 2000, Mbeki stated "As I listened and heard the whole story told about our own country, it seemed to me that we could not blame everything on a single virus."[41] Throughout his speech, Mbeki went on to question the link between HIV/AIDS and poverty and the AIDS rate in Africa, drawing fire from those who perceived his comments to be a direct challenge to the viral theory of AIDS. The resulting firestorm in the U.S. and international press was tremendous. Many delegates saw Mbeki's speech as a pledge to study the problem, rather than a call to action. "I am heartbroken," said Phil Wilson, executive director of the African American AIDS Policy and Training Institute of Los Angeles. "This was an opportunity to make a difference, and he decided not to."[42] Dr. William Blattner, cofounder of the Institute for Human Virology, a Baltimore-based company working on AIDS vaccines, left the stadium angry. "It's more than a lost opportunity. It is a travesty," he said.

Nevertheless, Mbeki struck a chord with many delegates by suggesting that all of Africa's health problems were the product of an economic imbalance. "Extreme poverty is the world's biggest killer and the greatest cause of ill health and suffering across the globe," he said, citing a 5-year-old WHO report.[41] Many in the media who had prior knowledge of Mbeki's interest in the Duesberg theories of HIV/AIDS overreacted to his comments, despite accuracies contained in the speech. These accuracies were further obscured by the overhaul of the South African pharmaceutical industry initiated by Health Minister Manto Tshabalala-Msimang, which placed a ban on the use of antiretroviral drugs in public hospitals. This ban was subsequently blamed for delays in distribution of critically needed drugs. Then, in November 2008, the *New York Times* reported that, due to Thabo Mbeki's rejection of scientific consensus on AIDS and his embrace of AIDS denialism, an estimated 365,000 people had perished in South Africa.[44]

These disparate viewpoints—fueled by the press—regarding the causes and factors relating to the transmission, control, and treatment of HIV/AIDS and TB highlight fundamental differences, on a global scale, which threaten to undermine existing programs and thwart development of new approaches and technologies targeting these interconnected diseases.

With respect to global diseases, fortunately and unfortunately, the public's memory fades quickly, as evidenced over the past 2 years in the U.S. and other countries confronted by a global economic meltdown and a looming health care crisis. As public focus shifts and memory fades on HIV/AIDS and TB, so does the momentum given to disease-specific initiatives. Thus, despite recent advancements in TB diagnosis and drug development supported largely by the U.S. government and the Bill & Melinda Gates Foundation, future efforts may become diluted if international political momentum is not maintained to address global problems, meet global health goals, and provide for future sustainable communities.

The World Health Organization

The World Health Organization, headquartered in Geneva, Switzerland, is the agency of the United Nations responsible for health; it is a huge organization with an enormous budget. The daily work of WHO is carried out by a secretariat consisting of thousands of staff at headquarters, regional offices, and in member countries. This bureaucracy is headed by a director-general, who is nominated by an executive board and elected by a general assembly. The World Health Assembly is the main ratifying body of WHO, and consists of delegates from each member state, of which there are currently 192. The assembly usually meets in Geneva in May; they review and approve the budget and policy and program directions for the coming year. If necessary, they elect a director-general and members of the executive board. Although said to be the main policy-making body for WHO, in actuality, the assembly actually typically rubber stamps recommendations proposed by the secretariat. Formed in 1948 during a period of aggressive and optimistic international organization-building, the objective of WHO then, and now, is nothing less than to facilitate "the attainment by all peoples of the highest possible level of health." The constitution of WHO defines health very broadly: "a state of complete physical, mental, and social well-being and not merely the absence of disease or infirmity." WHO works to attain this ambitious goal by guiding and coordinating international health efforts.

The executive board is made up of members (currently, 32), elected from among the assembly. Their main meeting is in January, at which they approve the agenda and directions for the coming year. If necessary, they nominate the director-general. Although they have more influence than the assembly on the directions WHO pursues, they are substantially guided by the work of the secretariat.

WHO also has regional offices for Africa, Europe, the Americas, Southeast Asia, the Eastern Mediterranean, and the Western Pacific. Some of these, notably the Pan-American Health Organization (PAHO), were existing regional entities when WHO was created. Unwilling to disband in favor of WHO, PAHO agreed to become part of the WHO/UN structure only if they retained a large degree of autonomy. Other regional centers were able to reach similar agreements when they joined or were formed. Such a degree of independence is rare in U.N. circles, and has meant that WHO cannot force regional organizations to work to the central organizations' priorities.

Interestingly, countries can choose which regional organization—if any—they want to join. This has resulted in some odd bedfellows: Thailand, for example, is a member of the Southeast Asia regional organization, but its immediate neighbor to the south, Malaysia, decided to join the Western Pacific region.

Finally, WHO designates academic or health institutions as collaborating centers for a period of 4 years. Although funded by national governments, these collaborating centers contribute to the research and program priorities of WHO (*www.who.int/en/immunisation. org.uk/index.html*).

WHO's budget consists of regular contributions from member—about $850 million USD in 2002/03—and voluntary contributions from members and others for specific, time-limited projects—about $1.38 billion USD for the same period. WHO publishes its prospective program budget each year (the budget for 2006–2007 is available at *apps.who.int/gb/ebwha/pdf_files/ AMTSP-PPB/a-mtsp_4en.pdf*).

In order to meet the greater demands being placed on WHO, the director-general proposed an increase in the overall level of the budget of $427 million USD for the biennium 2008–2009, will ideally include integration, with an ambitious plan for scaling up of treatment of drug resistant TB. Roll-out of adequate early diagnosis in TB is an intrinsic component of the mitigation of drug resistance.

References

1. Pneumocystis pneumonia—Los Angeles. MMWR Morb Mortal Wkl Rep 1981;30:250–252.

2. UNAIDS/WHO. AIDS epidemic update: November 2009. Geneva 2009 (UNAIDS/09.36E / JC1700E (English original, November 2009).

3. CDC: Global Tuberculosis. Proceedings of The Fourth National Conference on Laboratory Aspects of Tuberculosis. San Francisco, CA, USA 2002 .

4. Dye C, Scheele S, Dolin P, Pathania V, Raviglione MC: Consensus statement. Global burden of tuberculosis, estimated incidence, prevalence, and mortality by country. WHO Global Surveillance and Monitoring Project. JAMA 1999;282:677–686.

5. World Health Organization: Global Tuberculosis Control: Surveillance, Planning, Financing (WHO, Geneva, Switzerland) 2006.

6. World Health Organization. Global tuberculosis control:epidemiology, strategy, financing: WHO report 2009. Geneva 2009 (WHO/HTM/TB/2009.411).

7. Collins K, Quinones-Mateu M, Toossi Z, and Arts E. Impact of Tuberculosis on HIV-1 replication, diversity, and disease progression. AIDS 2002;Rev. 4:165–176.

8. Zumla A and Gandy M. Epilogue: Politics, Science and the New Tuberculosis. In eds. Zumla, A and Gandy, M., The return of the white plague: global poverty and the "new" tuberculosis. Verso Books, London, UK, and New York, USA 2003; p237.

9. CDC: Emergence of Mycobacterium tuberculosis with Extensive Resistance to Second-Line Drugs-Worldwide, 2000–2004. MMWR 2006;55(11):301–305.

10. CDC: Extensively drug-resistant tuberculosis-United States, 1993–2006. MMWR 2007;56(11):250–253.

11. Cohen T and Murray M. Modeling epidemics of multidrug-resistant M. tuberculosis of heterogeneous fitness. Nature Medicine 2004;10:1117–1121. (Provides an interesting model of multidrug-resistant TB which has implications for future control efforts.)

12. Dooley S, Jarvis W, Martone W, and Snider DE Jr: Multi-drug resistant tuberculosis. Ann Intern Med 1992;117:257–259.

13. Frieden T, Sterling T, Pablos-Mendez A, Kilburn JO, Cauthen GM, and Dooley SW: The emergence of drug resistant tuberculosis in New York City. N Engl J Med 1993;328:521–526.

14. Ghandi NR, Moll A, Sturm A et al. Extensively drug-resistant tuberculosis as a cause of death in patients co-infected with tuberculosis and HIV in a rural area of South Africa. Lancet 2006;368:1575–1580.

15. www.doctorswithoutborders.org/publications/alert...MSFAlert-Fall2006.pdf. (Details the high mortality associated with an outbreak of XDR-TB in South Africa and raises additional questions as to virulence of involved TB strains and the origin of extensive resistance101. Operational Outlook: the gathering storm of drug-resistant TB. Provides a 'view from the trenches' in combating the rising tide of MDR- and XDR-TB.)

16. MMWR: Notice to readers: revised definition of extensively drug resistant tuberculosis. JAMA 2006;296:2792.

17. World Health Organization. Global tuberculosis control: epidemiology, strategy, financing: WHO report 2009. Geneva 2009 (WHO/HTM/TB/2009.411)

18. STOP TB Activity Report 2008. International Union against Tuberculosis and Lung Disease; p12.

19. Jones K, Hesketh T, and Yudkin J: Extensively drug-resistant tuberculosis in sub-Saharan Africa: an emerging public health concern. Trans Soc Trop Med Hyg 2008;102:219–224.

20. Andrews JR, Shah NS, Gandhi N, Moll T, Friedland G, and Tugela Ferry Care and Research (TF CARES) Collaboration: Multidrug-resistant and extensively drug-resistant tuberculosis: implications for the HIV epidemic and antiretroviral therapy rollout in South Africa. J Infect Dis 2007;196 (Suppl 3):S482–490.

21. Bateman C. 'One shot' to kill MDR TB—or risk patient death. S Afr Med J 2007;97(12):1233–1236.

22. Goldman RC, Plumley KV, and Laughon BE: The evolution of extensively drug resistant tuberculosis (XDR-TB): history, status and issues for global control. Infect. Disord Drug Targets 2007;7(2):73–91.

23. Benatar SR. Prospects for global health: lessons from tuberculosis. Thorax 1995; 50:487–489.

24. World Health Organization. Global tuberculosis control : epidemiology, strategy, financing : WHO report 2009. Geneva 2009 (WHO/HTM/TB/2009.411).

25. Hopewell PC, Chaisson RE. Tuberculosis and Human Immunodeficiency Virus Infection. In eds. Reichmann LB, Hershfield ES, Tuberculosis. A Comprehensive International Approach (2nd revised and expanded edition). New York, Basel: Marcel Dekker; 2000;525–552.

26. Cantwell MF, Binkin NJ. Impact of HIV on tuberculosis in sub-Saharan Africa: a regional perspective. Int J Tuberc Lung Dis 1997;(1):205–214.

27. Raviglione MC, Snider DE Jr, Kochi A. Global epidemiology of tuberculosis in sub-Saharan Africa: a regional perspective. Jama 1995;273:220–226.

28. Selwyn PA, Sckell BM, Alcabes P, Friedland GH, Klein RS, Schoenbaum EE. High risk of active tuberculosis in HIV infected drug users with cutaneous anergy. Jama 1992;268:504–509.

29. Antonucci G, Girardi E, Raviglioni MC, Ippolito G, Gista. Risk Factors for tuberculosis in HIV infected persons. a prospective cohort study. Jama 1995;274:143–148.

30. Allen S, Batungwanayo J, Kerlikowski K, et al. Prevalence of tuberculosis in infected urban Rwandan women. Am Rev Respir Dis 1992;146:1439–1444.

31. Rieder HL. Epidemiologic basis of tuberculosis control. Paris 1999 (IUATLD).

32. Andrew Speaker's tuberculosis is multi-drug resistant, not extensively drug resistant, doctor's say (2007). www.medicinet.com.

33. World Health Organization. First meeting of the global working group on TB/HIV. Geneva 2001 (WHO/CDS/TB/2001.293)

34. UNAIDS. Joint action for results: UNAIDS outcome framework, 2009–2011. (UNAIDS/09.13E / JC1713E

35. World Health Organization. Strategic framework to decrease the burden of TB/HIV. WHO/CDS/TB/2002.296, WHO/HIV_AIDS/2002.2

36. Wells DW, Cegielski P, Nelson LJ et al. HIV Infection and Multidrug-Resistant Tuberculosis—The Perfect Storm. JID 2007;196:S86–107.

37. Schmidt Alice, "The Underfunding of TB Research across Europe" in Campaign for Access to Essential Medicines, Medecins Sans Frontiere, May, 2009.

38. STOP TB/WHO Blueprint for the Development of TB Diagnostics (2009).

39. Van Deun A, Martin A, Palomino JC. "Diagnosis of drug resistant tuberculosis: reliability and rapidity of detection (State of the Art Series. Drug resistant tuberculosis. Edited by C-Y Chiang, Number 3 in the series). Int J Tuberculosis and Lung Dis 2010;14(2):131–140.

40. Heim, K. Too much talk in cushy conferences, not enough action. Seattle Times, Thursday, June 18, 2009. Pacific Health Summit.

41. Thabo Mbeki. Speech at the Opening Session of the 13th International AIDS Conference, Durban, South Africa (July 9, 2000), http://www.anc.org.za/ancdocs/history/mbeki/2000/tm0709.html

42. San Francisco Chronicle, July 10, 2000.

43. WHO/Global Plan to Stop TB, 2006–2015 [103].

44. .Study Cites Toll of AIDS Policy in South Africa.. The New York Times, 25 Nov 2008. http://www.nytimes.com/2008/11/26/world/africa/26aids.html?_r=1&hp.

45. WHO/Stop TB Partnership. The Stop Tb Strategy 2006–2015; Building on and enhancing DOTS WHO/HTM/TB/2006.368 .

46. Van Kampen S, Ramsay A, Anthony R, Klatser P. Retooling National TB Control Programmes (NTPs) with New Diagnostics: The NTP Perspective. PLoS ONE 5(7), e11649.

Chapter 23 HIV-RELATED TUBERCULOSIS

WALKYRIA PEREIRA PINTO AND

MARCO ANTONIO DE ÁVILA VITÓRIA

Unfortunately, the environmental factor that is essential for the rising prevalence of drug-resistant tuberculosis around the globe is humankind...Our response to this challenge will reflect on whether we deserve the appellation "sapient"...

—MICHAEL D. ISEMAN

Introduction

Tuberculosis (TB) has been largely recognized as one of the most important causes of morbidity and mortality among HIV-infected individuals, particularly in resource-limited settings. According to WHO estimates, the risk for acquiring TB is 20 to 37 times greater among HIV-positive individuals than in the general population. In 2007, approximately 1.4 million cases and 456,000 deaths related to TB occurred in the HIV-infected population worldwide, which represented 15% of total TB cases, and almost 25% of global HIV-associated deaths occurred in that year.[1] Countries from Sub-Saharan Africa, the region most affected by the HIV epidemic and also with a high TB prevalence, accounted for approximately 80% of these cases and deaths projected in 2007 (**Figure 23–1**).

This strong bidirectional interaction between these two diseases causes HIV infection to accelerate TB disease progression and vice versa, presenting a significant challenge for successful global TB and HIV control.[2,3] HIV infection adds more difficulties for the systems where poverty and lack of health promotion hamper TB control. The crisis of health care represented by the superposition of HIV and TB in Sub-Saharan Africa may make it impossible in this region to reach the Millennium Development Goal of reducing TB prevalence and mortality by 50% by 2015.[4]

Another issue that deserves special attention is coinfection with drug-resistant TB (DRTB) and HIV. There are concerns that the critical overlap between the global HIV and multidrug-resistant TB (MDRTB) epidemics is emerging. This convergence increases the chance of nosocomial MDRTB transmission in places where resources for effective infection control are scarce and HIV treatment services are becoming more widely available.[5]

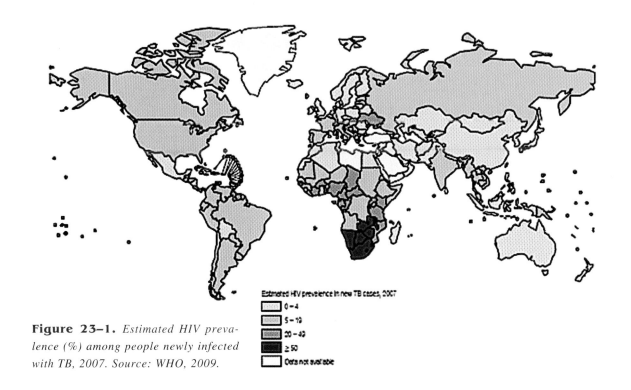

Figure 23–1. *Estimated HIV prevalence (%) among people newly infected with TB, 2007. Source: WHO, 2009.*

Antiretroviral Management of HIV-infected Individuals With Tuberculosis

The rollout of highly-active antiretroviral therapy (HAART) is increasingly seen as an essential component of TB control.[6] Several studies demonstrated that the introduction of HAART reduced TB incidence rates by up to 80% to 90% at the individual level and by 50% to 60% at the population level, and also promoted a significant decrease in case-fatality rates and recurrent TB (**Figures 23–2, 23–3, 23–4,** and **23–5**).[3,7–10]

However, studies have demonstrated that, despite the evident benefits of HAART on TB control, the mortality rate during the first months of therapy among TB-HIV coinfected individuals are elevated in resource limited settings when compared with industrialized countries (**Figure 23–5**).[11–16] This elevated early mortality has been frequently attributed to late patient presentation for HIV diagnosis and treatment, as well as the additional delay on ART initiation in these patients because of the challenges associated with the management of concomitant treatment of both infections (**Table 23–1**).

TABLE 23–1	Challenges on Treatment of TB in the Context of HIV Coinfection[a]
	• Complex drug interactions that can occur during concomitant TB and HIV therapies
	• Occurrence of immune reconstitution syndrome (IRIS)
	• High pill burden associated with concomitant TB and HIV treatment
	• Overlapping toxicities
	• Adherence issues

[a]Source: Kwara et al., 2005.[17]

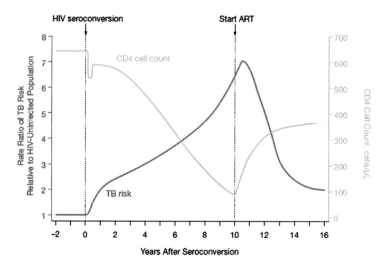

Figure 23–2. *Schematic of the risk of TB and change in CD4 cell count from onset of HIV and impact of ART. Source: Havlir et al., 2008.[3]*

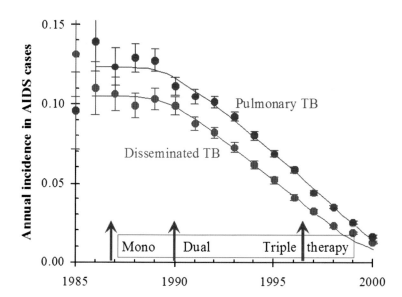

Figure 23–3. *TB among AIDS patients in Brazil (1986–2000). Source: Epidemiological Bulletin of Brazilian AIDS Programme, 2001.*

Therefore, considering the benefits and challenges associated with the expanded access to HAART and its management in the context of TB-HIV coinfection, WHO recently revised the global recommendations for antiretroviral treatment in adults and adolescents, outlining standardized and simplified recommendations to improve the delivery treatment for HIV-positive individuals with concomitant active TB, particularly for settings with limited resources.[18]

For patients with active TB in whom HIV infection is diagnosed and HAART is required, the first priority is to initiate standard antituberculosis treatment. However, in spite of potential challenges presented by comanagement of HIV and TB, HAART is now indicated for all HIV-infected individuals with active TB, irrespective of clinical immunologic parameters, and should be initiated as soon as possible (within the first 8 weeks) after starting TB treatment. In making these recommendations, WHO placed a high value on the reduction of early mortality from TB/HIV coinfection, potential reduction of TB transmission when the coinfected population is started early on HAART, and reduction of HIV morbidity/mortality and TB recurrence. Previous recommendations were more conservative, and early HAART initiation was recommended only in patients with more severe or advanced immunosuppression and in HIV-positive individuals with CD4 T lymphocyte counts >350 cells/mm^3. WHO also stated that HIV treatment should be

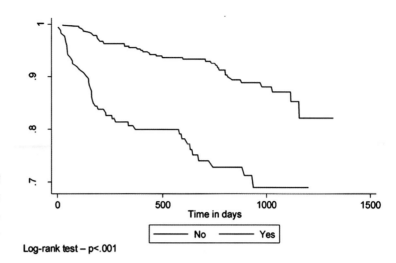

Figure 23–4. *Survival after a TB diagnosis, by exposure to HAART, in the THRio Cohort, Rio de Janeiro, Brazil. Source: Saraceni V. et al., 2008.*[10]

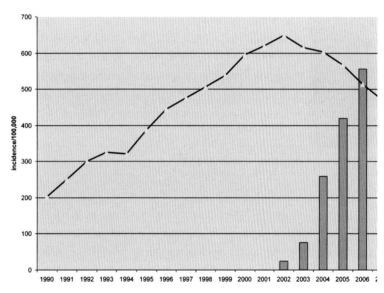

Figure 23–5. *TB incidence and ART uptake in Botswana (1990–2007). Source: Botswana MOH TB control program, 2010.*

postponed until after completion of TB treatment, and at that point HAART therapy should be revaluated.[19]

The current recommended standard initial HAART regimens in TB/HIV coinfected individuals are the same as those recommended for HIV-positive patients without TB and comprises two nucleoside analogs (NRTIs) plus one nonnucleoside analog (NNRTI). There are few drug interactions between TB drugs and current NRTI drugs. However, as stavudine (d4T) is associated with peripheral neuropathy, its concomitant use with isoniazid (INH) may lead to an additive or cumulative effect, increasing the risk for or the severity of this adverse event.[20] Therefore, the preferred NRTI options to be used in TB/HIV coinfection are zidovudine (AZT) or tenofovir (TDF), combined with lamivudine (3TC) or emtricitabine (FTC).

Regarding the NNRTI component, efavirenz (EFV) is recommended as the preferred option, because of fewer interactions with rifampin when compared with nevirapine (NVP). For those TB/HIV coinfected individuals who are unable to tolerate EFV, an NVP-based regimen or a triple nucleoside (AZT+3TC+abacavir [ABC] or AZT+3TC+TDF) are alternative options. **Table 23–2** summarizes the major recommendations.

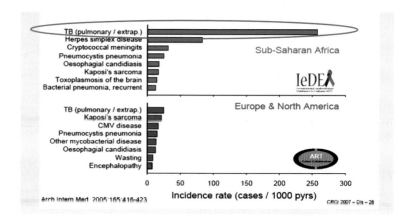

Figure 23–6. *Most common opportunistic illnesses (OIs) in the first 3 months.*

TABLE 23–2	Major WHO Recommendations for ART Use in TB/HIV Coinfection[a]
	• Start HAART in all HIV-infected individuals with active TB, irrespective of CD4 cell count.
	• Start TB treatment first, followed by HAART as soon as possible (within the first 8 weeks) after starting TB treatment
	• Use zidovudine or tenofovir combined with lamivudine or emtricitabine as the preferred NRTI backbone in patients starting HAART while on TB treatment
	• Use efavirenz as the preferred NNRTI component of in patients starting HAART while on TB treatment

[a]Source: WHO, 2009.[18]

In HIV-infected patients in whom an NNRTI regimen has failed, the recommendation is to switch therapy and introduce a ritonavir boosted protease inhibitor (bPI) in the new regimen. This approach is challenging in TB/HIV-coinfected patients, as all available bPIs at standard doses are contraindicated when used concomitantly with rifampin, due to significant drug interactions and reduction of standard dose of the majority of PIs by 75% to 90% secondary to rifampin.[21,22] Consequently, the HAART options are severely constrained for patients who develop TB and require PI-based therapy. Currently, this pharmacologic interaction can only be overcome by the use and "super-boosting" of specific PIs (lopinavir or saquinavir) with extra dosing of ritonavir (lopinavir 400 mg + ritonavir 400 mg twice daily or saquinavir 400 mg + ritonavir 400 mg twice a daily) in the ARV regimen, or by substitution of rifampin by rifabutin in the TB regimen. However, both options have important limitations in clinical practice. The use of lopinavir or saquinavir, with an adjusted dose of ritonavir ("superboosting" approach), is associated with high levels of toxicity, requiring close clinical and laboratory monitoring.[23–25] Unlike rifampin, rifabutin has minimal effects on plasma levels of PIs and, therefore, no restrictions or dose adjustments are required. Furthermore, a systematic review found no differences in TB cure or relapse rates between rifampin and rifabutin, and the incidence of side effects was low.[26] However, the current recommended dosing of rifabutin in the presence of bPIs is intermittent (150 mg three times a week), that precludes the development of fixed-dose combinations (FDC) and makes difficult the adoption of DOTS strategy. Current availability of rifabutin is limited, particularly in the public sector, and the cost is still high. Further research is urgently needed into the pharmacokinetics of rifabutin, 75 mg once daily in the presence of bPIs, which will permit the production of FDC and simplify therapy.

TABLE 23–3	Antituberculosis Drugs	
	Group 1	**First-line oral agents**: isoniazid (H); rifampin (R); ethambutol (E); pyrazinamide (Z); rifabutin (Rfb)[a]
	Group 2	**Injectable agents**[b]: kanamycin (Km); amikacin (Am); capreomycin (Cm);streptomycin (S)
	Group 3	**Fluoroquinolones(FQ)**[c]: ofloxacin (Ofx); moxifloxacin (Mfx); levofloxacin (Lfx).
	Group 4	**Oral bacteriostatic second-line agents**: ethionamide (Eto); protionamide (Pto); cycloserine (Cs); terizidone (Trd); p-aminosalicylic acid (PAS)
	Group 5	**Agents with unclear efficacy**[d]: clofazimine (Cfz); linezolid (Lzd); amoxicillin/clavulanate (Amx/Clv); imipenem/cilastatin (Ipm/Cln); high-dose isoniazid (high-dose H)[e] clarithromycin (Clr); thioacetazone (Thz).[f]

[a]Rifabutin is not on the WHO List of Essential Medicines. It has been added here as it is used routinely in patients on protease inhibitors in many settings.

[b]In MDRTB, should be used in the initial phase.

[c]Are the first choice in MDRTB.

[d]Not recommended by WHO for routine use in MDRTB patients.

[e]High-dose H is defined as 16–20 mg/kg/day.

[f]Thioacetazone is **contraindicated in HIV positive patients** because of life-threatening rash.

Source: Adapted from WHO, 2009.[27]

Treatment of HIV-Related Tuberculosis (TB/HIV)

The correct treatment of newly diagnosed cases of TB is the most effective measure for prevention of acquired resistance and one of the foundations of programs aimed at reducing the transmission and incidence of TB.

The general principles for treatment of TB/HIV are the same as for TB. The drugs most suitable for the vast majority of cases are the same that allowed the great progress in TB control in the last 3 decades of the 20th century. Considering the need for multidrug therapy for at least 6 months, it is necessary for health systems to continually evaluate and implement measures to ensure patient compliance and treatment efficacy. As directly observed treatment (DOT) has been credited with improved outcomes and with preventing the emergence of drug resistance in observational studies, it should always be recommended in national tuberculosis programs.[17] There are also recommendations that drug susceptibility testing should be performed in all cases of TB/HIV. These have not been implemented yet due to a lack of structure in many countries to perform culture in all cases. Because treatment should be started quickly, both for reasons of individual and public health, it is started on an empiric basis in most cases of TB and TB/HIV. The drugs available for treatment of TB and TB/HIV are listed in **Table 23–3**.

Patients who are TB/HIV treatment-naive, or who are presumed or known to have drug-susceptible TB should be treated with first-line drugs, using the scheme 2 (HREZ)/4 (HR), consisting of isoniazid (H), rifampin (R), ethambutol (E), and pyrazinamide (Z) for 2 months (intensive phase) and isoniazid (H) plus rifampin (R) (continuation phase), for 4 more months. Ethambutol is included to ensure the best treatment in cases with occult resistance to isoniazid, which is the most common form of initial resistance; it can be discontinued if susceptibility testing confirms

TABLE 23-4	Recommended Doses of First-Line Antituberculosis Drugs for Adults				
		Recommended dose			
		Daily		**3 times per week**	
Drug		**Dose & range (mg/kg)**	**Maximum (mg)**	**Dose & range (mg/kg)**	**Daily maximum (mg)**
Isoniazid		5 (4-6)	300	10 (8-12)	900
Rifampin		10 (8-12)	600	10 (8-12)	600
Pyrazinamide		25 (20-30)	—	35 (30-40)	—
Ethambutol		15 (15-20)	—	30 (25-35)	—
Streptomycin[a]		15 (12-18)	—	15 (12-18)	1000

[a] Patients aged over 60 years may not be able to tolerate more than 500–750 mg daily, so some guidelines recommend reduction of the dose to 10 mg/kg/day in patients in this age group. Patients weighing less than 50 kg may not tolerate doses above 500–750 mg/day. (*WHO Model Formulary 2008*, www.who.int/selection_medicines/list/en/). Source: WHO.[27]

no resistance of *M. tuberculosis* to drugs. When the treatment must be done with an intermittent regimen, it must be daily during the intensive phase and then intermittently, thrice weekly— [2(HRZE)/4(HR)3], with each dose being directly observed.

When intermittently used throughout therapy [2(HRZE)3/4(HR)3] was associated with relapse and failure rates 2–3 times higher than in patients who received the daily intensive phase and also carried a higher risk of acquired rifampin resistance (ARR).[27,28] It should not be used in patients with TB/HIV.

Pulmonary and extrapulmonary TB/HIV should be treated with the same drugs and regimens, but patients with central nervous system involvement need 9 months of therapy 2RHZE/7RH[29]—which can be prolonged to 12 months[30,31]—and corticosteroids such as IV dexamethasone (0.3–0.4 mg/kg, tapered over 6–8 weeks) or oral prednisone 1 mg/kg for 3 weeks, then tapered over 3–5 weeks.[30] Treatment with adjuvant corticosteroid is recommended only for TB/HIV meningitis and pericarditis.[27,29,30] For patients with cavitary pulmonary disease who remain sputum-culture–positive after 2 months of regular treatment, there are recommendations for extending the continuation phase with an additional 3 months to prevent relapse.[30,31] All authors are not in consensus regarding this recommendation. Some authors recommend only that, under these circumstances, drug susceptibility testing should be performed, keeping the basic schedule until completing 6 months in cases in which the test shows no resistance.[29] The recommended doses of first-line antituberculosis drugs for adults are shown in **Table 23–4**.

The effectiveness of this regimen is due to the high bactericidal activity of combination HR, and the sterilizing activity of the combination RZ. Under ideal conditions, in the intensive phase, the majority of bacilli are killed and the sputum becomes negative. There is clinical improvement and prevention of emergence of resistant strains. In the next phase, persisting bacilli are sterilized, increasing the chance of cure and reducing the risk for relapse.[32]

Some studies raise the possibility that TB/HIV therapy is impaired by the occurrence of enteropathies, which decrease absorption and thus lower the serum levels of antituberculosis drugs.[33–36] Potentially subtherapeutic levels of rifampin in patients with TB/HIV have been recorded, but its association with the emergence of resistance was not conclusive.[33] The comparison of the pharmacokinetics parameters of isoniazid, rifampin, and pyrazinamide from 12 healthy volunteers and HIV-positive patients who were at different stages of HIV infection found a correlation between more advanced disease and lower peak serum concentrations of isoniazid and rifampin. However, in all HIV-positive patients, the peak concentrations were higher than the minimum inhibitory concentration (MIC) for each drug.[35] A similar result was obtained in Nairobi, Kenya, in patients with TB who had malabsorption and consumptive disease (14 HIV-positive and 15 HIV-negative). There were observed decreased serum concentrations of isoniazid, rifampin, and pyrazinamide; however, peaks higher than the respective MICs for all drugs were reached in all patients. In this series, there was no correlation between the pharmacokinetic changes and HIV infection, CD4 count, or presence of diarrhea. The authors concluded that even patients with severe consumption and HIV infection have a good clinical response to antituberculosis therapy.[37]

Recently, low C_{max} values of pyrazinamide, although infrequent, were associated with an increased risk for poor treatment outcome (either treatment failure or death) among patients with TB, regardless of their HIV infection status.[36] Despite these observations, there is no evidence that malabsorption leads to poor outcomes of antituberculosis therapy in AIDS, and it seems that it has no major impact on clinical course in these patients.[37]

Even before the advent of HAART, despite the high and early mortality, the treatment of compliant patients with pansusceptible TB/HIV with the HRZ regimen for 6 or 9 months resulted in good clinical response and in rates of negative sputum smears similar to those of HIV-negative patients.[38–41]

The rates of recurrences were, in some records, similar in both groups,[39,40] but were generally higher in the HIV-positive group.[41,42] However, the use of recurrence rates for evaluation of therapy results in TB/HIV is impaired by the fact that it is unknown whether the recurrence is a true relapse (endogenous reactivation of the original strain that remained quiescent at the end of treatment) or a disease after exogenous reinfection. Most clinical investigation on outcomes in TB/HIV patients were carried out in areas of high rates of ongoing exposure to *M. tuberculosis* and did not compare the bacilli strains of initial and recurrent TB by means of restriction fragment-length polymorphism (RFLP). The few studies that use molecular techniques did find a high proportion of reinfection in this group of patients.[43] The increased rates of recurrence probably reflects both higher relapse and reinfection rates, as both are affected by the immunologic status of the coinfected patients,[42] but only relapses depend on antituberculosis treatment efficacy. One analytical review of cohort studies on the recurrence of pulmonary TB in adults cured by rifampin-based treatment showed that the HIV infection and a shorter duration of rifampin use independently increased the risk for recurrence of TB. The mean estimated recurrence rates were 4.5 and 1.9 cases/100 PY in HIV-infected and HIV-uninfected patients, respectively, and the additional risk incurred by HIV infection was large, especially in association with short durations (<6 mo) of rifampin prescription.[42] Increasing the total duration of treatment has been proposed to reduce recurrence in patients with TB/HIV,[44,45] but there is no consensus on this issue as it has not been adequately evaluated in clinical trials.[46] Moreover, although in HIV-negative patients the recurrence rate decreases with increased time since completion of treatment, in HIV-positive patients, no difference was detected in the recurrence rates over time.[42]

This lack of a time pattern, which may be related to the larger proportion of recurrences that are due to reinfection, raises questions about when the best time would be to add treatment.

Other limiting factors for increasing the total duration of treatment is to have to deal with drug interactions over a longer period. Different durations of TB treatment for HIV-positive and

HIV-negative individuals would be operationally difficult in resource-constrained and HIV-prevalent settings.

As for the use of rifampin for at least 6 months to reduce recurrence, this is largely accepted and is still being implemented nowadays. Until recently, an alternative regimen that uses rifampin only for 2 months–2HREZ/6HE—was the recommended initial therapy in 24 high-incidence countries to avoid the distribution of rifampin in unsupervised continuation phase treatment and minimize the risk of acquired rifampin resistance (ARR).[47] This 8-month regimen had higher rates of failure, relapse, and acquired drug resistance than did regimens that used rifampin throughout, particularly in TB with initial drug resistance to isoniazid, as demonstrated by a review of randomized controlled trials published between 1965 and 2008.[48] Unfavorable outcomes with 2HERZ/6HE, compared to 2HERZ/4HR, were also observed in an international multicenter, randomized trial with 1,355 TB patients.[49] Hence, the 2HERZ/6HE regimen was phased out by WHO in 2009.[27] Other predictors of TB/HIV treatment outcomes are prior AIDS diagnosis, baseline CD4 cell count,[50,51] HIV virus load in plasma, and, especially, the strength of immunologic recovery.[52] The patients diagnosed during the HAART era have a lower risk for death or having an AIDS event cumulative at 4 years compared to patients starting TB treatment during the pre-HAART era. However, even those on HAART have an event risk within the first 2 months of TB treatment that can be exceptionally high if the initial CD4 cell counts were <100 cells/mm^3 and declined thereafter.[21,51] Recently, data abstracted from medical records of 1,080 TB/HIV patients (that contributed 3,370 years of follow-up) treated with HRZ standard therapy showed, in multivariate modeling, that receipt of ART (that resulted in half the risk of recurrence) and CD4 cell counts of >200 cells/mm^3 any time after the initial diagnosis was associated with a significantly decreased hazard of recurrence.[52] Thus, probably a great improvement in the prognosis of TB/HIV should be achieved in the near future, with the more widespread use of the 6-month rifampin regimen and HAART.

As for tolerance, in TB/HIV patients there is great difficulty in identifying the cause of an adverse event as it may be associated with the drugs used to treat or prevent other infections, with anti-TB drugs, and/or with ART. In a retrospective study from England,[21] a total of 167 adverse events were recorded in 99 (54%) of 183 TB/HIV patients, leading to cessation or interruption of either TB or HIV therapy in 63 (34%) patients. Side effects usually occurred in the first 2 months of treatment: peripheral neuropathy in 21%, rash in 17%, gastrointestinal intolerance in 10%, hepatitis in 6%, and neurologic events in 7% of patients. In another retrospective study,[53] serious adverse events were significantly higher in HIV-infected than in HIV-uninfected individuals. Peripheral neuropathy and persistent vomiting were more common in coinfected patients. The authors considered that the large proportion of the excess adverse event rate in coinfected individuals coming from peripheral neuropathy could be due to the coadministration of d4T or ddI with isoniazid (which is now not recommended, due to a reported increase in neuropathy), but they observed that the removal from the analysis of those who received these drugs did not substantially reduce the observed incidence; this suggests the importance of other factors, such as HIV itself. All-cause interruptions of anti-TB treatment occurred with similar frequency in the two groups, and more than 85% of interruptions in both were due to hepatotoxicity, which typically presented within 2 months of starting treatment, with a median time off anti-TB treatment of 4 weeks. Thus, most interruptions necessitated full retreatment. The most common side effects in patients on treatment for TB and HIV were gastrointestinal symptoms, hepatotoxicity, rash, peripheral neuropathy,[21,53] and a variety of other symptoms (**Table 23–5**). This makes for difficult clinical management decisions, especially if ART is started concurrently. The coadministration of rifampin, isoniazid, pyrazinamide, NNRTIs, and cotrimoxazole can lead to similar

TABLE 23–5	Potential Overlying and Additive Toxicities of ART and Antituberculosis Therapy[a]			
	Toxicity	Antituberculosis Agent	Antiretroviral Agent	Comments
	Peripheral neuropathy	H; E; Eto/Pto; Lzd; Cs Aminoglycosides	D4T, ddl, ddC	Replace the ARV agent.
	CNS toxicity	H; Eto/Pto; Cs; FQ	EFV	EFV has a high rate of CNS adverse effects (confusion, impaired concentration, depersonalization, abnormal dreams, insomnia, and dizziness) in the first weeks, which typically resolve on their own. Frank psychosis is rare with EFV alone.
	Depression	H; Eto/Pto; Cs; FQ	EFV	Consider substituting for EFV if severe depression develops.
	Skin rash	H; R; Z; PAS; FQ; others	ABC, NVP, EFV, D4T, others	Do not rechallenge with ABC (can result in life-threatening anaphylaxis).
	Nausea and vomiting	H; E; Z; Eto/Pto; PAS; others	RTV,D4T,NVP and most others	Initiate antiemetic therapy. Discontinue suspected agent if this can be done (rarely necessary). Persistent vomiting and abdominal pain may be a result of developing hepatitis secondary to medications and/or lactic acidosis.
	Hepatotoxicity	H; R; E; Z; Eto/Pto; PAS; FQ	NVP, EFV, all protease inhibitors (RTV>), all NRTI	If with frank hepatitis, stop all therapy pending resolution. Consider suspending most likely agent permanently. Reintroduce remaining drugs one at a time, with the most hepatotoxic agents first, while monitoring liver function.
	Renal toxicity	Aminoglycosides; Cm	TDF (rare)	TDF may cause renal injury with the features of Fanconi syndrome, proteinuria, hypophosphatemia, hypouricemia, normoglycemic glycosuria, and acute renal failure. HIV-infected patients have an increased risk for renal toxicity and for electrolyte disturbances secondary to aminoglycosides and Cm.
	Optic neuritis	E; Eto/Pto (rare)	ddl	Suspend agent responsible for optic neuritis permanently.

[a]Adapted from WHO.[69]

adverse reactions.[31] These reactions are hard to predict and prevent. Thus, in patients with HIV, serologies for hepatitis B and C should always be performed because infection with hepatitis C virus and HIV are considered independent and additive risk factors for the development of drug-induced hepatitis (DIH).[54] DIH is defined as a serum AST or ALT > 3× upper limit of normal

(ULN) in the presence of symptoms, or serum AST or ALT > 5× ULN in the absence of symptoms.[31] Liver function must be monitored regardless of symptoms, before and especially in the first 2 months of treatment. Patients should be told to immediately report symptoms such as anorexia, nausea, vomiting, abdominal pain, or jaundice.[31] The anti-TB drugs should not be discontinued for mild gastrointestinal complaints. In the event of hepatitis, the drugs should be stopped. It may be necessary to deal with two or more anti-tuberculosis drugs, such as ethambutol, streptomycin, amikacin/kanamycin, capreomycin, or a fluoroquinolone.[31]

Once AST drops to less than twice the ULN and symptoms have improved, first-line medications can be restarted using a reintroduction regimen. If the drugs cannot be restarted or the initial reaction was life-threatening, then an alternative regimen should be used.[31]

Among the first-line TB drugs, pyrazinamide, isoniazid, and rifampin are all associated with hepatotoxicity, but scheme 2HREZ/4HR can be used in cases of chronic liver disease (even in patients who are carriers of hepatitis virus or who have a history of acute hepatitis or excessive alcohol habits), without clinical evidence of disease and with ALT and AST <3 times the ULN.[29] As for alternative regimens, there are differences between the schemes used in different countries, which follow recommendations of their own national tuberculosis programs, national AIDS programs, and medical societies.[27,29–31] See **Table 23–6** for examples of alternative schemes.

The Treatment of HIV-Related Drug-Resistant Tuberculosis (DRTB/HIV)

Isoniazid resistance is the most common form of antituberculosis drug resistance, whether in isolation or in combination with other drugs.[55] However, *M. tuberculosis* monoresistance to rifampin is rare, generally acting as a surrogate marker for dual resistance to isoniazid and rifampin—that is, multidrug-resistant TB (MDR-TB)—but it carries a worse prognosis, requiring, as recommended by the World Health Organization (WHO), the use of a fluoroquinolone and treatment for at least 12 months[55] (**Table 23–7**).

This treatment is also an attempt to prevent the development of a sequential pattern of resistance: from single-drug resistance to rifampin to multidrug resistance (MDR). The definitions of resistance are shown in **Table 23–8**.

HIV infection or AIDS are not risk factors for different forms of TB resistance,[56] but the association of coinfection with *M. tuberculosis* resistance have been recorded: (1) there is evidence that acquired rifampin resistance (ARR) is more common in HIV-positive patients,[57,58–60] and (2) higher vulnerability of HIV-positive patients to primary MDR TB has been documented.[59–62]

Possibly sporadic contact may cause the HIV-positive patient to be at risk for primary progressive TB,[61] but there is evidence that the strong predisposition to primary MDR TB or extensively drug-resistant TB (XDR TB) is given by the more advanced degree of immunodeficiency and by prolonged exposure in the nosocomial environment.[62–64] For instance, in an XDR-TB cluster in South Africa, most cases had not been previously treated for TB and two-thirds were recently hospitalized, suggesting the importance of nosocomial transmission. Among 53 patients with XDR TB, all 44 patients who underwent testing for HIV were infected, had a median CD4 cell count of 63 cells/mm^3, and were receiving antiretroviral therapy; 52 (98%) died in a median of 16 days after diagnosis.[64]

TABLE 23–6	TB/HIV Treatment: Examples of Alternatives Regimens	
	Events	**Therapeutic options**
	Intolerance to INH	2RZES$_5$/7RE[29] 2REZ/10RE[31]
	Intolerance to RMP	2HZES$_5$/10HE[29]
	Intolerance to EMB	2HRZ/4HR[29]
	Intolerance to PZA	2HRE/7HR[29]
	Baseline chronic hepatic disease without cirrhosis, with clinical stability, without symptoms and with AST or ALT > 3× USL	2HRF/7HR[29,31]
	Baseline chronic hepatic disease, with clinical symptoms, without jaundice and with AST or ALT > 3× USL	2HRE/6HE 2HSE/10HE 3SEOfx/9EOfx[29]
	Hepatic cirrhosis	RE + FQ (12–18 mo)[29] RE + Cs (12–18 mo)[29]
	Baseline acute hepatitis	3SEOfx / 6RH[29]
	Hepatotoxicity from treatment with ALT e AST> 5× USL *or* with jaundice *or* with other severe symptoms	3SEOfx / 9EOfx [29]

TABLE 23–7	Regimens for Mono- and Poly-Drug Resistance (DR)[a]	
	DR pattern	**Suggested regimens and duration (months)**
	H (± S)	R, Z, and E (6–9)
	H and Z	R, E, and FQ (9–12)
	H and E	R, Z, and FQ (9–12)
	R	H, E, FQ, plus at least 2 months of Z (12–18)
	R and E	H, Z, FQ, plus an injectable agent for at least the first 2–3 months (18)
	R and Z	H, E, FQ, plus an injectable agent for at least the first 2–3 months (18)
	H, E and Z	R, FQ, plus an oral second-line agent, plus an injectable agent for the first 2–3 months (18)

[a]Source: WHO.[69]

This scenario justifies the words of Chan and Iseman[63] to describe the threat posed by drug-resistant TB: "…highly drug-resistant strains—from multidrug-resistant tuberculosis (MDR-TB) to extensively drug-resistant TB (XDR-TB)—threaten to change the global stage of tuberculosis (TB) from largely a public health challenge to an incurable and, in collaboration with the HIV, a highly lethal disease." The effects of MDR/XDR-TB on the HIV epidemic can be listed as follows (readapted from Shenoi et al.[65]): (1) increased HIV mortality; (2) potential morbidity from drug toxicities of second-line TB drugs and ART; (3) nosocomial transmission to HIV patients; (4) risk to health care workers caring for HIV patients; (5) strain on national TB control programs and DOT programs; (6) unmet demand for laboratory services and specialized treatment

TABLE 23–11	Drug–Drug Interactions: TB Drugs vs. PIs[a]								
Color	**Interpretation**								
	No clinically significant interaction, or interaction unlikely based on knowledge of drug metabolism								
	Potential interaction that may require close monitoring, alteration of drug dosage or timing of administration								
	Interaction likely, do not use or use with caution								
	There are no clear data, actual or theoretical, to indicate whether an interaction will occur								
TB drug	**Protease Inhibitors**								
	ATV	DRV	FPV	IDV	LPV	NFV	RTV	SQV	TPV
Amikacin									
Capreomycin									
Cycloserine									
Ethambutol									
Ethionamide	No Data	No Data	No Data	No Data	No Data	No Data	No Data	No Data	No Data
Gatifloxacin									
Isoniazid									
Kanamycin									
Levofloxacin									
Moxifloxacin									
Ofloxacin									
P-Aminosalicylic Acid	No Data	No Data	No Data	No Data	No Data	No Data	No Data	No Data	No Data
Pyrazinamide									
Rifabutin									
Rifampin									
Rifapentine									
Streptomycin									

[a]Adapted from Khoo et al.[101]

TABLE 23–12	Drug–Drug Interactions: TB Drugs vs. NNRTIs and Newer ARVs[a]					
	Color	**Interpretation**				
		No clinically significant interaction, or interaction unlikely based on knowledge of drug metabolism				
		Potential interaction that may require close monitoring, alteration of drug dosage or timing of administration				
		Interaction likely, do not use or use with caution				
		There are no clear data, actual or theoretical, to indicate whether an interaction will occur				
	TB drug	**NNRTIs**			**Newer ARVs**	
		EFV	**ETV**	**NVP**	**MVC**	**RAL**
	Amikacin					
	Capreomycin					
	Cycloserine					
	Ethambutol					
	Ethionamide	No Data	No Data	No Data	No Data	No Data
	Gatifloxacin					
	Isoniazid					
	Kanamycin					
	Levofloxacin					
	Moxifloxacin					
	Ofloxacin					
	P-aminosalicylic acid	No Data	No Data	No Data	No Data	No Data
	Pyrazinamide					
	Rifabutin					
	Rifampin					
	Rifapentine					
	Streptomycin					

[a]Adapted from Khoo et al.[101]

Collaborative Activities to Reduce the Burden of TB and HIV: Isoniazid Preventive Therapy, Infection Control, Intensive Case Finding, and Cotrimoxazole Prophylaxis

Although ART has reduced the risk of TB among HIV-positive individuals,[8] more recent reports showed that even after ART initiation, the incidence of TB remains very high.[5,102] Therefore, prevention and treatment of TB in people living with HIV is an urgent priority for both HIV/AIDS and TB programs. In order to decrease the burden of TB and HIV in populations affected by both diseases, a set of collaborative activities that address the interface of TB and HIV were established by WHO[103] (**Table 23–14**).

TABLE 23–14	**Recommended Collaborative TB/HIV Activities**[a]

	A. Establish the mechanisms for collaboration
	  1. Set up a coordinating body for TB/HIV activities effective at all levels
	  2. Conduct surveillance of HIV prevalence among tuberculosis patients
	  3. Carry out joint TB/HIV planning
	  4. Conduct monitoring and evaluation

	B. Decrease the burden of tuberculosis in people living with HIV/AIDS
	  1. Establish intensified tuberculosis case-finding
	  2. Introduce isoniazid preventive therapy
	  3. Ensure tuberculosis infection control in health care and congregate settings

	C. Decrease the burden of HIV in tuberculosis patients
	  1. Provide HIV testing and counselling
	  2. Introduce HIV prevention methods
	  3. Introduce cotrimoxazole preventive therapy
	  4. Ensure HIV/AIDS care and support
	  5. Introduce antirctroviral therapy

[a]Source: Getahun et al.[103]

Among these 12 collaborative TB/HIV activities, there are three activities known as the *"Three I's,"* that those providing care to people with HIV should perform to protect them from TB infection, help prevent active disease from developing, and to identify active TB disease early and improve the chances of cure. These activities are the use of *isoniazid* preventive therapy, the adoption of TB *infection control* methods, and the promotion of *intensive case finding for TB.*[104]

Isoniazid preventive therapy (IPT) for TB can safely be given to people living with HIV without TB disease, reducing their risk for developing TB by 33%–67% for up to 48 months.[104] It is currently recommended for all people living with HIV in areas with a prevalence of latent TB infection >30%, and for all people living with HIV with documented latent TB infection or exposure to an infectious TB case, regardless of where they live.[105,106] More recently, evidence has shown that the combined use of isoniazid preventive therapy and antiretroviral therapy among people living with HIV significantly reduces the incidence of TB; and the use of IPT in patients who have successfully completed a course of TB therapy has been shown to markedly reduce the risk of subsequent TB cases[107–109] (**Figure 23–7**).

TB infection control (IC) measures are essential to prevent the spread of *M. tuberculosis* to vulnerable patients, health care workers, the community, and those living in congregate settings.[105,110] Fundamentally, TB infection control is about safety—people receiving or offering

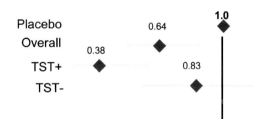

Figure 23–7. *Effect of IPT on TB: meta-analysis of clinical trials. Source: Woldehanna and Volmink, 2004.[107]*

TABLE 23–15	Five Steps for Patient Management to Prevent Transmission of TB in HIV Care Settings[a]		
Step	**Action**	**Description**	
1	Screen	Early **recognition** of patients with suspected or confirmed TB disease is the first step in the protocol. It can be achieved by assigning a staff member to screen patients for prolonged duration of cough immediately after they arrive at the facility. Patients with cough of more than two weeks duration, or who report being under investigation or treatment for TB,[a] should not be allowed to wait in the line with other patients to enter, register, or get a card. Instead, they should be managed as outlined below.	
2	Educate	Instructing the above mentioned persons identified through screening in **cough hygiene**. This includes instructing them to cover their noses and mouths when coughing or sneezing, and when possible providing face masks or tissues to assist them in covering their mouths.	
3	Separate	Patients who are identified as TB suspects or cases by the screening questions must be **separated** from other patients and requested to wait in a separate well-ventilated waiting area, and provided with a surgical mask or tissues to cover their mouths and noses while waiting.	
4	Provide HIV services	Triaging symptomatic patients to the front of the line for the services they are seeking (e.g. voluntary HIV counselling and testing, medication refills), to quickly provide care and reduce the amount of time that others are exposed to them is recommended. In an integrated service delivery setting, if possible, the patient should receive the HIV services they are accessing before the TB investigation.	

[a]Source: WHO & CDC,2006.[105]

HIV care should not have to worry about being exposed to and becoming infected with *M. tuberculosis* in the process. In light of the crisis of drug-resistant TB in countries with a high burden of HIV, establishing facilities that are safe from TB has become an emergency situation for health services, prisons, and other congregate settings, in general, but especially for HIV programs. **Table 23–15** summarizes the major steps for patient management to prevent TB transmission in HIV care settings.

TABLE 23–16	Key Messages on IPT, ICF, and IC[a]
	• TB preventive therapy with INH is safe and effective in people living with HIV, reducing the risk of TB by 33–62%.
	• Screening and diagnosing TB in people living with HIV can be challenging but TB is curable in people living with HIV.
	• TB infection control is essential to keep vulnerable patients, health care workers and their community safe from getting TB.

[a]Source: Date et al., 2008.[124]

Intensified case finding (ICF) for TB means regularly screening all people with or at high risk for HIV or in congregate settings (such as mines, prisons, military barracks) for the symptoms and signs of TB, followed promptly with diagnosis and treatment, and then doing the same for household contacts.[110–112] Simple questionnaires to screen for TB can be performed when people first seek HIV services (e.g., care, voluntary counseling and testing, etc.) and/or by community-based organizations supporting people with HIV.[113,114] A simplified algorithm using any one symptom consisting of cough, fever, night sweats, or weight loss can be used under programmatic conditions in resource-constrained settings to identify people living with HIV who are eligible for further diagnostic assessment for TB (**Figure 23–8**). In many clinical settings, absence of all four symptoms may adequately identify such individuals who are eligible for IPT.[115] Intensive case finding serves as the important gatekeeper for the two other I's (infection control and isoniazid preventive therapy), facilitating rapid identification of suspected cases of TB and acting as the necessary first step for healthcare providers to confidently prescribe IPT to people living with HIV who do not have active TB.[116]

Furthermore, the use of cotrimoxazole preventive therapy (CPT) is also a key TB/HIV activity promoted by WHO that decreases the burden of HIV among TB coinfected individuals.[117] Since the mid-1980s, CPT has been effective for the prevention of *Pneumocystis jiroveci* pneumonia and toxoplasmosis in HIV-positive individuals with advanced disease in industrialized countries and has also been used to avoid several secondary bacterial and parasitic infections in adults and children living with HIV/AIDS in resource-limited settings who present with symptomatic disease or CD4 cell counts <350 cells/mm^3.[117] Evidence from randomized clinical trials on CPT has shown reduced mortality among HIV-positive TB patients and reduced hospitalization and morbidity among persons living with HIV.[118,119] Other, nonrandomized and operational studies showed that CPT is feasible, safe, and results in reduced mortality rates patients with TB patients, even if they are already receiving ART.[120–122] Recently, an observational analysis of a study conducted in Africa (DART trial) showed that the use of CTX as prophylaxis halves mortality in severely immunosuppressed HIV-infected adults who have initiated ART, with benefits continuing for at least 72 weeks. Furthermore, CPT also reduces malaria incidence.[123] Considering this large body of evidence, WHO recommends that HIV/AIDS and TB programs should establish a system to provide CPT to eligible persons living with HIV who have active TB.[117]

Despite the considerable benefits, HIV programs have been slow to implement these TB-reducing services, resulting in missed opportunities to prevent many unnecessary cases of TB and related deaths.

In 2007, a global survey was conducted by WHO to assess progress in the development and implementation of CPT and IPT policy recommendations.[124] Data on national policies for CPT

	Yes	No
1. Prolonged cough > 3 weeks ?	[ ]	[ ]
2. Presence of night sweats > 3 weeks ?	[ ]	[ ]
3. Weight Loss > 3 kg of body weight in the last 4 weeks ?	[ ]	[ ]
4. Fever > 3 weeks ?	[ ]	[ ]

■ If "yes" to one or mo re questions : ←_____

Do sputum examination and continue evaluation according the TB

diagnostic algorithm of the national TB program   and according to clinical

signs

■ If "no" to all questions :

Stop TB investigations and repeat screening at the subsequent visit (every

3-6 months)

Figure 23–8. *Questionnaire for intensive TB screening in HIV patients. Source: Cain et al., 2010*

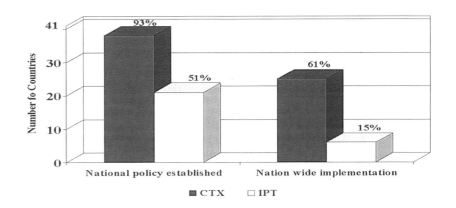

Figure 23–9. *Progress in development and implementation of CTX prophylaxis and IPT policy in respondent countries (n = 41). Source: Date et al., 2010.*

and IPT in HIV infection, current level of implementation at various facilities, and barriers to developing or implementing these policies were collected.

Of the 41 respondent countries 38 (93%) had developed a national policy regarding provision of CPT to persons living with HIV, but only 61% (25/41) had implemented the policy at a national scale (**Figure 23–9, Table 23–16**). Among 96% (24/25) of countries with nationwide implementation of CPT policy, >80% of ART facilities were also providing CPT, but provision of CPT in TB care services was very low. Provision of CPT in facilities providing services to HIV-infected children and HIV-exposed infants was also low. Erratic supply and stock-outs of CPT at health care facilities were the major obstacles to national scale-up of CPT policy for 70% (19/27) of these countries. Other barriers to national scale-up of the CPT policy included insufficient training and supervision of health care workers, lack of human resources, lack of a system to monitor provision of CPT, insufficient advocacy regarding CPT benefits, lack of integration of TB-HIV services, and fear of stigma.

41. el-Sadr WM, Perlman DC, Matts JP, et al. Evaluation of an intensive intermittent-induction regimen and duration of short-course treatment for human immunodeficiency virus-related pulmonary tuberculosis. Terry Beirn Community Programs for Clinical Research on AIDS (CPCRA) and the AIDS Clinical Trials Group (ACTG). Clin Infect Dis 1998;26:1148–1158.

42. Korenromp EL, Scano F, Williams BG, et al. Effects of Human Immunodeficiency Virus Infection on Recurrence of Tuberculosis after Rifampin-Based Treatment: An Analytical Review. Clin Infect Dis 2003;37:101–112.

43. Sonnenberg P, Murray J, Glynn JR, et al. HIV-1 and recurrence, relapse, and reinfection of tuberculosis after cure: a cohort study in South African mineworkers. Lancet 2001;358:1687–1693.

44. Pulido F, Peña JM, Rubio R, et al. Relapse of tuberculosis after treatment in human immunodeficiency virus-infected patients. Arch Intern Med 1997;157:227–232.

45. Perriëns JH, St Louis ME, Mukadi YB, et al. Pulmonary tuberculosis in HIV-infected patients in Zaire. A controlled trial of treatment for either 6 or 12 months. N Engl J Med 1995;332:779–784.

46. Dlodlo RA, Fujiwara PI, Enarson DA. Should tuberculosis treatment and control be addressed differently in HIV-infected and -uninfected individuals? Eur Respir J 2005; 25:751-7.

47. Mitchison DA. Antimicrobial Therapy of Tuberculosis: Justification for Currently Recommended Treatment Regimens. Semin Respir Crit Care Med 2004;25:307–315.

48. Menzies D, Benedetti A, Paydar A, et al. (2009) Effect of Duration and Intermittency of Rifampin on Tuberculosis Treatment Outcomes: A Systematic Review and Meta-Analysis. PLoS Med 2009;6(9):e1000146. Epub 2009 Sep 15.

49. Jindani A, Nunn AJ, Enarson DA. Two 8-month regimens of chemotherapy for treatment of newly diagnosed pulmonary tuberculosis:international multicentre randomised trial. Lancet 2004;364:1244–1251.

50. Panjabi R, Comstock GW, Golub JE. Recurrent tuberculosis and its risk factors:adequately treated patients are still at high risk. Int J Tuberc Lung Dis 2007;11:828–837.

51. Dheda K, Lampe FC, Johnson MA, et al. Outcome of HIV-Associated Tuberculosis in the Era of Highly Active Antiretroviral Therapy. J Infect Dis 2004;190:1670–1676.

52. Golub JE, Durovni B, King BS, et al. Recurrent tuberculosis in HIV-infected patients in Rio de Janeiro, Brazil. AIDS 2008;22:2527–2533.

53. Breen RA, Miller RF, Gorsuch T, et al. Adverse events and treatment interruption in tuberculosis patients with and without HIV coinfection. Thorax 2006;61:791–794.

54. Ungo JR, Jones D, Ashkin D, et al. Antituberculosis drug-induced hepatotoxicity. The role of hepatitis C virus and the human immunodeficiency virus. Am J Respir Crit Care Med 1998;157:1871–1876.

55. World Health Organization. 2008. Anti-tuberculosis drug resistance in the world: fourth global report. Geneva, Switzerland. World Health Organization; 2008. WHO/HTM/TB/2008.394.

56. Suchindran S, Brouwer ES, Van Rie A. Is HIV Infection a Risk Factor for Multi-Drug Resistant Tuberculosis? A Systematic Review. PLoS ONE. 2009;4(5):e5561. Epub 2009 May 15.

57. Bradford WZ, Martin JN, Reingold AL, et al. The changing epidemiology of acquired drug-resistant tuberculosis in San Francisco, USA. Lancet 1996;348:928–931.

58. Munsiff SS, Joseph S, Ebrahimzadeh A, et al. Rifampin-monoresistant tuberculosis in New York city, 1993–1994. Clin Infect Dis 1997;25:1465–1467.

59. Frieden TR, Sterling T, Pablos-Mendez A, et al. The emergence of drug-resistant tuberculosis in New York city. N Engl J Med 1993; 328:521–526

60. Moore M, Onorato IM, McCray E, et al. Trends in drug resistant-tuberculosis in the United States, 1993-1996. JAMA 1997;278:833–837.

61. Small PM, Hopewell PC, Singh SP, et al. The epidemiology of tuberculosis in San Francisco. A population—based study using conventional and molecular methods. N Engl J Med 1994;330:1703–1709.

62. Kent JK. The epidemiology of multidrug-resistant tuberculosis in the United States. Med Clin N Am. 1993;77:391–409.

63. Chan ED, Iseman MD. Multidrug-resistant and extensively drug-resistant tuberculosis:a review. Curr Opin Infect Dis 2008;21:587–595.

64. Gandhi NR, Moll A, Sturm AW, et al. Extensively drug-resistant tuberculosis as a cause of death in patients co-infected with tuberculosis and HIV in a rural area of South Africa. Lancet 2006;368:1575–580.

65. Shenoi S, Scott H, Moll A, et al. Multidrug-resistant and extensively drug-resistant tuberculosis:consequences for the global HIV community. Curr Opin Infect Dis 2009;22:11–17.

66. Yew WW and Leung CC. Management of multidrug-resistant tuberculosis: Update 2007. Respirology 2008;13:21–46.

67. Zhang Y and Yew WW. Mechanisms of drug resistance in Mycobacterium tuberculosis. Int J Tuberc Lung Dis 2009;13:1320–1330.

68. Mitchison DA, Nunn AJ. Influence of initial drug resistance on the response to short-course chemotherapy of pulmonary tuberculosis. Am Rev Respir Dis 1986;133:423–430.

69. World Health Organization. 2008. Guidelines for the programmatic management of drug-resistant tuberculosis. Geneva, Switzerland. WHO/HTM/TB/2008.402.

70. O'Donnell MR, Padayatchi N, Master I, et al. Improved early results for patients with extensively drug-resistant tuberculosis and HIV in South Africa. Int J Tuberc Lung Dis. 2009;13:855–861.

71. Shah S, McGowan J, Opulski B, et al. Interaction of drug interactions involving ART in New York City HIV specialty clinics. CROI 2007, Abstract 573.

72. De Maat M, De Boer A, Koks CH, et al. Evaluation of clinical pharmacist interventions on drug interactions in outpatient pharmaceutical HIV-care. J Clin Pharm Ther 2004;29:121–130.

73. Cottle LE, Evans-Jones JG, Khoo SH. Physician awareness of antiretroviral drug interactions. 15th Annual Conference of the British HIV Association, Liverpool, abstract P138. HIV Med April 2009;10(Suppl. 1):11–56.

74. Rastegar D, Knight A, Monolakis J. Antiretroviral errors among hospitalised patients with HIV infection. Clin Infect Dis 200;43:933–938.

75. Kigen G, Kimaiyo S, Owen A, et al. Prevalence of drug interactions between antiretroviral and co-administered drugs at the Moi Teaching and Referral Hospital (AMPATH), Eldoret-Kenya. 9th International Congress on Drug Therapy in HIV Infection, Glasgow, November 2008, abstract O-122.

76. Miller C, El-Kholi R, Faragon JJ, et al. Prevalence and risk factors for clinically significant drug interactions with antiretroviral therapy. Pharmacotherapy 2007; 27:1379–1386.

77. Yew W. Clinically Significant Interactions with Drugs Used in the Treatment of Tuberculosis. Drug Safety 2002;25:111-33.

78. Drugs.com. Rifampin drug interactions. Accessed February 2010 at, http://www.drugs.com/drug-interactions/rifampin.html

79. Ribera E, Lopez RM, Diaz M, et al. Steady-State Pharmacokinetics of a Double-Boosting Regimen of Saquinavir Soft Gel plus Lopinavir plus Minidose Ritonavir in Human Immunodeficiency Virus-Infected Adults. Antimicrob Agents Chemother 2004;48:4256–4262.

80. Doodley KE, Flexner C, Andrade AS. Drug Interactions Involving Combination Antiretroviral Therapy and Other Anti-Infective Agents: Repercussions for Resource-Limited Countries. J Inf Dis 2008;198:948–961.

81. Dean GL, Back DJ, de Ruiter A. Effect of tuberculosis therapy on nevirapine trough plasma concentrations. AIDS 1999;3:2489–2490.

82. Ribera E, Pou L, Lopez RM, et al. Pharmacokinetic interaction between nevirapine and rifampicin in HIV-infected patients with tuberculosis. J Acquir Immune Defic Syndr 2001;28:450–453.

83. Oliva J, Moreno S, Sanz J, et al. Coadministration of rifampin and nevirapine in HIV-infected patients with tuberculosis. AIDS 2003;17:637–638.

84. Nachega JB, Hislop M, Dowdy DW, et al. Efavirenz versus nevirapine-based initial treatment of HIV infection: clinical and virological outcomes in Southern African adults. AIDS 2008;22:2117–2125.

85. Manosuthi W, Sungkanuparph S, Vibhagool A, et al. Nevirapine- versus efavirenz-based highly active antiretroviral therapy regimens in antiretroviral- naive patients with advanced HIV infection. HIV Med 2004;5:105–109.

86. van Leth F, Phanuphak P, Ruxrungtham K, et al. Comparison of first-line antiretroviral therapy with regimens including nevirapine, efavirenz, or both drugs, plus stavudine and lamivudine: A randomised open-label trial, the 2NN Study. Lancet 2004; 363:1253-63.

87. de Beaudrap P, Etard JF, Guèye FN, et al. Long-Term Efficacy and Tolerance of Efavirenz- and Nevirapine-Containing Regimens in Adult HIV Type 1 Senegalese Patients. AIDS Res Hum Retroviruses 2008;24:753–760.

88. Cohen K, Meintjes G. Management of individuals requiring antiretroviral therapy and TB treatment. Curr Opinion HIV AIDS 2010;5:61–69.

89. López-Córtes LF, Ruiz-Valderas R, Viciana P, et al. Pharmacokinetic interactions between efavirenz and rifampicin in HIV infected patients with tuberculosis. Clin Pharmacokinet 2002;41:681–690.

90. Pedral-Sampaio DB, Alves CR, Netto EM, et al. Efficacy and safety of Efavirenz in HIV patients on Rifampin for tuberculosis. Braz J Infect Dis 2004;8:211–216.

91. Patel A, Patel K, Patel J, et al. Safety and antiretroviral effectiveness of concomitant use of rifampicin and efavirenz for antiretroviral-naive patients in India who are coinfected with tuberculosis and HIV-1. J Acquir Immune Defic Syndr 2004;37:1166–1169.

92. Friedland G, Khoo S, Jack C, et al. Administration of efavirenz (600 mg/day) with rifampicin results in highly variable levels but excellent clinical outcomes in patients treated for tuberculosis and HIV. J Antimicrob Chemother 2006;58:1299–1302.

93. Manosuthi W, Kiertiburanakul S, Sungkanuparph S, et al. Efavirenz 600 mg/day versus efavirenz 800 mg/day in HIV infected patients with tuberculosis receiving rifampicin: 48 weeks results. AIDS 2006;20:131–132.

94. Breen RA, Lipman MC, Johnson MA. Increased incidence of peripheral neuropathy with co-administration of stavudine and isoniazid in HIV-infected individuals. AIDS 2000;14:615.

95. Coyne KM, Pozniak AL, Lamorde M, et al. Pharmacology of second-line antituberculosis drugs and potential for interactions with antiretroviral agents. AIDS 2009;23:437–446.

96. Iwamamoto M, Wenning LA, Liou SY, et al. Rifampicin (RIF) modestly reduces plasma levels of MK-0518. 8th International Congress on Drug Therapy in HIV Infection, Glasgow, Scotland, November 2006, abstract P-299.

97. Wenning LA, Hanley WD, Brainard DM, et al. Effect of rifampin, a potent inducer of drug-metabolizing enzymes, on the pharmacokinetics of raltegravir. Antimicrob Agents Chemother 2009;53:2852–2856.

98. Isentress. US Prescribing Information, Merck & Co Inc, 2007. Accessed at, http://www.merck.com/product/usa/pi_circulars/i/isentress/isentress_pi.pdf

99. Selzentry [package insert]. Pfizer Inc, New York. August 2007

100. Videx US Prescribing Information, Bristol-Myers Squibb, 1991. Accessed at, http://packageinserts.bms.com/pi/pi_videx_ec.pdf

101. Khoo S, Gibbons S, Seden K, et al. Drug–drug Interactions between antiretrovirals and medications used to treat TB, Malaria, Hepatitis B&C and opioid dependence (systematic review). Accessed October 2009 at, www.who.int/hiv/topics/treatment/evidence/en.

102. Girardi E, Sabin CA, d'Arminio Monforte A, et al. Incidence of tuberculosis among HIV-infected patients receiving highly active antiretroviral therapy in Europe and North America. Clin Infect Dis 2005;41:1772–1782.

103. Getahun H, Van Gorkom J, Harries A, et al. Interim policy on collaborative TB/HIV activities. Geneva, Switzerland. Stop TB Department and Department of HIV/AIDS. World Health Organization 2004. Accessed at, http://www.who.int/hiv/pub/tb/en/Printed_version_interim-policy_2004.pdf

104. World Health Organization. 2008. WHO three "I"s meeting: Intensified Case Finding (ICF), Isoniazid Preventive Treatment (IPT) and TB Infection Control (IC) for People Living With HIV. Report of a Joint World Health Organization HIV/AIDS and TB Department Meeting, World Health Organization. HIV Department. Geneva, Switzerland, 2–4 April 2008. Accessed at, http://www.who.int/hiv/pub/meetingreports/WHO_3Is_meeting_report.pdf

105. World Health Organization (WHO), Centers for Disease Control and Prevention (CDC). Tuberculosis infection control in the era of expanding HIV care and treatment: an addendum to WHO guidelines for the prevention of tuberculosis in heath care facilities in resource-limited settings, 1999. Atlanta: CDC, 2006.

106. WHO Global Tuberculosis Programme, UNAIDS. Policy statement on preventive therapy against tuberculosis in people living with HIV. Report of a meeting held in Geneva, 18–20 February 1998. Weekly Epidemiological Record 1999;4(46):385–400.

107. Woldehanna S, Volmink J. Treatment of latent tuberculosis infection in HIV infected persons. Cochrane Database Syst Rev. 2004;(1):CD000171.

108. Grant AD, Charalambous J, Fielding KL, et al. Effect of routine isoniazid preventive therapy on tuberculosis incidence among HIV-infected men in South Africa: a novel randomized incremental recruitment study. JAMA 2005:293:2719–2725.

109. Golub JE, Saraceni V, Cavalcante SC, et al. The impact of antiretroviral therapy and isoniazid preventive therapy on tuberculosis incidence in HIV-infected patients in Rio de Janeiro, Brazil. AIDS 2007;21:1441–1448.

110. Golub JE, Mohan CI, Comstock GW, et al. Active case finding of tuberculosis: historical perspective and future prospects. Int J Tuberc Lung Dis 2005;9:1183–1203.

111. Kranzer K, Houben RM, Glynn JR, et al. Yield of HIV-associated tuberculosis during intensified case finding in resource-limited settings: a systematic review and meta-analysis. Lancet Infect Dis 2010;10:93–102.

112. Murray CJ Salomon JA. Expanding the WHO tuberculosis control strategy: rethinking the role of active case finding. Int J Tuberc Lung Dis 1998;2:S9–15.

113. Furin JJ, Rigodon J, Cancedda C, et al. Improved case detection of active tuberculosis associated with antiretroviral treatment program in Lesotho. Int J Tuberc Lung Dis 2007;11:1154–1156.

114. Bock NN, Jensen PA, Miller B, et al. Tuberculosis Infection Control in Resource-Limited Settings in the Era of Expanding HIV Care and Treatment. J Infect Dis 2007;196:S108-13.

115. Cain KP, McCarthy KD, Heilig CM, et al. An Algorithm for Tuberculosis Screening and Diagnosis in People with HIV. N Engl J Med. 2010;362:707–716.

116. World Health Organization. 2008. WHO three "I"s meeting: Intensified Case Finding (ICF), Isoniazid Preventive Treatment (IPT) and TB Infection Control (IC) for People Living With HIV. Report of a Joint World Health Organization HIV/AIDS and TB Department Meeting, World Health Organization. HIV Department. Geneva, Switzerland, 2–4 April 2008. Available at: http://www.who.int/hiv/pub/meetingreports/WHO_3Is_meeting_report.pdf

117. World Health Organization. Guidelines on co-trimoxazole prophylaxis for HIV-related infections among children, adolescents and adults. Geneva, WHO, 2006.

118. Wiktor SZ, Sassan-Morokro M, Grant AD, et al. Efficacy of trimethoprim-sulphamethoxazole prophylaxis to decrease the morbidity and mortality in HIV-1 infected patients with tuberculosis in Abidjan, Cote d'Ivoire: a randomised controlled trial. Lancet 1999;353:1469–1475.

119. Anglaret X, Chêne G, Attia A, et al. Early chemoprophylaxis with trimethoprim-sulphamethoxazole for HIV-1 infected adults in Abidjan, Cote d'Ivoire: a randomised trial. Cotrimo-CI study group. Lancet 1999;353:1463–1468.

120. Zachariah R, Harries AD, Arendt V, et al. Compliance with cotrimoxazole prophylaxis for the prevention of opportunistic infections in HIV-positive tuberculosis patients in Thyolo district, Malawi. Int J Tuberc Lung Dis 2001;5:843–846.

121. Zachariah R, Spielmann MP, Harries AD, et al. Cotrimoxazole prophylaxis in HIV infected individuals after completing antituberculosis treatment in Thyolo, Malawi. Int J Tuberc Lung Dis 2002;6:1046–1450.

122. Zachariah R, Spielmann MP, Chinji C, et al. Voluntary counselling, HIV testing and adjunctive cotrimoxazole reduces mortality in tuberculosis patients in Thyolo, Malawi. AIDS 2003;17:1053–1061.

123. Walker SA, Ford D, Gilks CF, et al. Daily co-trimoxazole prophylaxis in severely immunosuppressed HIV-infected adults in Africa started on combination antiretroviral therapy: an observational analysis of the DART cohort. Lancet 2010;375:1278–1286.

124. Date A, Vitória M, Granich R, et al. Progress in implementation of co-trimoxazole prophylaxis and isoniazid preventive policies for people living with HIV. Bull World Health Org 2010;88:253–259.

Chapter 24 AIDS-ASSOCIATED MALIGNANCIES AND THEIR TREATMENT

MARK BOWER AND JUSTIN STEBBING

It is difficult to determine whether the infectious agents play any role in inducing this lesion. We have recently seen numerous cases of Kaposi's sarcoma in young homosexual men, and it is our opinion that these lesions may well be induced by an infectious agent.

—BERNARD ACKERMAN, NYU, APRIL 23, 1981

Introduction

Acquired immunodeficiency syndrome (AIDS) following infection with human immunodeficiency virus (HIV) was brought to the world's attention in 1981 with the first case reports of *Pneumocystis carinii* pneumonia in homosexual men in Los Angeles.[1] These reports were quickly followed by descriptions of Kaposi's sarcoma (KS) in similar patient groups.[2,3] There followed a cornucopia of opportunistic infections and isolated reports of high- grade B-cell non-Hodgkin's lymphoma (NHL), both primary cerebral lymphomas and systemic NHL. By 1985, high-grade B cell NHL was included, along with Kaposi's sarcoma, as an AIDS-defining illness by the U.S. Centers for Disease Control and Prevention (CDC), following the publication of series of ninety homosexual men with NHL.[4–8] A final AIDS-defining malignancy, invasive cervical cancer, was added in 1993, although the incidence of this malignancy is not increased as dramatically in HIV-seropositive women.[9]

A number of other cancers occur at an increased frequency in people with HIV infection including Hodgkin's disease, anal cancer, lung cancer and testicular seminoma.[10] However, these malignancies have not been included in the definition of AIDS and they fall outside the scope of this chapter.

Dramatic improvements in the antiviral therapy of HIV infection occurred in the second half of the 1990s that have altered the natural history of HIV infection in those economies where these medicines are widely available. The introduction of highly-active antiretroviral therapy (HAART) has led to a fall in the incidence of both opportunistic infection and AIDS-associated malignancies.

Highly-Active Antiretroviral Therapy (HAART)

The development of effective antiretroviral therapies commenced with the introduction of nucleoside reverse transcriptase inhibitors (NRTIs), starting with zidovudine (AZT) in 1987. In the last decade, five new classes of antiretroviral agents have been introduced: protease inhibitors (PIs), including saquinavir, indinavir, ritonavir, nelfinavir, lopinavir, and atazanavir; nonnucleoside reverse transcriptase inhibitors (NNRTIs), including nevirapine, delaviridine, and efavirenz; nonnucleotide reverse transcriptase inhibitors (NRTIs), namely, tenofovir); integrase inhibitors, namely, raltegravir; and fusion inhibitors, namely, enfurvirtide. The introduction of the first two classes in the late 1990s led to the use of combination treatment referred to as HAART. HAART has had an enormous impact on the treatment of HIV in terms of overall survival, incidence of opportunistic infections and quality of life. In randomized studies HAART leads to a dramatic decline in the mortality and morbidity of HIV.[11] However, only 1.5 million of the estimated 42 million people infected with HIV worldwide are receiving HAART, as the majority of affected people live in developing countries.[12] In addition, even in the established market economies with access to medical treatment, many individuals remain undiagnosed and consequently do not receive HAART. For the most common AIDS-defining malignancy, Kaposi's sarcoma (KS), HAART remains an effective therapy,[13] although its effect on lymphoma has been more controversial.[14,15]

AIDS-Related Systemic Lymphoma

Epidemiology of AIDS-Related Lymphoma in Era of HAART

Non-Hodgkin's lymphomas (NHLs) are associated with both congenital and iatrogenic immunosuppression, and so it was perhaps not surprising that an increased incidence was demonstrated early in the AIDS epidemic. Registry linkage studies in the pre-HAART era found that the incidence of NHL in HIV-positive individuals was 60–200 times higher than in the matched HIV-negative population,[16,17] and the relative risk was even greater for primary cerebral lymphomas.[18] Following the introduction of HAART, the incidence of both Kaposi's sarcoma (KS) and primary cerebral lymphoma has fallen significantly in both registry linkage and cohort studies.[19–21] This is thought to be secondary to the immune reconstitution that occurs with HAART.[22,23]

In contrast, the effects of HAART on systemic NHL are less clear,[24,25] although some cohort studies suggest a modest, nonsignificant decline in the incidence,[26] including in the population of patients with hemophilia.[27] An international meta-analysis of 20 cohort studies compared the incidence of systemic NHL between 1992–1996 and 1997–1999. This meta-analysis confirmed an overall reduction in the incidence of both primary cerebral lymphoma (rate ratio = 0.42) and systemic immunoblastic lymphoma (rate ratio = 0.57), but not Burkitt's lymphoma (rate ratio = 1.18).[24]

Predictors of AIDS-Related Lymphoma. Genetic, infectious, and immunologic factors influence the development of AIDS-related lymphoma. For example, germ line chemokine and chemokine receptor gene variants have been found to influence the chance of developing these tumors. Acyclovir has mild activity against Epstein-Barr virus in vivo, and one case control study has shown that administration of high-dose acyclovir (≥800mg/d) for ≥1 year was associated with a significant reduction in the incidence of NHL.[28] However, data concerning the association between serum Epstein-Barr viral DNA loads and lymphoma development are controversial.[29,30]

chemotherapy, and even with the restarting HAART at the end of the chemotherapy, this took 12 months to recover to baseline levels.[46] This phase II study has been expanded to 39 selected patients now,[47] and EPOCH is currently under investigation in a multicenter study. As there are no comparative studies, it is difficult to recommend an optimal gold standard therapy and there are advocates of conventional CHOP as well as supporters of infusional therapies.

The high rate of leptomeningeal disease at presentation, which may be asymptomatic led to the widespread use of staging lumbar punctures and prophylactic intrathecal chemotherapy for patients considered to be at high risk of relapse in the cerebrosphial fluid. The prophylactic administration of intrathecal chemotherapy to patients with these risk factors but without meningeal disease at presentation prevented meningeal relapse in 81%.[48]

Chemotherapy results in a decline in CD4 cell counts in both the immunocompetent and immunocompromised and prophylaxis to prevent opportunistic infections particularly in this patient group requires careful attention. It is well established in the management of HIV infection that prophylaxis against *Pneumocystis carinii* pneumonia (PCP) should commence when the CD4 cell count falls below 200 cells/mm^3 and against *Mycobacterium avium* complex (MAC) when it falls below 50 cells/mm^3.[49,50]

The prolonged T cell depletion recorded following EPOCH was previously demonstrated for patients receiving chemotherapy in the pre-HAART era.[51] The concomitant use of chemotherapy and HAART has been widely practiced and when used together the CD4 cell count declines by 50% during chemotherapy but recovers rapidly within one month of completing chemotherapy. The CD8 and natural killer (CD16 and CD56) cell counts follow a similar profile whilst the B cell (CD19) count recovers more slowly but is restored to pre-chemotherapy levels by 3 months. There was no change in the HIV mRNA viral load during chemotherapy.[52] In view of the decline in CD4 cell count by 50%, PCP prophylaxis should commence at CD4 cell counts of 400 cells/mm^3 and MAC at CD4 counts of 100 cells/mm^3.

The improved survival described since the introduction of HAART and the preservation of immune function suggests that the combination of chemotherapy with HAART is an important step forward in the management of AIDS-related lymphomas. However, there are both toxicity and pharmacokinetic drawbacks to the concomitant administration of chemotherapy and HAART. For example, the potentiation of myelotoxicity with CDE combined with protease inhibitors may be a consequence of microsomal enzyme inhibition reducing the metabolism of cytotoxics in this regimen.[45]

Outcomes in the Era of HAART. The complete remission rates for regimens using the combination of chemotherapy and HAART are 48%–92% and the published 2 year overall survivals are 48–60%.[53–58] These response rates and survival duration statistics are starting to approach those seen in the general population with advanced-stage, high-grade lymphoma. Indeed, although the prognostic factors for survival in the pre-HAART era were predominantly immunologic (prior AIDS-defining illness and CD4 cell count), a more recent analysis of prognostic factors in AIDS-related lymphoma closely resembles that for the general population, with the international prognostic index being an equally valuable guide in both circumstances.[59] Recent data from our institution suggests the CD4 count to be an independent prognostic variable too, and a prognostic model has been established based solely on international prognostic index (IPI) scores and CD4 cell counts.

Future Developments for AIDS-Related Lymphomas. The improvements in the treatment of HIV infection have led to a more aggressive management strategy for AIDS-related lymphomas and this has resulted in better outcomes. Further refinements mirror those seen in immunocompetent patients with high-grade lymphoma, including the addition of anti-CD20 antibodies to first-line therapy and the use of high-dose chemotherapy with autologous stem cell transplantation at first relapse. Rituximab, in addition to chemotherapy, has yielded increased response rates (70% complete response, with a 59% 2-year survival).[36] Patients have also undergone successful autologous stem cell transplantation for AIDS-related lymphomas, despite predictions that myelodysplasia would make harvesting difficult.[60–63]

Primary Cerebral Lymphoma

Primary central nervous system lymphoma (PCL) is defined as non-Hodgkin's lymphoma that is confined to the craniospinal axis, without systemic involvement. This diagnosis is rare in immunocompetent patients, but occurs more frequently in patients with both congenital and acquired immunodeficiency. AIDS-related PCL occurs equally frequently across all ages and transmission risk groups, and the tumors are high-grade, diffuse large cell B-cell or immunoblastic non-Hodgkin's lymphomas. The presence of Epstein-Barr virus is a universal feature of HIV-associated PCL, but EBV is not found in other PCLs.[64] EBV may be detected by immunocytochemical staining of biopsy tissue or by polymerase chain reaction (PCR) amplification of cerebrospinal fluid using EBV specific oligonucleotide primers.[65,66]

Epidemiology

Registry linkage studies confirmed a markedly increased relative risk of PCL among patients with AIDS, with an incidence as high as 2%–6% in one early report.[67] This vastly elevated incidence of PCL was confirmed by both cohort and linkage studies. Patients who develop PCL generally have advanced immunosuppression and, for the most part, have had a prior AIDS-defining illness. Shortly after the introduction of HAART, a decline in the incidence of PCL was recognized by many clinicians, and a meta-analysis of cohort studies that compare the pre- and post-HAART eras confirmed a significant decline (RR 0.42; 99% CI, 0.24–0.75).[24] Indeed, this decrease is more dramatic than that seen for systemic AIDS-related lymphomas, and PCL is associated with more severe immunosuppression than is systemic AIDS-related lymphoma.

Clinical Presentation and Differential Diagnosis

The most common causes of cerebral mass lesions in HIV-seropositive patients are toxoplasmosis and primary cerebral lymphoma, and the differential diagnosis often proves difficult.[68] Both diagnoses occur in patients with advanced immunodeficiency (CD4 cell counts <50 cells/mm^3) and present with headaches and focal neurologic deficits. Clinical features that favor PCL include a more gradual onset over 2 to 8 weeks and the absence of a fever. CT and MRI scanning usually reveal solitary or multiple ring-enhancing lesions with prominent mass effect and edema. Again, these features occur in both diagnoses, although PCL lesions are usually periventricular whereas toxoplasmosis more often affects the basal ganglia. Thus, the combination of clinical findings and standard radiologic investigations rarely provide a definitive diagnosis. Moreover, toxoplasma serology (IgG) is falsely negative in 10% to 15% of patients with cerebral toxoplasmosis. More than 85% patients with cerebral toxoplasmosis will respond clinically and radiologically to 2 weeks of antitoxoplasma therapy, and this has become the cornerstone of the diagnostic algorithm for cerebral masses in severely immunodeficient patients.

In these patients, it has been standard practice to commence empiric antitoxoplasmosis treatment for 2 weeks' duration, and resort to a brain biopsy if there is no clinical or radiologic improvement. This strategy avoids the routine use of brain biopsy in these patients who frequently have a very poor performance status and prognosis. Although this algorithm avoids early surgical intervention, it is relatively ineffective in diagnosing PCL early and may compromise the outcome of therapy in these patients. In addition, there is a disinclination to treat patients with radiotherapy or chemotherapy empirically, based exclusively on the failure of antitoxoplasmosis treatment, without a definitive histologic diagnosis.

The discovery that all HIV-associated PCLs are associated with EBV infection has led to the development of a PCR method that can detect EBV-DNA in the cerebrospinal fluid. This has become established as a diagnostic test with a high sensitivity (83%-100%) and specificity (>90%).[69,70] In addition, radionuclide imaging by [201]thallium single photon emission computed tomography ([201]Th-SPECT) or ^{18}F-fluorodeoxyglucose positron emission tomography (FDG-PET) is able to differentiate between PCL and cerebral toxoplasmosis. PCLs are thallium-avid and demonstrate increased FDG uptake on PET scanning. However, although both techniques have high specificity for PCL, neither are highly sensitive and thus cannot be used alone; in combination with PCR, they are emerging as a diagnostic alternative to brain biopsy. The application of PCR and [201]Th-SPECT in the diagnosis of contrast-enhancing brain lesions in 27 patients was shown to result in a positive and a negative predictive value of 100% and 88%, respectively, which supports their combined value as an alternative to brain biopsy.[71] Further studies are now required to compare effectiveness of PCR with [201]Th-SPECT or FDG-PET.

Treatment

The standard treatment for PCL is whole-brain irradiation, but the median survival time associated with this modality is just 2.5 months or less. Although patients who were treated with radiotherapy or chemotherapy lived longer than those who received best supportive care only, no randomized studies have been conducted; it remains uncertain whether therapy improves survival.[72] There is increasing enthusiasm for the treatment of PCL in immunocompetent patients with both radiotherapy and chemotherapy, and recent results have been encouraging. The use of chemotherapy for PCL is limited by the poor penetration of cytotoxics into brain parenchyma (on account of the blood-brain barrier) and by the toxicity—especially myelosuppression—of these agents in patients with advanced immunosuppression and poor performance status. Combination chemotherapy prolongs survival in immunocompetent patients with PCL, but at the cost of severe myelotoxicity. Single-agent chemotherapy with intravenous high-dose methotrexate and folinic acid rescue was studied in AIDS patients with PCL in the context of a prospective uncontrolled study, which included 15 patients. The results showed a complete response in 47% of patients, a median survival of 19 months, a low relapse rate of approximately 14%, and no evidence of either neurologic impairment or treatment-limiting myelotoxicity.[73] A controlled trial of intravenous methotrexate versus whole-brain irradiation is needed to confirm these encouraging results. Now that antiretroviral therapies are improving survival, it may be necessary to reassess currently available diagnostic and treatment modalities aiming to cure HIV-associated PCL.

One intriguing development is the description of tumor regression of PCL with HAART therapy alone.[74] These case report observations require confirmation in cohort studies, but in our experience, very few patients with HIV-associated PCL are HAART-naïve at the time of diagnosis of PCL.

Kaposi's Sarcoma

Epidemiology, Virology, and Pathogenesis

Soon after the first events of the HIV epidemic, the *New York Times* headline "Rare cancer seen in 41 homosexuals" referred to cases of KS. This aggressive and frequently fatal epidemic variant of KS affected homosexual men with AIDS approximately 20 times as frequently as male patients with hemophilia and AIDS who had similar degrees of immunosuppression.[75–79] Although the incidence of KS in American men with AIDS decreased from 40% in 1981 to less than 20% in 1992, it remains today the most common AIDS-associated cancer in the U.S. and an important cause of morbidity and mortality worldwide, particularly in Sub-Saharan Africa.[80–87]

A total of four clinical variants of KS have now been described—classical, endemic, iatrogenic (post-transplant), and epidemic (AIDS-associated) forms[88]—but in the light of recent discoveries regarding the viral pathogenesis of KS, these variants are now thought to represent different manifestations of the same pathologic process.[89]

It was noted early in the HIV pandemic that AIDS-associated KS was more prevalent in gay men than in other transmission groups, and this observation lead Valerie Beral and Harold Jaffe to propose that a second infectious agent could account for the prevalence of KS in immunodeficient patients.[77,90] In 1994, Chang and colleagues[91] used representational difference analysis to identify DNA fragments of a previously unrecognized herpesvirus, which they called Kaposi's sarcoma–associated herpesvirus (KSHV), also known as human herpesvirus-8 (HHV-8).[91] This was the second oncogenic virus, after human papillomavirus, to be identified by molecular techniques. Soon after, KSHV was implicated in the etiopathology of primary effusion lymphoma (PEL)[92] and multicentric Castleman's disease (MCD),[93,94] the management of which will be discussed later. Although studies have been published on the contribution of cytokines as well as HIV-1 tat protein in the pathogenesis of KS, the presence of KSHV is a necessary factor in the development of this tumor, and it can be found in every KS lesion, at every stage of its development. In addition, immunosuppression in the host appears to be an important cofactor in the clinical expression of KS in KSHV-infected individuals.[95]

The 165Kb KSHV genome was sequenced within 2 years of the virus' discovery, and it provided initial clues about the way in which this virus might induce uncontrolled cellular proliferation.[96] Unusual to KSHV (among the herpesviruses) and its newly discovered primate cousins is the very large number of genes encoding homologs of host genes.[97–105] For example, KSHV encodes a homolog of cyclin D2, whereas the related gammaherpesvirus, EBV LMP-1, induces cyclin D2 in B-cells (which normally do not express this protein).[106] It is thought that the acquisition of host genes may enable KSHV to utilize many host cellular processes and avoid antiviral responses. The virus encodes proteins that are homologous to human oncoproteins, including another cyclin that inhibits the retinoblastoma protein, which controls the G1-to-S phase of cell growth, and a Bcl-2–like protein that prevents apoptosis.[107–110]

KSHV also encodes a viral homolog of interleukin-6 (IL-6), which is thought to act in a paracrine manner and stimulate a local acute phase response. Increased levels of IL-6 are found in tissues affected by KSHV, and IL-6 is thought to be an important growth factor in not only KSHV driven neoplasms[111–114] but also in lymphomas driven by Epstein-Barr virus.[115,116] As such, there are data that suggest that KS is not a clonal neoplasm, per se, but begins as a localized inflammatory response.[117]

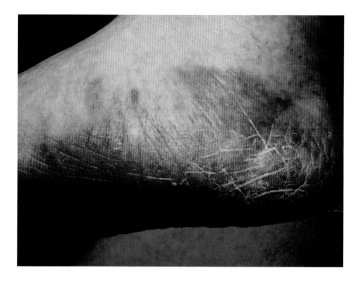

Figure 24–2. *Reddish-purple well demarcated plaque on the instep of an AIDS patient with Kaposi's sarcoma.*

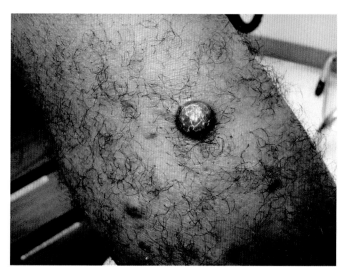

Figure 24–3. *Opposite of the same patient in* **Figure 24–4** *with purple color and induration of the entire lower extremity between the knee and the ankle representing extensive Kaposi's sarcoma.*

Clinical Features

The first cases of KS described in 1872 were observed to be "idiopathic pigmented multiple sarcomas of the skin."[118] AIDS-related KS exhibits a wide spectrum of clinical presentations, and some patients may have few lesions, others have many, and these sometimes develop rapidly.[82] The earliest cutaneous lesions are frequently asymptomatic, innocuous-looking, macular, pigmented lesions, which vary in color from faint pink (**Figure 24–2**) to vivid purple (**Figure 24–3**). Larger plaques occur, usually on the trunk, as oblong lesions following the line of skin creases. Lesions may develop to form large plaques and nodules (**Figure 24–4**) that can be associated with painful edema. Lymphatic infiltration is a common feature in the limbs and causes lymphedema and ulceration.

Oral lesions are a frequent accompaniment that may lead to ulceration, dysphagia, and secondary infection. Gastrointestinal lesions are usually asymptomatic but may bleed or cause obstruction. Pulmonary KS is a life-threatening complication that usually presents with dyspnea and a dry cough, with or without fever, and may cause hemoptysis. Chest radiographs typically reveal a diffuse, reticulonodular infiltrate and pleural effusion. The main differential diagnosis of

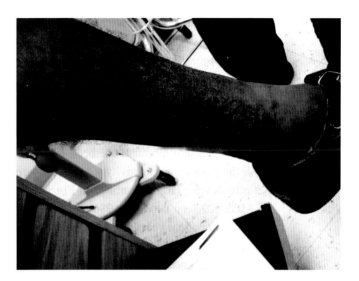

Figure 24–4. *Inner leg near the knee in an AIDS patient who stopped his medications on his own for several months He then developed purplish induration over both lower legs and this exophytic pink tumor. Both areas were positive for Kaposi's sarcoma.*

cutaneous KS is bacillary angiomatosis, a feline zoonosis caused by *Bartonella henselae*, a fastidious gram-negative bacterium of the Rickettsia family.[119–121]

Treatment of KS

The prognosis of patients with KS depends on the stage of the KS, the level of immunosuppression, and the response to anti-HIV therapy.[122] KS is staged using the AIDS clinical trials group modified staging classification (**Table 24–1**). For patients with symptomatic disease or life-threatening visceral disease, prompt effective therapy is usually merited; for patients with asymptomatic indolent lesions, HAART alone may result in complete regression.

HAART in KS

Current data suggest that there has been a fall in the incidence of KS, both as a first AIDS diagnosis and a subsequent manifestation in HIV-seropositive cohorts from established market economies. This decline in KS coincides with the introduction of HAART regimens, and in some cohort studies, the relative risk of developing KS is significantly lower among people receiving HAART.[21,25,124–126] A large number of case reports and small studies documenting responses of KS to HAART have been published, and regression of KS during monotherapy with zidovudine (AZT) has also been observed.[127]

TABLE 24–1	The Modified AIDS Clinical Trials Group Staging of KS (1997)[123]		
	Good risk (all of the following) T0 I0	**Poor risk (any of the following) T1 I1**
Tumor (T)	Confined to skin, lymph nodes or minimal oral disease	Tumor-associated edema or ulceration Extensive oral KS Gastrointestinal KS KS in other non-nodal viscera
Immune status (I)	CD4 count >150 cells/mm^3	CD4 <150 cells/mm^3

with the vehicle gel demonstrated an objective response ($p = 0.002$).[146] Application-site reactions (i.e. erythema, bruising, flaking) were common, but rarely severe.[147,148] Additional topical treatments available include liquid nitrogen.

Larger cutaneous or oral lesions may be treated with radiotherapy, and local control is generally achieved. For cutaneous lesions, either a single fraction of 8Gy or 16Gy in four fractions is routinely used. Although the response rate and duration of local control may be better with fractionated regimens compared to single-fraction treatment, toxicity and patient convenience are worse. Cosmetic improvement is usually achieved, although there may be a halo appearance due to the margin around treated lesions. Severe mucositis and acute edema reactions may follow radiation treatment of the oral cavity and feet, and for this reason, treatment is given in four fractions at weekly intervals. Recurrent tumor is common and, therefore, radiotherapy treatment is usually reserved for symptomatic and cosmetically disturbing lesions.[149]

Future Developments for AIDS-Related Kaposi's Sarcoma

KS has been recognized as a clinical entity for well over a century and has been a known complication of HIV infection for 3 decades. It is only in the last few years since the discovery of KSHV as its causative agent that the multiplicity of factors in KS pathogenesis are being unravelled. A wide variety of treatments appear able to inhibit KS growth, including antiretrovirals, cytotoxic chemotherapeutic agents, retinoids, thalidomide, and inhibitors of matrix metalloproteinases. There is also considerable interest in evaluating the role of antiherpes drugs for KS. The role of interferon-α, both pegylated and nonpegylated forms are being established in clinical trials following significant evidence of antineoplastic and antiviral activity in vitro.

An improved understanding of the functions of the KSHV genes, the identification of novel immune-evasion strategies, and the analysis of the KS microenvironment in the context of a viral infection, should lead to a better understanding of angiogenesis, the immune system and the interaction of viruses with their hosts. This will help us to design safer strategies to treat virus-induced pathology. As many cases of KS do not resolve with HAART and require treatment with cytotoxic chemotherapy, it is also important to reveal the underlying mechanisms involved in the response to treatment.

Cervical Cancer

Epidemiology

Invasive cervical cancer was included as an AIDS-defining diagnosis in 1993, although the incidence of cervical cancer was not then increased significantly in HIV-seropositive women.[9,150] Nonetheless there is good epidemiologic evidence that the precursor lesions—cervical intraepithelial neoplasia (CIN) or squamous intraepithelial lesion (SIL)—occur more frequently in women with HIV.[151] Human papilloma virus (HPV) has a central role in the pathogenesis of both CIN and invasive cervical cancer. HIV is associated with a higher prevalence of HPV in the cervix, a high frequency of multiple HPV genotypes, and persistence of HPV in the cervix, as well as a higher prevalence of CIN/SIL, a higher progression from low-grade SIL (LGSIL) to high-grade SIL (HGSIL), and a greater likelihood of relapse of CIN II/III after therapy. The risk for SIL is greatest amongst women with CD4 cell counts <200cells/mm^3. These findings mandate close colposcopic surveillance.[152]

Effects of HAART on Pre-Invasive Cervical Cancer

The effect of HAART on the natural history of CIN has been addressed in women with advanced HIV. Five months after starting HAART, the prevalence of CIN fell from 66% to 49%, regression of HGSIL to LGSIL occurred in 23%, and the regression from LGSIL to normal in 43%. These changes occurred without a significant change in the level of HPV DNA in cervical tissue.[153] In a recent Women's Interagency HIV study (WIHS) cohort from five U.S. cities, the effect of HAART on CIN was assessed by 6 monthly smear testings. After adjustment for CD4 cell count and Papanicolaou smear status, women on HAART were 40% (95% CI, 4–81) more likely to demonstrate regression and less likely (odds ratio, 0.68; 95% CI, 0.52–0.88) to demonstrate progression.[154] However, the benefits of HAART have not been reproduced in all studies, and HAART appears to have limited ability to clear HPV infection and induce regression of CIN in HIV-positive women. Current data suggest that frequent cervical smears should be offered to all HIV-positive women and that CIN should be aggressively treated in these women.

Invasive Cervical Cancer Management

In most centers, HIV-seropositive women with invasive cervical cancer are treated using the same protocols as are used in immunocompetent women. One retrospective series compared 28 HIV-positive women with 132 seronegative women treated at the same institution and during the same time period. The results demonstrated that women with HIV had more advanced cervical cancer at presentation.[155] A similar case control study from the same institution demonstrated that women with cervical cancer who were HIV-seropositive relapsed more frequently and had a worse median survival.[156] Although there is hope that the survival of invasive cervical cancer may improve with the introduction of HAART, there is scant data to support this optimism.[157]

As HPV also causes anal intraepithelial neoplasia (AIN), the precursor lesion for anal cancer, we have examined whether effective HAART leads to regression of AIN. Results were inconclusive,[158] although we did find in 99 men that anal cytology by the Palefsky method is simple to undertake, has a sensitivity and specificity comparable with cervical cytology, and can therefore be used as the basis of a pilot screening project in centers with large cohorts of HIV-positive homosexual men who have a high risk for developing anal carcinoma.[159] Unlike other HIV-associated cancers, there has been no significant change in the incidence, clinical features, or overall survival since the introduction of HAART.[160]

Primary Effusion Lymphoma (PEL)

PEL is an unusual lymphoproliferative disorder, accounting for 2% or less of HIV-associated lymphomas, and is even more rarely encountered in the HIV-seronegative patient. PEL is divided into classic and solid variants. Classic PEL is characterized by lymphomatous involvement of the serosal surfaces, whereas solid PEL manifests initially with tissue-based tumors and no malignant effusions.[161,162] They are similar by morphology, immunophenotype, and molecular analysis. KSHV, along with high levels of interleukin (e.g., IL-6) may be found in PEL tumor cells, and this is frequently necessary to aid in the diagnosis. The ramifications of large and typically recurrent pleural, pericardial, and peritoneal effusions are grave and are responsible for the high morbidity and mortality associated with this condition.[163]

PEL cells have a characteristic phenotype highlighted by CD45, CD30, CD38, CD138 and MUM1 coexpression.[161] Classic B-cell markers (CD19, CD20) and T-cell markers (CD2, CD3,

CD5, CD7) are not typically seen. Gene expression profiling has shown that PEL expresses a gene profile distinct from other lymphomas, but more akin to multiple myeloma cell lines.

There is no clear standard of care established in the treatment of PEL, and due to its low incidence, randomized clinical trials at present are not feasible. As with the other KSHV-associated diseases, if HIV coinfection is identified, antiretroviral therapy is critical. Spontaneous regression with the commencement of HAART has been described.[164] Traditionally, the use of standard cytotoxic regimens used for non-Hodgkin's lymphomas are suboptimal, and median survival in treated cohorts is poor. Induction of apoptosis with the inhibition of nuclear factor kappa B (NF-κB) in PEL cell lines has led to the investigation of proteasome inhibitors, which decrease the activation of NF-κB and its antiapoptotic effects.[165] Bortezomib, a proteosome inhibitor that is FDA-approved in the U.S. for use in multiple myeloma, has been shown to enhance the in vitro cytotoxic effects of doxorubicin and paclitaxel, and has been used successfully in combination with anthracycline-based cytotoxic chemotherapy regimens. Inhibition of mTOR with rapamycin is effective at decreasing in vitro PEL growth and in vivo mouse xenograft model tumor growth, and its increasing use in the treatment of PEL can be foreseen.[166] Cases of prolonged survival in persons treated adjunctively with antiviral therapy (ganciclovir or cidofovir) have also prompted the adjunctive use of these drugs in PEL. Valproate to treat PEL induces lytic KSHV replication and leads to apoptosis in combination with antiviral agents.

Multicentric Castleman Disease (MCD)

MCD is a rare lymphoproliferation, and we have calculated that in the HAART era it has an incidence of 4.3/10,000 patient years.[167] MCD is an aggressive lymphoproliferative disorder, characterized by constitutional symptoms, anemia, and generalized lymphadenopathy. Small series have shown that most MCD cases are driven by KSHV, including 100% of HIV-seropositive patients and the majority of HIV-negative patients.[168] The failure to identify KSHV in all MCD lesions may reflect technical limitations in KSHV detection, the ability for KSHV to induce MCD distant to the biopsied tissue, or an alternate etiology for a limited number of cases. On occasion, MCD may be associated with non-Hodgkin's lymphoma, particularly the plasmablastic variant. A key to making the diagnosis is to suspect MCD in high-risk individuals who present in the appropriate clinical context—that is, an immunosuppressed individual with KSHV infection or other KSHV-associated disease. A definitive diagnosis can only be made by pathologic examination of an involved lymph node or extranodal mass. Detection of KSHV in biopsied tissue or in the peripheral blood can aid in the diagnosis. C-reactive protein, KSHV viral load, and serum IL-6 levels, if available, may be useful as markers of disease activity and response to therapy.[169]

In patients with MCD and HIV infection, treatment with antiretroviral therapy is necessary, but caution should be taken as life-threatening flares of MCD have been reported as a manifestation of immune reconstitution. Splenectomy can be useful in establishing the diagnosis and can induce clinical remissions; however, these remissions are short-lived, and relapse typically occurs within a few months. Systemic therapy is the mainstay of treatment for patients with MCD, and ranges from aggressive remission-induction chemotherapy regimens—CHOP (cyclophosphamide-doxorubicin-vincristine-prednisone); ABV (doxorubicin-bleomycin-vincristine); single-agent maintenance chemotherapy (oral etoposide, cyclophosphamide, vinblastine); immunomodulatory agents (thalidomide, interferon-α); and monoclonal antibodies against the IL-6 receptor (altizumab) and CD-20 (rituximab).[170]

Among all of these treatments, rituximab has shown the most promise in inducing durable remissions. In a prospective study of 24 individuals with chemotherapy-dependent HIV-associated MCD, rituximab was associated with sustained remission off treatment at day 60 (the primary end point) in 22 patients (92%).[66] More recently, the efficacy and safety of four weekly infusions of rituximab in 21 consecutive patients with previously untreated plasmablastic HIV-associated MCD has been investigated.[171] All but one patient achieved clinical remission of symptoms, hematologic and serum chemistry normalization, and 70% achieved a radiologic response. In three patients who relapsed, retreatment with rituximab was successful.[172] The main adverse event seen in these patients is reactivation of KS, which is intriguing and may be due to a rapid B cell depletion that is observed during rituximab therapy, or an immune reconstitution inflammatory syndrome to hitherto latent antigens. Rituximab therapy in this study was shown to be associated with a decline in KSHV levels initially and at the successful treatment of relapse.

Given the lytic nature of KSHV in MCD, antiviral therapy is also a consideration. A recent randomized controlled trial demonstrated the efficacy of valganciclovir in reducing KSHV replication in individuals with KSHV infection but without evidence of KS, PEL, or MCD. In patients with MCD, ganciclovir and valganciclovir have been independently shown to induce remissions alone or in combination with other agents.[173]

Conclusion

In the 1960s, the U.S. Surgeon General at that time announced that infectious diseases would no longer be a problem. This followed the eradication of both smallpox and polio. Since the 1980s, approximately 22 million persons have died of AIDS, often as a result of ensuing cancers, which can, in some ways, be regarded as opportunistic infections themselves. The peak of the AIDS epidemic in the U.S. occurred in 1993, and by 1995 there was a decline in the incidence of new patients due to the widespread use of HAART (which, in resource-rich regions, resulted in a 73% decrease in the development of AIDS among HIV-infected people, and an equally remarkable 75% decline in mortality among patients with AIDS). Nonetheless, the prevalence of HIV continues to increase, driven by a stable number of new infections each year and longer survival of those infected.

HAART has also been associated with dramatic decreases in the incidence of Kaposi's sarcoma and, to a lesser extent, AIDS-related lymphoma. It is now clear that effective control of the underlying HIV and its related immunosuppression prevents development of these cancers. However, the vast majority of HIV-infected individuals do not have access to HAART because of financial and social circumstances. Thus, we are left with the stark reality that malignant disease may be preventable, but only in resource-rich areas of the world.

An understanding of the pathways that EBV, KSHV, and HPV utilize to induce cellular proliferation provides us an understanding of conserved pathways in cellular evolution. Their targeting will undoubtedly reveal new mechanisms involved in transformation, and the hope is that these will, in turn, reveal new drug targets that will help eradicate both HIV and cancer.

References

1. Gottlieb MS, Schroff R, Schanker HM, Weisman JD, Fan PT, Wolf RA, Saxon A. Pneumocystis carinii pneumonia and mucosal candidiasis in previously healthy homosexual men: evidence of a new acquired cellular immunodeficiency. N Engl J Med 1981;305:1425–1431.

2. Harris C, Small CB, Klein RS, Friedland GH, Moll B, Emeson EE, Spigland I, Steigbigel NH. Immunodeficiency in female sexual partners of men with the acquired immunodeficiency syndrome. N Engl J Med 1983;308:1181–1184.

3. Stebbing J, Bower M. What can oncologists learn from HIV? Lancet Oncol 2003;4:438–445.

4. Ziegler JL, Templeton AC, Vogel CL. Kaposi's sarcoma: a comparison of classical, endemic, and epidemic forms. Seminars in Oncology. 1984;11:47–52.

5. Boring CC, Brynes RK, Chan WC, Causey N, Gregory HR, Nadel MR, Greenberg RS. Increase in high-grade lymphomas in young men. Lancet 1985;1:857–859

6. Levine AM, Gill PS, Meyer PR, Burkes RL, Ross R, Dworsky RD, Krailo M, Parker JW, Lukes RJ, Rasheed S. Retrovirus and malignant lymphoma in homosexual men. JAMA 1985;254:1921–1925.

7. Stebbing J, Marvin V, Bower M. The evidence-based treatment of AIDS-related non-Hodgkin's lymphoma. Cancer Treat Rev 2004;30:249–253.

8. Thirlwell C, Sarker D, Stebbing J, Bower M. Acquired immunodeficiency syndrome-related lymphoma in the era of highly active antiretroviral therapy. Clin Lymphoma 2003,4.86–92

9. Phelps RM, Smith DK, Heilig CM, Gardner LI, Carpenter CC, Klein RS, Jamieson DJ, Vlahov D, Schuman P, Holmberg SD. Cancer incidence in women with or at risk for HIV. Int J Cancer 2001;94:753–757.

10. Powles T, Bower M, Daugaard G, Shamash J, de Ruiter A, Johnson M, Fisher M, Anderson J, Mandalia S, Stebbing J, Nelson M, Gazzard B, Oliver T. Multicenter study of human immunodeficiency virus-related germ cell tumors. J Clin Oncol 2003;21:1922–1927.

11. Palella FJ, Jr., Delaney KM, Moorman AC, Loveless MO, Fuhrer J, Satten GA, Aschman DJ, Holmberg SD. Declining morbidity and mortality among patients with advanced human immunodeficiency virus infection. HIV Outpatient Study Investigators. N Engl J Med 1998;338:853–860

12. Stebbing J, Gazzard B. Stemming the epidemic: prevention and therapy go hand-in-hand. J HIV Therapy 2003;8:51–55.

13. Jacobson L. Impact of highly effective anti-retroviral therapy on the incidence of malignancies among HIV infected individuals. Bethesda: J AIDS Hum Retrovirol;1998:A39.

14. Matthews GV, Bower M, Mandalia S, Powles T, Nelson MR, Gazzard BG. Changes in acquired immunodeficiency syndrome-related lymphoma since the introduction of highly active antiretroviral therapy. Blood 2000;96:2730–2734.

15. Beral V, Newton R, Reeves G, collaborators. obotsa. International collaboration on HIV and cancer. J AIDS 2000;23:A8.

16. Beral V, Peterman T, Berkelman R, Jaffe H. AIDS-associated non-Hodgkin lymphoma. Lancet 1991;337:805–809.

17. Biggar RJ, Rosenberg PS, Cote T. Kaposi's sarcoma and non-Hodgkin's lymphoma following the diagnosis of AIDS. Multistate AIDS/Cancer Match Study Group. Int J Cancer 1996;68:754–758.

18. Auperin I, Mikolt J, Oksenhendler E, Thiebaut JB, Brunet M, Dupont B, Morinet F. Primary central nervous system malignant non-Hodgkin's lymphomas from HIV-infected and non-infected patients: expression of cellular surface proteins and Epstein-Barr viral markers. Neuropathol Appl Neurobiol 1994;20:243–252.

19. Ledergerber B, Telenti A, Egger M, Study ftSHC. Risk of HIV related Kaposi's sarcoma and Non-Hodgkin's lymphoma with potent antiretroviral therapy: prospective cohort study. British Med J 1999;319:23–24.

20. Inungu J, Melendez MF, Montgomery JP. AIDS-related primary brain lymphoma in Michigan, January 1990 to December 2000. AIDS Patient Care STDS. 2002;16:107–112.

21. Portsmouth S, Stebbing J, Gill J, Mandalia S, Bower M, Nelson M, Gazzard B. A comparison of regimens based on non-nucleoside reverse transcriptase inhibitors or protease inhibitors in preventing Kaposi's sarcoma. AIDS 2003;17:17–22.

22. Autran B, Carcelain G, Debre P. Immune reconstitution after highly active anti-retroviral treatment of HIV infection. Adv Exp Med Biol 2001;495:205–212.

23. Lederman M. Immune restoration and CD4+ T-cell function with antiretroviral therapies. AIDS 2001;15 Suppl 2:S11–S15.

24. International Collaboration on HIV and Cancer: Highly Active Antiretroviral Therapy and Incidence of Cancer in Human Immunodeficiency Virus-Infected Adults. J Natl Cancer Inst 2000;92:1823–1830.

25. Rabkin CS. AIDS and cancer in the era of highly active antiretroviral therapy (HAART). Eur J Cancer 2001;37:1316–1319.

26. Stebbing J, Gazzard B, Mandalia S, Teague A, Waterston A, Marvin V, Nelson M, Bower M. Antiretroviral treatment regimens and immune parameters in the prevention of systemic AIDS-related non-Hodgkin's lymphoma. J Clin Oncol 2004;22:2177–2183.

27. Wilde JT, Lee CA, Darby SC, Kan SW, Giangrande P, Phillips AN, Winter M, Spooner R, Ludlam CA. The incidence of lymphoma in the UK haemophilia population between 1978 and 1999. Aids 2002;16:1803–1807.

28. Fong IW, Ho J, Toy C, Lo B, Fong MW. Value of long-term administration of acyclovir and similar agents for protecting against AIDS-related lymphoma: case-control and historical cohort studies. Clin Infect Dis 2000;30:757–761.

29. Bossolasco S, Cinque P, Ponzoni M, Vigano MG, Lazzarin A, Linde A, Falk KI. Epstein-Barr virus DNA load in cerebrospinal fluid and plasma of patients with AIDS-related lymphoma. J Neurovirol 2002;8:432–438.

30. Van Baarle D, Wolthers KC, Hovenkamp E, Niesters HG, Osterhaus AD, Miedema F, Van Oers MH. Absolute level of Epstein-Barr virus DNA in human immunodeficiency virus type 1 infection is not predictive of AIDS-related non-Hodgkin lymphoma. J Infect Dis 2002;186:405–409.

31. Scadden DT, Zeira M, Woon A, Wang Z, Schieve L, Ikeuchi K, Lim B, Groopman JE. Human immunodeficiency virus infection of human bone marrow stromal fibroblasts. Blood 1992;76:317–322.

32. Sitalakshmi S, Srikrishna A, Damodar P. Haematological changes in HIV infection. Indian J Pathol Microbiol 2003;46:180–183.

33. Sarker D, Thirlwell C, Nelson M, Gazzard B, Bower M. Leptomeningeal disease in AIDS-related non-Hodgkin's lymphoma. AIDS 2003;17:861–865.

34. Massarweh S, Udden MM, Shahab I, Kroll M, Sears DA, Lynch GR, Teh BS, Lu HH. HIV-related Hodgkin's disease with central nervous system involvement and association with Epstein-Barr virus. Am J Hematol 2003;72:216–219.

35. Desai J, Mitnick R, Henry D, Llena J, Sparano J. Patterns of central nervous system recurrence in patients with systemic human immunodeficiency virus-associated non-Hodgkin lymphoma. Cancer 1999;86:1840–1847.

36. Spina M, Jaeger U, Sparano JA, Talamini R, Simonelli C, Michieli M, Rossi G, Nigra E, Berretta M, Cattaneo C, Rieger AC, Vaccher E, Tirelli U. Rituximab plus infusional cyclophosphamide, doxorubicin, and etoposide in HIV-associated non-Hodgkin lymphoma: pooled results from 3 phase 2 trials. Blood 2005;105:1891–1897.

37. Navarro JT, Ribera JM, Oriol A, Vaquero M, Romeu J, Batlle M, Flores A, Milla F, Feliu E. Influence of highly active anti-retroviral therapy on response to treatment and survival in patients with acquired immunodeficiency syndrome-related non-Hodgkin's lymphoma treated with cyclophosphamide, hydroxydoxorubicin, vincristine and prednisone. Br J Haematol 2001;112:909–915.

38. Spina M, Carbone A, Vaccher E, Gloghini A, Talamini R, Cinelli R, Martellotta F, Tirelli U. Outcome in patients with non-hodgkin lymphoma and with or without human immunodeficiency virus infection. Clin Infect Dis 2004;38:142–144.

39. Antinori A, Cingolani A, Alba L, Ammassari A, Serraino D, Ciancio BC, Palmieri F, De Luca A, Larocca LM, Ruco L, Ippolito G, Cauda R. Better response to chemotherapy and prolonged survival in AIDS-related lymphomas responding to highly active antiretroviral therapy. AIDS 2001;15:1483–1491.

40. Besson C, Goubar A, Gabarre J, Rozenbaum W, Pialoux G, Chatelet FP, Katlama C, Charlotte F, Dupont B, Brousse N, Huerre M, Mikol J, Camparo P, Mokhtari K, Tulliez M, Salmon-Ceron D, Boue F, Costagliola D, Raphael M. Changes in AIDS-related lymphoma since the era of highly active antiretroviral therapy. Blood 2001;98:2339–2344.

41. Bower M, Stern S, Fife K, Nelson M, Gazzard BG. Weekly alternating combination chemotherapy for good prognosis AIDS-related lymphoma. Eur J Cancer 2000;36:363–367.

42. Sparano JA, Lee S, Henry DH, Ambinder RF, von Roenn J, Tirelli U. Infusional cyclophosphamide, doxorubicin and etoposide in HIV associated non-Hodgkin's lymphoma: A review of the Einstein, Aviano and ECOG experience in 182 patients. J AIDS 2000;23:A11.

43. Sparano JA, Wiernik PH, Hu X, Sarta C, Schwartz EL, Soeiro R, Henry DH, Mason B, Ratech H, Dutcher JP. Pilot trial of infusional cyclophosphamide, doxorubicin and etoposide plus didanosine and filgrastim in patients with HIV associated non-Hodgkin's lymphoma. J Clin Oncol 1996;14:3026–3035.

44. Sparano JA, Anand K, Desai J, Mitnick RJ, Kalkut GE, Hanau LH. Effect of highly active antiretroviral therapy on the incidence of HIV-associated malignancies at an urban medical center. J Acquir Immune Defic Syndr 1999;21 Suppl 1:18–22.

45. Bower M, McCall-Peat N, Ryan N, Davies L, Young AM, Gupta S, Nelson M, Gazzard B, Stebbing J. Protease inhibitors potentiate chemotherapy-induced neutropenia. Blood 2004;104:2943–2946.

46. Little R, Pearson D, Gutierrez M, Steinberg S, Yarchoan R, Wilson W. Dose-adjusted chemotherapy with suspension of antiretroviral therapy for HIV-associated non-Hodgkin's lymphoma. J AIDS 2000;23:A11.

47. Little RF, Pittaluga S, Grant N, Steinberg SM, Kavlick MF, Mitsuya H, Franchini G, Gutierrez M, Raffeld M, Jaffe ES, Shearer G, Yarchoan R, Wilson WH. Highly effective treatment of acquired immunodeficiency syndrome-related lymphoma with dose-adjusted EPOCH: impact of antiretroviral therapy suspension and tumor biology. Blood 2003;101:4653–4659.

48. Levine AM, Wernz JC, Kaplan L, Rodman N, Cohen P, Metroka C, Bennett JM, Rarick MU, Walsh C, Kahn J. Low dose chemotherapy with central nervous system prophylaxis and zidovudine maintenance in AIDS-related lymphoma. J Am Med Assoc 1991;266:84–88.

49. Kaplan JE, Masur H, Holmes KK. Guidelines for preventing opportunistic infections among HIV-infected persons--2002. Recommendations of the U.S. Public Health Service and the Infectious Diseases Society of America. MMWR Recomm Rep 2002;51:1–52.

50. Yeni PG, Hammer SM, Hirsch MS, Saag MS, Schechter M, Carpenter CC, Fischl MA, Gatell JM, Gazzard BG, Jacobsen DM, Katzenstein DA, Montaner JS, Richman DD, Schooley RT, Thompson MA, Vella S, Volberding PA. Treatment for adult HIV infection: 2004 recommendations of the International AIDS Society-USA Panel. JAMA 2004;292:251–265.

51. Zanussi S, Simonelli C, D'Andrea M, Comar M, Bidoli E, Giacca M, Tirelli U, Vaccher E, De Paoli P. The effects of antineoplastic chemotherapy on HIV disease. AIDS Res Hum Retroviruses 1996;12:1703–1707.

52. Powles T, Imami N, Nelson M, Gazzard BG, Bower M. Effects of combination chemotherapy and highly active antiretroviral therapy on immune parameters in HIV-1 associated lymphoma. AIDS 2002;16.531–330.

53. Vaccher E, Spina M, di Gennaro G, Talamini R, Nasti G, Schioppa O, Vultaggio G, Tirelli U. Concomitant cyclophosphamide, doxorubicin, vincristine, and prednisone chemotherapy plus highly active antiretroviral therapy in patients with human immunodeficiency virus-related, non-Hodgkin lymphoma. Cancer 2001;91:155–163.

54. Ratner L, Lee J, Tang S, Redden D, Hamzeh F, Herndier B, Scadden D, Kaplan L, Ambinder R, Levine A, Harrington W, Grochow L, Flexner C, Tan B, Straus D. Chemotherapy for human immunodeficiency virus-associated non-Hodgkin's lymphoma in combination with highly active antiretroviral therapy. J Clin Oncol 2001;19:2171–2178.

55. Cortes J, Thomas D, Rios A, Koller C, O'Brien S, Jeha S, Faderl S, Kantarjian H. Hyperfractionated cyclophosphamide, vincristine, doxorubicin, and dexamethasone and highly active antiretroviral therapy for patients with acquired immunodeficiency syndrome-related Burkitt lymphoma/leukemia. Cancer 2002;94:1492–1499.

56. Thirlwell C, Stebbing J, Nelson M, Gazzard B, Bower M. CDE chemotherapy plus HAART for AIDS-related non-Hodgkin's lymphoma. 6th International Congress on Drug Therapy in HIV infection. Glasgow; 2002:94.

57. Lascaux AS, Hemery F, Goujard C, Lesprit P, Delfraissy JF, Sobel A, Lepage E, Levy Y. Beneficial effect of highly active antiretroviral therapy on the prognosis of AIDS-related systemic non-Hodgkin lymphomas. AIDS Res Hum Retroviruses 2005;21:214–220.

58. Lester R, Li C, Galbraith P, Vickars L, Leitch H, Phillips P, Shenkier T, Gascoyne R. Improved outcome of human immunodeficiency virus-associated plasmablastic lymphoma of the oral cavity in the era of highly active antiretroviral therapy: a report of two cases. Leuk Lymphoma 2004;45:1881–1885.

59. Rossi G, Donisi A, Casari S, Re A, Cadeo G-P, Carosi G. The International Prognostic Index can be used as a guide to treatment decisions regarding patients with human immunodeficiency virus-related non-Hodgkin lymphoma. Cancer 1999;86:2391–2397.

60. Molina A, Krishnan AY, Nademanee A, Zabner R, Sniccinski I, Zaia J, Forman SJ. High dose therapy and autologous stem cell transplantation for human immunodeficiency virus-associated non-Hodgkin lymphoma in the era of highly active antiretroviral therapy. Cancer 2000;89:680–689.

61. Gabarre J, Azar N, Autran B, Katlama C, Leblond V. High-dose therapy and autologous haematopoietic stem-cell transplantation for HIV-1-associated lymphoma. Lancet 2000;355:1071–1072.

62. Kentos A, Vekemans M, Van Vooren JP, Lambermont M, Liesnard C, Feremans W, Farber CM. High-dose chemotherapy and autologous CD34-positive blood stem cell transplantation for multiple myeloma in an HIV carrier. Bone Marrow Transplant 2002;29:273–275.

63. Re A, Cattaneo C, Michieli M, Casari S, Spina M, Rupolo M, Allione B, Nosari A, Schiantarelli C, Vigano M, Izzi I, Ferremi P, Lanfranchi A, Mazzuccato M, Carosi G, Tirelli U, Rossi G. High-dose therapy and autologous peripheral-blood stem-cell transplantation as salvage treatment for HIV-associated lymphoma in patients receiving highly active antiretroviral therapy. J Clin Oncol 2003;21:4423–4427.

64. MacMahon EM, Glass JD, Hayward SD, Mann RB, Becker PS, Charache P, McArthur JC, Ambinder RF. Epstein-Barr virus in AIDS-related primary central nervous system lymphoma. Lancet 1991;338:969–973.

65. Larocca LM, Capello D, Rinelli A, Nori S, Antinori A, Gloghini A, Cingolani A, Migliazza A, Saglio G, Cammilleri-Broet S, Raphael M, Carbone A, Gaidano G. The molecular and phenotypic profile of primary central nervous system lymphoma identifies distinct categories of the disease and is consistent with histogenetic derivation from germinal center-related B cells. Blood 1998;92:1011–1019.

66. Ivers LC, Kim AY, Sax PE. Predictive value of polymerase chain reaction of cerebrospinal fluid for detection of Epstein-Barr virus to establish the diagnosis of HIV-related primary central nervous system lymphoma. Clin Infect Dis 2004;38:1629–1632.

67. Snider WD, Simpson DM, Nielsen S, Gold JW, Metroka CE, Posner JB. Neurological complications of acquired immune deficiency syndrome: analysis of 50 patients. Ann Neurol 1983;14:403–418.

68. Cheung TW. AIDS-related cancer in the era of highly active antiretroviral therapy (HAART): a model of the interplay of the immune system, virus, and cancer. "On the offensive--the Trojan Horse is being destroyed"—Part B: Malignant lymphoma. Cancer Invest 2004;22:787–798.

69. Cinque P, Brytting M, Vago L, Castagna A, Parravicini C, Zanchetta N, D'Arminio Monforte A, Wahren B, Lazzarin A, Linde A. Epstein-Barr virus DNA in cerebrospinal fluid from patients with AIDS-related primary lymphoma of the central nervous system. Lancet 1993;342:398–401.

70. Arribas J, Clifford D, Fichtenbaum C, Roberts R, Powderly W, Storch G. Detection of Epstein-Barr virus DNA in cerebrospinal fluid for diagnosis of AIDS-related central nervous system lymphoma. J Clin Microbiol 1995;33:1580–1583.

71. Castagna A, Cinque P, d'Amico A, Messa C, Fazsio F, Lazzarin A. Evaluation of contrast-enhancing brain lesions in AIDS patients by means of Epstein-Barr virus detection in cerebrospinal fluid and 201thallium single photon emission tomography. AIDS 1997;11:1522–1523.

72. Bower M, Fife K, Sullivan A, Kirk S, Phillips RH, Nelson M, Gazzard BG. Treatment outcome in presumed and confirmed AIDS-related primary cerebral lymphoma. Eur J Cancer 1999;35:601–604.

73. Jacomet C, Girard P, Lebrette M, Farese V, Monfort L, Rozenbaum W. Intravenous methotrexate for primary central nervous system non-Hodgkin's lymphoma in AIDS. AIDS 1997;11:1725–1730.

74. McGowan JP, Shah S. Long-term remission of AIDS-related primary central nervous system lymphoma associated with highly active antiretroviral therapy. AIDS 1998;12:952–954.

75. Friedman-Kien A, Laubenstein L, Marmor M, al. e. Kaposi's sarcoma and pneumocystis pneumonia among homosexual men-New York and California. MMWR 1981;30:250–254.

76. Friedman-Kien A, Saltzman B. Clinical manifestations of classical, endemic African, and epidemic AIDS-associated Kaposi's sarcoma. J Am Acad Dermato 1990;22:1237–1250.

77. Beral V, Peterman TA, Berkelman RL, Jaffe HW. Kaposi's sarcoma among persons with AIDS: a sexually transmitted infection? Lancet 1990;335:123–128.

78. Frisch M, Biggar RJ, Engels EA, Goedert JJ. Association of cancer with AIDS-related immunosuppression in adults. JAMA 2001;285:1736–1745.

79. Friedman-Kien AE, Saltzman BR, Cao Y, Nestor MS, Mirabile M, Li JJ, Peterman TA. Kaposi's sarcoma in HIV-negative homosexual men. Lancet 1990;335:168–169.

80. Hermans P, Clumeck N. Kaposi's sarcoma in patients infected with human virus (HIV): an overview. [Review]. Cell Mol Biol 1995;41:357–364.

81. Herman PS, Shogreen MR, White WL. The evaluation of human herpesvirus 8 (Kaposi's sarcoma-associated herpesvirus) in cutaneous lesions of Kaposi's sarcoma: a study of formalin-fixed paraffin-embedded tissue. Am J Dermatopathol 1998;20:7–11.

82. Hermans P. Epidemiology, etiology and pathogenesis, clinical presentations and therapeutic approaches in Kaposi's sarcoma: 15-year lessons from AIDS. Biomed Pharmacother 1998;52:440–446.

83. Hermans P, Clumeck N, Picard O, Vooren JP, Duriez P, Zucman D, Bryant JL, Gill P, Lunardi-Iskandar Y, Gallo RC. AIDS-related Kaposi's sarcoma patients with visceral manifestations. Response to human chorionic gonadotropin preparations [In Process Citation]. J Hum Virol 1998;1:82–89.

84. Hermans P, Lundgren J, Sommereijns B, Katlama C, Chiesi A, Goebel FD, Gonzales LJ, Proenza R, Barton SE, Pedersen C, Clumeck N. Survival of European patients with Kaposi's sarcoma as AIDS-defining condition during the first decade of AIDS. AIDS 1997;11:525–531.

85. Herndier B, Ganem D. The biology of Kaposi's sarcoma. Cancer Treat Res 2001;104:89–126.

86. Mueller N, Hatzakis A. Opportunistic malignancies and the acquired immunodeficiency syndrome. Princess Takamatsu Symp 1987;18:159–171.

87. Mueller BU. Cancers in human immunodeficiency virus-infected children. J Natl Cancer Inst Monogr 1998:31–35.

88. Franceschi S, Geddes M. Epidemiology of classic Kaposi's sarcoma, with special reference to mediterranean population. Tumori 1995;81:308–314.

89. Stebbing J, Portsmouth S, Gotch F, Gazzard B. Kaposi's sarcoma--an update. Int J STD AIDS. 2003;14:225–227.

90. Beral V, Bull D, Darby S, Weller I, Carne C, Beecham M, Jaffe H. Risk of Kaposi's sarcoma and sexual practices associated with faecal contact in homosexual or bisexual men with AIDS. Lancet 1992;339:632–635.

91. Chang Y, Cesarman E, Pessin M, Lee F, Culpepper J, Knowles D, Moore P. Identification of herpesvirus-like DNA sequences in AIDS-associated Kaposi's sarcoma. Science 1994;266:1865–1869.

92. Cesarman E, Chang Y, Moore PS, Said JW, Knowles DM. Kaposi's sarcoma-associated herpesvirus-like DNA sequences in AIDS-related body-cavity-based lymphomas. N Engl J Med 1995;332:1186–1191.

93. Soulier J, Grollet L, Oskenhendler E, Cacoub P, Cazals-Hatem D, Babinet P, d'Agay M-F, Clauvel J-P, Raphael M, Degos L, Sigaux F. Kaposi's sarcoma-associated herpesvirus-like DNA sequences in multicentric Castleman's disease. Blood 1995;86:1276–1280.

94. Waterston A, Bower M. Fifty years of multicentric Castleman's disease. Acta Oncol 2004;43:698–704.

95. Stebbing J, Portsmouth S, Bower M. Insights into the molecular biology and sero-epidemiology of Kaposi's sarcoma. Curr Opin Infect Dis 2003;16:25–31.

TABLE 25–1 | **Interventions to Prevent Mother-to-Child Transmission of HIV[a]**

Elective Cesarean Section	Antiretroviral Drugs	Infant Feeding Interventions
Mechanisms		
Intrapartum transmission may occur through: • ascending HIV infection from the genital tract to the amniotic fluid and the fetus after rupture of membranes • microtransfusions between maternal and fetal blood circulation during uterine contractions • exposure to contaminated maternal blood and genital secretions during passage through the birth canal. Elective CS before labor starts and before rupture of membranes eliminates these exposures.	Maternal viral load is the pre-eminent risk factor for MTCT Use of ARV drugs reduces viral load in the plasma, genital tract, and breast milk.	HIV particles are present in the cellular and cell-free compartments of breast milk; the portal of entry is the infant's GI tract, possibly through breaches in the mucosal surface or via cells such as M-cells or enterocytes. Breast milk is thought to maintain or enhance the infant's intestinal barrier function, while nonhuman substances may damage the bowel wall integrity. It is postulated that "mixed feeding" with breast milk and other fluids/foods results in damage to the intestinal wall and entry of HIV. Complete avoidance of breastfeeding eliminates the risk of transmission postnatally. Compared to prolonged "mixed" breastfeeding, exclusive breastfeeding (EBF) and stopping breastfeeding at 6 months carries less risk of postnatal transmission. Other mechanisms to reduce transmission include maternal ARV during breastfeeding to reduce viral load and ARV to the breastfeeding infant (postexposure prophylaxis).
Efficacy/Effectiveness		
• In the European Mode of Delivery trial: 1.8% MTCT rate in the elective CS arm versus 10.5% in the vaginal delivery arm, representing 80% efficacy[4] • 50% reduction in MTCT rate in meta-analysis of > 8,500 mother-child pairs (mainly receiving zidovudine monotherapy)[5]	• The seminal ACTC076 trial demonstrated effectiveness of ARVs in MTCT prevention for the first time: 8.3% MTCT rate in intervention arm (antenatal, intrapartum and neonatal zidovudine) versus 25.5% in the placebo arm.[6] • Antenatal HAART is associated with >90% decreased MTCT risk.	• 3 studies (South Africa, Zimbabwe and Cote d'Ivoire)[7] have shown that exclusive breastfeeding is associated with >50% reduced risk of transmission compared to nonexclusive breastfeeding ("mixed feeding"). • Maternal or infant ARV during pregnancy and breastfeeding further reduces postnatal transmission through breastfeeding to ≤2%.
Coverage/Uptake		
• In Europe, elective CS rates peaked in 2000 at around 70%, but remain high, at ~50%. • Not recommended as a safe public health approach to PMTCT in resource-limited settings.	• In resource-rich settings, >90% of diagnosed pregnant women receive ARVs for PMTCT. • Globally, coverage is around 33%.	• In Europe, most HIV-infected women formula-feed. • In the developing world, risks for transmission with breastfeeding need to be weighed against the hazards of not breastfeeding on an individual basis. For women who choose to breastfeed, exclusive breastfeeding for the first 6 months is recommended. • Although breastfeeding is the cultural norm in resource-limited settings, EBF is rare unless support is given.

[a]ARV=antiretroviral; CS=cesarean section delivery; GI=gastrointestinal; MTCT=mother-to-child transmission; EBF=exclusive breastfeeding.

pathogenesis of postnatal transmission via breast milk is not fully understood, but risk factors include the pattern and duration of breastfeeding and severe breast pathology. Some risk factors are modifiable, and their identification has resulted in development and evaluation of a range of interventions for prevention of MTCT (PMTCT). The three main interventions are use of antiretroviral (ARV) drugs for mother and baby to reduce viral load, elective cesarean section (CS) delivery (which takes place before labor begins and before rupture of membranes), and safe alternatives to breastfeeding (**Table 25–1**). However, despite substantial advances in PMTCT, the complex, multifactorial mechanisms and timing of transmission remain poorly understood.

PMTCT Programs. The World Health Organization (WHO) promotes a comprehensive, strategic approach to the prevention of HIV infection in infants and young children, consisting of four components (**Table 25–2**). Reducing the number of HIV infections among women of childbearing age will have a profound effect in reducing the number of infants at risk for infection, as for each and every avoided HIV infection in a woman of childbearing age there is an avoided infection in any child she might have. Primary prevention will also have an indirect impact on the well-being of children, if HIV infections are prevented in parents. Estimates from models indicate that a decrease in antenatal HIV prevalence of 10% (e.g., from 30% to 20%) would result in a 33% reduction in the annual number of HIV infections in infants. The addition of family planning services to PMTCT programs to prevent unintended pregnancy in HIV-infected women is a highly cost-effective approach to preventing new infections in infants. Furthermore, preventing unwanted pregnancies not only prevents MTCT, but also has the potential to reduce the number of social or "traditional" orphans due to abandonment or to maternal death.

TABLE 25–2	UN Strategic Approach to the Prevention of HIV Infection in Infants		
	Prevention of primary HIV infection	Prevention of unintended pregnancies among women infected with HIV	Prevention of HIV transmission from women infected with HIV to their infants
	Provision of treatment, care, and support to women infected with HIV and to families		

In resource-rich settings, high antenatal coverage, good access to and uptake of a combination of PMTCT interventions and widespread HAART use have contributed to the very low MTCT rates now reported (<1–2%) and small numbers of perinatally-acquired AIDS cases in recent years (**Figures 25–1a** and **25–1b**). However, there are still missed opportunities for PMTCT in these settings particularly among vulnerable groups of women, mainly relating to late or lack of identification of HIV infection in pregnancy. Some infants are infected as a result of missed opportunities for antenatal HIV diagnosis and/or PMTCT, while others are infected despite PMTCT interventions.

In resource-limited settings, while reliable, simple and inexpensive PMTCT regimens such as single-dose nevirapine for mother and infant and abbreviated antenatal ARV prophylaxis are available, estimated global coverage remains below 10%. Although this varies between countries, overall there has been no noticeable impact on the number of infected children born annually[8]. MTCT rates continue to be high, reaching up to 40% if children are exposed to long term breastfeeding into the second year of life, and more than 20% in some places even where

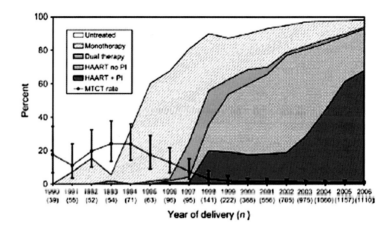

Figure 25–1a. *Use of ART and MTCT rates in 1990–2006 in the UK and Ireland National Study of HIV In Pregnancy and Childhood (NSHPC).*[9]

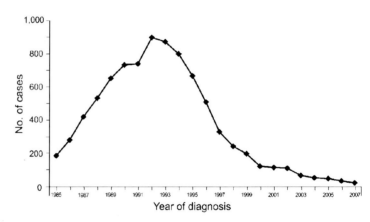

Figure 25–1b. *Estimated numbers of perinatally acquired AIDS cases by year of diagnosis, 1985–2007—United States and dependent area. (Note: Data have been adjusted for reporting delays and missing risk factor information.)*

Source: U.S. Centers for Disease Control and Prevention. Available at: http://www.cdc.gov/hiv/topics/ surveillance/resources/slides/pediatric.

PMTCT programmes are in place. New guidelines for the use of ARV drugs for treating pregnant women and preventing HIV infection in infants were published late in 2009 which should lead to fewer vertically infected infants (**Table 25–3**).

The Role of Infant Feeding in Transmission and Survival. Breastfeeding and HIV has been a subject of debate and disagreement for the past two decades. Prolonged breastfeeding by an HIV-infected woman can double the overall risk of MTCT of HIV from less than 20% to about 40%. Formula feeding has eliminated postnatal transmission via breastfeeding in resource-rich settings; however, this intervention is problematic in many areas of the world where avoidance of all breastfeeding exposes children to different risks including increased mortality risks from infectious diseases and malnutrition due to inadequate replacement feeding. Balancing these risks was difficult without rigorous scientific data. However, new research findings this century have led to our ability to quantify more precisely the transmission risks associated with both the pattern and duration of breastfeeding, and the risks associated with not breastfeeding.

Duration of Breastfeeding[10]. The longer a woman breastfeeds, the greater the risk of HIV transmission. In a meta-analysis of randomized controlled trials from sub-Saharan Africa conducted by the Breastfeeding and HIV International Transmission Study Group (BHITS) in 2004, the cumulative probability of late postnatal transmission at 18 months was 9.3% (95% CI 3.8–14.8%), with an estimated risk of approximately 1% per month of breastfeeding, constant over time from 4 weeks to 18 months (i.e., late postnatal transmission). While breastfeeding

TABLE 25-3	WHO Key Recommendations for the Use of ARV Drugs for Treating Pregnant Women and Preventing HIV Infection in Infants (November 2009)
	• In pregnant women with confirmed HIV serostatus, initiation of ART for her own health is recommended for all HIV-infected pregnant women with CD4 cell count <350 cells/mm^3, irrespective of WHO clinical staging; and for all HIV-infected pregnant women in WHO clinical stage 3 or 4, irrespective of CD4 cell count
	• HIV-infected pregnant women in need of ART for their own health should start ART irrespective of gestational age and continue throughout pregnancy, delivery and thereafter
	• In pregnant women in need of ART for their own health, the preferred first-line ART regimen should include an AZT + 3TC backbone: AZT + 3TC + NVP or AZT + 3TC + EFV. Alternative regimens that are recommended include TDF + 3TC (or FTC) + NVP and TDF + 3TC (or FTC) + EFV
	• Infants born to HIV-infected women receiving ART for their own health should receive: (a) for breastfeeding infants: daily NVP from birth until 6 weeks of age; (b) for nonbreastfeeding infants: daily AZT or NVP from birth until 6 weeks of age
	• All HIV-infected pregnant women who are not in need of ART for their own health require an effective ARV prophyaxis strategy to prevent HIV transmission to the infants. ARV prophylaxis should be started from as early as 14 weeks gestation or as soon as possible when women present late in pregnancy, during labor, or at delivery
	• For all HIV-infected pregnant women who are not in need of ART for their own health, ARV prophylaxis options are: (A) antepartum daily AZT, sd-NVP at onset of labor, AZT + 3TC during labor and delivery, AZT + 3TC for 7 days postpartum. In breastfeeding infants, maternal prophylaxis should be coupled with daily administration of NVP to the infant from birth until one week after all exposure to breast milk has ended; in nonbreastfeeding infants, maternal prophylaxis should be coupled with daily administration of AZT or NVP from birth until 6 weeks of age to the infant; (B) Option B consists of triple ARV drugs starting from as early as 14 weeks of gestation until one week after all exposure to breast milk has ended. In breastfeeding infants, the maternal triple ARV prophylaxis should be coupled with daily administration of NVP to the infant from birth until 6 weeks of age; in non-breastfeeding infants, the maternal triple ARV prophylaxis should be coupled with the daily administration of AZT or NVP to the infant from birth until 6 weeks of age.

transmission may take place from birth to 4 weeks (early postnatal transmission), it is difficult to quantify this risk, as a positive PCR test at around 4 weeks could indicate transmission during delivery or via early breastfeeding. In a pooled analysis of data from South African and West African cohorts, the overall risk of postnatal transmission was greater in children breastfed for more than 6 months, compared to those who ceased breastfeeding early (<6 months 3.9% vs. >6 months 8.7%; adjusted hazard ratio: 1.8).

Pattern of Breastfeeding. The pattern or type of breastfeeding has been shown to be a significant risk factor in MTCT. Most women "mix-feed", introducing other fluids and feeds in addition to breast milk to their children's diets from the first few months of life. Early studies examining risks of MTCT did not distinguish between exclusive breastfeeding (i.e., giving only breast milk to an infant) and mixed breastfeeding. A randomized controlled trial from Kenya,

obstetrics/gynaecology[45]. Management of transition of care from pediatric to adult services varies between and within countries. Careful long-term follow-up of vertically-infected adults is needed, given their life-long HIV infection and complex treatment histories.

Conclusions

Mother-to-child transmission is the dominant mode of acquisition for children. Vertically-acquired pediatric HIV has been almost eliminated in many parts of the developed world, with universal antenatal screening offering infected women the chance of reducing in utero/ perinatal transmission to <2% and safe formula feeding removing any risk of postnatal transmission. The few children who do acquire HIV infection are usually followed from birth and are offered treatment at an early stage, which has reduced mortality from 46% at age ten years with no treatment, to 30% with any ART; further reductions in mortality are achieved with HAART, although the numbers alive at age 10 are not yet available.

In the developing world the situation is less positive, with only 10% of women estimated to access PMTCT interventions, which, with rising antenatal HIV prevalence, results in an estimated 400,000–700,000 children becoming infected each year. HAART and other supportive therapies have been shown to have a similar impact on survival of infected children as in developed countries with substantial improvements seen in survival and general morbidity. The problem of limited resources is compounded by poor health infrastructures and limited laboratory facilities, making diagnosing, monitoring and treating infected children on the scale required problematic.

References

1. UNAIDS. 2008 Report on the Global AIDS Epidemic. Geneva: UNAIDS.
2. ibid.
3. Thorne C, Newell ML. Mother-to-child transmission of HIV infection and its prevention. Curr HIV Res 2003 October;1(4):447–462.
4. European Mode of Delivery Collaboration. Elective caesarean-section versus vaginal delivery in prevention of vertical HIV-1 transmission: a randomised clinical trial. Lancet 1999 March 27;353(9158):1035–1039.
5. The International Perinatal HIV Group. The mode of delivery and the risk of vertical transmission of human immunodeficiency virus type 1—a meta-analysis of 15 prospective cohort studies. N Engl J Med 1999 April 1;340(13):977–987.
6. Connor EM, Sperling RS, Gelber R, Kiselev P, Scott G, O'Sullivan MJ, et al. Reduction of maternal-infant transmission of human immunodeficiency virus type 1 with zidovudine treatment. Pediatric AIDS Clinical Trials Group Protocol 076 Study Group. N Engl J Med 1994 November 3;331(18):1173–1180.
7. HIV Transmission Through Breastfeeding. A Review of Available Evidence. 2007 Update. WHO, UNAIDS, Unicef, UNFPA. ISBN 978 92 4 159659 6. http://www.who.int/child_adolescent_health/documents/9789241596596/en/index.html
8. Ibid UNAIDS 2008.
9. Townsend CL, Cortina-Borja M, Peckham CS, Tookey PA. Trends in management and outcome of pregnancies in HIV-infected women in the UK and Ireland, 1990–2006. BJOG 2008;115(9):1078–1086.
10. The Breastfeeding and HIV International Transmission Study Group (BHITS). Late postnatal transmission of HIV in breast-fed children: an individual patient data meta-analysis. J Infectious Dis 2008;189(12):2154–2166.
11. Nduati R, Mbori-Ngacha D, Richardson B, Overbaugh J, Mwatha A, et al. Effect of breastfeeding and formula feeding on transmission of HIV-1: a randomized clinical trial. JAMA 2000;283(9):1167–1174.
12. Coovadia HM, Rollins N, Bland RM, Little K, Coutsoudis A, Bennish M, Newell ML. Mother-to-child transmission of HIV-1 infection during exclusive breastfeeding in the first 6 months of life: an intervention cohort study. Lancet 2007;369(9567):1107–1116. Illiff PJ, Piwoz EG, Tavengwa NV,

Zunguza CD, Marinda ET, Nathoo KJ, et al. Early exclusive breastfeeding reduces the risk of postnatalHIV-1 transmission and increases HIV-free survival. AIDS 2005;19(7):699–708.

13. Taha T, KumwendaN, Hoover D, Kafulufula G, Fiscus S, Nkhoma C, et al. The impact of breastfeeding on the health of HIV-positive mothers and their children in sub-Saharan Africa. Bull World Health Organization 2006;84(7):546–554. Thior I, Lockman S, Smeaton L, Shapiro R, Wester C, Heymann S. Breastfeeding plus infant zidovudine prophylaxis for 6 months vs formula feeding plus infant zidovudine for 1 month to reduce mother-to-child HIV transmission in Botswana: a randomised trial: the Mashi Study. JAMA 2006;296(7):794–805. Kuhn L, Aldrovandi G, Sinkala M, Kankasa C, Semrau K, Mwiya M, et al. Effects of early, abrupt weaning on HIV-free survival of children in Zambia. N Eng J Med 2008;359(2):130–141.

14. Becquet R, Bequet L, Ekouevid, Vihol, Sakarovitch C, Fassinou P, et al. Two-year morbidity-mortality and alternatives to prolonged breast-feeding among children born to HIV-infected mothers in Cote d'Ivoire. PLoS Med 2007;4(1):e17.

15. Rollins N, Becquet R, Bland RM, Coutsoudis A, Coovadia H, Newell ML. Infant feeding, HIV transmission and mortality at 18 months: the need for appropriate choices by mothers and prioritization within programmes. AIDS 2008;22(17):2349–2357.

16. Bland RM, Little K, Coovadia H, Coutsoudis A, Rollins N, Newell ML. Intervention to promote exclusive breast-feeding for the first 6 months of life in a high HIV prevalence area. AIDS 2008;22(7):883–891.

17. Coovadia HM, Bland RM. Preserving breastfeeding practice through the HIV pandemic. Trop Med Int Health 2007;12(9):1116–1133.

18. Sherman GG, Stevens G, Jones SA, Horsfield P, Stevens WS. Dried blood spots improve access to HIV diagnosis and care for infants in low-resource settings. J Acquir Immune Defic Syndr 2005;38(5):615–617.

19. Blanche S, Newell ML, Mayaux MJ, Dunn DT, Teglas JP, Rouzioux C, et al. Morbidity and mortality in European children vertically infected by HIV-1. The French Pediatric HIV Infection Study Group and European Collaborative Study. J Acquir Immune Defic Syndr Hum Retrovirol 1997;14(5):442–450.

20. European Collaborative Study. Fluctuations in symptoms in human immunodeficiency virus-infected children: the first 10 years of life. Pediatrics 2001;108(1):116–122.

21. European Collaborative Study. Weight, height and human immunodeficiency virus infection in young children of infected mothers. Pediatr Infect Dis J 1995;14(8):685–690.

22. de Martino M, Tovo PA, Galli L, Gabiano C, Chiarelli F, Zappa M, et al. Puberty in perinatal HIV-1 infection: a multicentre longitudinal study of 212 children. AIDS 2001;15(12):1527–1534.

23. Arpadi SM. Growth failure in children with HIV infection. J Acquir Immune Defic Syndr 2000;25 Suppl 1:S37–S42.

24. Dunn D, HIV Paediatric Prognostic Markers Collaborative Study Group. Short-term risk of disease progression in HIV-1-infected children receiving no antiretroviral therapy or zidovudine monotherapy: a meta-analysis. Lancet 2003;362(9396):1605–1611.

25. Obimbo EM, Mbori-Ngacha DA, Ochieng JO, Richardson BA, Otieno PA, Bosire R, et al. Predictors of early mortality in a cohort of human immunodeficiency virus type 1-infected african children. Pediatr Infect Dis J 2004;23(6):536–543; Dabis F, Elenga N, Meda N, Leroy V, Viho I, Manigart O, et al. 18-Month mortality and perinatal exposure to zidovudine in West Africa. AIDS 2001;15(6):771–779.; Newell ML, Coovadia H, Cortina-Borja M, Rollins N, Gaillard P, Dabis F. Mortality of infected and uninfected infants born to HIV-infected mothers in Africa: a pooled analysis. Lancet 2004 ;364(9441):1236–1243.

26. de Martino M, Tovo PA, Balducci M, Galli L, Gabiano C, Rezza G, et al. Reduction in mortality with availability of antiretroviral therapy for children with perinatal HIV-1 infection. Italian Register for HIV Infection in Children and the Italian National AIDS Registry. JAMA 2000;284(2):190–197.

27. Gibb DM, Duong T, Tookey PA, Sharland M, Tudor-Williams G, Novelli V, et al. Decline in mortality, AIDS, and hospital admissions in perinatally HIV-1 infected children in the United Kingdom and Ireland. BMJ 2003;327(7422):1019.

28. The Collaboration of Observational HIV Epidemiological Research Europe Study Group. Response to combination antiretroviral therapy: variation by age. AIDS 2008;22(12):1463–1473.

29. De Rossi A, Walker AS, Klein N, De FD, King D, Gibb DM. Increased thymic output after initiation of antiretroviral therapy in human immunodeficiency virus type 1-infected children in the Paediatric European Network for Treatment of AIDS (PENTA) 5 Trial. J Infect Dis 2002;186(3):312–320; Walker AS, Doerholt K, Sharland M, Gibb DM. Response to highly active antiretroviral therapy varies with age: the UK and Ireland Collaborative HIV Paediatric Study. AIDS 2004 ;18(14):1915–1924.

30. Goetghebuer T, Haelterman E, Le CJ, Dollfus C, Gibb D, Judd A, et al. Effect of early antiretroviral therapy on the risk of AIDS/death in HIV-infected infants. AIDS 2009; 23(5):597–604.

31. European Collaborative Study. CD4 cell response to antiretroviral therapy in children with vertically acquired HIV infection: is it associated with age at initiation? J Infect Dis 2006;193(7):954–962.

32. Violari A, Cotton MF, Gibb DM, Babiker AG, Steyn J, Madhi SA, et al. Early antiretroviral therapy and mortality among HIV-infected infants. N Engl J Med 2008 November 20;359(21):2233–2244.

33. UNICEF. Children and AIDS 3rd Stock-taking report 2008, Geneva: UNICEF.

34. Bolton-Moore C, Mubiana-Mbewe M, Cantrell RA, Chintu N, Stringer EM, Chi BH, et al. Clinical outcomes and CD4 cell response in children receiving antiretroviral therapy at primary health care facilities in Zambia. JAMA 2007;298(16):1888–1899.

35. KIDS-ART-LINC Collaboration. Low risk of death, but substantial program attrition, in pediatric HIV treatment cohorts in Sub-Saharan Africa. J Acquir Immune Defic Syndr 2008;49(5):523–531.

36. Sutcliffe CG, van Dijk JH, Bolton C, Persaud D, Moss WJ. Effectiveness of antiretroviral therapy among HIV-infected children in sub-Saharan Africa. Lancet Infect Dis 2008;8(8):477–489, ibid KIDS-ART-LINC 2008

37. Rekha B, Swaminathan S. Childhood tuberculosis—global epidemiology and the impact of HIV. Paediatr Respir Rev 2007 June;8(2):99–106; Newton SM, Brent AJ, Anderson S, Whittaker E, Kampmann B. Paediatric tuberculosis. Lancet Infect Dis 2008;8(8):498–510.

38. Gray DM, Zar H, Cotton M. Impact of tuberculosis preventive therapy on tuberculosis and mortality in HIV-infected children. Cochrane Database Systematic Review 2009(1).CD006418.

39. Jaquet D, Levine M, Ortega-Rodriguez E, Faye A, Polak M, Vilmer E, et al. Clinical and metabolic presentation of the lipodystrophic syndrome in HIV-infected children. AIDS 2000;14(14):2123–2128.

40. Leonard EG, McComsey GA. Metabolic complications of antiretroviral therapy in children. Pediatr Infect Dis J 2003;22(1):77–84.

41. McComsey GA, O'Riordan M, Hazen SL, El-Bejjani D, Bhatt S, Brennan ML, et al. Increased carotid intima media thickness and cardiac biomarkers in HIV infected children. AIDS 2007;21(8):921–927.

42. Chintu C, Bhat GJ, Walker AS, Mulenga V, Sinyinza F, Lishimpi K, et al. Co-trimoxazole as prophylaxis against opportunistic infections in HIV-infected Zambian children (CHAP): a double-blind randomised placebo-controlled trial. Lancet 2004; 364(9448):1865–1871.

43. Gibb DM, Masters J, Shingadia D, Trickett S, Klein N, Duggan C, et al. A family clinic--optimising care for HIV infected children and their families. Arch Dis Child 1997;77(6):478–482; Prendergast A, Tudor-Williams G, Jeena P, Burchett S, Goulder P. International perspectives, progress, and future challenges of paediatric HIV infection. Lancet 2007; 370(9581):68–80.

44. Thorne C, Townsend CL, Peckham CS, Newell ML, Tookey PA. Pregnancies in young women with vertically acquired HIV infection in Europe. AIDS 2007;21(18):2552–2556; Brogly SB, Watts DH, Ylitalo N, Franco EL, Seage GR, III, Oleske J, et al. Reproductive health of adolescent girls perinatally infected with HIV. Am J Public Health 2007;97 (6):1047–1052.

45. Foster C, Judd A, Tookey P, Tudor-Williams G, Dunn D, Shingadia D, et al. Young people in the United Kingdom and Ireland with perinatally acquired HIV: the pediatric legacy for adult services. AIDS Patient Care STDS 2009;23(3):159–166.

Chapter 26 MEETING THE UNIQUE NEEDS OF HIV-POSITIVE WOMEN

SHARON L. WALMSLEY AND MONA R. LOUTFY

Often the most vulnerable women in our society are women living with AIDS; how accountable we have been to their needs will be the yard stick that future generations will measure us against.

—GUSTAAV WOOLDVART, Acting Chairman
AIDS Accountability International

Introduction

As the HIV and AIDS pandemic continues, it is increasingly devastating for women in particular. Women account for more than half of the prevalent HIV cases globally, and more than 60% of prevalent cases in Sub-Saharan Africa. We will review how the feminization of HIV results from multiple factors, including the increased risk for acquisition of HIV by women for both biologic and social reasons. There are also important issues related to the natural history, virology, response to and adverse events related to antiretroviral therapy (ART) in women that will be reviewed. Furthermore, there are other women's health issues that are important to consider in the context of HIV infection, including contraception, pregnancy, and gynecologic issues including cervical diseases, cancer, and menopause. A topic of increasing importance is aging and how this affects HIV-positive women. Finally, HIV-positive women carry a significant burden of mental health issues along with other psychosocial considerations, including those that affect the social determinants of health—critical issues to consider when reviewing the topic of women and HIV.

Although the complex, deeply rooted and multifaceted structural inequalities that condition women's risk and constrain their access to treatment are increasingly recognized, responses rarely address them. There is still no licensed prevention method women can use without partners' involvement and cooperation. Emerging evidence around sex differences suggest that the treatment guidelines and regimens being rolled out may not be optimal for women. Much of the biomedical research related to HIV does not provide answers that are applicable to women and many clinical trials are not designed with women in mind, nor powered to address gender-specific issues.

In this chapter, we review what is known and emphasize what is not known, and call for action to improve research to enable us to make wiser and more informed decisions in care.

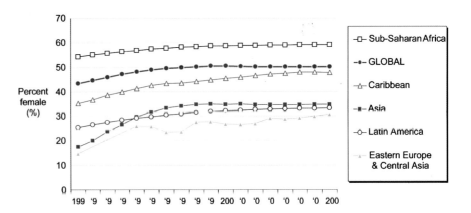

Figure 26–1. *Percentage of HIV cases being female over the last two decades. Source: UNAIDS/WHO Epidemic Update, 2008 Report;[1] used by permission.*

Epidemiology and Transmission Risk

As of the end of December 2008, there were 33.4 million individuals living with HIV, including 31.3 million adults and 2.1 million children.[1] Of the adults, 15.7 million are women, reflecting the fact that the HIV epidemic has now met gender parity. The observation of an increased number of women infected with HIV and the increasing proportion of new cases in this gender are similar throughout the world, not just in the developing world where the number of HIV-infected individuals is greater (**Figure 26–1**). Unfortunately, another disturbing trend is that an increased proportion of these new cases in the developing world are occurring in young women. Of the 12 million young persons between 15 and 24 years of age living with HIV, 7.3 million have occurred in young women; this is particularly apparent in Sub-Saharan Africa. In short, the current global response to the HIV epidemic is clearly not working for women.

Women acquire HIV predominantly through heterosexual intercourse or through injection drug use and the sharing of contaminated needles. In Sub-Saharan Africa the most common mode of transmission is through heterosexual intercourse.

In all countries, including those in Africa, the Caribbean, Latin America, Europe, Asia, and North America, the proportion of women living with HIV has continued to increase, and the proportion of new cases that are attributable to women has also increased (**Figure 26–2**). For example, in Western Europe, the proportion of new cases attributable to women increased from 25% in 1997 to 38% in 2002. In Canada,[2] 27.8% of newly registered HIV cases in 2006 were women. 33% of all newly diagnosed HIV cases in North America are from high risk heterosexual intercourse. In many countries of Europe and North America, many of the newly diagnosed women with HIV are immigrants. This has been particularly apparent in the United Kingdom, Spain, and Canada. In Eastern Europe and Central Asia, 40% of newly registered HIV cases in 2006 were women. In this circumstance, however, injection drug use and sex work are the main methods of HIV transmission to women, with 35% of HIV-positive women infected through injecting drugs themselves and 50% acquiring HIV through unprotected sex with drug-injecting partners. Similarly, in the United States,[3] the proportion of AIDS cases that are women has significantly increased over time. Women accounted for 27% of all cases in 2007 and only 7% in 1985. The other alarming factor in the U.S. is the degree to which women of color are disproportionately affected. In the reporting of the 2007 AIDS diagnosis rate, the rate for black/African American females (39.8/100,000) were 22 times higher than the rate for white females (1.8/100,000).[3]

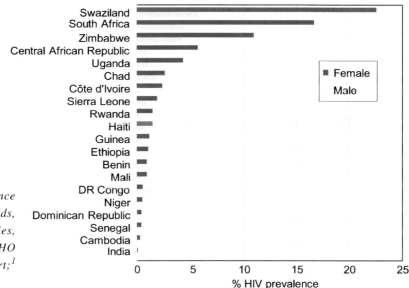

Figure 26–2. *HIV prevalence (%) among 15- to 24-year-olds, by sex, and selected countries, 2005–2007. Source: UNAIDS/WHO Epidemic Update, 2008 Report;[1] used by permission.*

Risk of HIV Acquisition for Women

Women have several factors that may increase their vulnerability to HIV, and it is generally accepted that women are more susceptible than men to HIV infection. Biologic factors play an important role in a woman's risk.[4] It is felt that the delicate tissue in the female sexual organs is vulnerable to tears, creating a direct transmission route for the virus. The ejaculate of an HIV-positive male comes into direct contact with vaginal and cervical mucosa, which contains numerous cells for the virus to infect. Also, compared to female genital secretions, male ejaculate is released in greater quantities and contains a higher viral content.

Sexual HIV transmission risk depends on a number of factors, including the infectivity of the source (which could be related to the viral load in plasma or semen)[5] and the presence of genital ulcers or other sexually transmitted diseases (STDs) that could cause breakdown of the genital mucosa and increase the risk for a sexual exposure.[6] As demonstrated in **Table 26–1**, it has been estimated that the risk of HIV transmission through insertive vaginal sex is <0.1% per exposure and receptive vaginal sex 0.01%–1.5%, in contrast to a risk of <0.1% per act of insertive anal sex and 3% for an act of receptive anal intercourse.[7,8] A study in 16 Italian clinical centers that included 524 female partners of-HIV infected men and 206 male partners of HIV infected-women demonstrated that the efficiency of male-to-female transmission was 2.3 times greater than that of female-to-male transmission (95% CI, 1.1–4.8).[9] It was thought that gender differences in the contact surfaces and the intensity of exposure to HIV during sexual intercourse could account for the difference in the efficacy of transmission.

Social factors play an important role in leading to the increasing vulnerability of women to HIV.[10] Throughout the world, there are a number of gender inequalities, and in many parts of the world, women have limited control over the ability to practice or to negotiate low-risk sexual behaviors. Frequently, the social standing and the inability of the women to control the frequency or the nature of sexual interactions could put them at increased risk. In addition, many women are exposed to violence, and forced sex may result in genital tears and lacerations that contribute to viral transmission. This violence similarly prevents women from safe sex negotiation and

TABLE 26–1	Estimated Risk of HIV Transmission Based on Various Routes of Exposure (Per-Act Risk[7,8])	
	Type of exposure (from a source known as HIV-positive)	Risk of HIV transmission per exposure
	Accidental needle stick	0.2%–0.4%
	Mucosal membrane exposure	0.1%
	Receptive oral sex	Varied from 0 to 6.6%
	Insertive vaginal sex	≤ 0.05%
	Insertive anal sex	≤ 0.1%
	Receptive vaginal sex	0.1%–0.15%
	Receptive anal sex	≤ 3%
	Sharing injecting drug user's needle	0.7%
	Transfusion	90–100%

access to treatment, and may also prevent women from getting tested for HIV or disclosing their HIV status. This could have implications not only for transmission but for disease progression, as well as access to therapy.

Natural History of HIV Disease in Women

In the initial years of the HIV epidemic, it was thought that the disease in women progressed at a much more rapid rate than in men. However, it is likely that these studies were biased. Men were much more likely to present because of Kaposi's sarcoma, which can occur at a relatively preserved CD4 count.[11,12] In addition, men who have sex with men (MSM) frequently perceived themselves to be at risk and often would get tested early, leading to lead-time bias in the determination of outcomes. In contrast, many women would not get tested because of unperceived risk, or would not be tested until they presented late with an opportunistic infection such as esophageal candidiasis or Pneumocystis pneumonia when the CD4 count was much lower. In addition, many of the cohorts of women that were studied in the early part of the epidemic were largely comprised of injection drug users who had co-infection with Hepatitis C, did not have access to medical care, and had confounding issues of drug abuse, alcohol, homelessness, poverty etc. which may have impacted outcomes.[13-16]

More recently, there have been a number of cohort studies which have followed individuals prospectively from the presumed date of seroconversion. These data sets include the Johns Hopkins Clinical Cohort,[17] the Swiss HIV Cohort,[18] the London Clinic Cohort,[19] the Italian Antiretroviral Treatment Group,[20] and the EuroSIDA Cohort.[21] Follow-up of seroconverters between 2 and 6 years have not demonstrated any differences between the sexes with regard to clinical progression, and any differences that did occur were due to differences in access to treatment.

There does appear to be a difference in baseline HIV viral load between men and women, particularly at preserved CD4 counts, where the viral load in women is typically 0.5 log lower than that of their male counterparts (**Figure 26–3**).[22] As HIV disease progresses, however, and

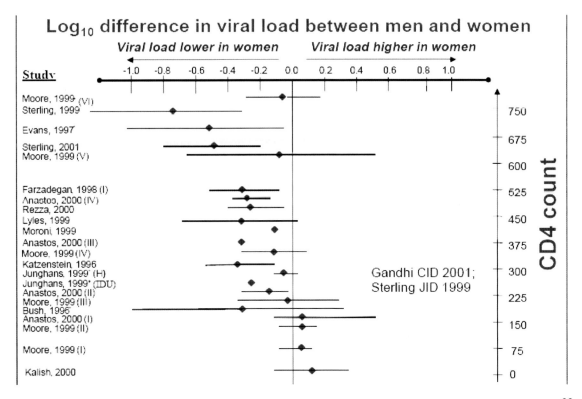

Figure 26–3. *Difference in baseline viral load between men and women. Source: Gandhi CID, 2001.*[22]

CD4 counts fall below 500 cells/mm³, the viral load difference between men and women disappears. The biologic reason for such a difference is not known.[23–26]

Response to Antiretroviral Therapy

Virology

Globally, HIV-1 is divided into three groups: M (major), O (outliers), and N (new, or non-M, non-O). Group M includes 10 subtypes (clades): A, B, C, D, F1, F2, G, H, J, K.[27] There also exist recombinant clades that are becoming increasingly recognized. Most of the world is infected with non-B clade virus, with clades C and A being most prevalent in Africa. The efficacy of ART has been studied predominately in men in North America and Europe with a predominance of HIV-1 clade B. Concern has been raised about differences in efficacy of ART against non-B clade HIV and how this may affect initial response to ART, as well as the resistance patterns with treatment failure.[28] It is important to consider the impact of gender on response to ART. Especially because a high proportion of HIV-positive women are from Africa or Asia, and many of the infected women living in North America and Western Europe are of African ancestry, the predominant viral clades will potentially be different in women than in men.

One study assessing ART response in non-B clade virus in 79 Africans infected with subtypes A, C, and D found no difference in antiretroviral efficacy, measured by the proportion of patients achieving undetectable HIV RNA.[29] Notably, nearly 90% of the 23 patients with

counterparts.[88] In the GRACE study cited above, nausea, but not diarrhea, was reported more commonly in women than in men.[68]

Unfortunately, very little is known at this time about the relative toxicity of the newer agents in women. Etravirine, a second-generation NNRTI, has been reported to be associated with an increased risk for rash (although not statistically significant) in women relative to men.[70] Tipranavir/r has been associated with higher drug levels in women relative to men, but this did not result in any differences in viral load reduction or the rate of adverse events in the RESIST clinical trials.[89] For maraviroc, no gender differences have yet been evaluated. No gender differences have been noted with raltegravir.

A number of cohort studies have demonstrated more pronounced metabolic abnormalities in women on ART compared to those seen in men—specifically, higher levels of serum triglyceride and low-density lipoprotein, higher levels of glucose and measures of insulin resistance, and higher markers of cardiovascular disease (CVD) risk such as C-reactive protein (CRP).[90–94] In the large collaborative DAD cohort, CVD was found to be increased in individuals on cART, specifically, PI/r and abacavir. The relative risk for the association of cumulative use of cART with CVD in this cohort was even higher for women than for men.[95] As premenopausal women in the general population are thought to have a lower incidence of CVD, it is important that this potential relationship be better elucidated. These data also provide greater support for the current trends to decrease other CVD risk factors for both men and women living with HIV.

Another toxicity of increasing concern is the potential for adverse effects on bone mineral density (BMD), particularly as the HIV population ages. It remains controversial as to whether the increased risk for osteoporosis and osteopenia observed in cross-sectional and prospective cohorts is related to HIV itself, ART or certain elements of it, or from an increased risk associated with traditional risk factors, such as smoking.[96] Whether or not it affects the genders differentially is also unclear. In the Women Interagency HIV Study, an association was found between BMD, HIV infection, and treatment, demonstrating that HIV-infected women were more likely to have osteopenia and osteoporosis compared to HIV-negative women, and rates further increased in those on cART.[97] This is further supported by data from the SMART study, in which there was an improvement in BMD during periods of drug therapy interruption,[98] although this management strategy is no longer recommended. These data were not analyzed by gender. In the Canadian Women's study, there was no difference in BMD between HIV-infected women and age- and sex-matched controls, although there was an increased risk for fragility fractures among the women with HIV infection.[99a] It is unclear whether the fractures were related to trauma, or whether or not the current technology is inadequate to determine BMD. A population based study demonstrated an overall fracture prevalence of 2.49% in women with HIV versus 1.72% in non-HIV infected women $p=.002$ with the risk increasing with age.[99b] Small, randomized trials have shown that increases in BMD can be observed in HIV-infected women receiving standard osteoporosis therapies such as alendronate, but guidelines for the appropriate use of these agents in the setting of HIV are not available.[100]

Lipodystrophy, or body fat redistribution, is one of the major side effects of greatest concern for patients initiating ART. Some of the lipodystrophy characteristics may be different in women than in men.[101–106] In the case definition for lipodystrophy developed by Carr and colleagues,[107] female gender was a significant risk factor for lipodystrophy and is a variable included in the score. There are no good data to determine whether rates or extent of fat redistribution vary by gender, or whether certain antiretrovirals may differentially impact the genders more than others. However, a number of smaller cohort studies have demonstrated that HIV-infected women are more likely to complain of fat gain in the breasts and abdomen than are their male counterparts, and that women have fewer concerns about peripheral lipoatrophy. The impact of race may however confound the data. In the DEXA substudy of the WIHS cohort, the majority of participants—both HIV-infected and -uninfected—were overweight or obese, and the majority of cases from ethnic minorities. Leg fat was found to be significantly lower in the women on ART.[103]

In switch studies from thymidine analogs to nonthymidine analogs, the general trends were for an improvement in peripheral fat. Too few women were included to assess the gender element, and no study was analyzed by gender.[108,109]

The unanswered question—and one that remains poorly studied—is why there may be sex differences in adverse outcomes.[110] The existing hypothesis is that there may be differences in pharmacokinetic parameters relative to the antiretroviral drugs.[111] This could affect all aspects of pharmacokinetics, including bioavailability, distribution, metabolism, and elimination.[112] Women are known to have decreased stomach acid and, therefore, may have slower gastric emptying time, which may be magnified with oral contraceptives or during pregnancy. There may be differences in their diets that may affect the bioavailability of many medications. Drug metabolism could vary, but to date there have not been any consistent differences found in gut cytochrome enzymes or in P-glycoproteins. Women tend to weigh less and have more proportional fat with varying plasma volumes, which could affect free drug distribution. There also may be less organ flow, and estrogen may affect plasma binding proteins, which, in turn, could affect the free level of drugs.[113,114] Progesterone in women may increase CYP2A4 activity, whereas hepatic G-glycoprotein may be increased in men—both factors potentially affecting drug metabolism. Finally, a proportion of HIV-infected women have underlying hepatitis C, which could affect liver function and the elimination of drugs. It is important to remember that the coadministration of other medications can affect each stage of any metabolism, which may vary by sex.

There is an increasing need for a better understanding of this issue. It is important to determine whether or not certain agents are associated with increased toxicity in women relative to men, not only to ensure that the best agents are chosen for therapy, but because the development of toxicity could affect antiretroviral efficacy.[115-120] Toxicity-related discontinuation or intermittent adherence could lead to less-than-optimal antiretroviral response, and the emergence of drug resistance could compromise future treatment options. Data from the ICONA cohort study suggest that this may be occurring.[121,122] In this cohort, in which 3,142 patients started a first ART regimen, 721 interrupted ART for at least 12 weeks. Women, injection drug users, and patients with a higher current CD4 count were more likely to interrupt over a median clinical follow-up of 41 months. In the multivariate hazards model, women were more likely to interrupt than men (RH 1.59; 95% CI, 1.15–2.19). ART interruption was associated with an increased rate of clinical progression in this cohort and in a Swiss HIV cohort reported in a recent study.[123]

Pharmacokinetics and Pharmacogenomics

Pharmacokinetics

Sex-related differences in the pharmacokinetic disposition of certain ARVs have been observed, and may have important implications in the treatment of HIV-positive women, in terms of both efficacy and toxicity. Specific studies describing sex differences in the pharmacokinetics of ARVs are summarized in **Table 26–3**.

In a study involving 157 men and 29 women, the mean 24-hour area under the concentration curve (AUC) of saquinavir was found to be 30.2 mg × h/L in women and 18.5 mg × h/L in men

TABLE 26–3	Sex Differences in Antiretroviral Pharmacokinetics[a]		
	Drug	**Findings**	**Refs.**
	Abacavir	No observed sex differences in PK	238
	Emtricitabine	No observed sex differences in PK	239
	Lamivudine	Higher triphosphate concentrations in women	86
	Stavudine	No observed sex differences in PK	240
	Tenofovir	No observed sex differences in PK	241
	Zidovudine	Higher triphosphate concentrations in women	86
	Efavirenz	Higher mean plasma concentration in women	136,144
	Nevirapine	Higher mean plasma concentration in women	133,135,136
	Amprenavir	No observed sex differences in PK	242
	Atazanavir	No observed sex differences in PK	131
	Fosamprenavir	No observed sex differences in PK	243
	Indinavir	Increased oral clearance in men	127
	Lopinavir/r	No observed sex differences in PK	242
	Nelfinavir	No observed sex differences in PK	129
	Ritonavir	No observed sex differences in PK in healthy volunteers	242
	Saquinavir	Higher mean serum AUC (56%) in women; higher C_{min} in women	124,125
	Tipranavir/r	No data available	89
	Darunavir	Exposure 16.8% higher in females (n=68), not thought clinically important	67

[a]PK, pharmacokinetics; AUC, area under the curve; C_{min}, trough concentration.

$(p = 0.004)$.[124] In addition, higher trough (C_{min}) values of saquinavir were observed among women. In contrast, a smaller study in HIV-negative individuals found no sex differences in saquinavir AUC.[125] Several studies have observed an increase in oral clearance of indinavir in men compared to women.[126,127] In children older than 12 years of age, a 39% increase in lopinavir plasma clearance was observed in boys compared to girls, but no significant difference was seen in children under the age of 12.[128] Clinically important sex-related pharmacokinetic variability has not been observed for either nelfinavir or atazanavir.[129–132a] However in a recent study we found that approximately 20% of women had C_{min} to Atazanavir >1.5% the population mean despite no difference in C_{max}.[132b] For tipranavir/r, in the RESIST studies, women had higher steady-state plasma tipranavir/r trough concentrations than did men (adjusted means, 38.75 µM vs 45.3 µM for men and women, respectively), but this did not affect efficacy rates or rates of adverse events.[89]

In terms of NRTIs, Anderson et al.[86] observed a 2.3- and 1.6-fold higher triphosphate concentration of zidovudine and lamivudine, respectively, in women compared to men. Sex-related differences have also been described with the NNRTIs nevirapine and efavirenz, with women in general having higher plasma levels of each relative to men.[133] Regazzi et al.[134] observed a 20%

increase in mean AUC of nevirapine in women compared to men, although when corrected for body weight, the results were no longer statistically significant.

A relationship between low body weight and high plasma concentrations of nevirapine was also reported in a separate observational study.[135] In another study, mean efavirenz plasma concentrations of 4.0 mg/L and 2.8 mg/L have been observed in women and men, respectively. Higher plasma concentrations of these NNRTIs may increase the risk of drug-specific toxicities in women.[136,137]

Although the aforementioned studies highlight the potential pharmacokinetic variability observed between women and men for certain ARVs, the under-representation of women in clinical trials makes it difficult to achieve sufficiently powered analyses on these differences.[110,138,139] The paucity of data on sex-related differences in ARV pharmacokinetics complicates the management of HIV in women, and ensuring plasma drug concentrations within the acceptable therapeutic range becomes an added concern when treating women. Although therapeutic drug monitoring (TDM) is a potential tool for the adjustment of ARV doses, further research defining appropriate plasma thresholds of ARVs in women is necessary.[40]

Pharmacogenomics

Pharmacogenomics, the study of how genomic variations influence the response to drugs, is a topic of increasing interest in the context of HIV.[141,142] Since a high proportion of HIV-positive women in the world are from Africa or Asia, pharmacogenomics is emerging as an important consideration in the response of women to ART.

Host genetics may play an important role in antiretroviral drug metabolism. For instance, polymorphisms in the cytochrome P450 enzyme, CYP2B6, have been found to influence the metabolism of efavirenz.[143] A novel allele, identified as CYP2B6*16, is found commonly among individuals of African origin and has been linked to reductions in efavirenz metabolism and, consequently, higher steady-state plasma levels.[144] In addition, the T/T genotype at position 516 of CYP2B6 and the resultant increase in efavirenz AUC is more frequently seen in African-Americans relative to European-Americans (20% vs. 3%; $p<0.0001$). Patients with these polymorphisms may be at higher risk for efavirenz-related central nervous system toxicity.[145] Although other polymorphisms have been identified that may influence the pharmacokinetics of certain ARVs, the functional importance of these changes and impact on either efficacy or toxicity requires further research.

The most recent application of pharmacogenomics is the association between the HLA-B*5701 allele and abacavir hypersensitivity.[146,147] The abacavir hypersensitivity reaction is a serious adverse reaction to the NRTI abacavir, which is characterized by a complex of symptoms including rash, fever, and flulike complaints. The reaction occurs in approximately 4% to 8% of patients who receive abacavir, and requires that affected patients permanently discontinue this agent as rechallenge can be potentially fatal. The presence of the HLA-B*5701 gene is associated with an increased risk for developing the abacavir hypersensitivity reaction, and genetic testing has emerged as a potentially useful new tool for avoiding this reaction.[148] The distribution of HLA-B*5701 is highest among Caucasian populations in northern Europe, North America, and Australia. Interestingly, certain Asian and African populations have a prevalence of HLAB*5701 that is <1%, explaining the lower risk for abacavir hypersensitivity among these individuals relative to other ethnicities. Abacavir may therefore be a safe ARV option for most women of African or Asian ancestry.

Women's Health Topics

Contraception and Protection From Sexually Transmitted Infections

The ideal contraceptive for an HIV-infected women would: (1) be reliable and safe; (2) not increase the risk for pelvic inflammatory disease; (3) be reversible if a pregnancy was planned; (4) prevent transmission of HIV to a seronegative partner; (5) not interfere with ART; and (6) not be user-dependent.[149] Despite its high failure rate at birth control (12%), the major form of contraception for HIV-infected women at this time is the condom, which depends on male agreement to participate.[150] Condoms are also important as consideration of contraception due to the importance they play in the prevention of HIV and other STD transmission. However, due to the relatively high contraceptive failure rate, other methods of birth control are often recommended in addition to condoms, adding to the cost and complexity of the situation. In many parts of the world, women do not have the ability to control safe sex practices and, thus, may need to depend on hormonal contraception in order to prevent pregnancy. There are a number of issues with this approach. First, drug interactions may occur between the hormonal contraceptives and many of the ART agents.[151] Those that are inducers my render certain components of ART ineffective and result in a lack of virologic control (**Table 26–4**). HIV medications may be CYP3A4 inducers, decreasing hormonal contraceptive levels and, therefore, increasing the risk for pregnancy.

Also of concern is whether or not hormonal contraception may affect HIV acquisition or disease progression.[152] A commonly used method of hormonal contraception in the global setting of HIV is depot medroxyprogesterone acetate (DMPA) injection (Depo-Provera), as it is less expensive, has a prolonged effect, and is not known to interact with other drugs. However, DMPA does have its drawbacks, including the potential to increase the risk for osteoporosis. Furthermore, a recent study has demonstrated that the use of DMPA by HIV-negative women was associated with a two-fold hazard ratio of HIV acquisition (95% CI, 1.3-3.1; p = .003). The reason for this remains unclear, but it is possible that the hormonal contraceptives, through the development of cervical ectopy and the upregulation of CCR5, may create a more vulnerable mucosal surface to HIV exposure. Furthermore, the use of DMPA might affect disease progress in HIV-infected women. In the subanalysis of a recent controlled clinical trial in which 599 HIV infected women were randomized to either intrauterine devices (IUDs) or hormonal contraception (either the oral contraceptive pill or DMPA), it was found that exposure to the oral contraceptive or DMPA was associated with an increased risk for HIV disease progression among women not yet on ART.[153] Mortality among women who started on the IUD was 2/100 women years, 3.2/100 woman years in those starting DMPA, and 2.4/100 women years in those starting the oral contraceptive pill. Furthermore, 148 women were found to have their CD4 count fall below 200 cells/mm³ and needed to initiate ART during follow-up. The rates were 11.2/100 women years of follow-up in the IUD arm, 17.5/100 women years in the DMPA arm, and 14.3/100 women years in the oral contraceptive arm. Although the results of this study need confirmation, it does raise some concern over the appropriate contraceptive for women.

IUDs are another commonly used option.[154] WHO does not recommend use of the copper IUD in women with HIV because of the associated increased risk for cervical and endometrial infection and complications. However, the newer IUD, Mirena, is being used with increasing frequency in the HIV-negative population and may hold promise for the future for HIV-positive women. Mirena is an IUD system containing levonorgestrel, which slowly releases the hormone

TABLE 26–4	Pharmacokinetic Interactions between Antiretrovirals and Hormonal Contraceptives[a, 244]		
	Antiretroviral	**Interaction**	**Recommendation**
	Delavirdine	Ethinyl estradiol levels may increase	Clinical significance unknown
	Efavirenz	37% increase in ethinyl estradiol No interaction with depo-medroxyprogesterone.	Use alternative or additional method of contraception if using oral contraceptives
	Nevirapine	~20% decrease in ethinyl estradiol No interaction with depo-medroxyprogesterone.	Use alternative or additional method of contraception if using oral contraceptives
	Amprenavir	Increase in ethinyl estradiol and norethindrone levels observed with amprenavir; 20% decrease in amprenavir levels	Do not coadminister; use alternate method of contraception
	Atazanavir	48% increase in ethinyl estradiol AUC, 110% increase in norethindrone AUC	Use lowest effective dose or alternative methods
	Darunavir/ritonavir	Potential decrease in ethinyl estradiol	Use alternative or additional method of contraception
	Fosamprenavir	Increase in ethinyl estradiol and norethindrone levels observed with amprenavir; 20% decrease in amprenavir levels	Do not coadminister; use alternate method of contraception
	Indinavir	26% increase in norethindrone, 24% increase in ethinyl estradiol	No dose adjustment
	Lopinavir/ritonavir	42% decrease in ethinyl estradiol	Use alternative or additional method of contraception
	Nelfinavir	18% decrease in norethindrone, 47% decrease in ethinyl estradiol No interaction with depo-medroxyprogesterone	Use alternative or additional method of contraception if using oral contraceptives
	Ritonavir	40% decrease in ethinyl estradiol	Use alternative or additional method of contraception
	Saquinavir	No data	No data
	Tipranavir/r/ritonavir	~50% decrease in ethinyl estradiol C_{max}	Use alternative or additional method of contraception
	Raltegravir	No anticipated drug interaction	No dose adjustment
	Maraviroc	No anticipated drug interaction	No dose adjustment

[a]AUC, area under the curve; C_{max}, peak concentration.

partner is also infected. This must be considered in the setting whether the baby itself is infected or non-infected.

Risk Factors for Increased Mother-to-Child Transmission. A number of factors may increase the risk for HIV transmission from mother to fetus. In general, the maternal factors relate to advanced maternal disease and can include high viral load, late HIV disease, and low CD4 count.[175,176] Other factors that have been shown to increase transmission include maternal injection drug use, coinfection with hepatitis C, or the presence of other sexually transmitted diseases such as gonorrhea, chlamydia, herpes, or syphilis. Therefore, it is important to monitor the mother for these coinfections so that she can be managed appropriately. Pregnancy should be considered earlier rather than later in the course of HIV disease. There is no absolute viral load below which HIV transmission does not occur, but a number of studies have demonstrated that the higher the HIV viral load in the mother, the greater the increased risk for HIV transmission to babies; the percentage is extremely small for viral loads <1,000 copies/mL.

Obstetric factors that have been associated with the increased risk for transmission include ruptured membranes for greater than 4 hours and chorioamnionitis, and any invasive procedures (such as scalp electrodes) that may increase bleeding.[177]

Virologic factors for transmission could include the particular clade with which the mother has been infected, and HLA discordance between mother and fetus.

Antiretroviral Therapy in Pregnancy. The prevention of mother-to-child transmission was revolutionized with PACTG076, which was a double-blind, placebo-controlled, randomized trial to determine the efficacy of AZT in reducing the risk for mother-to-child HIV transmission.[166] This involved 490 HIV-infected women between 14 and 34 weeks' gestation who had a CD4 count >200 cells/mm^3 and who were antiretroviral-naïve. AZT was given to the mother antepartum at a dose of 100 mg 5 times a day then intrapartum as a 2-mg/kg IV drip during labor and delivery, with a 2-mg/kg IV loading dose, and then 1 mg/kg per hour until delivery. The newborn was then given oral AZT syrup, 2 mg/kg every 6 hours, for a period of 6 weeks. In total, there were 415 births, of which 363 had known HIV status; 25.5% were HIV-positive in the placebo group compared to 8.3% in the AZT group, for a relative risk reduction of 69%.

There has not been any prospective, controlled trial of combination ARV in this setting. However, a number of retrospective cohort studies of combination ART have found that, for cART therapy, the current observational risk of transmission is approximately 1%.

One of the major considerations for the management of HIV-infected women is the safety of antiretroviral drug use during pregnancy.[178–185] The FDA has classified drugs into a number of categories based on the risk observed in animal and human models. The FDA classifications of the HIV medications[186] are listed in **Table 26–5**. No drug currently meets the FDA classification of A in pregnancy (shown to be safe in randomized studies in humans). Drugs in the B category include DDI, tenofovir, atazanavir, nelfinavir, saquinavir, and enfuvirtide. Drugs in class C include abacavir, 3TC, D4T, AZT, delavirdine, nevirapine, amprenavir, fosamprenavir, lopinavir, and tipranavir/r. Category B implies that no risks have been demonstrated in animal studies but studies have been done to substantiate lack of risk in humans. Category C implies that the animal studies either are lacking or show risk, and that there are no human studies. The only drug in category D—that is, contraindicated during pregnancy—is efavirenz, which is currently contraindicated in pregnancy because it has been shown to cause encephaly and other neural tube defects in macaque models. A number of case reports have appeared in the literature of neural tube defects in human fetuses exposed in the first trimester to efavirenz.[187] It remains unclear whether this

TABLE 26-5	U.S. Food and Drug Administration (FDA) Pregnancy Categories for Currently Approved Antiretrovirals[186]

Drug	FDA Category[a,]
Abacavir	C
Didanosine	B
Emtricitabine	B
Lamivudine	C
Stavudine	C
Tenofovir	B
Zalcitabine	C
Zidovudine	C
Delavirdine	C
Efavirenz	D
Nevirapine	C
Etravirine	B
Amprenavir	C
Atazanavir	B
Darunavir	B
Fosamprenavir	C
Indinavir	C
Lopinavir/r	C
Nelfinavir	B
Ritonavir	B
Saquinavir	B
Tipranavir/r	C
Enfuvirtide	B
Maraviroc	B
Raltegravir	C

[a]FDA categories defined as: **A**, adequate and well-controlled studies of pregnant women fail to demonstrate a risk to the fetus during the first trimester of pregnancy (and no evidence exists of risk during later trimesters). **B**, animal reproduction studies fail to demonstrate a risk to the fetus, and adequate but well-controlled studies of pregnant women have not been conducted. **C**, safety in human pregnancy has not been determined; animal studies are either positive for fetal risk or have not been conducted, and the drug should not be used unless the potential benefit outweighs the potential risk to the fetus. **D**, positive evidence of human fetal risk that is based on adverse reaction data from investigational or marketing experiences, but the potential benefits from the use of the drug among pregnant women might be acceptable despite its potential risks. **X**, studies among animals or reports of adverse reactions have indicated that the risk associated with the use of the drug for pregnant women clearly outweighs any possible benefit.

incidence is truly above the rate seen in the general population.[188] Until more information is available, other agents are recommended, if available. Also contraindicated during pregnancy include is combination treatment with D4T and DDI. In January 2001, Bristol Myers Squibb—which manufactures both drugs—announced that there were three maternal deaths due to lactic acidosis in pregnant women on this combination. All cases occurred late in gestation; there were two cases of pancreatitis and two cases of fetal death.[189]

The public health services task force for the antiretroviral drugs in pregnant women has updated their recommendations. In terms of the NNRTI class, the recommended agent is nevirapine, provided the maternal CD4 count is <250 cells/mm³. In terms of the protease inhibitors, lopinavir/ritonavir is the recommended agent. Alternatives include indinavir and saquinavir. The recommended NRTI include AZT and 3TC. Alternative agents include abacavir, DDI, D4T, and FTC. At this time, data are insufficient to make a recommendation for tenofovir, but a recent presentation from the U.S. Pregnancy Registry would suggest it is safe.[190]

It is important to recognize that changes can occur in drug disposition during pregnancy. Some of the changes that could affect this include decreased gastrointestinal motility from progesterone, increased total body water and plasma volume, increased cardiac output and renal plasma flow, increased body fat stores, changes in protein binding due to decreased albumin, and increased alpha and beta globulins. An observation from small pharmacokinetic studies with certain agents—namely, lopinavir/r, nelfinavir and atazanavir—is that drug levels, particularly trough levels, may decrease in the third trimester of pregnancy.[191–194] This may result from a change in the volume of distribution. Although treatment guidelines at this time do not routinely recommend increasing the dose of these agents in the third trimester, consideration should be made for doing this in patients with inadequate virologic suppression, frequent blips, or those with virologic rebound in the last trimester of pregnancy. These decisions could be guided by therapeutic drug monitoring, where available.

Prevention of Mother-to-Child Transmission in the Developing World. The best means of preventing mother-to-child transmission is through the use of cART in the pregnant woman, with the goal of achieving suppression of viral replication prior to delivery. Unfortunately, for economic reasons, this approach is currently not available for many women in resource-limited settings. Numerous clinical trials have been conducted in this setting to address shorter-term (more economical) approaches to therapy. These studies on prevention of maternal-to-child transmission during pregnancy and breastfeeding have been the subject of recent Cochrane reviews.[195,196] The discussion of these protocols and limitations are beyond the scope of this chapter. None of these approaches result in as low a risk of transmission to the mother as cART does, but they are associated with a decreased risk for transmission. However, the use of incompletely suppressive regimens has resulted in increased rates of viral resistance in the mother and in infected babies. This has further consequences on the effect of subsequent use of ARV for maternal health.

Cesarean Section. A prospective, randomized, controlled trial was conducted by the European Mode of Delivery Collaboration, which included HIV-infected pregnant woman who were randomized at 38 weeks to elective caesarean section or vaginal delivery. Of the 436 that were randomized 370 were analyzed.[172] The risk of transmission was 3/170 (1.8%) in those who received elective cesarean section compared to 21/200 (10.5%) in those randomized to a vaginal delivery, for a relative risk reduction of 83% (*p* = 0.001). Subsequently, a meta-analysis of 15 cohort studies that individually included at least 100 infected women, for a total of 8,533 mother-child pairs.[173] The adjusted odds ratio for C-section was 0.43 (95% CI, 0.33–0.56). In those who are also on ART, the risk for transmission in those with elective cesarean section was 2% compared to 7.3% for other modes of delivery. It is important to note that none of these studies involved patients who used cART, and in the current era, cART may reduce the rate of vertical transmission, such that the added benefit of cesarean section is minimal.

Breastfeeding. HIV DNA is present in breast milk and HIV transmission can occur through breastfeeding.[197] The risk also increases with the duration of breastfeeding, although the exact mechanism of transmission is still not well understood. A randomized trial involving 425 women from Nairobi, Kenya, examined breastfeeding versus formula feeding.[198] The compliance with breastfeeding was 96% and with formula feeding was 70%; the results demonstrated that the risk for transmission was 36.7% in the breastfeeding group and 20.5% in the formula feeding group. More recently, however, a study presented at the International AIDS Society Conference demonstrated that mother-to-baby transmission was less than 1% among HIV-infected women and baby in the developing world treated with cART therapy not only during labor and delivery but also postpartum for 6 months of breastfeeding.[174] This study has had significant impact on the possible management of HIV-infected pregnant women throughout the world, and it is important at this time for us to advocate for cART therapy for mothers to allow safe breastfeeding.

Gynecologic Issues in HIV

Menstrual Cycle. Data on the influence of HIV on the menstrual cycle are conflicting.[199–203] Older studies demonstrated a prolongation of the cycle, whereas the WHIS study suggested an increase in short cycles. Some studies have reported an increase in menstrual abnormalities. Some of the abnormalities in cohort studies could be related to confounders such as malnutrition, wasting, advanced disease, or opportunistic infections. Some data also are available from small populations suggesting that HIV is associated with an earlier onset of menopause.

Sexually Transmitted Diseases and Gynecologic Infections. Several studies have shown that HIV-infected women are more likely than those without HIV to exhibit higher prevalence, severity, and range of gynecologic infections, including vulvovaginal candidiasis, sexually transmitted infections (such as chlamydia, gonorrhea, and herpes simplex), and pelvic inflammatory disease, along with other vulvar and vaginal diseases such as bacterial vaginosis.[204]

Minkoff and colleagues[205] found that in a sample of minority women in New York City, 66% of those with HIV had at least one gynecologic disorder, compared with 41% of uninfected women. Infected women also were more likely to acquire a new disorder within 1 year.[205] The frequency of disorders that are strongly linked to behavioral factors was not associated with women's HIV status, but conditions with primarily biologic causes were more common among HIV-infected women.

Bacterial Vaginosis

Persistence and severity of bacterial vaginosis increases with the progression of immune deficiency, and effective cART has been associated with a lowering of the risk for vaginosis. Bacterial vaginosis increases the expression of HIV in the genital tract and may promote HIV transmission.[206]

Psychosocial and Mental Health Considerations

It is important to recognize that women living with HIV have a number of psychological issues that may affect their diagnosis and ability to adhere to ART. Unlike gay and bisexual men, women do not necessarily form natural, gender-related support groups, and many women experience their HIV diagnosis in isolation, not knowing anyone else who is HIV-infected. Furthermore, given the stigma associated with an HIV diagnosis, many of these women fail to disclose their HIV status to others and live in isolation and often in a state of depression. It is also important to remember that a woman with HIV infection may be just one member of an infected family; in many such cases, the woman puts her energies into managing an affected child or infected partner before taking care of her own health. In some parts of the world, women who are diagnosed with HIV are at very high risk for domestic violence, and in these environments, many women choose to not get tested or, if they do get tested and are found to have the infection, they will fail to disclose their HIV diagnosis to their partners. Therefore, it is important to explore whether or not a woman perceives herself to be at physical or emotional risk when informing her of a positive diagnosis for HIV.[222–223]

Furthermore, many women living with HIV are also living in poverty, and often do not have access to health care. In many parts of the world, women are not empowered to make their own health care decisions and are often influenced by partners as to whether or not they can accept therapy or consider participation in a clinical trial.[224] It is important to recognize that women often have other responsibilities related to their children, family, and housekeeping, and may not be able to attend clinics during normal working hours; they will often need some assistance with child care.[225] Competing family and health commitments often result in women mismanaging their own disease. Furthermore, women may be ashamed of their HIV diagnosis and so may hide their medications; this may result in lower treatment adherence rates. It is important also to be aware that any medications that may need to be kept in a communal setting (such as in a refrigerator) could affect a patient's ability to take medications: she may be fearful of others identifying the medications, concerned about a possible breach in confidentiality about her HIV status, or worried that these drugs might be within reach of children, posing the risk for accidental poisoning.

Injection drug use is a major risk factor for HIV infection in women in North America, Eastern Europe, Central Europe, South America, and Southeast Asia, with seroprevalence rates as high as 30% in some series. Therefore, it is important for clinicians working with HIV-infected women with histories of illicit drug use to have a familiarity not only with the diagnosis and treatment of substance abuse but also with the special clinical manifestations of HIV seen among drug users—including hepatitis B and C, tuberculosis, endocarditis, and community-acquired methicillin-resistant *Staphylococcus aureus*.[226–228] In addition, several drug interactions are known to occur between methadone and therapies used for HIV. Furthermore, such patients also present a number of challenging issues related to housing, poverty, abuse, depression, adherence, violence, and psychiatric illness.

In many parts of the developing world, an increased proportion of HIV-infected patients are new immigrants, often women. These women often have considerable struggles with language barriers, and issues related to food and housing and immigration status; consequently they may not have the ability or time to access appropriate health care.[229] Many women living with HIV also have very strong religious ties focusing on their faith and belief in God to help them with their disease rather than relying medical care. Cultural barriers may also prevent many women from seeking medical care. The decision whether or not to become pregnant often presents a considerable dilemma for women. On the one hand, a women may wish to behave according to cultural norms, but on the other hand may be fearful about the risk for transmitting HIV to a child or about having her diagnosis disclosed to her family or to others.[230]

In addition to the importance of social, drug use, and abuse history as described above, depressive symptoms have been shown to be increased in HIV-positive women; these symptoms are and independently associated with ART adherence and HIV disease progression.[231-235] Cook[236] and colleagues reported that women living with HIV had rates of severe depressive symptoms as high as 47%. These high levels of depressive symptoms significantly reduced the probability of using ART. Women receiving treatment for depression were more likely to be taking their ART medications. Depression in women with HIV has also been shown to be associated with increased mortality. Analysis of depressive symptoms, mortality, and CD4 decline in the HIV Epidemiology Research Study showed that women with chronic depressive symptoms were twice as likely to die than were women with mild or no depressive symptoms.[237] In order to achieve better mental health as well as to decrease the rate of HIV disease progression and other negative health outcomes in women with HIV who are depressed, HIV care needs to include sensitive and effective mental health treatment.

Finally, we cannot stress enough the importance of social determinants of health and how they affect the well-being of HIV-positive women. In many settings, women in general—and those living with HIV, even more so—tend to live in poverty, have insecure housing, have poorer education and lower income, and live in violence. If these social issues are not at the forefront of their care, it is extremely difficult to mange all the other issues.

Conclusion

As women continue to represent a growing proportion of the individuals infected with HIV, it is crucial to consider sex-specific issues when attempting to meet their needs. Increased risks for HIV acquisition, differences in antiretroviral pharmacokinetic profiles, pharmacogenomic variability, and different and increased risks for antiretroviral-related adverse events in women as compared to men merit more research. Data indicating that women and men experience variable types and severities of adverse events to some antiretrovirals can be used to help select the most tolerable regimen for female patients. Although antiretroviral trials have not demonstrated gender differences in the virologic responses of women compared to men, it is hoped that more women will be included in future drug trials, increasing the power of such studies to assess gender differences. Specific women's health issues are important to address when caring for HIV-positive women, including contraception, pregnancy, gynecologic disorders, and menopause. All of these women's health topics are associated with specific, important issues as they relate to HIV. As an example, how many antiretrovirals can influence drugs levels of hormonal contraceptives? Fertility and pregnancy planning options are becoming increasingly important, as the majority of women living with HIV are of reproductive age and current therapy allows HIV to be treated as a chronic infection. Additional research as well as global advocacy are needed on reproductive assistance methods for HIV-positive women. Issues including access to sperm banks and in vitro fertilization services must be addressed. A topic of increasing importance is aging in HIV-positive women, including all of the age-related health issues, and particularly osteoporosis, breast cancer, dementia, and cardiovascular disease. Finally, addressing the mental health problems, psychosocial issues, and other determinants of health that influence the lives of HIV-infected women at all levels should be considered as one of the first steps in the care of

150. Weller D, Davis K. Condom effectiveness in reducing heterosexual HIV transmission. Cochrane Database Syst Rev. 2002; CD003255.

151. Cohn SE, Park JG, Watts DH, et al. Depo-medroxyprogesterone in women on antiretroviral therapy: effective contraception and lack of clinically significant interactions. Clin Pharmacol Ther 2007;81(2):222–227.

152. Morrison CD, Richardson BA, Mmiro F, et al. Hormonal contraception and the risk of HIV acquisition. AIDS 2007;21(1):85–95.

153. Stringer EM, Levy J, Sinkala M, et al. HIV disease progression by hormonal contraceptive method; secondary analysis of randomized trial. AIDS 2009;23:1377–1382.

154. Steen R, Shapiro K. Intrauterine contraceptive devices and risk of pelvic inflammatory disease: standard of care in high STI prevalence settings. Reprod Health Matters. 2004;12(23):136–143.

155. Van Damme L, Govinden R, Mirembe FM, et al. Lack of effectiveness of cellulose sulphate gel for the prevention of vaginal HIV transmission. N Engl J Med 2008;359:463–472.

156. Abdool-Karim S. ART containing vaginal microbicides in the clinical pipeline: A status of the studies Symposium, Presented at the XVII International AIDS Conference, Mexico City. 3–8 August 2008; #THSY0602.

157. Rosenberg Z. ARV-based microbicides: cause for optimism. Symposium, Presented at the XVII International AIDS Conference, Mexico City. 3-8 August 2008; #MOSY0106.

158a. Van Damme L, Ramjee G, Alary M, et al. Effectiveness of COL-1492, a nonoxynol-9 vaginal gel, on HIV-1 transmission in female sex workers: a randomised controlled trial. Lancet 2002;360(9338):971–977.

158b. Abdool Karim Q et al. 18th IAC; Vienna, July 18–23, 2010, Abstract TUSS0502.

158c. Kashuba A, et al. 18th IAC; Vienna, July 18–23, 2010, Abstract TUSS0503.

158d. Sokal D, et al. 18th IAC; Vienna, July 18–23, 2010, Abstract TUSS0504.

158e. Abdool Karim Q, et al. Effectiveness and safety of tenofovir gel, an antiretroviral microbicide, for the prevention of HIV infection in women. Science 2010 Sep 3;329(5996):1168–1174.

159. Loutfy M, Hart TA, Mohammed SS, DeSheng S, Walmsley SL, et al. Fertility desires and intentions of HIV-positive women of reproductive age in Ontario, Canada: a Cross-sectional Study. PLoS ONE 2009, Dec 7;4(12):e7925.

160a. Finer LB, Henshaw, SK. Disparities in rates of unintended pregnancy in the United States, 1994 and 2001. Perspect Sex Reprod Health 2006;38(2):90–96.

160b. Loutfy M, Hart TA, Mohammed SS, DeSheng S, Walmsley SL, et al. Fertility desires and intentions of HIV-positive women of reproductive age in Ontario, Canada: a Cross-sectional Study. PLoS ONE 2009, Dec 7;4(12):e7925.

160c. Raboud J, Li M, Walmsley S, et al. Factors associated with HIV-positive women carrying pregnancies to term. J Obstet Gynaecol Can 2010 Aug; 32(8):756–762.

161. Massad LS, Springer G, Jacobson L, et al. Pregnancy rates and predictors of conception, miscarriage and abortion in US women with HIV. AIDS 2004;18:281–286.

162. Sedgh F, Larsen U, Spiegelman D, et al. HIV-1 disease progression and fertility in Dar es Salaan, Tanzania. JAIDS. 2005 Aug 1;39(4):439–445.

163. Gray RH, Wawer MJ, Serwadda D, et al. Population-based study of fertility in women with HIV-1 infection in Uganda. Lancet 1998;351(9096):98–103.

164. Kim LU, Johnson MR, Barton S, et al. Evaluation of sperm washing as a potential method of reducing HIV transmission in HIV-discordant couples wishing to have children. AIDS 1999;13(6):645–651.

165. Sauer MV, Wang JG, Douglas NC, et al. Providing fertility care to men seropositive for human immunodeficiency virus: reviewing 10 years of experience and 420 consecutive cycles of in vitro fertilization and intracytoplasmic sperm injection. Fertil Steril 2009;91(6):2455–2460.

166. Sperling RS, Shapiro DE, Coombs RW, et al. Maternal viral load, zidovudine treatment, and the risk of transmission of human immunodeficiency virus type 1 from mother to infant: Pediatric AIDS Clinical Trials Group Protocol 076 Study Group. N Engl J Med 1996;335(22):1621–1629.

167. Cooper ER, Charurat M, Mofenson L, et al. Combination antiretroviral strategies for the treatment of pregnant HIV-1-infected women and prevention of perinatal HIV-1 transmission. J AIDS; 29:484–494.

168. National Guideline Clearinghouse. Public Health Service Task Force for Recommendations for Use of Antiretroviral Drugs in Pregnant HIV-Infected Women for Maternal Health and Interventions to Reduce Perinatal HIV Transmission in the United States. 2008. Accessed December 14, 2009 at, http://www.guideline.gov/summary/summary.aspx?ss=15&doc_id=14451&nbr=7241.

169. World Health Organization. Antiretroviral Drugs for Treating Pregnant Women and Preventing HIV Infection in Infants: Towards Universal Access: Recommendations for a Public Health Approach, 2006 Version. Accessed December 10, 2009 at, http://www.who.int/hiv/pub/mtct/antiretroviral/en/.

170. Loutfy MR and Walmsley SL. Treatment of HIV infection in pregnant women: antiretroviral management options. Drugs 2004;64(5):471–488.

171. Paredea R, Cheng, I, Kuritzkes DR, et al. Postpartum antiretroviral drug resistance in HIV-1infected women receiving pregnancy-limited antiretroviral therapy. AIDS 2010;24(1):45–43.

172. The European Mode of Delivery Collaboration. Elective caesarean-section versus vaginal delivery in prevention of vertical HIV-1 transmission: a randomised clinical trial. Lancet 1999;353(9158):1035–1039.

173. The International Perinatal HIV Group. The mode of delivery and the risk of vertical transmission of human immunodeficiency virus type 1: a meta-analysis of 15 prospective cohort studies. N Engl J Med 1999;340(13):997–987.

174. Shapiro R, Hughes M, Ogwu A, et al. A randomized trial comparing highly active antiretroviral therapy regimens for virologic efficacy and the prevention of mother-to-child HIV transmission among breastfeeding women in Botswana (The Mma Bana Study). Presented at the 5th IAS Conference on HIV Pathogenesis, Treatment and Prevention, Cape Town, Africa, 19–22 July 2009;Abstract #WELBB101.

175. Garcia PM, Kalish LA, Pitt J, et al. Maternal levels of plasma human immunodeficiency virus type 1 RNA and the risk of perinatal transmission. N Engl J Med 1999;341(6):394–402.

176. Nair P, Alger L, Hines S, et al. Maternal and neonatal characteristics associated with HIV infection in infants of seropositive women. J AIDS1993;6(3):298–302.

177. The International Perinatal HIV Group. Duration of ruptured membranes and vertical transmission of HIV-1: a meta-analysis from 15 prospective cohort studies. AIDS 2001;15(3):357–368.

178. Townsend CL, Willey BA, Cortina-Borja M, et al. Antiretroviral therapy and congenital abnormalities in infants born to HIV-infected women in the UK and Ireland, 1990–2007. AIDS 2009 Feb 20;23(4):519–524.

179. Morris AB, Rua Dobles A, Cu-Uvin S, et al. Protease inhibitor use in 233 pregnancies. J AIDS 2005;40:30–33.

180. Covington DL, Conner SD, Doi PA, et al. Risk of birth defects associated with Nelfinavir exposure during pregnancy. Obstet Gynecol 2004;103(6):1181–1189.

181. Zuk DM, Hughes CA, Foisy MM, et al. Adverse effects of antiretrovirals in HIV-infected pregnant women. Ann Pharmacother 2009;43:1028–1035.

182. Floridia M, Tamburrini E, Ravizza M, et al. Lipid profile during pregnancy in HIV-infected women. HIV Clin Trials 2006;7(4):184–193.

183. Desmit M, Willems B, Dom P, et al. Absence of a teratogenic potential from a novel next-generation NNRTI, TMC278. Presented at the 12th European AIDS Conference, Cologne, Germany, 11–14 November 2009; Poster PE7.1/4.

184. Lzurieta P, Kakuda TN, Clark A, et al. Safety and pharmacokinetics of Etravirine in pregnant HIV-infected women. Presented at the 12th European AIDS Conference, Cologne, Germany, 11–14 November 2009; Poster PE4.1/6.

185. Hanlon M, O'Dea S, Clarke S, Mulcahy F. Maternal hepatotoxicity with boosted Saquinavir as part of combination ART in pregnancy. Presented at the 14th Conference on Retroviruses and opportunistic Infection, Los Angeles February 25–28 2006; Poster 753.

186. Antiretroviral Pregnancy Steering Committee Registry. Antiretroviral Pregnancy Registry International Interim Report for 1 January 1989 through 31 July 2009. Wilmington NC; Registry coordination center, 2009. http://www.apregistry.com/forms/interim_report.pdf. Accessed December 10, 2009.

187. Fundaro C, Genovese O, Rendeli C, et al. Myelomeningocele in a child with intrauterine exposure to efavirenz. AIDS 2002;16:299–300.

188. Bussmann H, Wester CW, Wester CN, et al. Pregnancy rates and birth outcomes among women on efavirenz-containing highly active antiretroviral therapy in Botswana. JAIDS Syndr 2007; 45:269–273.

189. Marcus K, Truffa M, Boxwell D, et al. Recently indentified adverse events secondary to NRTI therapy in HIV-infected individuals: cases from the FDA's Adverse Events Reporting Systems (AERS). Presented at the 9th Conference of Retroviruses and Opportunistic Infections, Seattle, WA 24–28 February 2002; Abstract LB14. Alexandra, VA: Foundation for Retrovirolog and Human Health, 2002.

190. Squires K, Olmscheid B, Guyer B, and Zhang Z. TDF-containing antiretroviral regimens in pregnancy: finding from the antiretroviral pregnancy registry. Presented at the 49th Interscience Conference on Antimicrobial Agents and Chemotherapy, San Francisco, California, 12–15 September 2009; Poster H-917.

191. Stek AM, Mirochnick M, Capparelli E, et al. Reduced lopinavir exposure during pregnancy. AIDS 2006;20(15):1931–1939.

192. Unadkat JD, Wara DW, Hughes MD, et al. Pharmacokinetics and safety of indinavir in HIV-infected pregnant women. Antimicrob Agents Chemother 2007;51(2):783–786.

193. Villani P, Floridia M, Pirillo MF, et al. Pharmacokinetics of nelfinavir in HIV-1-infected pregnant and nonpregnant women. Br J Clin Pharmacol 2006;62(3):309–315.

194. Eley T, Vandeloise E, Child M, et al. Pharmacokinetics and clinical outcomes with atazanavir 300 mg QD/ritonavir 100 mg (ATV/r) QD + ZDV/3TC during the 3rd trimester of pregnancy in HIV + women:

interim results from BMS AI424182. Presented at the XVII International AIDS Conference, Mexico City 3–8 August 2004; Abstract TUPE0121.

195. Suksomboon N, Poolsup N, Ket-aim S. Systemic review of the efficacy of antiretroviral therapies for reducing the risk of mother-to-child transmission of HIV infection. J Clin Pharm Ther. 2007;32(3):293–311.

196. Horvath T, Madi BC, Iuppa IM, et al. Interventions for preventing late postnatal mother-to-child transmission of HIV. Cochrane Database of Syst Rev 2009 Jan 21;(1):CD006734.

197. Ghosh MK, Kuhn L, West J, et al. Quantitation of human immunodeficiency virus type 1 in breast milk. J Clin Microbiol 2003;41(6):2465–2470.

198. Nduati R, Richardson BA, John G, et al. Effect of breastfeeding on mortality among HIV-1 infected women: a randomised trial. Lancet 2001;357(9269):1651–1655.

199. Harlow SD, Schuman P, Cohen M, et al. Effect of HIV infection on menstrual cycle length. J Acquir Immune Defic Syndr 2000;24(1):68–75.

200. Massad LS, Evans CT, Minkoff H, et al. Effects of HIV infection and its treatment on self-reported menstrual abnormalities in women. J Womens Health (Larchmt) 2006;15(5):591–598.

201. Reichelderfer PS, Coombs RW, Wright D, et al. Effect of menstrual cycle on HIV-1 levels in the peripheral blood and genital tract. AIDS 2000;29;14(14):2101–2107.

202. Villanueva JM, Ellerbrock TV, Lennox JL, et al. The menstrual cycle does not affect human immunodeficiency virus type 1 levels in vaginal secretions. J Infect Dis 2002;185:170–177.

203. Greenblatt RM, Ameli N, Grant RM, et al. Impact of the ovulatory cycle on virologic and immunologic markers in HIV-infected women. J Infect Dis 2000;181:82–90.

204. Sobel JD. Gynecologic infections in human immunodeficiency virus-infected women. Clin Infect Dis. 2000;31(5):1225–1233.

205. Minkoff HL, Eisenberger-Matityahu D, Feldman J, et al. Prevalence and incidence of gynecologic disorders among women infected with human immunodeficiency virus. Am J Obstet Gynecol 1999;180:824–836.

206. Warren D, Klein RS, Sobel J, et al. A multicenter study of bacterial vaginosis in women with or at risk for HIV infection. Inf Dis Obst Gyn 2001;9:133–141.

207. Rebbapragada W, Wachihi C, Pettengell C, et al. Negative mucosal synergy between herpes simplex type 2 and HIV in the female genital tract. AIDS 2007;21:589–598.

208. Watson-Jones D, Weiss HA, Rusizoka M, et al. Effect of herpes simplex suppression on incidence of HIV among women in Tanzania. N Engl J Med 2008;358:1560–1571.

209. Celum C, Wald A, Lingappa J, et al. Twice-daily acyclovir to reduce HIV-1 transmission from HIV-1/HSV-2 co-infected persons within HIV-1 serodiscordant couples: a randomized, double-blind, placebo-controlled trial. Presented at the 5th IAS Conference on HIV Pathogenesis, Treatment and Prevention, Cape Town, Africa, 19–22 July 2009; Abstract #WELBC101.

210. Watts DH, Springer G, Minkoff H, et al. Occurrence of vaginal infections among HIV-infected and high-risk HIV-uninfected women: longitudinal findings of the Women's Interagency HIV Study. J AIDS 2006;43:161–68.

211. Hoegsberg B, Abulafia O, Sedis A, et al. Sexually transmitted disease and human immunodeficiency virus infection among women with pelvic inflammatory disease. Am J Obstet Gynecol 1990;163:1135–1139.

212. Schuman P, Ohmit SE, Klein RS, et al. Longitudinal study of cervical squamous intraepithelial lesions in human immunodeficiency virus (HIV)-seropositive and at risk HIV-seronegative women. J Infect Dis 2003;188:128–136.

213. Sun XW, Kuhn L, Ellerbrock TV, et al. Human papillomavirus infection in women infected with the human immunodeficiency virus. N Engl J Med 1997;337:1343–1349.

214. Hankins C, Coutee F, Lapointe N, et al. Prevalence of risk factors associated with human papillomavirus infection in women living with HIV. Can Med Assoc J 1999;160:185–191.

215. Franceschi S and Jaffe H. Cervical cancer screening of women living with HIV infection: a must in the era of antiretroviral therapy. Clin Infect Dis 2007;45(4):510–513.

216. Kenneth HF, Wu JW, Squires KE, et al. Prevalence and persistence of cervical human papillomavirus infection in HIV-positive women initiating highly active antiretroviral therapy. JAIDS;2009;51:274–282.

217. Massas LS, Fazzari MJ, Anastos K, et al. Outcomes after treatment of cervical intraepithelial neoplasia among women with HIV. J Low Genit Tract Dis. 2007;11(2):90–97.

218. Robinson WR, Hamilton CA, Michaels SH, Kissinger P, et al. Effect of excisional therapy and highly active antiretroviral therapy on cervical intraepithelial neoplasia in women infected with human immunodeficiency virus. Am J Obstet Gynecol 2001;184:538–543.

219. Fantry LE, Zhan M, Taylor GH, et al. Age of menopause and menopausal symptoms in HIV-infected women. AIDS Patient Care STDS 2005;19(11):703–711.

220. Schoenbaum EE, Hartel D, Lo Y, et al. HIV infection, drug use, and onset of natural menopause. Clin Infect Dis 2005;41(10):1517–1524.

Prevent

221. Office of the Medical Director, New York State Department of health AIDS Institute in collaboration with the John Hopkins University, Division of Infectious Diseases. Medical care for menopausal and older women with HIV infection. March 2008. Accessed December 10, 2009 at, http://www.hivguidelines.org.

222. Cohen M, Deamant C, Barkan S, et al. Domestic violence and childhood sexual abuse in women with HIV infection and women at risk for HIV. Am J Public Health 2000; 90:560–565.

223. Vlahov D, Wientge D, Moore Et al. Violence among women with or at risk for HIV infection. AIDS Behav 1998;2:53–60.

224. Ojikutu BO and Stone VE. Women, inequality, and the burden of HIV. N Engl J Med 2005;;352(7):649–652.

225. Stein MD, Crystal S, Cunningham WE, et al. Delays in seeking HIV care due to competing caregiver responsibilities. Am J Public Health 2000; 90(7):1138–1140.

226. Selwyn PA, O'Connor R, Schottenfeld RS. Female drug users with HIV infection: Issues for medical care and substance abuse treatment. Chapter 13 in HIV Infection in Women (Minkoff H, DeHovitz JA, Duerr A), Raven Press, 1995;241–262.

227. Cohen MH, Cook JA, Grey D, et al. Medically eligible women who do not use HAART: the importance of abuse, drug use, and race. Am J Public Health 2005;94(7):1147–1151.

228. Lucas GM, Cheever LW, et al. Detrimental effects of continued illicit drug use on the treatment of HIV-1 infection. J AIDS;2001; 27(3):251–259.

229. Gielen AC, McDonnell KA, Wu AW, et al. Quality of life among women living with HIV: the importance of violence, social support and self care behaviors. Soc Sci Med 2001;52:315–322.

230. Gruskin S, Ferguson L, O'Malley J. Ensuring sexual and reproductive health for people living with HIV: an overview of key human rights, policy, and health systems issues. Reprod Health Matters 2007;15:4–26.

231. Haug NA, Sorensen JL, Gruber VA, et al. HAART adherence strategies for methadone clients who are HIV-positive. Behav Modif 2006;30(6):752–781.

232. Cook JA, Grey D, Burke-Miller J, et al. Effects of treated and untreated depressive symptoms on highly active antiretroviral therapy use in a US multi-site cohort of HIV-positive women. AIDS Care 2006;18(2):93–100.

233. Turner BJ, Laine C, Cosler L, Hauck WW. Relationship of gender, depression, and health care delivery with antiretroviral adherence in HIV-infected drug user. J Gen Intern Med 2003;18(4):248–257

234. Ouimette PC, Brown PJ, Najavits LM. Course and treatment of patients with both substance use and posttraumatic stress disorders. Addict Behav 1998;23(6):785–795.

235. Mellins CA, Kang E, Leu CS, et al. Longitudinal study of mental health and psychosocial predictors of medical treatment adherence in mothers living with HIV disease. AIDS Patient Care STDS 2003;17(8):470–416.

236. Cook, JA, Cohen MH, Burke, J, et al. Effects of depressive symptoms and mental health quality of life on use of highly active antiretroviral therapy among HIV-seropositive women. J AIDS; 2002;30:401–409.

237. Ickovics JR, Hamburger ME, Vlahov D, et al. HIV Epidemiology Research Study Group. Mortality, CD4 cell count decline, and depressive symptoms among HIV-seropositive women: longitudinal analysis from the HIV Epidemiology Research Study. JAMA 2001;285:1466–1474.

238. Weller S, Radomski KM, Lou Y, et al. Population pharmacokinetics and pharmacodynamic modeling of Abacavir (159U89) from a dose-ranging, double-blind, randomized monotherapy trial with human immunodeficiency virus-infected subjects. Antimicrob Agents Chemother 2000;48(8):2052–2060.

239. Emtriva™ (emtricitabine capsules) product monograph. Foster City, CA: Gilead Sciences Inc., November 2005

240. Zerit® (satvudine) product monograph. Princeton, NJ: Bristol-Myers Squibb Company, August 2006.

241. Kearney BP, Gill SC, Flaherty JF, et al. Effect of demographic variables on the pharmacokinetics of Tenofovir DF in HIV-infected patients and healthy subjects. Presented at the 41st Interscience Conference on Antimicrobial Agents and Chemotherapy, Chicago, Ill, 16–19 December 2001; Abstract 504.

242. Fletcher C. Gender differences in antiretroviral therapy pharmacokinetics and pharmacodynamics. Presented at the 11th Conference on Retroviruses and Opportunistic Infections, San Francisco, CA, 8-11 February 2004; Webcast session, Thursday, February 12, 2004. Accessed January 7, 2007 at, http://www.retroconference.org/ 2004/pages/webcast.htm.

243. Shelton MJ, Wire MB, Lou Y, et al. Pharmacokinetic and safety evaluation of high-dose combinations of fosamprenavir and ritonavir. Antimicrob Agents Chemother 2006;50(3):928–934.

244. Toronto General Hospital, Immunodeficiency Clinic. www.hivclinic.ca. Accessed November 28, 2009.

1% of global funding for HIV prevention was dedicated to sex work.[10] The latter statistics indicate a lost opportunity to affect the spread of the disease. The most effective way to combat this scourge is a combined, culturally sensitive approach carefully adapted to local needs. Antiretroviral therapy (ART) reduces viral load in body fluids of those infected and was remarkably effective in stemming the tide of transmission in Brazil. Recent practical approaches to reduce transmission are the application of antimicrobial gels, ART prophylaxis, and serosorting of HIV status in men who have sex with men.[20, 29, 47]

Structural Barriers

The limited resources that are devoted to the commercial sex industry are impeded by several structural barriers that increase HIV vulnerability among workers and inhibit prevention measures from realizing their full potential. Sex workers face stigma and discrimination when seeking health services. As seen in Ghana, stigma discourages sex workers from seeking health services and getting tested for fear of becoming known as being HIV positive.[48]

As stated in 2010 by a commercial sex worker in Ghana, "This is not a good business. It's dirty money. You don't tell people if you are in this line of work or if you are HIV-positive. You go to another town or village to get tested and to get treatment. That way no one knows if you have AIDS."

Society blames them for the epidemic, and many workers endure discrimination from staff in health clinics. These issues contribute to the fact that, as stated earlier, the majority of sex workers do not have access to prevention services. Violence toward sex workers is as high as 70% percent in many areas and prevents safe-sex practices, increasing the risk for HIV transmission.[49] Many sex workers experience sexual coercion by clients when the men are asked to use a condom.[50] Government regulation and legality of the commercial sex industry is a delicate balance in terms of HIV prevention in sex work. Multiple studies conclude that the illegal status of the industry has negative effects on prevention efforts. Evidence concludes that the criminalization of commercial sex exposes workers to increased violence and human rights violations.[51, 52] Legal status also affects the effectiveness of health promotion programs in the sex industry. One study shows that the unlicensed sector is isolated from peer-education and support.[53] However, this complex problem is not solved by simply legalizing prostitution; rather, governments need to be aware of the competing factors that must be considered in programs. For one, history indicates that the legalization of commercial sex allows for growth of the industry and sex tourism to flourish, increasing the HIV risk and degree of mobility.[50]

Conclusions

In the 21st century, even in developing countries, more sex workers are connecting with clients using cell phones or Internet social media such as Facebook or Twitter.[8] As modern technology evolves, so must our approach to HIV prevention and control within this industry. This communication technology affords government agencies and international agencies such as the World Health Organization (WHO) unique opportunities to impact with a high cost/benefit ratio. Many developing countries such as Africa and India are experiencing an explosive growth of Internet access, making this an ideal time to adapt HIV prevention programs to these new social medias. Harnessing available technology to dissolve the existing structural barriers and mitigate the isolating nature of sex work is key to groundbreaking programs.[54] For example, with the use of cell phone and Internet targeting, sex workers can access prevention education privately, thus removing or reducing the stigma a worker endures when visiting a health clinic. The sex worker can also be the conduit to the clientele, who can be educated simultaneously. A recent study in China supports this approach: 75% of female sex workers studied were Internet users and 64% were willing to participate in online HIV/STD prevention programs, if available.[55] Evidence shows that this technology offers many benefits such as high mobility, low cost, and the ability to reach a large number of people.[56] Innovative strategies using cell phones, text messaging, social media, and other communication methods using mobile devices are being rapidly accepted.

References

1. Aral SO, Mann JM. Commercial sex work and STD: the need for policy interventions to change society patters. Sex Transm Dis 1998;25(9):451–454.

2. UNAIDS, 2006. HIV and sexually transmitted infection prevention among sex workers in Eastern Europe and Central Asia. UNAIDS/06.10E. Joint United Nations Programme on HIV/AIDS.

3. Padilla MB, Guilamo-Ramos V, Bouris A, Reyes AM. HIV/AIDS and tourism in the Caribbean: an ecological systems perspective. Am J Public Health 2010;100(1):70–77.

4. Black S, et al. A social marketing approach for de-marketing sex tourism. Business Review 2010;15(2):33–41.

5. Gyys P, Jenkins C, Pisani E. HIV surveillance among female sex workers. AIDS 2001 Apr;15 (Suppl 3):S33–40.

6. Commission on AIDS in Asia 2008 Redefining AIDS in Asia. Crafting an effective response. New Delhi: Oxford University Press;2008.

7. UNAIDS, Technical Update, 2002 (*better source #50*).

8. Author unknown. Increase in condom use and decline in HIV and sexually transmitted diseases among female sex workers in Abidjan, Cote d'Ivoire, 1991–1998. AIDS 2003;17(18s).

9. Piot P. Setting new standards for targeted HIV prevention: the Avahan Initiative in India. Sex Transm Infect. 2010 Feb;86(Suppl 1):i1–2.

10. UNAIDS, 2009 AIDS epidemic update. UNAIDS/09.36E/JC1700E. Geneva, Joint United Nations Programme on HIV/AIDS AND World Health Organization. 2009

11. UNAIDS, Guidance note on HIV and sex work. UNAIDS/09.09E/JC1696E. Joint United Nations Programme on HIV/AIDS AND World Health Organization. 2009.

12. UNAIDS, 2002 AIDS epidemic update. UNAIDS/02.26E. Joint United Nations Programme on HIV/AIDS AND World Health Organization. 2002.

13. Guo HY, Duan S, Xiang LF, et al. Cost-effectiveness of female sex worker interventions by using sex 2.0 tool in Dehong prefecture, Yunnan province. Pubmed 2010;44(8):717–720 (Chinese).

14. International Committee on the Rights of Sex Workers in Europe. The Sex Workers in Europe Manifesto. 2005. European Conference on Sex Work, human rights, labour and migration. October 15–16; Brussels, Belgium (pp. 1–11).

15. Global AIDS Monitoring and Evaluation Team. West African HIV/AIDS epidemiology and response synthesis. 2008.

16. Dandona R, Dandona L, Gutierrez JP et al. High risk of HIV in non-brothel based female sex workers in India. BMC Public Health 2005;5:87

17. Panchanadeswaran S, Johnson SC, Sivaram S, et al. A descriptive profile of abused female sex workers in India. J Health Popul Nutr 2010;28(3):211–220

18. Sirotin N, et al. Effects of government registration on unprotected sex amongst female sex workers in Tijuana; Mexico. Pubmed 2010;21(6):466–470.

19. Chen MY, Donovan B, Harcourt C, et al. Estimating the number of unlicensed brothels operating in Melbourne. Aust N Z J Public Health 2010 Feb;34(1):67–71.

20. Eaton LA , Cherry C, Cain D. et al. A Novel Approach to Prevention for At-Risk HIV-Negative Men Who Have Sex With Men:Creating a Teachable Moment to Promote Informed Sexual Decision-Making. Am J Public Health 2011 (Jan 13).

21. UNAIDS 2002. Sex work and HIV/AIDS: UNAIDS technical update. Geneva, Joint United Nations Programme on HIV/AIDS. 2002.

22. Estes, R. J. and Weiner, N. A. The Commercial Sexual Exploitation of Chilren in the U.S., Canada and Mexico. Philadelphia, PA: University of Pennsylvania School of Social Work 2001.

23. Kumar, P. Sex trafficking and STI/HIV in Southeast Asia: connections between sexual exploitation, violence and sexual risk. United Nations Development Programme, 2009.

24. Piot, P., Greener, and Russell, S. Squaring the circle: AIDS, poverty and human development. PLoSMedicine 2007;4(10):e314

25. Le M., D'Onofrio C., and Rogers J. HIV Risk Among Three Classes of Female Sex Workers in Vietnam. 2010. Journal of Sex Research 47(1), 38–48.

26. mapnetwork.org AIDS in Asia 04 page 87

27. Todd CS., Alibayeva G., Khakimov MM. et al. Prevalence and Correlates of Condom Use and HIV Testing Among Female Sex Workers in Tashkent, Uzbekistan: Implications for HIV Transmission. AIDS and Behavior 2007;11:435–442. Accessed at http://www.ncbi.nlm.nih.gov/pubmed/16909325.

28. Vanwesenbeek I. Another decade of social scientific work on sex work: a review of research 1990–2000. Annu Rev Sex Res 2001;12:242–289.

29. Sonder GJ, Prins JM, Regez RM et al. Comparison of two HIV post-exposure prophylaxis regimens among men having sex with men. Sex Transm Dis 2010;37(11):681–686.

30. Rushing R, Watts C, Rushing S. Living the reality of forced sex work: perspectives from young migrant women sex workers in northern Vietnam. J Midwifery Womens Health. 2005 Jul Aug;50(1):e41–44

31. Bandyopadhyay M and Thomas J. Women migrant workers' vulnerability to HIV infections in Hong Kong. AIDS Care 2002;14(4): 509–521

32. 2006 Annual Review the International AIDS Alliance.

33. Celentano DD, Nelson KE, Supraser S, et al. Behavioral and sociodemographic risks for frequent visits to commercial sex workers among northern Thai men. AIDS 1993 Dec;7(12):1647–652.

34. Madhivanan P, Hernandez A, Gogate A. et al. Alcohol use by men is a risk factor for the acquisition of sexually transmitted infections and human immunodeficiency virus from female sex workers in Mumbai, India.Sex Transm Dis. 2005 Nov;32(11):685–690.

35. Alam, Mohammad Khairul. AIDS in India: sex workers and truck drivers playing vital roles. Global Health Council. Accessed at http://www.globalhealth.org/reports/report.php3?id=257.

36. Vickerman P, Foss AM, Pickles M, et al. To what extent is the HIV epidemic in southern India driven by commercial sex? AIDS 2010;24(16):2563–2572.

37. Leggett T. Drugs, sex work, and HIV in three South African cities. Published online. SA Health Info 2008 www.sahealthinfo.org/admodule/drugs.htm.

38. Hong Y, Li X. Behavioral studies of female sex workers in China: a literature review and recommendation for future research. AIDS Behav 2008 Jul;12 (4):623–636.

39. Mack N, Grey TG, Amsterdam A, et al. Central American sex workers' introduction of the female condom to different types of sexual partners. AIDS Educ Prev. 2010 Oct;22(5):466–481.

40. Mack N, Grey TG, Amsterdam A, Matta Cl, Williamson N. Introducing female condoms to female sex workers in Central America. Int Perspect Sex Reprod Health. 2010 Sep;36(3):149–155.

41. Rojanapithayakorn, W. The 100% Condom Use Programme in Asia. Reprod Health Matters. 2006 Nov;14(28):41–52.

42. Hanenberg, RS, Sokal DC, Rojanapithayakorn W, et al. Impact of Thailand's HIV-control programme as indicated by the decline of sexually transmitted diseases. Lancet 1994 July;344(8917):243–245.

43. UNAIDS Summary Booklet of Best Practices in Africa. UNAIDS/00.34E. Geneva, Joint United Nations Programme on HIV/AIDS. 2000

44. Vuylsteke B, Das A, Dallabetta G, et al. Preventing HIV among sex workers. In: Mayer K, Pizer HF, eds. HIV Prevention. London UK: Academic Press; 2008 (pp. 376–406).

45. Laga M, Galavotti C, Sundaramon S, et al. The Importance of Sex-Worker Interventions: The Case of Avahan in India. Sex Transm Infect 2010;86:250.

46. Monitoring the AIDS Pandemic Network 2004 AIDS in ASIA: Face the Facts, UNAIDS 2006.

47. van Griensven F, Thienkrua W, Sukwicha W et al. Sex frequency and sex planning among men who have sex with men in Bangkok, Thailand: implications for pre- and post-exposure prophylaxis against HIV infection. J Int AIDS Soc 2010;14(13):13.

48. Raingruber B, Uwazie E, Bowie, S. Women's Voices: Attitudes and Behaviors of Female Ghanaian Sex workers regarding HIV prevention and AIDS-related stigma. ssues Ment Health Nurs. 2010 Aug;31(8):514–519.

49. Garcia-Morena C, Watts C. Violence against women:its important for HIV/AIDS. AIDS 2000;14(30):S253–S265.

50. Sanchez, L. Boundaries of legitimacy: sex, violence, citizenship, and community in a local sexual economy. Law and Social Inquiry 1999;22:543–580.

51. Durojaye E, Oluduro O, Okeke U. Sex work, HIV/AIDS and sexual rights in Africa: the Nigerian experience. Indian Journal of Human Rights and the Law 2009;6:13–58.

52. Rekart M. L Sex-work harm reduction. Lancet. 2005 Dec 17;366(9503):2123–2134.

53. Harcourt C, O'Connor J, Egger S, The decriminalization of prostitution is associated with better coverage of health promotion programs for sex workers. Aust N Z J Public Health 2010;24(5):482–486.

54. Ybarra ML and Bull SS. Current trends in Internet- and cell phone-based HIV prevention and intervention programs. Curr HIV/AIDS Rep. 2007;4:201–207.

55. Hong, Y., Li, X., Fang, X et al. Internet Use Among Female Sex Workers in China: Implications for HIV/STI Prevention. AIDS Behav. Published online 17 November 2010.

56. Swendeman D, Rotheram-Borus MJ. Innovation in sexually transmitted disease and HIV prevention: internet and mobile phone delivery vehicles for global diffusion. Curr Opin Psychiatry. 2010;23(2):139–144.

57. Tran TN, Detels R, Lan HP Condom use and its correlates among female sex workers in Hanoi, Vietnam AIDS Behav 2006;10(2):159–167.

Chapter 28

AFRICAN AMERICANS AND HIV: EPIDEMIOLOGY, CONTEXT, BEHAVIORAL INTERVENTIONS, AND FUTURE DIRECTIONS FOR PREVENTION*

DARIGG C. BROWN, DONNA HUBBARD MCCREE, AND AGATHA N. EKE

In America today, AIDS is virtually a black disease, by any measure.

—PHIL WILSON, Executive Director of the Black AIDS Institute, Los Angeles, California

Introduction

Significant inequities exist in rates of HIV and other sexually transmitted infections (STIs) in the United States, with racial and ethnic minority communities (e.g., blacks/African Americans and Hispanics/Latinos) being severely impacted. Among racial and ethnic minority populations, African American communities, based on the available data, are the most disproportionately impacted and affected.[1,2] Further, the causes of these inequities and other health disparities—including cancer, cardiovascular diseases, and STIs among African Americans—are interrelated and are primarily due to contextual and structural factors such as higher poverty rates, lack of access to adequate health care, higher incarceration rates, lower income, lower educational attainment, and racism.[3–7] Therefore, strategies for tackling HIV should be based on an integrated approach and specific intervention strategies should address the social, structural, and contextual environments in which all health inequities occur among African Americans.

A complete review of the complexities and history of the HIV epidemic among African Americans is beyond the scope of this volume. In this chapter, the authors explore the epidemiology and context of HIV and AIDS among African Americans, provide a brief summary of the state of the science regarding behavioral interventions for HIV prevention, and offer suggestions for future directions.

The contents of this article are solely the responsibility of the authors and do not necessarily represent the views of the Centers for Disease Control and Prevention.

Epidemiology of HIV and AIDS in African Americans

Since the HIV epidemic was first recognized in 1981,[8] when only AIDS was reported through surveillance, the distribution of AIDS diagnoses among racial/ethnic groups has shifted from predominantly affecting non-Hispanic whites to disproportionately affecting people of color in the United States. Cases reported in the first year among blacks/African Americans included 23 gay men, 6 heterosexual men and women, and 9 injection drug users.[8,9] Although the U.S. Centers for Disease Control and Prevention (CDC) has collected surveillance data on AIDS cases since 1981, this national system for the surveillance of HIV infection has evolved over time as understanding of the epidemic has advanced. The most recent surveillance report[1] from the CDC provides estimated numbers and rates of diagnoses of HIV infection, including cases that progressed to AIDS, from the 42 areas (37 states and 5 U.S.-dependent areas) that have had confidential, name-based HIV infection reporting for a sufficient length of time—that is, since at least January 2005—to allow for stabilization of data collection and for adjustment of the data in order to monitor trends. Unless cited otherwise, the data that follow are reported from the HIV Surveillance Report, Diagnoses of HIV Infection and AIDS in the United States and Dependent Areas, 2008.[1]

From 2005 through 2008, the estimated annual rate of diagnoses of HIV infection among black/African Americans increased from 68/100,000 population to 74/100,000 population. In 2008, black/African Americans accounted for 52% of all diagnoses of HIV infection. The 2008 estimated rate of diagnoses for black/African Americans was greater than three times the rate for the Hispanic/Latino population and more than nine times the rate in the white population. Additionally, the estimated rate of AIDS diagnoses among black/African Americans remained stable from 2005 through 2008. In 2008, the estimated rates of AIDS diagnoses among black/African Americans—49.3 per 100,000 population—was approximately three times the rate in the Hispanic/Latino population and 10 times the rate in the white population. Finally, in 2007 (the last year for which data are available), the rate of deaths among persons with a diagnosis of HIV infection was highest among black/African Americans, 331.2 per 100,000 population, and between 2005–2007, the annual rate of deaths among African Americans with an AIDS diagnosis remained stable.

Regarding rates by gender within the African American community, estimated rates of diagnosis of HIV infection are highest in men. By transmission category, estimated rates of diagnosis of HIV infection are the highest among those reporting male-to-male sexual contact. Further, significant inequities exist in rates of new HIV infection for black/African American men and women compared to men and women of other races/ethnicities.[10–13] The rate of new HIV infection for black/African American men is six times that of white men and three times that of Hispanic/Latino men.[13] The rate for black/African American women is almost 15 times the rate for white women and approximately four times the rate for Latino/Hispanic women.[13] The data suggest that lifetime risk for HIV infection is 1 in 16 for black/African American men and 1 in 30 for black women.[13,14]

By age group, 13- to 29-year-old African Americans are also disproportionately affected by HIV compared to other racial/ethnic group members of the same age.[13] Although African Americans represent only 14% of the United States population between 13 and 29 years of age,[15] they account for half of all new infection in this age group.[13] Further, young black/African American gay and bisexually active men are particularly affected, as they represent about 55% of new infections among African Americans 13 to 29 years of age.[13,16]

Context of HIV in African Americans

Behavioral Risk for HIV in African Americans

Partner Characteristics. There is evidence that the observed racial and ethnic inequities in HIV infection rates are not solely accounted for by risk behaviors (for example, multiple partnerships, condom use, and other individual-level sexual behaviors).[17] Rates of HIV and other STIs are higher among African American women despite their risk behavior. A more general look at this trend shows that African Americans have a higher likelihood of acquiring HIV and other STIs, even with lower-risk behaviors.[4]

Prevalence in the African American population is high,[17] leading to an increased probability of sex with an infected individual. One population determinant considered to be a significant contributor to HIV racial disparities is sexual network characteristics.[18] For African Americans, multiple partnerships and high levels of sexual mixing between high-risk and low-risk individuals facilitate the spread of HIV and other STIs.[4] In their research, Laumann and Youm[19] found that black and white Americans participate in largely separate sexual networks and have different numbers of concurrent partnerships. Both groups tend to mix assortatively—that is, to form partnerships between people with similar characteristics. Although blacks are more likely than whites to mix assortatively by race, they are less likely than whites to mix assortatively by risk, thereby perpetuating the risk and maintaining infection within their communities.[19] Black Americans are more likely than white Americans to report concurrent partnerships. Evidence of this difference was found in the 1995 National Survey of Family Growth, where 21% of black women reported concurrent partnerships in the previous 5 years compared with 12% of women in the general population.[4,20] Similarly, the 2002 National Survey of Family Growth showed that black men in the U.S. were more than twice as likely as white men to have concurrent partnerships.[4,21] Inherently, multiple concurrent sexual partnerships tend to spread HIV and other STIs more rapidly than the same number of partnerships held separately. A recent study conducted by Adimora and colleagues[21] showed that having a partner who has had concurrent partnerships was a risk factor for heterosexual HIV transmission among African Americans who were otherwise at low risk.

Unprotected Sex. The risk for transmitting HIV, whether during concurrent sexual partnerships or separate sequential partnerships, becomes exponentially greater if individuals engage in unprotected sex. Previous studies show that a majority of people living with HIV report reduced sexual risk behaviors after diagnosis.[22,23] However, studies and other media sources[24,27] reveal that a substantial minority of HIV-positive persons continue to engage in risky sexual behaviors. In fact, Kalichman[24] estimated from a U.S. sample that approximately 33% of HIV-positive individuals continued to have unprotected sexual intercourse.

A timely example of how HIV continues to devastate the African American community is the high incidence of infection among blacks in the District of Columbia,[25] which has transformed into a "Modern HIV Epidemic."[26] Heterosexual transmission is a leading cause of infection, and black women are at a disproportionately high risk, their infection rate approaching those of women in some developing countries such as Tanzania (7.0%) and Uganda (7.1%).[28] Of all black residents in the city, more than 4% are known to have HIV, while more than three-quarters (76%) of all HIV-infected persons in the District are black.[25] In a recent study conducted by Magnus and colleagues,[29] the authors sought to examine the risk factors of Washington, D.C.'s emerging epidemic among heterosexuals. The study participants—most (92.3%) of whom were black—reported low condom use (71.2% of most recent vaginal sex and 100% of most recent anal sex were unprotected).[29] The statistics regarding the lack of condom use are similar to those found in other studies.[20,30,31] Although this study confirms what research has suggested for quite some time—that HIV risk is perpetuated through behaviors such as having unprotected sex—it also suggests that such behaviors cannot be disassociated from what are seen today as normative heterosexual sexual behaviors.[29] Therefore, in addition to those that are race and gender specific, the African American community might be better served by prevention strategies that are network-based rather than individually-based.[29]

Role of Alcohol and Substance Abuse. Related to unprotected sex and other sexual risk behaviors is the use of alcohol and illicit drugs. The leading causes of HIV infection among African American men and women are exacerbated by high-risk behaviors such as drug and alcohol use and engaging in unprotected sex while under the influence of these substances.[32,33] A number of studies have highlighted an association between the increased prevalence of crack cocaine use and increased risk for HIV.[23,34–38] African American communities experience high rates of crack cocaine use and an increasingly disproportionate burden of HIV prevalence and HIV-related mortality.[39,40] Alcohol consumption has also been shown to lead to risky sexual behavior and, consequently, has a strong correlation to HIV infection.[41–44] In a study by Hines and colleagues,[45] the relationship between acculturation (the extent of adaptation to U.S. mainstream society), alcohol consumption, and HIV-related risky sexual behavior among African American women was examined. The study showed that women who were most likely to engage in risky sexual behavior—multiple partners, nonmonogamous or in a nonmonogamous relationship and inconsistent condom use—were more highly acculturated. Alcohol use proved related to risky sexual behavior when considered in conjunction with respondents' level of acculturation. In essence, those women at risk for contracting HIV were highly acculturated women.[45] Additionally, in qualitative studies conducted by Essien and colleagues,[46] African American men stated that they were aware that their drinking and drug use had, at times, impaired their judgment and created HIV risk situations. Despite this knowledge and the motivation to reduce their risky behaviors, many African American men in the study reported not using condoms or not avoiding antecedent activities—such as drinking and drug use—thereby continuing the cycle.

The Context of Behavioral Risk for HIV in African Americans

Individual Factors. Based on historical patterns, black sexuality was, for centuries, socially constructed as different than "normal" sexuality (i.e., associated with being white, middle-class, and heterosexual).[47,48] The framing of black sexuality as deviant and immoral, as well as the characterization of black men as sexual predators, became socially ingrained before the emergence of the HIV epidemic in the early 1980s.[49] Such inaccurate social constructions influence individual attitudes and behaviors and may contribute to an increase in the HIV prevalence among African Americans.[49] Further, these constructions may also lead to a decrease in self-esteem and an increase in emotional stress if they continue as part of the normative belief.

The identity of African Americans as individuals and as a population was often challenged and shaped by negative social constructs of the Black body.[50] For example, race has been used as a basis of justification for conducting studies to determine a genetic predisposition of violence among blacks, in general, compared to white Americans. However, such a study might seem disingenuous without a comparable study that examines the predisposition of white American men to violence compared with white British or Canadian men.[50] This may all be predicated on the notion that violence is indeed believed to be the result of a gene.

A strategy often utilized by African Americans to cope with such negative constructs is *resiliency*. The concept of resiliency and its association with HIV among African Americans has been discussed in the literature, mostly from the standpoint of adolescent health and experiences with or tendencies toward risky sexual behaviors or substance use.[51–53] However, in more general terms, Airhihenbuwa[50] suggests that resiliency might actually normalize a problem condition for blacks in a way that suggests that normal behavior is an exception. For example, black men are often portrayed as inferior to other races, but are socialized within their own spheres to be dominant and to demonstrate their sexual prowess by having intercourse with as many women as possible without regard to emotional linkage or disease transmission. Black women, on the other hand, are expected to be submissive, but are often stigmatized and labeled as promiscuous when they contract an STI. The pressure to deal with such sexual expectations and stigmatization may cause black women to employ resiliency techniques that leave them feeling disempowered. Moreover, resiliency is based on the notion that the onus of change is on the individual rather than on addressing the institutional and structural forces that produce emotional distress. This allows for the proliferation of linkages that are often hastily made between race and observed disease patterns, leading to one of the most enduring and tenacious psychosocial factors that continues to advance disparities in HIV–stigma.

Stigma is a major obstacle to controlling the HIV epidemic among African Americans.[54] Notions about maintaining health are steeped in cultural norms that are often invalidated at the research level when a group (e.g., African Americans) is associated with a particular disease. Stigma works as a separatist force to divide "normal" individuals from the diseased or inferior subpopulation. Encompassing its numerous variations in definition,[55–57] stigma is essentially a negative social label that has the power to marginalize and to turn people's perceptions and attitudes against those who are viewed as otherwise unfit or threatening by their very presence.

In the early days of the epidemic, HIV was commonly attributed to homosexual white men and, therefore, was associated solely with that group. Because of the stigma associated with homosexual behavior, African Americans distanced themselves from HIV. However, when research revealed the emergence of HIV among blacks, stigmatizing beliefs started to take hold and African Americans became quite sensitive to how the emerging characterizations of HIV were to those historically attributed to blacks.[49] The rise of HIV in the black community had lasting implications for HIV prevention in the U.S. Not only did stigma fester in the minds of white Americans and others who distanced themselves from "diseased" blacks (i.e., *externalized stigma*), it also infiltrated the relationships that African Americans had with each other, in their families and communities, and how they viewed themselves (i.e., *internalized stigma*). The adverse effects of these types of stigmas, especially when it came to HIV and mental health, have been reported elsewhere.[58,59] Although much progress has been made over the last several decades, there are still countless instances where family members shun and communities close their doors and fail to provide adequate support to those who are HIV-positive. This is done partly out of fear and partly out of ignorance.[60,61] The blaming and labeling only fuels the epidemic by causing HIV-infected individuals to feel isolated, resulting in a failure to disclose their seropositive status to partners.[62] The effects of stigma can be far more damaging at the institutional level. For instance, at school or in the workplace, HIV-positive persons can be ostracized and mistreated as a result of unfair policies that provide no protections or resources for the affected individual.[63,64] Although it occurs less often now than it once did, HIV-positive persons are still subjected to resistance and discrimination in health care settings, or, worse yet, such facilities may not be accessible to them or provide adequate types of services.[65,66] In African American communities, churches may also play a role in isolating individuals with HIV and have been reluctant to respond to the epidemic.[67,68] Even inmates with HIV report experiences with stigmatization in prison and how it affects their decisions about disclosure.[69] Stereotypes and prejudicial attitudes are often held by other inmates as well as prison staff. Fortunately, there is a national recognition of the epidemic and a call to action to help stem the spread of HIV.[28,70,71]

African Americans' negative attitudes about HIV and efforts to prevent its spread—and about the American medical care system in general—are also greatly influenced by the history of medical atrocities committed against blacks in the U.S. The impact of the infamous Tuskegee Syphilis Study, during which black sharecroppers and day laborers—many of whom had syphilis—were denied treatment once it became available and were not given the opportunity to provide informed consent to the study,[72] is often cited as a source of distrust of the medical system by African Americans.[50] In an effort to highlight a critical historical point, Vanessa Northington Gamble[73] uncovered experiences of medical distrust that predated public revelations about the Tuskegee Syphilis Study. The point she was making was that describing the Tuskegee Syphilis Study as the singular reason behind African American distrust of the medical institution failed to explain deeply entrenched attitudes within the black community. Gamble[73] articulated that it was important to examine the Tuskegee study within a broader social and historical context so as to recognize that many factors influenced, and continue to influence, African Americans' views of the medical and public health communities. One example offered by Gamble describes how Georgia physician Thomas Hamilton conducted studies to test the duration of prolonged exposure to sun as the cause for heatstroke by burying black men up to their necks in the ground and watching and waiting until they fainted. In another example, Gamble reveals that between 1845 and 1849, three Alabama slave women were used by Dr. J. Marion Sims—the father of modern gynecology—to develop an operation to repair vesicovaginal fistulas by subjecting the women to 30 painful operations without anesthesia.[50] With the history of such medical misdeeds indelibly imprinted on the African American experience, it is conceivable that distrust of medical science, researchers, and government institutions exist in the community. This can make it difficult for health care professionals or social service workers to convince African Americans to seek appropriate care and treatment for HIV. As numerous reports have shown, these preconceived notions about modern medicine and the lack of value placed on one's life can be a barrier that is not easily overcome.[74–79]

Social Factors. Social factors (also referred to as *social determinants*) affect the distribution of HIV through their effects on behavior, networks, and risk of exposure to infection.[4] The effect of these social factors on the HIV epidemic among African Americans has been understudied. In general, key underlying social factors of HIV transmission among African Americans are social networks, partner selection, cultural norms, discrimination, socioeconomic status, and incarceration.

It is empirically valid that poverty creates and maintains vulnerability to HIV and AIDS.[50] There are a disproportionate number of African Americans living in poverty; therefore, it is not difficult to reason that a disproportionate number of African Americans are infected and affected by HIV due to poverty. However, to address poverty, one must address issues of social inequity and social injustice associated with poverty, which is to confront a history of racism.[50] African Americans have lacked opportunities that were afforded other racial and ethnic groups, particularly in the areas of employment and education.[80] This has only served to reinforce a lack of economic resources and stability for blacks in the United States. As a result of such economic instability, blacks may find it more difficult to secure adequate housing in safe environments. Lack of housing or the availability of only unstable housing have been identified as key contributors to rising HIV rates among blacks.[80,81] Further, lower-income African Americans often do not prioritize sexual health and disease prevention in the same way they prioritize other personal issues. Daily struggles, such as paying the rent or mortgage, providing for children, and obtaining and maintaining employment, all may reduce the perceived importance of HIV.[82,83] Additionally, lack of access to resources and inequitable resource distribution have been linked with risky sexual behaviors, lack of access to health care, and an increase in STI rates.[80,84,85] These factors, combined with a high unemployment rate, low mean income, and low education levels, can heavily influence sexual patterns and networks,[80] as people tend to interact with others of similar backgrounds and circumstances.

Another important social factor is incarceration. Instances of incarceration are an unfortunate reality for many African American families. In 2005, over 2.2 million persons were in U.S. prisons.[86] Although only 12% of the U.S. population at that time was considered black or African American, 40% of persons in correctional institutions were black.[87] The disproportionate number of black men compared to white men who spend time in jail or prison can lead to a host of social challenges for black families in the U.S., not the least of which is a negative effect on health outcomes and HIV. The causes of these negative effects are linked to a disruption in sexual networks, or what Thomas and Torrone[88] called "forced migration." When incarceration is high, there is a greater likelihood of disproportionate sex ratios, wherein the women who are left behind lose the financial, social, and emotional support of the incarcerated partner. Therefore, women may begin sexual relationships with other, unincarcerated men while their partners are behind bars.[4] The danger is that multiple women begin vying for the attention of a much smaller pool of "available" men. Additionally, incarcerated men may become involved in same-sex intercourse with others who have a high probability of HIV infection,[4] and upon their release, return to their partners and increase the potential spread of HIV.[89,90]

The crack epidemic that occurred in the U.S. during the latter part of the 20th century also had a severe effect on the incarceration of African Americans, especially those living in poor communities. Socially, the African American community experienced high mortality from crack and other illicit drug activity. A sense of hopelessness gripped many African American communities as they became more destabilized. Legally, these communities became the targets of toughened drug legislation and enforcement, leading to an especially high rate of incarceration for black men. By 2001, 16.6% of black men had been incarcerated.[80,91] From 1995 to 2003, arrests related to illicit drugs were responsible for nearly half of the increase in the number of prison inmates.[86] In summary, high levels of incarceration often lead to increased partner concurrency and increased exposure of incarcerated men to high-risk sex and drug-using behaviors which, in turn, fuel the HIV epidemic in African American communities.[92]

Contribution of Other STIs. African Americans are also disproportionately affected by other STIs. African Americans represented more than 48% of the 1 million cases of chlamydia, and 70% of the 356,000 cases of gonorrhea diagnosed in 2007.[93–95] These data translate into a chlamydia rate eight times as high as the rate among Caucasians and a gonorrhea rate 19 times the rate in Caucasians.[93–95] Significant racial inequities also exist for African Americans in syphilis rates. In 2007, the syphilis rate among African Americans (2.0 per 100,000 population) was seven times that among Caucasians.[94]

The inequities in STI diagnoses among African Americans are significant because of evidence linking an increasing risk for HIV acquisition to the presence of STIs such as chlamydia, gonorrhea, and syphilis,[96,97] as well as transmission of these STIs.[98–100] Additional research is needed to better understand how the presence of other STIs may facilitate ongoing sexual transmission of HIV among African Americans.

Experiences with Racism and Discrimination. Kessler[101] defines *racial* or *ethnic discrimination* as unfair, differential treatment on the basis of race or ethnicity[101] and suggests that African American adults are disproportionately affected by racism compared to other ethnic or racial groups. Additionally, the available literature suggests a link between experiences with racial discrimination and negative health outcomes, including infection with HIV.[102–113] For example, there is a link between racial discrimination in mortgage rates by realtors and residential segregation in lower-income, urban areas.[114] This segregation tends to concentrate the social influences of poverty in a particular area and predispose individuals to social and economic isolation, violence, and illicit drug use.[114] Further, residence among African Americans contributes to sexual risk behaviors because African Americans tend to choose partners from the neighborhoods in which they live.[115] Discrimination also contributes to unequal distribution of health care among African Americans compared to whites. African Americans tend to be more likely to be uninsured and/or underinsured than whites and more likely to encounter barriers to obtaining health insurance and access to care even when they have insurance.[116] Lack of or limited access to care can result in not seeking care for HIV and subsequently to higher rates of transmission.[117] Additionally, because of racial segregation, African Americans may be more likely to seek care in areas where the quality of health care is low.[118] This may result in substandard care and greater health inequities.

Homophobia. Homophobia, the fear or hatred of same-sex attraction or behavior on the basis of negative beliefs and attitudes, has been associated with HIV risk behavior among African Americans.[119] The literature[120] suggests that homophobia is part of the African American culture and is driven by religious and political forces. As such, African American gay, bisexual, and transgender persons—who occupy a dual minority status based on race and sexual orientation—report discrimination from both the African American and gay communities as well as negative health outcomes, such as depression.[121,122] Further, the literature suggests that experiences with homophobia may put individuals at greater risk for isolation, physical violence, psychological distress, and mental health disorders such as depression. Regarding HIV risk, data suggest an association between depressive symptoms and HIV risk behaviors in African American adolescents.[123–125] One study[125] found an association between psychological distress and high-risk sexual behavior, including inconsistent condom use, sex while under the influence of drugs or alcohol, sex with high-risk sexual partners, and STIs.

Behavioral Interventions for HIV Prevention Among African Americans

Significant progress has been made in behavioral and biomedical interventions since the beginning of the epidemic.[126] Antiretroviral drugs (ARVs) have been successful in prolonging and improving the quality of life of those infected with HIV. Despite this progress, the lack of a cure or vaccine leaves implementation of effective and sustainable behavioral interventions the only proven prevention strategy to date for combating the HIV epidemic.[127,128]

The goal of behavioral interventions is to alter behaviors that make individuals more vulnerable to becoming infected or infecting others with HIV.[129,130] The scientific literature and evidence from community providers have shown that behavioral interventions reduce risk behaviors in a wide range of populations, including men who have sex with men (MSM), injection drug users (IDUs), women, adolescents, patients being treated for STIs or seen in health clinics, and persons with other risk factors.[131,132]

Types of Behavioral Interventions

Most behavioral interventions are based on theories that link risk behavior to individual psychological processes such as cognition, beliefs, attitudes, self-efficacy, skills, and perceptions.[129,133] Although such interventions have been shown to be effective in reducing HIV risk behaviors, their effects may not be sustainable, given competing pressures from processes external to the individual. Many studies have established that risk behaviors are ultimately influenced by the larger environmental and community contexts in which individuals live.[134,135] Behavioral interventions are often classified based on the various levels at which they are delivered to positively influence individual, group, and community factors.

Individual-Level Interventions (ILI). Many of the existing behavioral interventions for HIV prevention are individual-level interventions (ILI) that are delivered to single individuals, one at a time. These interventions are designed to motivate individuals to reduce behaviors that put them at risk for acquiring and/or transmitting HIV. They include strategies such as personal risk assessment, risk-reduction counseling, and skills development, including condom use and condom negotiation skills. In addition, they may provide access to information or educational materials that improve the individual's knowledge and attitudes toward HIV acquisition or transmission, and may link or refer individuals to community resources, such as clinics and other health services.[129] An example of individual-level interventions is Project RESPECT.

> ***Project RESPECT*** *is a one-on-one, client-focused HIV/STI prevention counseling intervention, consisting of either 2 (Brief) or 4 (Enhanced) interactive counseling sessions. In the first session (20 minutes) of both Brief and Enhanced Counseling interventions, HIV counselors help STD clinic patients identify personal risk factors and barriers to risk reduction and work with patients to develop an achievable personalized risk reduction plan. HIV-antibody testing is offered at the end of the first session. The second session of the Brief Counseling intervention (20 minutes) includes a discussion of the HIV test result and additional counseling to support patient-initiated behavior change and to help patients develop a longer-term risk reduction plan. Participants in the Enhanced Counseling intervention receive three weekly 60-minute counseling sessions in addition to the first session. (http://www.cdc.gov/hiv/topics/ research/prs/resources/factsheets/RESPECT.htm*

Group-Level Interventions (GLI). Group-level interventions (GLIs) employ the same strategies as ILIs, but are delivered to groups of varying sizes. The use of a small-group format in behavioral interventions enables participants to learn with and from each other in a "safe" environment,[129] thus encouraging interactions among members and helping to normalize and reinforce participants' behavior change. GLIs seek to change individual behavior within the context of a group by assisting participants, as part of a group setting, in identifying, adopting, and maintaining behaviors that reduce their risk for transmission and/or acquisition of HIV.[129] These interventions are usually delivered face-to-face and in one or more sessions (1–32), with durations that vary based on the nature and goal of the intervention.[136] An example of a small-group intervention program is Healthy Relationships:

> ***Healthy Relationships*** *is a multisession, small-group, skills-building program for men and women living with HIV. The program is designed to reduce participants' stress related to safer sexual behaviors and disclosure of their serostatus to family, friends, and sex partners. It consists of five 120-minute sessions during which participants learn problem-solving and decision-making skills to address coping with stress related to safer sexual behaviors and disclosure of serostatus. Participants observe while the facilitators model the skills; they watch scenes from popular movies portraying characters using similar skills, and role-play the scenes as though the situation pertained to safer sex negotiation or serostatus disclosure. Participants receive feedback from the facilitators and each other to encourage self-efficacy, self-evaluation, and behavior change. (http://www.cdc.gov/hiv/topics/research/prs/resources/ factsheets/ healthy-relationship.htm)*

Dyad- and Family-Level Interventions. Dyad- and family-level interventions are delivered in the context of interpersonal relationship dynamics involving family members or partners within a dyad, and focus on communication patterns between or among these groups.[129] Dyadic interventions differ from individual or small-group–focused HIV prevention programs in that they address the ongoing dynamic and interactional forces within dyads that contribute to sexual risk behavior, including gender roles, power imbalances, communication styles, childbearing intentions, and quality of relationship issues (such as commitment, satisfaction, and intimacy).[137] The goal of dyadic interventions is to promote safer sexual behaviors for both members of the dyad. An example of couple or dyadic interventions is Project Connect:

> ***Project Connect*** *was a six-session relationship-based intervention for women in a heterosexual relationship that emphasized communication, negotiation and how gender roles affect relationship dynamics and helped to decrease risky behaviors for couples receiving the intervention together and for couples where the woman attended alone. There were no differences in effects for couples receiving the intervention together or where the woman received the intervention alone. (http://www.cdc.gov/hiv/topics/ research/prs/resources/factsheets/Connect.htm.)*

Family-level HIV interventions are designed to promote behavior change by utilizing the family as the target of intervention. This may include the nuclear family, a family of choice, or a network of individuals who are mutually committed to one another.[138] Family-level interventions are often aimed at helping adolescents deal with problems that may put them at risk for HIV. Families are mobilized to communicate important values, model appropriate behaviors, monitor adolescents' behaviors, and encourage the adoption of HIV-preventive practices.[138,139]

An example of a family-level HIV prevention intervention is REAL Men:

> ***REAL (Responsible, Empowered, Aware, Living) Men*** *is a group-level, skill-building intervention for fathers (or father figures) of adolescent boys*

ages 11–14. The outcomes are to encourage communication between fathers and sons about sexuality, to promote delay of sexual debut, and to promote condom use among sexually active boys[140] (http://www.cdc.gov/hiv/topics/ research/prs/resources/factsheets/REALmen.htm).

Community-Level Interventions (CLIs). In community-level interventions (CLIs), the community is recognized as a unit of identity. The health status characteristics of the community rather than individual or small group behaviors and characteristics are targeted.[138,139] CLIs seek to improve the HIV risk conditions and behaviors in a community by changing social norms regarding risk behaviors, and increasing the social acceptability and support for safer behaviors.[129,141] CLIs may involve altering social policies or characteristics of the environment that constitute barriers to adopting safer behaviors by members of the community. Using concepts and theories such as Diffusion of Innovation and Community Empowerment, CLIs have the advantage of reaching large numbers of individuals who are at risk and empowering community members to take an active role in addressing HIV risk problems and issues.[129,141] Although CLIs are more likely to have smaller intervention effects, they have the potential for broader reach, longer-lasting effects, and to be less costly.[135,142] Examples of CLIs include community mobilization, social marketing campaigns, community-wide events, policy interventions, and structural interventions. One such CLI is Community PROMISE:

> ***Community PROMISE*** *is a community-level intervention designed to promote progress toward consistent HIV prevention through community mobilization and distribution of small-media materials and risk reduction supplies, such as condoms and bleach. It uses role model stories and peer advocates from the community to collect and assess community information, including HIV/STI risk behaviors and influencing factors, and to appropriately tailor the intervention to different populations at risk in the community. Communities that received Community PROMISE showed significant movement toward consistent condom use with their main and non-main partners, and increased condom carrying among members of the communities (http://www.cdc.gov/hiv/topics/ research/prs/resources/factsheets/promise.htm).*

Evidence-Based Interventions. Early HIV interventions began with care providers, family members, and communities who made extraordinary efforts to provide for the medical and psychological needs of their friends and family members affected by the new epidemic.[143] As the state of the science has developed, time and resources have been devoted to developing and rigorously evaluating behavioral interventions for their efficacy in reducing behavioral risk of acquiring HIV infection.[143,144] Meta-analytic studies lend confidence in the results of evidence-based interventions over the alternatives, including no intervention.[145,146]

The term "evidence-based" is often used in the literature to connote the use of research and scientific studies as a base for determining the best practices in a field.[143] Evidence-based practice, a term initially used in the field of medicine, is a broader term that reflects not just evidence from research but also lessons learned over time from practice and consensus among experts regarding existing evidence.[147] Thus, an evidence-based HIV prevention intervention refers to an intervention that has been rigorously evaluated, and has demonstrated efficacy in reducing HIV or STI incidence or HIV-related risk behaviors.[148]

A range of HIV prevention interventions now exist with varying characteristics, such as their theoretical foundation, targeted risk group, manner of delivery, content, length, intensity, method of evaluation, and type and strength of the scientific evidence.[143] The CDC developed a framework for classifying HIV behavioral interventions, Tiers of Evidence, to guide prevention providers in selecting the best interventions for the risk populations they serve. More information on CDC's tiers of evidence can be found at *http://www.cdc.gov/hiv/topics/research/prs/tiers-of-evidence.htm*. **Table 28–1** lists examples of behavioral interventions that have met CDC's standards for evidence of efficacy, included in Tiers I and II of the evidence framework. These interventions were specifically (100% participation) developed for African Americans or were evaluated with a study population consisting of a majority of African Americans (i.e., ≥50% in the study sample).[143]

Gaps in Intervention Strategies for African American Risk Populations. Gaps in intervention research exist despite the progress that has been made as African Americans continue to be disproportionately affected by HIV.[149–151] As previously stated, the majority of the interventions are focused on what individuals can do to change their risk behaviors, regardless of setting and level (individual, group, dyad/family or community) at which the intervention is delivered. Although these strategies have been shown to reduce risk, they may not address the myriad contextual and social factors that many African Americans face. These factors have the potential of undercutting efforts to reduce risk, resulting in higher rates of HIV transmission, and must be addressed in behavioral interventions. Existing interventions targeting African American MSM do not intervene on issues such as stigma and homophobia that may be associated with HIV risk behavior in this group. Some EBIs address these issues—examples are Many Men, Many Voices (*http://www.cdc.gov/hiv/topics/research/prs/resources/factsheets/3mv.htm*) and d-up: Defend Yourself (*http://www.effectiveinterventions.org/en/Interventions/d-up.aspx*) — but there are no proven interventions or strategies to address these issues in the community or at the structural level. Therefore, more interventions are needed for black MSM that employ strategies to address these issues and other barriers that black MSM encounter from the social and cultural environments in which risk behavior occurs.

Similarly, interventions for African American women may not adequately address the social and environmental contexts that impede efforts aimed at behavioral risk reduction among women. High-risk sex—that is, unprotected sex with an HIV-positive partner or partner of unknown status—is well established as the main route of HIV transmission for African American women.[152] However, few of the available behavioral interventions specifically target heterosexual couples.[152,153] Women are often left with the burden of convincing their male partners to adopt prevention strategies such as condom use, which may be challenging to disadvantaged African American women.[149] Recognizing the intersections of these factors and HIV prevention and minimizing their negative influence on women's ability to adopt safe behaviors should be important components of future intervention research targeting African American women. More couple-based interventions are needed that create a safe environment for both men and women to discuss their relationship dynamics and how to reduce associated risks for HIV.[153] Additionally, although evidence-based interventions are available for heterosexually active African American men—for example, Nia (http://www.cdc.gov/hiv/topics/research/prs/resources/factsheets/nia.htm) and Focus on the Future (*http://www.cdc.gov/hiv/topics/research/prs/resources/factsheets/focus-future.htm*)—more interventions are needed in which male gender perspectives are channeled into positive strategies for men to protect both themselves and their female partners from HIV.[153] Adolescents generally are vulnerable to HIV and other STIs due to their physical, psychological, and social attributes. However, African American youth are exposed to risk factors—including early age at sexual initiation, substance abuse, high rates of STIs and HIV in

TABLE 28–1	Evidence-Based Interventions by Level and Subpopulation			
	Evidence-Based Intervention	Population	% African American	Description
Level of Intervention: Individual-Level				
	Positive Choice: Interactive Video Doctor	HIV+	50	An interactive, computer-based intervention aims to improve screening and counseling about ongoing sex risk and substance use among HIV-positive patients; delivered during clinic visit; includes positive risk assessment on a laptop computer, viewing of a 24-minute video clip on doctor counseling session based on the positive risk assessment; followed by a booster video session at 3 months to reflect any changes in risk behaviors since last visit.
	RESPECT	General clinic patients	59	Consists of either two (Brief) or four (Enhanced) interactive counseling sessions; increases clients' perception of personal risks; emphasizes incremental risk-reduction strategies.
	Project START	Incarcerated heterosexual adult men	52	Multisession intervention for people being released from a correctional facility; increases clients' awareness of personal risk; emphasizes incremental risk-reduction strategies; provides clients with tools and resources to reduce their risk.
	Focus on the Future	Heterosexual young adult men	100	Clinic-based, 45- to 50-minute single-session; addresses common errors and problems associated with young men's use of condoms; provides information, motivation, and skills to increase men's ability to use condoms correctly and consistently; delivered by lay health advisors who are African American male.
	Female and Culturally Specific Negotiation Intervention	Heterosexual adults; drug users; women	100	An *Enhanced Negotiation* intervention includes four 20- to 40-minute sessions delivered over a 3- to 4-week time span; focuses on the social context of women's daily lives, including gender-specific behaviors and social interactions, norms and values, and power and control; teaches women risk-reduction strategies, including correct condom use, safer injection, and communication and assertiveness skills.
	Sister-to-Sister (also Small-Group Intervention)	Heterosexual adult women clinic patients	100	A brief (20-minute), one-on-one, skill-based HIV/STD risk-reduction behavioral intervention for sexually active African American women 18 to 45 years old; delivered during routine medical visit; provides intensive, culturally sensitive health information and skills to empower and educate women and help them reduce HIV/STD risk.

TABLE 28–1	Evidence-Based Interventions by Level and Subpopulation *(continued)*			
	Evidence-Based Intervention	Population	% African American	Description
Level of Intervention: Group-Level				
	VOICES/VOCES	Heterosexual adult men and women; STD clinic patients	62	A single-session video-based intervention; designed to increase condom use among STD clinics patients; facilitated group discussion following video on HIV risk behaviors and condom negotiation; provides participants with samples of condoms. (Video available in both English and Spanish.).
	Street Smart	Youth/ runaways, homeless	53	A multisession, skills-building program; helps youth practice safer sexual behaviors and reduce substance use. Sessions address improving youths' social skills, assertiveness and coping through exercises on problem solving, identifying triggers, and reducing harmful behaviors; also provides individual counseling and trips to community health providers.
	Healthy Relationships	HIV +	74	A 5-session program based on Social Cognitive Theory; focuses on developing skills, self-efficacy, and positive expectations about new behaviors through modeling behaviors and practicing new skills.
	Women Involved in Life Learning from Other Women (WILLOW)	HIV+, heterosexual adult women	84	An adaptation of the SISTA intervention; consists of four sessions delivered by two female facilitators, one of whom is living with HIV; emphasizes gender pride, supportive social networks, coping strategies to reduce stress, STD transmission and HIV re-infection risk behaviors, and skills for negotiating safer sex.
	Sisters Informing Healing Living and Empowering (SIHLE)	High-risk youth	100	A peer-led, social-skills training intervention aimed at reducing HIV sexual risk behavior among sexually active, African American teenage females, ages 14–18; consists of four 3-hour, gender-specific and culturally relevant sessions, delivered by two peer facilitators (ages 18-21) and one adult facilitator in a community-based setting; strategies include skills practice, group discussions, lectures, role-playing, and take-home exercises.
	Sisters Informing Sisters on Topics about AIDS (SISTA)	Heterosexual adult women	100	Five peer-led group sessions; designed to increase condom use; focuses on ethnic and gender pride; provides HIV knowledge, coping, and skills training around sexual risk reduction behaviors and decision-making.

TABLE 28–1	Evidence-Based Interventions by Level and Subpopulation (*continued*)			
	Evidence-Based Intervention	Population	% African American	Description
Level of Intervention: Group-Level				
	Nia	Heterosexual men	100	A 2- to 4-session (6 hours total), video-based, small-group–level intervention; based on the Information-Motivational-Behavioral Skills (IMB) model; aims to bring groups of men together, increase motivation to reduce risks, and help men learn new skills to promoting condom use and increase intentions to use condoms
	Self-Help in Eliminating Life-threatening Diseases (SHIELD)	Drug users	94	A 6-session (plus pre-program contact) intervention that trains current and former drug users to be Peer Educators who share HIV prevention information with people in their social networks (e.g., friends, family, sex partners). The target population is male and female adults (18 years and older) who are current or former "hard" drug users (heroin, cocaine, and crack) who interact with other drug users.
	Many Men, Many Voices (3MV)	MSM	100	A 7-session intervention for gay men of color; addresses behavioral factors specific to gay men of color, including cultural/social norms, sexual relationship dynamics, and the social influences of racism and homophobia.
	HORIZONS	High risk youth; females	100	A gender- and culturally-tailored STD/HIV intervention for African American adolescent females seeking sexual health services; consists of two interactive group sessions (4 hours each) and four individual telephone calls (15 minutes each); fosters a sense of cultural and gender pride and emphasize diverse factors contributing to adolescents' STD/HIV risk,.
	Living In Good Health Together ("light")	Heterosexual adults	74	A 7-session, HIV-risk reduction intervention; aimed to stimulate motivation for behavior change along with individualized skill building required to accomplish personal HIV-related goals.
	Project FIO (The Future Is Ours)	Heterosexual adult women	73	Consists of 8 interactive sessions that allow women to connect with each other by sharing their feelings about relationships with men, values and personal vulnerability; understand and personalize their risk for HIV and other STDs, identify barriers to safer sex, and gain practical knowledge about a range of risk-reduction strategies, including male and female condoms and mutual HIV testing; provides women with the skills necessary to communicate and negotiate safer sex with their partners and how to solve problems to avoid relapses.

TABLE 28-1	Evidence-Based Interventions by Level and Subpopulation (*continued*)			
	Evidence-Based Intervention	Population	% African American	Description
Level of Intervention: Dyad- and Family-Level Interventions				
	Connect	Heterosexual adult men and women	55	A 6-session, relationship-based intervention, intended for heterosexual men and/or women and their main sexual partners; teaches couples techniques and skills to enhance the quality of their relationship, communication, and shared commitment to safer behaviors.
	Focus on Youth with Informed Parents and Children Together (FOY+ImPACT)	High-risk youth	100	An 8-session group intervention that provides youth with the skills and knowledge they need to protect themselves from HIV and other STDs. Plus ImPACT, a single-session intervention delivered to each youth and his/her parent or guardian; emphasizing parental monitoring and communication.
	Responsible, Empowered, Aware, Living Men (REAL Men)	High-risk youth	96	A group-level, skill-building intervention for fathers (or father figures) of adolescent boys ages 11-14; encourages communication between fathers and sons about sexuality and to promote delay of sexual intercourse in youth and condom use among sexually active youth. Activities include: 6 group sessions for fathers only; video modeling and practice of fathers talking to sons about sexual topics; a take-home activity is given to be completed with sons; a joint session with sons to discuss peer pressure and parental monitoring

their communities, poverty, and higher school dropout rates—that make them more vulnerable than adolescents of other races/ethnicities.[154]

To better address the risk faced by African American youth and to sustain changes in their sexual behavior, future interventions should employ strategies that address the individual, social, and environmental factors that influence youth risk behaviors. Also important is the need to recognize the diversity of youth, particularly African American youth, and to tailor interventions to the different groups based on age, gender, level of sexual experience, sexual orientation and gender identity, level of risk, and setting of risk.[151,154]

Future Directions for HIV/AIDS Prevention Among African Americans

Based on the available literature and current state of the HIV epidemic, the authors suggest the following for future HIV prevention strategies targeting African Americans:

- Continued education to improve understanding of HIV as a sexually transmitted infection and to improve understanding of the behavioral risk factors—for example, early sexual debut, multiple and concurrent partners, and unprotected sex—for HIV transmission among African Americans

- Additional research to identify the pathways through which social, contextual, and structural factors such as poverty, racism, lower educational attainment, homophobia, higher incarceration rates, and discrimination affect HIV risk behavior among African Americans
- Evidence-based structural interventions based on theories that address social determinants of health and are designed for, and specifically target, the HIV-risk behaviors of African Americans.

Additionally, although not highlighted in this volume, the authors also offer the following strategies as future initiatives:

- Broader dissemination of current, evidence-based interventions to African American populations (for example, MSM and women) at highest risk for HIV transmission and acquisition
- Increased efforts with HIV testing, knowing one's status, and linkage to appropriate care, treatment, and preventive services
- Increased screening and treatment for other STIs as part of a comprehensive plan to stop the ongoing sexual transmission of HIV
- Additional research on biomedical interventions such as pre-exposure (PrEP—providing medication to HIV-negative persons to prevent HIV transmission) and postexposure (PEP—providing medication to partners of HIV-positive persons to prevent HIV transmission) prophylaxis and male circumcision, to determine their effectiveness in HIV prevention efforts targeting African Americans
- Identification and integration of successful strategies for combating health inequities in other diseases into HIV prevention efforts among African Americans.

These strategies will require a sustained, concentrated, collaborative approach from a multidisciplinary team of providers, researchers, academicians, advocates, community partners, and individuals living with HIV, as well as coordination between federal and nonfederal agencies, community-based organizations, universities, health departments, and health care systems. With this effort and input and commitment from the community, inequities in rates of new HIV infections among African Americans can be eliminated.

References

1. CDC. HIV Surveillance Report, 2008; vol. 20. http://www.cdc.gov/hiv/topics/surveillance/resources/reports/. Published June 2010. Accessed July 1, 2010.
2. CDC. Sexually Transmitted Disease Surveillance, 2007. Atlanta, GA: US Department of Health and Human Services: 2008. http://www.cdc.gov/std/stats07/toc.htm. Accessed July 15, 2010.
3. Adimora AA, Schoenbach VJ, Martinson FE, Martinson FE, Coyne-Beasley T, Doherty I, Stancil RG, Fullilove RE. Heterosexually transmitted HIV infection among African Americans in North Carolina. J Acq Immunodeficiency Syndrome 2006;41:616–623.
4. Aral SO, Adimora AA, Fenton KA. Understanding and responding to disparities in HIV and other sexually transmitted infections in African Americans. Lancet 2008;372:337–340.
5. Chu C, Selwyn PA. Current health disparities in HIV/AIDS. AIDS Reader 2008;18(3):144–146, 152–158.
6. Gehlert S, Sohmer D, Sacks T, Mininger C, McClintock M, Olopade O. Targeting Health Disparities: A Model Linking Upstream Determinants to Downstream Intervention. Health Affairs 2008:27(2):339–349.
7. LaVeist T, Thorpe R, Bowen-Reid T, Jackson J, Gary T, Gaskin D, Brown D. Exploring Health Disparities in Integrated Communities: Overview of the EHDIC Study. J Urban Health: Bull NY Acad Med 2007;85(1):11–32.
8. CDC. Update on Kaposi's sarcoma and opportunistic infections in previously healthy persons—U.S. MMWR 1982;31:294–301.

9. Smith DK, Gwinn M, Selik RM, Miller KS, Dean-Gaitor H, Ma'at PI, De Cock KM, Gayle H. HIV/AIDS among African Americans: progress or progression? AIDS 2000;14:1237–1248.

10. Hall HI, Song R, Rhodes P, et al. Estimation of HIV incidence in the United States. JAMA 2008;300 (5):520–529.

11. CDC. Subpopulation estimates from the HIV Incidence Surveillance System—United States, 2006. MMWR 2008;57(35): 985–989. Accessed September 22, 2008.

12. CDC. HIV prevalence estimates —United States, 2006. MMWR 2008;57(39): 1073–1076 .

13. Hall HI, An Q, Hutchinson A, et al. Estimating the lifetime risk of a diagnosis of the HIV infection in 33 states, 2004–2005. J Acquir Immune Defic Syndr 2008;49(3): 294–297..

14. CDC. HIV/AIDS Facts HIV/AIDS among African Americans. CDC, 2009; www.cdc.gov/hiv.

15. U.S. Census Bureau. Public Use Microdata Sample. 2006. Accessed July 7, 2010 at, hppt://dataferrett.census.gov/.

16. CDC. HIV and AIDS among African American Youth. CDC, 2010. Accessed July 5, 2010 at, www.cdc.gov/ .

17. Hallfors DD, Iritani BJ, Miller WC, & Bauer, DJ. (2007). Sexual and drug behavior patterns and HIV and STD racial disparities: the need for new directions. American Journal of Public Health, 97, 125–132.

18. Newman LM & Berman SM. Epidemiology of STD disparities in African American communities. Sex Trans Dis 2008;35(12):S4–S12.

19. Laumann EO & Youm, Y. Racial/ethnic group differences in the prevalence of sexually transmitted diseases in the United States: a network explanation. Sex Trans Dis 1999;26:250–261.

20. Adimora A, Schoenbach V, Bonas D, Martinson F, Donaldson K, Stancil T. Concurrent sexual partnerships among women in the United States. Epidemiology 2002;13:320–327.

21. Adimora AA, Schoenbach VJ, & Doherty IA. HIV and African Americans in the southern United States: sexual networks and social context. Sex Trans Dis 2006;33(7 Suppl), S39–S45.

22. Weinhardt LS, Care MP, Johnson BT & Bickman NL. Effects of HIV counseling and testing on sexual risk behavior: A meta-analytic review of published research 1999;1985–1997.

23. Campsmith ML, Nakashima AK & Jones JL. Association between crack cocaine use and high-risk sexual behaviors after HIV diagnosis. J Acq Imm Deficiency Syndromes 2000;25(2):192–198. doi: 10.1097/00126334-200010010-00015. American Journal of Public Health 89(9):397–1405.

24. Kalichman SC. HIV transmission risk behaviors of men and women living with HIV-AIDS: Prevalence, predictors, and emerging clinical interventions. Clin Psych: Science and Practice 2000;7(1): 32–47. doi: 10-1093/clipsy/7.1.32.

25. Vargas JA, & Fears D. At least 3 percent of DC residents have HIV or AIDS, city study finds; rate up 22% from 2006. The Washington Post. 2009, March 15.

26. District of Columbia Department of Health, HIV/AIDS Administration District of Columbia HIV/AIDS Epidemiology Annual Report 2007.

27. Crepaz N & Marks G. Towards an understanding of sexual risk behavior in people living with HIV: A review of social, psychological, and medical findings. AIDS 2002;16(2):135–149.

28. Joint United Nations Programme on HIV/AIDS (UNAIDS) and World Health Organization (WHO). AIDS epidemic update 2007.

29. Magnus M, Kuo I, Shelley K, Rawls A, Peterson J, Montanez L, West-Ojo T, Hader S, Hamilton F, & Grenberg AE. Risk factors driving the emergence of a generalized heterosexual HIV epidemic in Washington, District of Columbia networks at risk. AIDS 2009;23:1277–1284.

30. Adimora AA & Schoenbach VJ. Contextual factors and the black–white disparity in heterosexual HIV transmission. Epidemiology 2002;13:707–712.

31. Forna FM, Fitzpatrick L, Adimora AA, McLellan-Lemal E, Leone P, Brooks JT, et al. A case-control study of factors associated with HIV infection among black women. J Nat Med Assoc 2006;98:1798–1804.

32. Leigh B & Stall R. Substance use and risky sexual behavior for exposure to HIV: Issues in methodology, interpretation, and prevention. Am Psychol 1993;48(10):1035–1045.

33. Centers for Disease Control and Prevention. (2002). HIV surveillance report, 14.

34. Fullilove MT, Fullilove RE, Haynes K, Gross S. Black women and AIDS prevention: a view towards understanding the gender rules. J Sex Res 1990;27:47–64.

35. Hoffman JA, Klein H, Eber M & Crosby H. Frequency and intensity of crack use as predictors of women's involvement in HIV-related sexual risk behaviors. Drug Alcohol Dependence 2000;58(3):227–236. doi: 10.1016/S0376-8716(99)00095-2.

36. Daniulaityte R, Carlson RG & Siegal HA. "Heavy users", "controlled users", and "quitters": understanding patterns of crack use among women in a mid-western city. Substance Use and Misuse, 2007;42(1);129–152. doi: 10.1080/10826080601174678.

37. Harzke AJ, Williams ML & Bowen AM. Binge use of crack cocaine and sexual risk behaviors among African-American, HIV-positive users, AIDS Behavior 2009;13:1106–1118.

38. MacMaster SA, Rasch RFR, Kinzly ML, Cooper RL & Adams SM. Perceptions of sexual risks and injection for HIV among African American women who use crack cocaine in Nashville, Tennessee, Health & Social Work 2009;34(4):283–291.

39. Centers for Disease Control and Prevention Research. HIV/AIDS surveillance report, 2005. 2007a;Vol. 17:pp. 1–46. Atlanta, GA: US Department of Health and Human Services, CDC.

40. Centers for Disease Control and Prevention Research. Update to racial/ethnic disparities in diagnoses of HIV/AIDS—33 states, 2001–2005. Morbidity and Mortality Weekly Report 2007b;56(9):189–193.

41. Spikes PS, Purcell DW, Williams KW, Chen Y, Ding H & Sullivan PS. Sexual risk behaviors among HIV-positive black men who have sex with women, with men, or with men and women: implications for intervention development. Am J Public Health 2009;99(6);1072–1078.

42. Shuper PA, Neuman M, Kanteres F, Baliunas D, Joharchi N & Rehm, J. Causal considerations on alcohol and HIV/AIDS – a systematic review. Alcohol & Alcoholism 2010;45(2):159–166.

43. Wells BE, Kelly BC, Golub SA, Grov C & Parsons JT. Patterns of alcohol consumption and sexual behavior among young adults in nightclubs. Amer J Drug and Alcohol Abuse 2010;36(1):39–45.

44. Amaro H, Raj A, Vega RR, Mangione TW & Perez LN. Racial/ethnic disparities in the HIV and substance abuse epidemics: communities responding to the need. Public Health Reports 2001;116;434–448.

45. Hines AM, Snowden LR & Graves KL. Acculturation, alcohol consumption and AIDS-related risky sexual behavior among African American women. Women and Health 1998;27(3):17–35.

46. Essien EJ, Meshack AF, Peters RJ, Ogungbade GO, & Osemene NI. Strategies to prevent HIV transmission among heterosexual African-American men. BMC Public Health 2005;5(3),

47. Roberts, D. Killing the black body: Race, reproduction, and the meaning of liberty. New York, NY: Pantheon Books. 1997.

48. Hill Collins P. Black sexual politics: African Americans, gender, and the new racism. New York: Routledge. 2004.

49. Ford CL, Whetten KD, Hal SA, Kaufman JS & Thrasher AD. Black sexuality, social construction, and research targeting 'the Down Low' ('the DL'). Ann Epidemiology 2007;17:209–216.

50. Airhihenbuwa CO. Healing our differences: The global crisis of health and politics of identity. Maryland: Roman and Littlefield. 2007.

51. Dutra R, Forehand R, Armistead L, Brody G, Morse E, Morse PS, & Clark, L. Child resiliency in inner-city families affected by HIV: the role of family variables. Behaviour Research and Therapy 2000;38(5): 471–486.

52. Rosenblum A, Magura S, Fong C, Cleland C, Norwood C, Casella D, Truell J & Curry P. Substance use among young adolescents in HIV-affected families: resiliency, peer deviance, and family functioning. Substance Use and Misuse 2005;40(5);581–603.

53. Fisher HH, Eke AN, Cance JD, Hawkins SR & Lam WK. Correlates of HIV-related risk behaviors in African American adolescents from substance-using families: patters of adolescent-level factors associated with sexual experience and substance use. J Adolescent Health 2007;42(2):161–169.

54. Darrow WW, Montanea JE & Gladwin H. AIDS-related stigma among black and Hispanic young adults. AIDS Behavior 2009;13;1178–1188.

55. Goffman E. Stigma: notes on the management of spoiled identity. Englewood Cliffs, NJ: Prentice-Hall. 1963.

56. Johnson AG. Stigma. The Blackwell Dictionary of Sociology: A user's guide to sociological language. Malden, MA: Blackwell Publishers. 2000;313.

57. Herek, GM. Thinking about AIDS and stigma: a psychologist's perspective. J Law Med Ethics 2002;30:594–607.

58. Crandall C & Coleman, R. AIDS-related stigmatization and the disruption of social relationships. J Soc Pers Rel 1992;9:163–177.

59. Lee, R, Kochman, A, & Sikkema, K. Internalized stigma among people living with HIV/AIDS. AIDS Behavior 2002;6:309–319.

60. Herek GM & Glunt EK. An epidemic of stigma: public reactions to AIDS. Amer Psychol 1988;43:886–891.

61. Herek GM & Capitanio JP. Conspiracies, contagion, and compassion: trust and public reactions to AIDS. AIDS Education and Prevention 1994;6(4):365–375.

62. Clark HJ, Lindner G, Armistead L & Austin B. Stigma, disclosure, and psychological functioning among HIV-infected and non-infected African-American women. Women & Health, 2004;38(4):57–71.

63. Farnham, PG. Defining and measuring the costs of the HIV epidemic to business firms. Public Health Reports 1994;109(3):311–318.

64. Rao D, Angell B, Lam C & Corrigan, P. Stigma in the workplace: employer attitudes about people with HIV in Beijing, Hong Kong, and Chicago. Soc Sci Med 2008;67(10):1541–1549.

65. Foster PH. Use of stigma, fear, and denial in development of a framework for prevention of HIV/AIDS in rural African American communities. Family Community Health 2007;30(4):318–327.

66. Auerbach C & Beckerman NL. HIV/AIDS prevention in New York City: identifying sociocultural needs of the community. Social Work Health Care 2010;49(2):109–133.

67. Baker, S. HIV/AIDS, nurses, and the black church: a case study. Journal of the Association of Nurses in AIDS Care 1999;10(5):71–79.

68. Smith J, Simmons E & Mayer KH. HIV/AIDS and the black church: what are the barriers to prevention services? J Nat Med Assoc 2005;97(12):1682–1685.

69. Derlega VJ, Winstead BA, Gamble KA, Kelkar K & Khuanghlawn P. nmates with HIV, stigma, and disclosure decision-making. J Health Psychol 2010;15(2):258–268.

70. Levi J. An HIV agenda for the new administration. Am J Publ Health 2001;91:1015–1016.

71. Sutton MY, Jones RL, Wolitski RJ, Cleveland JC, Dean HD & Fenton KA. A review of the Centers for Disease Control and Prevention's response to the HIV/AIDS crisis among blacks in the United States. Am J Publ Health 2009;99(Suppl 2): S351–S359.

72. Jones J. Bad blood: The Tuskegee syphilis experiment. The Free Press, New York. 1981.

73. Gamble VN. Under the shadow of Tuskegee: African Americans and health care. Am J Publ Health 1997;87:1773–1778.

74. Gamble VN. A legacy of distrust: African Americans and medical research. Am J Prev Med 1993;9:35–38.

75. Kadaba LS. Minorities in research. Chicago Tribune. 1993 September 13.

76. Wong J. Mistrust leaves some blacks reluctant to donate organs. Sacramento Bee. 1993 February 17.

77. Lyles C. Blacks hesitant to donate; cultural beliefs, misinformation, mistrust make it a difficult decision. The Virginian-Pilot. 1994 August 15.

78. Stevens C. Research: distrust runs deep; medical community seeks solution. The Detroit News. 1995 December 10.

79. Wickham D. Why blacks are wary of white MDs. The Tennessean, 13A. 1997 May 21

80. Hogben M & Leichliter, JS. Social determinants and sexually transmitted disease disparities. Sex Trans Diseases 2008;35(12);S13–S18.

81. Nicholas SW, Jean-Louis B & Ortiz B et al. (Addressing the childhood asthma crisis in Harlem: The Harlem children's zone asthma initiative. Am J Publ Health 2005;95:245–249.

82. de la Cancela, V. Minority AIDS prevention: Moving beyond cultural perspectives towards sociopolitical empowerment. AIDS Education Prevention 1989;1(2):141–153.

83. Braithwaite RL & Taylor SE. Health issues in the black community, 2nd Edit. San Francisco, CA: Jossey-Bass. 2001.

84. Moran JS, Aral SO & Jenkins WC et al. The impact of sexually transmitted diseases in minority populations. Public Health Rep, 1989;104:560–565.

85. Fullilove, RE. African Americans, health disparities and HIV/AIDS: recommendations for confronting the epidemic in black America. A report from the National AIDS Minority Council 2006. Available at: http://www.nmac.org/public_policy/4616.cfm. Accessed December 29, 2009.

86. Okie, S. Sex, drugs, prisons, and HIV. N Engl J Med 2007;356:105–108.

87. Doherty IA, Leone PA & Aral SO. Social determinants of HIV infection in the Deep South. Ame J Publ Health, 2007;97;391.

88. Thomas JC & Torrone E. Incarceration as forced migration: Effects on selected community health outcomes. Am J Publ Health, 2006;96:1762–1765.

89. Adimora AA, Schoenbach, VJ, Martinson, F, Donaldson, KH, Stancil, TR, & Fullilove, RE. Concurrent sexual partnerships among African Americans in the rural south. Ann Epidemiology 2004;14:155–160.

90. Adimora AA, Schoenbach VJ, Martinson FE, Donaldson KH, Stancil TR & Fulllilove RE. Concurrent partnerships among rural African Americans with recently reported heterosexually transmitted HIV infection. J Acquire Immune Def Syndr 2003;34, 423–429.

91. Bonczar TP. Prevalence of imprisonment in the U.S. population, 1974–2001. Washington, DC: US Department of Justice, Bureau of Justice Statistics, 2003.

92. Gaiter JL, Potter RH & O'Leary A. Disproportionate rates of incarceration contribute to health disparities. Amer J Publ Health 2006;96(7):1148–1149. CDC. Trends in Reportable Sexually Transmitted Diseases in the United States, 2006.

93. National Surveillance Data for Chlamydia, Gonorrhea, and Syphilis. Atlanta, GA: US Department of Health and Human Services: November 2007, http://www.cdc.gov/std/

94. CDC. Trends in Reportable Sexually Transmitted Diseases in the United States, 2007. National Surveillance Data for Chlamydia, Gonorrhea, and Syphilis. Atlanta, GA: US Department of Health and Human Services: January 2009, http://www.cdc.gov/std/.

95. CDC. Most Widely Reported, Curable STDs Remain Significant Health Threat. Atlanta, GA: US Department of Health and Human Services: March 2009, http://www.cdc.gov/std/.

96. Cohen M. Perspective HIV and Sexually Transmitted Diseases: Lethal Synergy. Topics in HIV Medicine, 2004;12(4):104–107.

97. Gavin SR, Cohen MS. The role of sexually transmitted diseases in HIV transmission. Nat Rev Microbiol 2004;2:33–34.

98. Reynolds, SJ, Risbud, AR, Shepherd M, et al. Recent herpes simplex virus type 2 infection and the risk of human immunodeficiency virus type 1 acquisition in India. J Infect Dis 2003;187:1513–1521.99.

99. CDC. Health Disparities Experienced by Black or African Americans—United States. MMWR, January 14, 2005;54(1): 1–3.

100. CDC. IIIV prevention through early detection and treatment of other sexually transmitted diseases – United States recommendations of the Advisory Committee for HIV and STD Prevention. MMWR, 1998;47(RR-12):1–24.

101. Kessler, R. C., Michelson, K. D., & Williams, D. R. The prevalence, distribution, and mental health correlates of perceived discrimination in the United States. J Health Social Behavior 1999;40:208–230.

102. Brondolo E, Brady ver Halen N, Pencille M, Beatty D, Contrada RJ. Coping with racism: A selective review of the literature and a theoretical and methodical critique. J Behavioral Medicine 2009;32:64–68.

103. Harrell JP, Hall S, Taliferro J. Physiological responses to racism and discrimination: Assessment of the evidence. Am J Public Health 2003;93:243–248.

104. Jones CP Levels of racism: A theoretic framework and a gardener's tale. Am J Public Health 2000;90(8):1212–1215.

105. Jones CP. Confronting institutionalized racism. Phylon 2003;50:7–22.

106. Krieger N. Discrimination and health. In Berkman L & Kawachi I, Eds., Social Epidemiology. Oxford, England: Oxford University Press. 2000;36–75.

107. Krieger N. Embodying inequality: A review of concepts, measures, and methods for studying health consequences of discrimination. In N. Krieger, Ed., Embodying inequality: Epidemiologic perspectives. New York: Baywood Publishing Co. 2005;101–158.

108. Krieger N, Rowley D, Hermann AA, Avery B, Phillips MT. Racism, sexism and social class: Implications for studies of health, disease and well-being. Am J Prev Med 1993;9:82–122.

109. Kwate NO, Valdimarsdottir HB, Guevarra JS, Vovbjerg DH. Experiences of racist events are associated with negative health consequences for African American women. J Natl Med Assoc 2003;95:450–460.

110. Mays VM, Cochran SD, Barnes NW. Race, race-based discrimination and health outcomes among African Americans. Ann Rev Psychol 2007;58, 201–225.

111. Williams, D. R. African-American health: the role of the social environment. J Urban Health 1998;75(2):300–321.

112. Randall V. Dying while black: An in-depth look at a crisis in the American healthcare system. Dayton, OH: Seven Principles Press. 2006.

113. William D. R. & Williams-Morris R. Racism and mental health: the African American experience. Ethnicity Health 2000;5(34):243–268.

114. Massey DS, Denton NA. American Apartheid: Segregation and the Making of the Underclass, Cambridge, MA: Harvard University Press.1993.

115. Zenilman J.M., Ellish N., Fresia A., & Glass G. The geography of sexual partnerships in Baltimore: Applications of core theory dynamics using a geographic information system. Sex Trans Diseases 1999;26:75–81

116. Doty MM & Holmgren AL. Health care disconnect: Gaps in coverage and care for minority adults. findingsFindings from the commonwealth fund biennial health insurance survey (2005). Issue Brief (Commonwealth Fund), 2008;21:12.

117. Kaufmann GR, Zaunders JJ, Cunningham P, Kelleher AD, Grey P, et al. Rapid restoration of CD4 T cell subsets in subjects receiving antiretroviral therapy during primary HIV-1 infection. AIDS 2000;14:2643–2651.

118. Baicker K, Chandra A, & Skinner JS Geographic variation in health care and the problem of measuring racial disparities. Perspectives on Biological Medicine 2005;48:S42–53.

119. Spikes P, Willis L, Koenig L. Violence, Trauma, and Mental Health Disorders in McCree DH, Jones K, and O'Leary A, Eds. African Americans and HIV; Understanding and Eliminating the Crisis. Springer, 2010, in press.

120. Kennamer JK, Honnold J, Bradford J & Hendricks M. Differences in disclosure of sexuality among African American and white gay/bisexual men: Implications for HIV/AIDS prevention. AIDS Education and Prevention 2000;12:519–531.

121. Cochran SD. Emerging issues in research on lesbians' and gay men's mental health: Does sexual orientation really matter? Amer Psychol 2001;932–937.

122. Cochran SD, Sullivan JG& Mays VM. Prevalence of mental disorders, psychological distress and mental health services use among lesbian, gay and bisexual adults in the United States. J Consul Clin Psychol 2003;71(1):53–61.

123. Brown LK, Tolou-Shams M, Lescano C, Houck C, Zeidman J, Pugatch D, Lourie KJ. Depressive symptoms as a predictor of sexual risk among African American adolescents and young adults. J Adolescent Health 2006;39(3):444.e1–444.e8.

124. DiClemente RJ, Wingood GM, Crosby RA, Sionean C, Brown L, Rothbaum B, Zimand E, Cobb BK, Harrington K & Davies S. A prospective study of psychological distress and sexual risk behavior among Black adolescent females. Pediatrics 2001;108(5):e85.

125. Seth P, Raiji PT, DiClemente RJ, Wingood GM & Rose E. Psychological distress as a correlate of a biologically confirmed STI, risky sexual practices, self efficacy and communication with male sex partners in African-American female adolescents. Psychol Health Med 2009;14:291–300.

126. Global HIV Working Group. Behavioral change and HIV prevention 2008. Retrieved May 21, 2010 from http://www.globalhivprevention.org/pdfs/PWG_behavior%20report_FINAL.pdf

127. Fishbein M. The role of theory in HIV prevention. AIDS CARE 2000;12(3):273–278

128. Lagakos SW, Gable AR. Challenges to HIV Prevention — Seeking Effective Measures in the Absence of a Vaccine. N Engl J Med, 2008;358;15:1543–1545.

129. McCree D, Eke A, Williams S. Dyadic. Small Group, and Community -Level interventions for STD/HIV Prevention. In Aral SO, Douglas JM, Lipshutz JA, Eds. Behavioral Interventions for prevention and control of sexually transmitted diseases. New York, NY: Springer Science. 2007;105–125.

130. Bonell C, Imrie J. Behavioral interventions to prevent HIV infection: rapid Evolution, increasing rigor, moderate success. Br Med Bull 2001;58:155–170.

131. Kelly JA, Spielberg F, McAuliffe TL. Defining, Designing, Implementing, and Evaluating Phase 4 HIV Prevention Effectiveness Trials for Vulnerable Populations. J Acquir Immune Def Syndr 2008;1(47) (Suppl 1):S28–S33.

132. Satcher D. The Importance of Behavioral Science in HIV Prevention. Public Health Reports 1996;111(Suppl 1):S1–S2.

133. St Lawrence J. Behavioral Interventions for STDS: Theoretical Models and Intervention Methods. In S.O. Aral, J.M. Douglas, and J.A. Lipshutz (Eds.), Behavioral Interventions for prevention and control of sexually transmitted diseases. New York, NY: Springer Science. 2007;105–125.

134. DiClemente, R. J., Salazar, L. F. and Crosby, R.A. A Review of STD/HIV Preventive Interventions for Adolescents: Sustaining Effects Using an Ecological Approach. J Ped Psychol 2007;32(8)888–906.

135. Kelly J. Challenges in the Development of Community-Level Interventions. Am J Public Health 1999;89(3):299–301.

136. Texas Department of State Health Services; Basics of Evidence-Based interventions and the Programs Review Panel. Retrieved May 21, 2010, from www.dshs.state.tx.us/hivstd/kickoff/0911_EBI_PMRP.ppt

137. Burton J, Darbes, LA, Operario D. Couples-Focused Behavioral Interventions for Prevention of HIV: Systematic Review of the State of Evidence. AIDS Behavior 2008;14:1–10.

138. DiClemente RJ, Wingood GM. Expanding the Scope of HIV Prevention for Adolescents: Beyond Individual-level Interventions. J Adolescent Health 2000;26(6);377–378.

139. University of California, San Francisco 2004. How does HIV prevention work on different levels? Retrieved May 21, 2010, from http://www.caps.ucsf.edu/pubs/FS/pdf/LevelsFS.pdf

140. DiIorio C, McCarty F, Resnicow K, Lehr S, Denzmore P. REAL Men: A Group-Randomized Trial of an HIV Prevention Intervention for Adolescent Boys. Am J Public Health 2007;97(6):1084–1089.

141. Valdiserri RO, Ogden LL, McCray E. Accomplishments in HIV prevention science: implications for stemming the epidemic. Nature Medicine 2003;9(7);881–886.

142. Pinkerton SD, Kahn JG, Holtgrave DR. Cost-Effectiveness of Community-Level Approaches to HIV Prevention: A Review. J Primary Prevention 2002;23(2);175–198.

143. Centers for Disease Control and Prevention The 2009 Compendium of Evidence-Based HIV prevention Interventions, 2009. Accessed May 21, 2010 at, http://www.cdc.gov/hiv/topics/research/prs/index.htm

144. Norton WE, Amico KR, Cornman DH, Fisher WA, Fisher JD. An Agenda for Advancing the Science of Implementation of Evidence-Based HIV Prevention Interventions. AIDS Behavior 2009;13:424–429.

145. Crepaz N, Marshal KJ, Aupont LW, Jacobs ED, Mizuno Y, Kay LS, Jones P, McCree DH, O'Leary A. The Efficacy of HIV/STI Behavioral Interventions for African American Females in the United States: A Meta-Analysis. Am J Public Health 2009;99(11);2069–2078.

146. Johnson BT, Scott-Sheldon LAJ, Smoak ND, LaCroix JM, Anderson JR, Carey MP. Behavioral Interventions for African Americans to Reduce Sexual Risk of HIV: A Meta-Analysis of Randomized Controlled Trials. J Acquir Immune Def Syndr 2009;51;492–501.

147. National Association of Social Workers (NASW) Evidence-Based Practice. Retrieved May 21, 2010, from http://www.socialworkers.org/research/naswresearch/0108evidencebased/default.asp.

148. CDC. http://www.cdc.gov/hiv/topics/research/prs/evidence-based-interventions.htm. Accessed June 15, 2010.

149. El-Bassel, N.A., Caldeira, L.M., and Gilbert, L. Addressing the Unique Needs of African American Women in HIV Prevention. Am J Public Health 2009;99(6);996-1001.

150. Beatty L, Wheeler D, Gaiter J. HIV Prevention Research for African Americans: Current and Future Directions. J Black Psychol 2004;30:40-58.

151. Purcell DW, McCree DH. Recommendations From a Research Consultation to Address Intervention Strategies for HIV/AIDS Prevention Focused on African Americans. Am J Public Health 2009;99(11):1937–1940.

152. Dworkin SL, Fullilove RE, Peacock D. Are HIV/AIDS Preventions for Heterosexually Active Men in the United States Gender Specific? Am J Public Health 2009;99(6);981–984.

153. Elwy AR, Hart GJ, Hawkes S, Petticrew M. Effectiveness of Interventions to Prevent Sexually Transmitted Infections and Human Immunodeficiency Virus in Heterosexual Men. Arch Internal Med 2002;162:1818–1830.

154. Miller KS, Boye CB, Cotton G. The STD and HIV Epidemic in African American Youth: Reconceptualizing Approaches to Risk Reduction. J Black Psychol 2004;30:124-137.

Chapter 29 HIV/AIDS in Hispanic/Latino Communities*

JEFFREY H. HERBST, JOANA M. STALLWORTH,
ROBERTO MEJIA, JOSÉ A. BAUERMEISTER,
AND ANTONIA M. VILLARRUEL

*La salud es un bien que consiste en proporción y en armonía
de cosas diferentes y es como un concierto de música
que hacen entre sí los humores del cuerpo.*

*[Health is a good that is in proportion and harmony of different things
and is like a music concert that together makes the body's humors.]*

—FRAY LUÍS DE LEÓN, 16th Century

Introduction

As the largest, youngest and fastest growing ethnic minority group in the United States, Hispanics/Latinos† are adversely and disproportionately affected by the HIV/AIDS epidemic. Many Latinos living in the U.S. share Spanish as a common language, but this group of people are diverse in terms of demographic characteristics, cultural values, and socioeconomic circumstances.[1] Other factors contributing to the diversity of Latinos include: race and religion; country of origin; migration status (documented, undocumented, and refugee status); generational status or length of residence in the U.S.; cultural influences on familial and interpersonal relationships; acculturation to the mainstream U.S. culture; socioeconomic status, including employment, housing status, income level, and education; and health status and access to quality health care.

Despite this rich and vibrant diversity of the U.S. Latino population, combinations of the above-mentioned factors can place Latinos at increased risk for acquiring or transmitting HIV/AIDS. Further, the growing U.S. Latino population poses challenges to the provision of linguistically and culturally competent HIV/AIDS prevention services, care, and treatment.

The findings and conclusions in this chapter are those of the authors and do not necessarily represent the views of the U.S. Centers for Disease Control and Prevention (CDC).

†*Hispanics or Latinos are people who classify themselves in one of the specific Spanish, Hispanic, or Latino categories listed on the Census 2000 questionnaire—"Mexican, Mexican American, Chicano," "Puerto Rican," or "Cuban"—as well as those who indicate that they are "other Spanish/Hispanic/Latino." Persons who indicated that they are "other Spanish/Hispanic/Latino" include those whose origins are from Spain, the Spanish-speaking countries of Central or South America, and the Dominican Republic. Starting with Census 2000, the question on race asked respondents to report the race or races they consider themselves to be. Thus, Hispanics may be of any race. For the purposes of this chapter, the terms Hispanic and Latino are used interchangeably.*

679

account for a growing share of persons diagnosed with HIV/AIDS. In fact, Latinos have the second highest rate of HIV/AIDS diagnoses among all racial/ethnic groups. From the beginning of the epidemic through 2007, 17% of the total number of AIDS cases reported to the U.S. Centers for Disease Control and Prevention (CDC) were among Latinos.[5] As illustrated in **Figure 29–1**, the percentage of AIDS diagnoses reported from 1985 to 2007 decreased among whites, while the percentages among blacks/African Americans and Latinos increased during that same time period.[5]

Figure 29–2 illustrates rates of HIV/AIDS diagnoses among Hispanic/Latino adults and adolescents from 2004 to 2007 in the 34 states with confidential name-based HIV infection reporting.[5] The average rates of HIV/AIDS ranged from as high as 71.6 per 100,000 persons in New York to as low as 6.1 per 100,000 persons in North Dakota. Other states with particularly high rates of HIV/AIDS diagnoses among Latinos include Mississippi (52.9 per 100,000 persons), Florida (49.1 per 100,000 persons), and New Jersey (49.0 per 100,000 persons). It is important to note, however, that states with sizeable Latino populations (i.e., California, Connecticut, Illinois, and Massachusetts) and the Commonwealth of Puerto Rico do not yet have mature, confidential name-based HIV infection reporting systems. The current exclusion of these areas result in an underrepresentation of HIV/AIDS cases reported for all Latinos in the U.S.

Hispanic/Latino men and women experience higher rates of new HIV infections and AIDS cases than do non-Hispanic whites. In 2007, the rate of HIV/AIDS among Latino males (56.2 per 100,000) was three times the rate for white males (18.7 per 100,000), and the rate of HIV/AIDS among Latino females (16.0 per 100,000) was nearly four times the rate for white females (3.3 per 100,000).[5] According to the CDC's National Center for Health Statistics, HIV/AIDS was the fourth leading cause of death among Latino men and women aged 35 to 44 years in 2006.[6] In

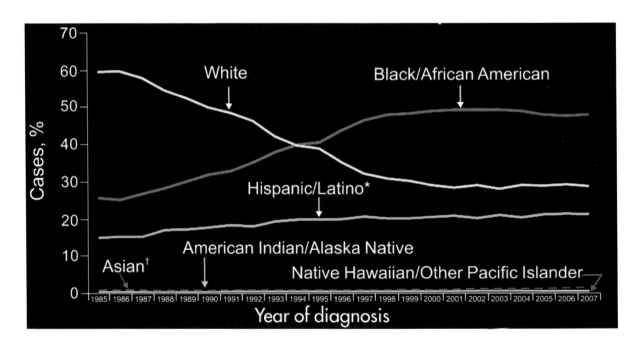

Figure 29–1. *Percentages of AIDS cases among adults and adolescents, by race/ethnicity and year of diagnosis; 1985–2007, United States and dependent areas. Source: Centers for Disease Control and Prevention. HIV/AIDS Surveillance Report, 2007. Vol 19. Atlanta, GA: US Department of Health and Human Services, Centers for Disease Control and Prevention, 2009.[5] Also available online at: http://www.cdc.gov/hiv/topics/surveillance/resources/slides/race-ethnicity/index.htm. In the public domain.*

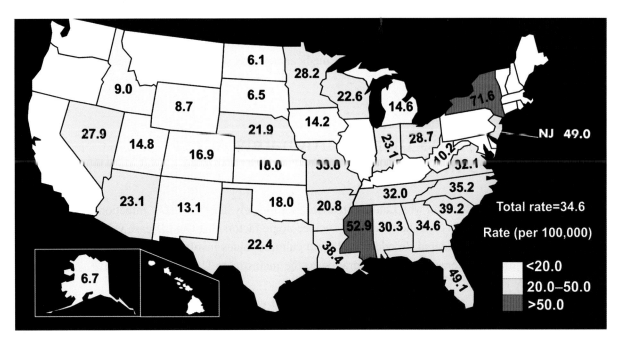

Figure 29–2. *Diagnosis rates of HIV/AIDS for Hispanic/Latino adults and adolescents, 2004–2007, 34 states (Hispanics/Latinos can be of any race). Source: Centers for Disease Control and Prevention. HIV/AIDS Surveillance Report, 2007. Vol 19. Atlanta, GA: US Department of Health and Human Services, Centers for Disease Control and Prevention, 2009.[5] Also available online at: http://www.cdc.gov/hiv/topics/surveil-lance/resources/slides/race-ethnicity/index.htm. In the public domain.*

addition, Latinos under the age of 24 make up more than half of the total U.S. Latino population. Latino young adults aged 20 to 24 years accounted for 24% of new AIDS cases, even though they only comprised 18% of the total young adult population.[5]

The CDC's HIV/AIDS surveillance data reveals that the modality of transmission among Latinos in the U.S. varies according to their place of birth.[5,7] From 2001 to 2005, the most common routes of HIV transmission among U.S.-born Latino men included male-to-male sexual contact (46%), injection drug use (15%) and high-risk heterosexual contact (10%). Similarly male-to-male sexual contact was the most common transmission category among Latino men born in South America, Cuba and Mexico (65%, 62%, and 54% respectively). In contrast, injection drug use (29%) and high-risk heterosexual contact (21%) were the most common transmission risk categories among Latino men born in Puerto Rico. Among Latino women, high risk heterosexual sex and injection drug use were the most common modalities of HIV transmission regardless of place of birth.

Latinos are also more likely than all other racial/ethnic groups to be tested for HIV after their disease has already progressed to AIDS. Although the incubation period of untreated HIV to AIDS is generally considered to be about 10 years, the CDC reported that from 1996 to 2006, 48.4% of Latinos were diagnosed with AIDS within 3 years after learning their initial HIV diagnosis compared to 37.1% of non-Hispanic whites.[8] Rates of progression to AIDS also varied by place of birth. Latinos born in Mexico and Central America exhibited a faster progression to AIDS than Latinos born in the U.S..[9] According to HIV testing data reported to the CDC in 2007 by state and local health departments, Latinos were more likely than non-Hispanic whites to receive a positive HIV test result (1.2% versus 0.8%), and to have received their test results and post-test counseling more than 2 weeks after testing (24.3% versus 21.5%).[10] Information on linkage to care opportunities among Latinos diagnosed with HIV/AIDS is limited. In one national probability study of persons infected with HIV, the likelihood of a 3-month delay between HIV diagnosis and first HIV medical care was significantly higher among Latinos than among non-Hispanic whites.[11]

Why Does HIV/AIDS Disproportionately Affect Latinos in the U.S.?

To better understand why Latinos are disproportionately at risk for HIV infection and experience greater delays in care and treatment, socioecologic factors that can increase vulnerability to HIV need to be considered. In addition, Latino cultural values involving sexuality and gender roles, familial involvement, and acculturation to the mainstream U.S. culture can have an impact on HIV risk.

Early in the epidemic, HIV prevention and care efforts were informed by individualistic models of health promotion. In 1990, for example, the National Institute of Mental Health (NIMH) Task Force to improve HIV prevention efforts concluded that HIV is "...*first and foremost a consequence of behavior. It is not who you are but what you do that determine(s) whether or not you expose yourself to HIV, the virus that causes AIDS.*"[12] Literature reviews have found evidence to support that behavior change interventions work, whether delivered one-on-one, to groups, or entire communities.[13–15] Some reviews have noted that intervention effects tend to only work in the short term, often due to the absence of intervention components addressing social and environmental forces that can shape and reinforce individual behavior.[16,17] A paradigm shift from *individualistic* to *socioecologic* approaches has been proposed where public health interventions intervene at multiple levels.[18] This shift is especially relevant as a potential long-term strategy to eliminate HIV/AIDS disparities among Latinos and other racial/ethnic minority groups.[19,20] However, this paradigm shift has not yet occurred.

A decade after the NIMH Task Force recommendations, Díaz and Ayala,[21] who conducted a critical review of the HIV/AIDS research with Latino men who have sex with men (MSM), concluded that the NIMH Task Force recommendations failed to highlight how the presence of social inequalities limit the enactment of risk-reduction behaviors. Acknowledging that Latinos in the U.S. do not live in a social vacuum, Díaz and Ayala highlighted the need to reconceptualize HIV/AIDS risk among Latinos as a "*characteristic of socially produced contexts [...] where individuals lose their power to enact their protective intentions, or where unsafe practices are perhaps the only viable and adaptive survival strategy*" (p. 24).[21] Socioecologic factors that can impact Latinos' risk of HIV infection include immigration status, socioeconomic position, discrimination, sexual prejudice, and gender inequalities. Each of these factors are obstacles that can hinder Latino communities from protecting themselves effectively against HIV.[22]

Rather than addressing the shared risks confronted by multiple social groups—for example, injection drug users and men who have sex with men (MSM)—we next focus on the role that cultural values and norms can play in exacerbating HIV/AIDS risk among all Latinos.

Cultural Factors and HIV/AIDS Inequalities

Cultural influences on behaviors and expectations can have both direct and indirect influences on sexual behavior.[23] For example, a woman's self-efficacy to negotiate condom use is often framed by Latino cultural values. These cultural values serve as indirect influences on sexual decisions and may include the effects of a broader societal context, such as the unequal distribution of social power between men and women. For Latinos, the cultural values of *respeto*,[24] *simpatia*,[25] *familismo*,[26] and culturally prescribed gender-roles—that is, *machismo* and *marianismo*[23,24]— are hypothesized to influence sexual behavior.‡ Given the paucity of studies that include specific measures of these concepts in research, we focus our attention on two concepts most often studied. gender roles and *familismo*.

Gender Roles. Gender roles among Latinos can serve as both risk and protective factors for sexual behaviors.[27] For women, expectations center on devotion and duty to the family, virginity, fidelity in relationships, and surrendering decision-making (including sexual decision-making) to males. These prescribed values can serve to support safer sex behaviors, especially those related to virginity, abstinence, and fidelity. Female gender norms have also been shown to be a barrier to the successful negotiation of condom use and other safer sex practices. Among U.S.- and Mexican-born Latina adolescents, later initiation of sexual intercourse, failure to use contraception, and fear or failure to negotiate safer-sex practices have been attributed to female gender-role expectations.[28] Moreover, Latina women may be more likely to experience intimate partner violence than women from other races/ethnicities.[29] Exposure to intimate partner violence has direct implications for HIV/AIDS prevention programs, as most programs assume that women are able to regain or negotiate their sexual relationship power with their partners.[28] In the context of intimate partner violence, however, women may be unable to enact safer sex behaviors due to fear of physical or emotional abuse;[30] and increased psychological distress and/or substance abuse behaviors.[31]

For men, gender role expectations are characterized by the concept of *machismo*, and can include traits such as strength, virility, aggressiveness, and acting as a spokesperson and protector of the family.[23] Risk behaviors consistent with male gender-role expectations include engaging in unprotected sexual behavior and having multiple sexual partners.[32] In contrast, the "protector" component of *machismo* can serve as a prompt for safer sexual behavior.

Among Latino MSM, the adoption of a homosexual identity may lead to alienation, and stigmatization. Within the context of traditional Latino gender norms, gay and bisexual men are often confronted with sexual discrimination in their communities. Deviation from pre-specified behaviors and characteristics belonging to a male Latino can result in violence, stigmatization, and abandonment from the individual's social network.[33] The silencing of same-sex attractions and behaviors at work, school, home, and other social venues may hinder opportunities to have open discussions regarding HIV/AIDS risk among Latino MSM.

As many Latinos are of the Catholic faith, Latino MSM also struggle with HIV prevention messages that may be contrary to traditional Catholic positions against the use of condoms and homosexual sex. In addition, negative experiences and expectations of rejection and discrimination because of a Latino MSM's sexual identity and same-sex behaviors may increase feelings of

---

‡*Simpatia and respeto are values that guide interpersonal communication and relationships. Simpatia mandates politeness and respect and discourages criticism, confrontation, and assertiveness. Respeto refers to the need to maintain and defend one's personal integrity and that of others and to allow for face-saving strategies whenever conflict or disagreements evolve.*

Familialism or familismo refers to the importance or significance of the family to the individual. Attitudes and behaviors include giving and receiving emotional and support to extended family, feelings of loyalty, and reciprocity.

The term machismo refers to a strong sense of masculine pride and an exaggerated sense of power and strength. Marianismo is the female gender role that expects women to be sexually pure and passive.

homonegativity (e.g., sexual prejudice and internalized homophobia) and psychological distress.[34,35] In some cases, Latino MSM may revert to maladaptive coping mechanisms, including the use and abuse of substances and/or increased sexual risk behaviors, as strategies to create perceived social connections.[36–39]

Although gender roles ascribed to Latino men and women are important, an acknowledgement of the continuous shaping and reshaping of these norms is required. Recent findings suggest that Latino men and women expect more balanced and reciprocal exchanges within their intimate relationships, including greater emphasis on companionship, intimacy, pleasure, and shared decision-making.[40] Consequently, gender roles within Latino populations must be consistently re-examined, by understanding both their expression among individuals and the social contexts that enable and reinforce them.

Familialism. Familialism, or *familismo*, is seen as one of the most important cultural values among all Latino subgroups.[24] From a network perspective, *familismo* involves strong identification with the family, attachment to the family, and feelings of loyalty, reciprocity, and solidarity with family members.[26] Among Latino migrants, *familismo* may serve as a protective buffer to racial/ethnic discrimination as well as to the hardships that result from navigating a new language, culture, and social system.

Familismo can also help mitigate economic adversity within lower income Latino communities through pooling of resources and creating local kinship networks in the U.S. Access to a strong, supportive family network has been found to be a protective factor against Latino migrant men having extramarital partners[40] and against Latino MSM engaging in substance abuse.[41] The construct of *familismo* also has protective effects on HIV-related risk behaviors among Latino youth. A study of Mexican, Puerto Rican, and Dominican eighth graders found that a dimension of *familismo* referred to as "subjugation to the family"—defined as respect for one's family, respect for parents and parental authority, and placing value of being a good person for one's family—had protective effects against sexual risk-taking among girls.[42] For the boys in this study, rates of sexual risk behaviors were unrelated to *familismo*.

Summary. Latino culture values involving sexuality and gender roles and familial involvement exert both positive and negative influences on risk for HIV/AIDS. Additional research is needed to explore how specific Latino cultural influences can be maximized for purposes of HIV prevention. Next, we review existing HIV prevention interventions for at-risk Latino populations.

Existing HIV Prevention Interventions for Latinos

To review existing HIV prevention interventions for Latinos, we use Frieden's 5-tier health impact pyramid as a conceptual framework (**Figure 29–3**).[18] The framework includes interventions that address social determinants of health at the base of the pyramid, followed by interventions that change the context of risk behaviors or protective actions, long-lasting protective interventions, clinical or biomedical interventions, and, at the top of the pyramid, counseling and educational interventions. Interventions toward the top of the pyramid address individual-level behavior change, while those toward the bottom of the pyramid address entire populations and have the greatest potential for public health impact. We frame our review of HIV prevention interventions for Latinos by first describing behavioral approaches—the top tier of pyramid—

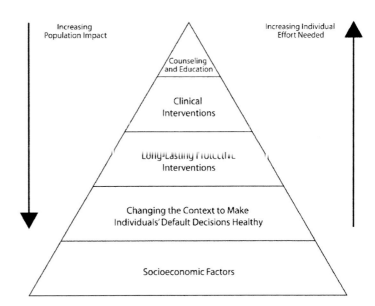

Figure 29-3. *The Health Impact Pyramid. Source: Frieden TR.[18] Reproduced with permission of the American Public Health Association.*

and work our way down to socioeconomic interventions. We begin at the top of the pyramid considering the majority of available interventions involving individual behavior change approaches.

Counseling and Educational Interventions: Individual Behavior Change Approaches

The top tier of the health impact pyramid involves traditional approaches to behavior change, including counseling and health education interventions (**Figure 29-3**).[18] A comprehensive systematic review and meta-analysis of the HIV behavioral prevention literature identified 20 studies that rigorously evaluated behavioral interventions for Latinos in the United States and Puerto Rico.[43] The meta-analysis found that interventions were efficacious in reducing sex risk behaviors (e.g., unprotected sex and multiple sex partners), increasing condom use, and decreasing the acquisition of new sexually transmitted infections. Further, interventions targeting injection drug users significantly reduced drug injection behaviors and sharing of drug injection paraphernalia—such as cookers and cotton—but not sharing of needles. The meta-analysis also found that interventions that directly addressed the Latino cultural belief of *machismo,* and those developed from formative ethnographic research with affected Latino communities, had the greatest efficacy in reducing sexual-risk behaviors. The meta-analysis also found that non-peer–delivered interventions were more efficacious, which is noteworthy given the popularity and frequency with which peer-based approach has been used in Latino communities.[44] Next, we review findings of HIV behavioral interventions for specific at-risk Latino subgroups, including MSM, injection drug users, heterosexual men and women, and youth (**Table 29-2**).

Interventions for MSM. The primary HIV transmission risk behavior among Latino men involves sexual contact with other men. However, to date, only one intervention developed exclusively for Latino MSM has been rigorously evaluated in a randomized trial. Carballo-Dieguez and colleagues[45] evaluated an 8-session intervention based on empowerment theory among 180 gay and bisexual Latino men in New York City. Unfortunately, men randomized to the intervention, *Latinos Empowering Ourselves,* did not report greater reductions in unprotected

TABLE 29–2   Description of HIV Behavioral Intervention for Hispanic/Latino Populations in the United States and Puerto Rico[a]

Study, Location, Study Dates	Design	Sample Characteristics	Intervention Description	Behavioral Findings
Men who have sex with men (MSM):				
Diaz (1998)[46] San Francisco, CA 1995–1996	1-group pre-post	87 gay and bisexual men; 3% transgender Age: 45% < age 30 Ethnicity: 62% Mexican, 14% Caribbean, 14% Central American	Name: Hermanos de Luna y Sol Unit of delivery: Individual and group Theory: Empowerment, self-regulation, psycho-cultural model of HIV risk, action contro Content: HIV information, safer sex intentions, group support/pride, and health-promotion Deliverer: Peer health educator Duration: 4 sessions (8 hrs); 1 outreach encounter Setting: Health center	CU increased for anal insertive sex (46% at BL to 64% at 4 mo) and anal receptive sex (55% at BL to 63% at 4 mo) at 4-month follow-up. Limitation: No statistical tests or comparison group.
Toro-Alfonso et al. (2002)[48] San Juan, Ponce, Mayaguez and Arecibo, Puerto Rico 1992–1995	1-group pre-post	587 gay men Age: 96% < age 40. Ethnicity: 100% Puerto Rican	Name: Conversations Among Men Unit of delivery: Group Theory: Health belief model Content: HIV/STI information, perception of risk, intimacy and self-concept, eroticizing safer sex, and safer sex negotiation skills Deliverer: Peer educator Duration: 5 sessions (15 hrs) Setting: CBO	Significant reduction in insertive UAI and receptive UAI. Limitation: Immediate post-intervention assessment and no comparison group.
Carballo-Dieguez et al. (2005)[45] New York City, NY 1998–2002	RCT with comparison group	180 gay or bisexual men Age: mean 32.9 ± 8.6 yrs Education: 13.9 ± 2.7 yrs % HIV+: 36 Ethnicity: 100% Hispanic/Latino	Name: Latinos Empowering Ourselves (LEO) Unit of delivery: Group Theory: Empowerment Content: Self-efficacy; delay gratification, goal setting, and problem solving skills; exploration of emotions; and changing popular cultural norms Deliverer: Gay-identified bilingual peer counselor Duration: 8 weekly sessions (16 hrs) Setting: NR	No significant intervention effects on sex risk behaviors at 2, 8 or 14-month follow-ups.

[a]Note: ARRM indicates AIDS Risk Reduction Model; CBO, community-based organization; CU, condom use; C&T, counseling and testing; ESOL, English for Speakers of Other Languages; HS, high school; IDU, injection drug use; MSM, men who have sex with men; NA, not applicable; NR, not reported; OR, odds ratio; post-tx, post-intervention; SCT, Social Cognitive Theory; STI, sexually transmitted infection; UAI, unprotected anal intercourse. Table adapted from Herbst et al. (2007).[43]

[b]Identified by the Centers for Disease Control and Prevention as an evidence-based HIV prevention intervention.

See http://www.cdc.gov/hiv/topics/research/prs/evidence-based-interventions.htm.[71]

TABLE 29–2 Description of HIV Behavioral Intervention for Hispanic/Latino Populations in the United States and Puerto Rico[a] *(cont'd)*

Study, Location, Study Dates	Design	Sample Characteristics	Intervention Description	Behavioral Findings
Somerville et al. (2006)[47] California and Texas 2003–2004	Pre-post assessments	766 young migrant MSM *Age:* 79% aged 18 to 25 yrs. *Education:* 68% some HS or HS graduates *Ethnicity:* 100% Mexican	*Name:* Young Latino Promotores *Unit of delivery:* Community *Theory:* Diffusion of innovation *Content:* Adaptation of Popular Opinion Leader intervention where cadres of opinion leaders relay HIV prevention messages to social networks *Deliverer:* Young Latino lay health advisors *Duration:* 2 yrs *Setting:* Community venues	Significant increase in CU for receptive anal sex. *Limitation:* Immediate post-intervention assessment and no comparison community.
Injection Drug Users (IDUs)				
Birkel et al. (1993)[49] Laredo, TX 1988–1991	1-group pre-post	519 out-of-treatment IDU *Sex:* 92.9% male *Age:* mean age 30 (SD=9) *Ethnicity:* 96% Hispanic (91.2% Mexican, 4.8% Other Caribbean)	*Name:* Horizontes AIDS Education Project *Unit of delivery:* Individual *Theory:* NR *Content:* Standard (HIV assessment, education, referral, provision of preventive materials) and enhanced intervention (outreach) *Deliverer:* Counselor for HIV C&T and indigenous outreach worker *Duration:* Continuously up to 3 yrs *Setting:* Community outreach	Significant reduction in sex risk ($p < 0.001$) and needle risk ($p < 0.001$) at 6-month follow-up. *Limitation:* Standard and enhanced groups combined; analyzed as pre-post.
Colon et al. (1993)[50] San Juan, Puerto Rico 1989–1991	RCT with standard outreach and HIV C&T comparison	1,866 out-of-treatment IDU *Sex:* 79.7% male *Age:* mean 32.5 years *Education:* 61% < HS % HIV+: 46 *Ethnicity:* 100% Puerto Rican	*Name:* Puerto Rico AIDS Prevention Project (PRAPP) *Unit of Delivery:* Group and individual *Theory:* NR *Content:* Standard outreach, HIV C&T, referral to drug treatment plus HIV information, CU and needle cleaning skill building, discussion of risk reduction strategies *Deliverer:* Outreach worker, social worker *Duration:* 3 sessions (1.5–3 hrs) *Setting:* Community outreach and HIV assessment center	No significant reduction in sex partners, injection drug use frequency or needle sharing and no significant increase in CU. Significant reduction in cooker sharing at 7-month follow-up ($p < 0.05$).

TABLE 29–2 Description of HIV Behavioral Intervention for Hispanic/Latino Populations in the United States and Puerto Rico[a] *(cont'd)*

Study, Location, Study Dates	Design	Sample Characteristics	Intervention Description	Behavioral Findings
Gonzalez et al. (1993)[51] San Francisco, CA 1991	1 group pre-post	37 in-treatment IDU Sex: 82% men Age: mean age 47.6 Serostatus: 45% HIV+ Ethnicity: 55% Mexican, 27% Puerto Rican, 18% Nicaraguan	Name: NR Unit of delivery: Group Theory: Cognitive-behavioral theory Content: Depression prevention skills and cognitive-behavioral tasks to modify mood-related thoughts and activities Deliverer: Bilingual co-therapists Duration: 6 weekly sessions (12 hrs) Setting: Methadone clinic	Among 11 patients, CU increased from 45% ($n=5$) at BL to 64% ($n=7$) at immediate post assessment. Limitation: Immediate post-intervention assessment and no comparison group.
Grella et al. (1995)[52] Los Angeles, CA 1990–1994	RCT with methadone only comparison	51 IDU women Age: mean 36.4 ± 7 years Education: 63% < HS Ethnicity: 100% Latino (sub-sample)	Name: UCLA Enhanced Methadone Maintenance Project Unit of Delivery: Group and individual Theory: NR Content: Methadone treatment; HIV/AIDS and drug risk information; change attitudes, behaviors, quality of life; group support Deliverer: Methadone counselor, case worker Duration: 4 sessions and 2 counselor contacts per month (min. 4 hrs) Setting: Methadone clinic	Reduced reporting of 2 or more sex partners ($p < 0.05$); decreased inconsistent CU ($p < 0.05$) at 18–24-month follow-up. No significant reduction in needle sharing partners and no increase in safer injection use.
Castro et al. (1997)[53] Southwest, USA Dates NR	Non-RCT with methadone comparison	35 in-treatment IDU Sex: 69% male Age: mean 39 years Education: 11.9 ± 2.1 yrs Ethnicity: 100% Mexican-American	Name: AIDS Prevention Program Unit of Delivery: Group and individual Theory: NR Content: Methadone treatment, AIDS and HIV testing information, exploration of feelings for recovery, personal skills, referrals to social services and job placement Deliverer: Counselor and speakers from drug treatment and narcotics anonymous programs Duration: Continuously over 18 weeks Setting: Methadone clinic	Significant reduction in unprotected sex ($p < 0.01$) and injection drug use ($p < 0.05$). No significant reduction in needle sharing.

TABLE 29–2	Description of HIV Behavioral Intervention for Hispanic/Latino Populations in the United States and Puerto Rico[a] (cont'd)				
	Study, Location, Study Dates	Design	Sample Characteristics	Intervention Description	Behavioral Findings
	Robles et al. (2004)[54,b] Vega Baja, Puerto Rico 1998–2001	RCT with standard NIDA comparison	557 IDU Sex: 89.4% male Age: 18 to 65 years Education: 57% < HS % HIV+: 11.3 Ethnicity: 100% Puerto Rican	Name: Modelo de Intervención Psicomédica Unit of Delivery: Individual Theory: Motivational interviewing Content: Comparison intervention plus self-efficacy, negotiating safe sex encounters, and case management Deliverer: Registered nurse, social worker (case manager), and outreach worker Duration: 8 sessions plus outreach Setting: Study site and outreach in community	No significant decrease in unprotected sex at 6-month follow-up. Significant decrease in injection drug use, and needle sharing at 6-month follow-up (p's < 0.05). No significant decrease in sharing cotton.
Women					
	Nyamathi et al. (1994)[55] Los Angeles, CA, dates NR	RCT with HIV/AIDS education comparison group	213 impoverished women Age: mean 31.3 ± 9.5 years Education: 9.8 ± 3.6 years Ethnicity: 43.9% Mexican, 9.4% Central American, 2.8% South American, 2.4% Puerto Rican	Name: UCLA AIDS Nursing Network Unit of Delivery: Group Theory: Comprehensive health seeking and coping paradigm Content: HIV C&T, AIDS education, role model stories, CU and needle cleaning skill building, self-esteem and interpersonal relationships Deliverer: Nurse counselor and outreach worker Duration: 1 session (2 hrs) Setting: Drug treatment program, homeless shelter	No significant reduction in sex partners at 2-week follow-up. Significant reduction in injection drug use at 2-week follow-up
	Flaskerud et al. (1997)[56] Los Angeles, CA 1991–1993	Non-RCT with no treatment control	508 low-income, immigrants Age: mean 29 ± 9.6 years Education: 9.2 ± 4.1 years Ethnicity: 44% Mexican, 43% Central American, 4% South American	Name: Psychoeducational Intervention Unit of Delivery: Group Theory: Cultural competence, women as caregivers Content: HIV information, risk-reduction strategies, health promotion, referrals, HIV C&T, CU and needle cleaning skills, negotiation skills Deliverer: Peer educator and health worker Duration: 2 sessions (2 wks) Setting: Women, Infants and Children office	Significant reduction in unprotected sex at 2-month follow-up. Limitation: Did not compare intervention and comparison groups.

TABLE 29–2	Description of HIV Behavioral Intervention for Hispanic/Latino Populations in the United States and Puerto Rico[a] (cont'd)			
Study, Location, Study Dates	**Design**	**Sample Characteristics**	**Intervention Description**	**Behavioral Findings**
Shain et al., 1999;[57,b] Korte et al., 2004[102] San Antonio, TX, 1993–1995	RCT with standard HIV and STI C&T	424 women with nonviral STI *Percent Hispanic:* 100% (stratified data) *Ethnicity:* 100% Mexican	*Name:* Sexual Awareness for Everyone (SAFE) *Unit of Delivery:* Group and individual *Theory:* ARRM *Content:* HIV and STI C&T; self-efficacy and risk awareness; group support; CU skills; and decision-making, communication and negotiation skills *Deliverer:* Hispanic female facilitator or nurse *Duration:* 3 weekly sessions (9–12 hrs) *Setting:* Study research clinic	Significant decrease in unprotected sex with partners having untreated or incompletely treated STIs ($p = 0.001$) at 1-year follow-up. Significant reduction in the acquisition of a new STI during the 1st year follow-up ($p = 0.006$), 2nd year follow-up ($p = 0.03$), and over the entire 2-year follow-up ($p < 0.008$).
Suarez-Al-Adam et al. (2000)[58] New Jersey, 1992–1993	RCT with health promotion control	46 Latinas *Age:* mean 34.5 years (range 20 to 59) *Education:* 46% < HS *Ethnicity:* 60% Puerto Rican, 18% Latin American, 4% Caribbean	*Name:* NIMH Collaborative *Unit of Delivery:* Group *Theory:* Social Cognitive Theory *Intervention content:* HIV information, social efficacy, CU skills, safe sex negotiation skill *Deliverer:* Facilitator *Duration:* 7 biweekly sessions (10.5 hrs) *Setting:* NR	No significant increase in CU at 3-month follow-up
Raj et al. (2001); Amaro et al. (2002)[59,b] Boston, MA dates NR	Non-RCT with no treatment comparison	162 women *Age:* mean 28.6 years; range 18 to 35 *Ethnicity:* 55% Dominican, 13% Puerto Rican, 13% Central American or Mexican	*Name:* HIV Intensive Prevention for Latinas *Unit of Delivery:* Group *Theory:* Social Cognitive Theory, Empowerment, Self-in-relation, Diffusion of Innovation, Theory of Gender and Power *Content:* HIV and STI education, HIV risk, partner violence, body image *Deliverer:* Community health educator, facilitator *Duration:* 12 weekly sessions (18 to 24 hrs) *Setting:* Community center	Significant increase in CU during vaginal sex with main male partner at the 3-month follow-up ($p < .05$).

TABLE 29–2 Description of HIV Behavioral Intervention for Hispanic/Latino Populations in the United States and Puerto Rico[a] (cont'd)

Study, Location, Study Dates	Design	Sample Characteristics	Intervention Description	Behavioral Findings
Harvey et al. (2004)[60] Los Angeles, CA 2000–2002	RCT with information only comparison	146 heterosexual couples Age: mean 22 ± 3.2 years Education: 12.5 ± 2.9 years Ethnicity: 86% Mexican	Name: The PARTNERS Project Unit of Delivery: Couples (alone or in group) Theory: Information-Motivation-Behavior Content: HIV and STI information, referral to HIV C&T, perceived vulnerability, control triggers for risky sex, condom skills, and safe sex communication skills. Deliverer: Male and female bilingual facilitator Duration: 1 session (2 hrs) Setting: Community-based clinic	No significant increase in CU at 3 or 5-month follow-ups.
Shain et al. (2004)[61,b] San Antonio, TX 1996–2000	RCT with HIV C&T, STI C&T, and risk information comparison	775 women Age: mean 20.9 ± 0.4 years Education: 10.7 ± 0.1 years Baseline STD: 100% Ethnicity: 77% Hispanic (100% Mexican)	Name: Sexual Awareness for Everyone (SAFE) – 2 Unit of Delivery: Group and individual Theory: AIDS Risk Reduction Model Content: HIV C&T, STI C&T, self-efficacy, perception of risk, CU skills, decision-making, communication and negotiation skills, support groups Deliverer: Nurse clinician, female facilitator Duration: 8 sessions (min. 17 hrs over 23 wks) Setting: STI clinic and study research clinic	No significant decrease in >1 sex partners at follow-ups. Significant reduction in STI re-infection at 24-month follow-up
Peragallo et al. (2005)[62,b] Chicago, IL 1999–2001	RCT with no treatment comparison	657 women Age: range 18 to 44 years Education: 61.9% < HS Ethnicity: 85% Mexican, 15% Puerto Rican	Name: Salud, Educacion, Prevencion y Autocuidado (SEPA) Unit of Delivery: Group Theory: Social Cognitive Theory Content: HIV/AIDS awareness, STI information, self-efficacy, misperceptions of condoms, CU skills, assertiveness and safer sex negotiation skills Deliverer: Red Cross-certified counselor and instructor Duration: 6 weekly sessions Setting: NR	Significant increase in consistent CU during vaginal sex (p=0.006).

TABLE 29-2 Description of HIV Behavioral Intervention for Hispanic/Latino Populations in the United States and Puerto Rico[a] (cont'd)

Study, Location, Study Dates	Design	Sample Characteristics	Intervention Description	Behavioral Findings
Heterosexual Men				
Mishra & Conner (1996)[63] San Diego, CA dates NR	RCT with no treatment comparison	89 male farm workers Age: mean 24.3 ± 5.6 years Education: 6.4 ± 4.2 years Ethnicity: 100% Mexican	Name: Tres Hombres sin Fronteras (Three Men without Borders) Unit of Delivery: Group Theory: NR Content: CU skills, where to obtain condoms, sexual abstinence, needle sharing risk Deliverer: Fotonovela, radionovela Duration: 15 radionovela segments over 3 weeks (1.25 hrs) Setting: Farm worker camps	Significant increase in CU at immediate post-intervention follow-up
Rhodes et al. (2009)[64] North Carolina 2003–2007	Non-RCT with wait list control	222 recent immigrant men Age: mean 29.8 ± 8.3 years Education: 53% 8th grade or less Ethnicity: 60% Mexico, 14% El Salvador, 7% Guatemala, 6% Honduras, 2% Colombia.	Name: HoMBReS: Hombres Manteniendo Bienestar y Relaciones Saludables (Men Maintaining Well-being and Healthy Relationships) Unit of Delivery: Group Theory: Social cognitive theory; empowerment education Content: Increase knowledge about HIV and STIs and testing, increase CU skills, reframe negative sociocultural expectations about being a man Deliverer: Navegante or lay health advisor Duration: 4 session training delivered over 2 weekends (16 hrs); intervention delivered over 18 months Setting: Male soccer leagues	Significant increases in consistent CU and HIV testing immediately after the intervention. Limitation: immediate post-intervention assessment only.

TABLE 29–2	Description of HIV Behavioral Intervention for Hispanic/Latino Populations in the United States and Puerto Rico[a] *(cont'd)*			
Study, Location, Study Dates	**Design**	**Sample Characteristics**	**Intervention Description**	**Behavioral Findings**
Youth				
Sellers et al. (1994)[68] Boston, MA and Hartford, CT 1990–1991	Non-RCT with no treatment comparison	586 urban adolescents *Sex:* 47.6% male *Age:* range 14 to 20 years *Ethnicity:* 94% Puerto Rican	*Name:* Poder Latino *Unit of Delivery:* Community and group *Theory:* NR *Content:* Increase HIV awareness, condom promotion and distribution *Deliverer:* Peer leaders and outreach worker *Duration:* Continuously over 18 mo. *Setting:* Community (CBOs, health centers, residences)	Significant reduction in number of sex partners among females ($p < 0.01$), but no significant reduction in number of partners among males.
Villarruel et al. (2006)[65,b] Philadelphia, PA, 2000–2003	RCT with health promotion control	553 adolescents *Sex:* 55% male *Ethnicity:* 85.4% Puerto Rican	*Name:* ¡Cuídate! (Take Care of Yourself) *Unit of Delivery:* Group *Theory:* SCT, theory of reasoned action *Intervention content:* HIV/AIDS/STI information, self-efficacy with abstinence, normative beliefs, CU skills, communication and negotiation of CU and abstinence *Deliverer:* Adult bilingual facilitator *Duration:* 6 sessions (8 hrs over 2 weeks) *Setting:* Schools on the weekend	Across the three follow-ups, significant reductions in sexual intercourse, multiple sex partners and days of unprotected sexual intercourse (all $p < 0.05$). Among sexually active youth at baseline, significant increase in consistent CU across the three follow-ups ($p < 0.05$).
Prado et al., (2007)[67] Miami-Dade County, Florida 2001–2005	RCT with 2 non-HIV controls (ESOL+PATH and ESOL+HEART)	266 adolescents and their primary caregivers *Sex:* 52% female *Age:* youth: mean 13.4 ± 0.68 yrs; caregivers: mean 40.9 ± 6.2 yrs *Ethnicity:* 40% Cuban, 25% Nicaraguan, 9% Honduran, 4% Colombian, 22% Other Latino	*Name:* Familias Unidas and Parent Preadolescent Training for HIV Prevention (PATH) *Unit of Delivery:* Adolescent and caregiver dyad *Theory:* Ecodevelopmental theory *Content:* Prevention of substance use and sexual risk behaviors by increasing family functioning and parental leadership *Deliverer:* 3 Hispanic facilitators with clinical experience *Duration:* 15 sessions (30 hrs), 8 family visits (8 hrs), 2 parent-adolescent circles *Setting:* NR	No significant intervention effects on reducing unprotected sex. Post-hoc analyses revealed significant intervention effects on engaging in unsafe sex at last sex.

Latino men. The intervention was associated with significant increases in consistent condom use and testing for HIV infection. It is noteworthy that the only interventions for Latino men focus on migrants, and there are currently no interventions developed and tested among heterosexual Latino men who are longer-term residents of the U.S.

Interventions for Youth. Latino youth are at high risk for early sexual debut, teen pregnancy, and STIs, including HIV. To date, five interventions have been developed and evaluated among Latino youth and/or their parents (**Table 29–2**).[65–70] Villarruel et al.[65] conducted a randomized trial of a culturally tailored intervention for Latino youth. The 6-session intervention called *¡Cuídate!* (Take Care of Yourself!) includes Latino cultural aspects of *familismo* and gender roles to frame abstinence and condom use as culturally accepted ways to prevent HIV. *¡Cuídate!* participants reported significantly greater reductions in sexual-risk behaviors across three follow-up assessments than control participants. *Poder Latino,* a community-level intervention evaluated in two northern U.S. cities, found that female adolescents in the intervention city (Boston, Massachusetts) reported significantly greater reductions in number of sex partners relative to females in the control city (Hartford, Connecticut).[68] No significant intervention effects were found among adolescent males.

Two interventions have been developed for both Latino youth and their parents. Prado and colleagues[67] evaluated *Familias Unidas*, a parent-centered HIV prevention intervention for adolescents and their parents in Miami-Dade County, Florida. The intervention did not significantly reduce HIV-related sexual risk behaviors, but did significantly reduce illicit drug use. *Familias Unidas* was also evaluated in a separate study of Latino youth with mild behavioral problems.[66] In this study, sexually active youth who participated in the intervention reported significant increases in condom use compared to youth in a control group. Another family-based intervention, *Respeto/Proteger: Respecting and Protecting Our Relationship*, was evaluated among Latino adolescent parents in Los Angeles, California.[70] The intervention significantly reduced episodes of unprotected sex among young mothers and fathers relative to a control intervention. Additional analyses revealed that male parental protectiveness significantly moderated intervention effects among mothers, whereas there was no significant moderating effect of female parental protectiveness on the intervention effects among adolescent fathers. These studies indicate that culturally appropriate, family-based approaches are effective ways to reduce HIV risk behaviors and increase protection actions among Latino youth.

Summary. Behavioral interventions that include counseling or health education approaches reduce HIV-related risk behaviors and increase protective actions.[43] The incorporation of Latino cultural beliefs in many of these interventions may be associated with greater efficacy in certain Latino subgroups.[23,43] Several of the behavioral interventions described above and in **Table 29–2** have been designated by the CDC as evidence-based—that is, they demonstrated the strongest evidence of efficacy in reducing HIV-related risk behaviors or STIs.[71] The evidence-based behavioral interventions developed exclusively for Latinos include one intervention for injection drug users,[54] three interventions for Latino women,[57,59,62] and one intervention for Latino youth.[65] Many of these interventions have been packaged by the CDC and are being nationally diffused through the Diffusion of Effective Behavioral Interventions (DEBI) project.[72]

As we are now in the third decade of the U.S. HIV/AIDS epidemic, there still remain gaps in our portfolio of efficacious behavioral interventions for at-risk Latinos. Research is still needed to develop and test the efficacy of interventions for Latino MSM, heterosexual men, and persons living with HIV/AIDS.

Clinical Interventions

Directly below counseling and health education interventions on the health impact pyramid are clinical interventions (**Figure 29–3**). Clinical interventions involve the use of medical treatment or devices to improve health outcomes.[18] Several clinical interventions for HIV/AIDS prevention are currently being studied, and these approaches may be appropriate for at-risk Latinos. These interventions include HIV treatment adherence interventions, antiretroviral therapy (ART) as pre-exposure prophylaxis (PrEP), the use of vaginal or rectal microbicides, and HIV vaccine trials.

ART Adherence Interventions. Adherence to combination ART is critical to controlling viral replication, maintaining immunologic function, and long-term survival in people living with HIV. Several randomized controlled trials have evaluated the impact of ART adherence on virologic and immunologic response; however, only one trial specifically targeted Latinos. In that trial, the efficacy of an adherence enhancement program for low-income, HIV-infected, Spanish-speaking Latinos was evaluated for improvements in health literacy, patient-provider relationships, and adherence to combination ART.[73] The intervention was associated with significant improvements in HIV health literacy and perceptions of the quality of relationship and communication with physicians, and a weak trend for increased self-efficacy for medication adherence management. However, the intervention did not improve actual medication adherence. More research is needed to understand the quality of health care and treatment provided to HIV-positive Latinos, and adherence to life-saving ART.

PrEP. Another biomedical intervention is PrEP for HIV prevention. PrEP involves the use of antiretroviral medications—for example, tenofovir and emtricitabine—before an individual is exposed to HIV. The hypothesis is that individuals at high risk for exposure to HIV will be protected from infection through daily ART use. Several trials are currently under way to test the efficacy of daily or intermittent PrEP use.[74] In one multinational trial, iPrEx, the efficacy of daily oral tenofovir and emtricitabine use is being tested among 3,000 MSM in six countries, including three in South America (Brazil, Ecuador, and Peru). Although the efficacy of PrEP has not yet been proven at the time of this writing, the approach holds promise in reducing the spread of HIV infection within high-risk Latino populations.

Vaginal and Rectal Microbicides. Topical microbicides are preparations (for example, gels, creams, or foams) that are applied either vaginally or rectally to prevent STIs, including HIV. Several microbicides are being developed, with the majority being intended for use immediately before intercourse. Although early clinical trials failed to demonstrate that microbicides protect against HIV infection,[75,76] recent studies have shown promising findings with the use of vaginal microbicide gels.[77] Few studies have investigated rectal microbicides use among Latino MSM. In one study, Latino men were asked to report how often they use rectal lubricants, their opinions about microbicidal gels, and their willingness to participate in rectal microbicidal trials. Latino men reported that they would use a lubricant containing an anti-HIV microbicide agent during anal sex, and expressed willingness to participate in a microbicide acceptability trial.[78] In contrast, there are no studies researching the acceptability and use of vaginal microbicides among Latino women.

HIV Vaccine Research. A safe and effective vaccine is one of the most important priorities in the field of HIV/AIDS prevention. Consequently, it is imperative to ensure that the vaccine itself, and the acceptability and uptake of the vaccine, is applicable across a variety of at-risk populations. Although Latinos are disproportionately affected by HIV/AIDS, to date they remain underrepresented in several large-scale vaccine trials. For example, the VaxGen Phase III efficacy trial included more than 5,400 men and women; however, only 7% of enrollees were Latino.[79] Studies have explored ways to improve recruitment of Latinos into vaccine trials. One study assessed HIV vaccine acceptability in a sample of Latino men in Los Angeles.[80] Participants were asked to rate the acceptability of eight hypothetical vaccines, and to report postvaccination risk behavior intentions. HIV vaccine acceptability was moderate, with ratings influenced by degree of efficacy, side effects, and cost. With regard to risk behaviors, only 10% of participants reported that they would decrease their use of condoms after receiving a vaccination. This study also suggested approaches to increase the cultural relevance of trial recruitment can facilitate Latino participation in such trials. If a single-dose vaccine can be developed to induce a long-lasting, HIV-specific immune response, then that vaccine would be listed as a long-lasting protective intervention.

Long-Lasting Protective Interventions: The Case for Male Circumcision

Several randomized trials conducted in Africa found that male circumcision has a strong protective effect against HIV infection among men.[81] In these studies, the protective effects of male circumcision chiefly concerned HIV transmission from females to their uninfected male partners. Nevertheless, male circumcision may be a promising biomedical approach for HIV prevention among Latinos due to low rates of circumcision among Latino men. A national probability sample of U.S. adults surveyed between 1999 and 2004 found that Latino men had lower rates of circumcision (42%) than non-Hispanic white (88%) or non-Hispanic black (73%) men.[82]

One study of immigrant Latino MSM living in New York City found that uncircumcised men were almost twice as likely to be HIV-positive as circumcised men.[83] In contrast, a large-scale cross-sectional study of black and Latino MSM in three major U.S. cities found that male circumcision offered no protection against incident HIV infection.[81] More importantly, this study did not find an association between circumcision status and reduced likelihood of HIV infection among black or Latino men who only engaged in unprotected insertive anal sex, a group that would clearly benefit from the intervention. The research findings available to date suggest that the benefits of male circumcision may only benefit a small proportion of Latino men who engage in unprotected sex with infected women. Further, the benefits of circumcision among Latino MSM and women are unsubstantiated.[81]

Changing the Context to Encourage Healthy Decisions: The Case of Social Marketing

Immediately beneath clinical interventions on the health impact pyramid are interventions that seek to change the context of risk behaviors and healthy decision-making (**Figure 29–3**). According to Frieden, interventions in this tier seek to change "*the environmental context to make healthy options the default choice, regardless of education, income, service provision, or other societal factors*" (p. 591).[18] Social marketing interventions fall within this tier as they encourage individual-level and community-level changes for improved health decision-making.[84] Social marketing often involves the use of mass media—radio, television, print media, and, more recently, the Internet—and advertising techniques to promote greater knowledge and behavioral and social change.

Social marketing has been used to bolster the recruitment of hard-to-reach Latinos into HIV prevention programs. *Proyecto Solaar* involved a social marketing campaign for recruiting gay and bisexual Latino men into a culturally based HIV prevention program.[85] The campaign included the publication of distinctive images in popular magazines read by the target population, a toll-free number and Web site for contacting the program, and innovative use of media to reinforce connection with the program. The campaign resulted in improved recruitment of participants into the HIV prevention program and strengthened the community-based agency's capacity to implement and evaluate their program.

Two campaigns that specifically targeted Latinos have been reported in the literature. The *Tú No Me Conoces* (You Don't Know Me) campaign sought to increase HIV awareness and testing among Latinos living along the U.S.-Mexico border in California.[86] The 8-week campaign included Spanish-language radio, print media, Web sites, and a toll-free HIV-testing referral hotline. Evaluation of the campaign revealed a significant increase in HIV testing at clinics affiliated with the study. In addition, over one-quarter of people seeking an HIV test had either heard or saw an HIV advertisement from the campaign. Martínez-Donate and colleagues[87] reported the impact of a campaign called *Hombres Sanos* (Healthy Men) to reduce HIV risk among heterosexually identified Latino men who have sex with men and women (MSMW). The campaign was conducted in northern San Diego County and was successful in contacting very hard-to-reach Latino men. Data on campaign exposure revealed 85.9% of heterosexual men and 86.8% of heterosexually identified MSMW reported awareness of the campaign. In addition, the campaign was associated with increased intentions to get tested for HIV and increased testing behavior. These studies suggest that social marketing can be a viable technique to provide HIV prevention to populations of Latinos who are difficult to reach and can lead to promising increases in protective behaviors. However, both studies were conducted in Southern California, and the generalizability of these findings to Latinos residing in other regions in the U.S. is limited. Additional research is needed to develop, implement, and evaluate culturally relevant social marketing campaigns on a national scale for at-risk Latino populations.

In 2009, the CDC launched a 5-year, multiphased social marketing campaign called Act Against AIDS (or, in Spanish, *Actúa contra el SIDA*). The goal of the campaign was to refocus attention on the U.S. HIV/AIDS crisis and to address complacency by reminding all Americans, including Latinos, of the significant health threat posed by HIV.[88] *Act Against AIDS* features public service announcements, online communications, and targeted messages and outreach to populations most severely affected by HIV (*www.nineandahalfminutes.org*). The campaign will be evaluated in terms of reaching at-risk populations, including Latinos, and level of awareness of the domestic HIV/AIDS crisis.

Socioeconomic Interventions

The bottom tier of the health impact pyramid represents interventions targeting social and economic factors that impact health and well-being (**Figure 29–3**).[18] Interventions in this tier of the pyramid address social determinants of health, and these interventions have the greatest potential for wide-scale public health impact. Various socioeconomic problems directly or indirectly increase Latinos' risk for HIV infection. These factors can include poverty, homelessness, illiteracy, and immigration status to name a few. As mentioned previously, Latinos are more likely than non-Hispanic whites to receive a diagnosis during the late stages of HIV infection, or when they already have AIDS, suggesting that they are not accessing testing or health care services through which HIV can be diagnosed earlier.[8] In addition, migration patterns, social structure, and language barriers, particularly among transient Latino migrants, can hinder access to HIV/AIDS prevention and care.[89] Recent immigrants face additional challenges, such as social isolation and lack of information about HIV/AIDS, that can further increase their risk of exposure to HIV.[90] Few interventions address social determinants of health,[91] and to our knowledge none have been evaluated within Latino communities. Next, we explore structural and systems-level approaches as future directions for HIV/AIDS prevention research among Hispanics/Latinos.[41]

Future Directions for HIV/AIDS Prevention Among Latino Populations

Structural and Systems-Level Approaches

The current state of the epidemic calls for innovative, multilevel approaches for HIV/AIDS prevention. These approaches require not only individual action, but also changes in societal-level determinants of risk.[20] For example, research can determine the association between immigration status and level of acculturation with the acquisition of STIs.[92] Prevention approaches should also be considered as a beginning point and not an end point and, as such, must take into account the impact of prevention, testing, and counseling in relation to access to care and treatment.

Three decades into the epidemic, stigma is still ever-present among health professionals[93] and within the larger Latino community.[94–96] HIV/AIDS stigma may hinder provision of and participation in HIV prevention services or access to care and treatment, and can increase mental health issues that can lead to risky behavior.[22] HIV/AIDS stigma reduction programs can address HIV-specific stigma (that is, living as an HIV-positive individual) as well as HIV-related stigma (being an injection drug user or experiencing sexual prejudice). Policies that encourage acceptance of nonheterosexual sexual identity—such as legalization of same-sex marriage and enforcement of antidiscrimination laws—may also contribute to the reduction of sexual prejudice, sexual identity stigma, and HIV-related risk behaviors. Consistent with lifting the federal ban on needle exchange programs and travel restrictions for people living with HIV/AIDS, policies are needed that earmark funds to incorporate and scale-up stigma-reduction programs.

Mechanisms are also needed to facilitate the integration of HIV/AIDS prevention interventions into primary care settings, faith-based communities, and other culturally and linguistically accessible health care locations for Latinos. HIV/AIDS prevention activities can be combined with other relevant prevention services (including mental health and substance abuse treatment) to maximally affect the epidemic. Furthermore, Latino cultural factors need to be targeted within integrated health care strategies as they increase the risk for Latinos not getting tested for hepatitis, HIV, and other STIs.[97] HIV/AIDS-related policies must also consider the unique characteristics and challenges confronted by two important Latino subgroups, namely, migrant workers and recent immigrants.[90]

Additional structural interventions include national, state and local policies to ensure that HIV/AIDS prevention for Latinos is viewed as a priority. Optimally, earmarked funds for

HIV/AIDS research, surveillance, and community-based programs that are focused on Latinos are needed to test the adequacy of existing interventions, to develop new interventions where appropriate, and to scale-up ongoing prevention and care efforts among Latinos.[98] At a minimum, a coordinated strategy is needed to provide more comprehensive epidemiologic data and projections through the inclusion all state-based HIV/AIDS cases. Such data will guide the allocation of HIV prevention resources based on a more accurate assessment of the epidemic.

Structural barriers must be surmounted to ensure Latinos are in leadership positions in academia, service, and government in order to design and implement necessary changes. A major barrier affecting the development of effective prevention, treatment, and policy approaches are the low numbers of Latinos with mature programs of research,[99] as well as the low numbers of Latinos in governmental research agencies. A concerted effort must be made to increase the number of Latinos in positions to advance an HIV prevention agenda. Their participation alongside other stakeholders, including politicians, religious leaders, and community members, have the potential to enrich ongoing HIV/AIDS prevention efforts within the Latino community.

Operational Research

As highlighted in this chapter, the number and scope of HIV prevention interventions developed for certain high-risk Latino subgroups are limited. Future research must address the need to develop and adapt interventions that target the spectrum of behaviors (such as risky sex and drug-injection practices) and subgroups most affected by the epidemic (for example, MSM).[41,72] Ways to advance the field include: incorporating community knowledge about at-risk populations and approaches into the development and adaptation of interventions; evaluating HIV prevention interventions developed and evaluated in Latin American and the Spanish-speaking Caribbean for use among U.S. Latinos; and determining the efficacy of promising interventions in more diverse Latino populations and settings.[98]

There is a paucity of information related to the process, barriers, and facilitators of scale-up and dissemination of existing evidence-based interventions in Latino communities. Formative operational research must be undertaken to determine the type of prevention approaches used by service providers in Latino communities, including mechanisms of intervention delivery—such as health professionals, community-based workers, or *promotoras* (community members who serve as liaisons between their communities and service providers)[100]—and settings (for example, home-, community-, or faith-based institutions).[101] Operational research must also identify the types of support and capacity-building assistance needed to effectively scale up interventions in Latino communities. Future dissemination efforts should not only ensure a sufficient infrastructure to provide technical assistance and capacity building for Latino-serving community-based organizations in relation to using interventions, but also provide training in cultural and linguistic competence to facilitate dissemination to diverse Latino communities.[72]

Conclusion

Since its inception nearly 30 years ago, the HIV/AIDS epidemic has been and continues to be strongly felt within diverse Latino communities throughout the U.S. and Puerto Rico. This chapter highlights the HIV/AIDS prevention needs of a burgeoning U.S. Latino population. Latinos continue to be disproportionately affected by HIV/AIDS compared to non-Hispanic whites, confront unique sociocultural and socioeconomic challenges, and are currently underserved for HIV-related treatment and care. As documented in this chapter, the determinants of HIV/AIDS risk among Latinos are complex and include factors such as gender, sexual orientation, language proficiency, literacy, level of acculturation, nation of origin, immigration status, and experience with racism and other forms of marginalization.[22,34] In addition, Latino cultural beliefs are critical considerations for effective HIV prevention efforts.

More importantly, structural and systems-level interventions are needed to address the problems of poverty, low education levels, and limited access to appropriate medical and mental health care.[18,41,86] As the U.S. Latino population continues to grow over the next few decades and continues to bear a heavy burden of the HIV/AIDS epidemic, multilevel approaches to HIV prevention for Latinos are needed to achieve a maximum impact on the epidemic.

References

1. U.S. Census Bureau. Hispanics in the United States. Washington, DC: U.S. Census Bureau; 2009. Accessed October 19, 2009 on http://www.census.gov/population/www/socdemo/hispanic/hispanic_pop_presentation.html.

2. U.S. Census Bureau. An older and more diverse nation by midcentury. Washington, DC: U.S. Census Bureau; 2008.

3. Pew Hispanic Center. Latinos account for half US population growth since 2000. Accessed October 19, 2009 at, http://pewhispanic.org/reports/report.php?ReportID=962008.

4. Pew Hispanic Center. Country of origin profiles. Accessed October 19, 2009 at, http://pewhispanic.org/data/origins/2009.

5. Centers for Disease Control and Prevention. HIV/AIDS Surveillance Report, 2007. Vol 19. Atlanta, GA: US Department of Health and Human Services, Centers for Disease Control and Prevention; 2009. Accessed February 9, 2010 at, http://www.cdc.gov/hiv/topics/surveillance/resources/reports/.

6. National Center for Health Statistics. WISQARS [Web-based Injury Statistics Query and Reporting System] Leading causes of death reports, 2006. Hyattsville, MD: US Department of Health and Human Services, Centers for Disease Control and Prevention. Accessed February 19, 2010 at, http://www.cdc.gov/injury/wisqars/index.html.

7. Centers for Disease Control and Prevention. HIV/AIDS among Hispanics—United States, 2001-2005. MMWR. 2007;56:1052–1057.

8. Centers for Disease Control and Prevention. Late- HIV testing—34 states, 1996 to 2005. MMWR. 2009;58(24):661–665.

9. Espinoza L, Hall HI, Selik RM, Hu X. Characteristics of HIV infection among Hispanics, United States 2003-2006. J Acquir Immune Defic Syndr. 2008;49(1):94–101.

10. Duran D, Usman HR, Beltrami J, Alvarez ME, Valleroy L, Lyles CM. HIV counseling and testing among Hispanics at CDC-funded sites in the United States, 2007. Am J Public Health. 2010;E-published ahead of print 10 February 2010.

11. Turner B, Cunningham W, Duan N, et al. Delayed medical care after diagnosis in a US national probability sample of persons infected with human immunodeficiency virus. Arch Intern Med. 2000;160:2614–2622.

12. Fishbein M, Bandura A, Triandis HC. Factors influencing behavior and behavior change: Final report to NIMH. Rockville, MD: National Institute on Mental Health;1991.

13. Coates T, Richter L, Caceres C. Behavioural strategies to reduce HIV transmission: how to make them work better. Lancet 2001;372(9639):669–684.

14. Albarracín D, Gillette JC, Earl AN, Glasman LR, Durantini MR, Ho MH. A Test of Major Assumptions About Behavior Change: A Comprehensive Look at the Effects of Passive and Active HIV-Prevention Interventions Since the Beginning of the Epidemic. Psychol Bull. 2005;131:856–897.

15. Herbst JH, Beeker C, Mathew A, et al. The effectiveness of individual-, group-, and community-level HIV behavioral risk reduction interventions for adult men who have sex with men: A systematic review. Am J Prev Med 2007;32 (Suppl. 4):S38–67.

16. Blankenship KM, Friedman SR, Dworkin S, Mantell JE. Structural interventions: concepts, challenges and opportunities for research. J Urban Health 2006;83:59–72.

17. Dworkin SL, Pinto RM, Hunter J, Rapkin B, Remien RH. Keeping the spirit of community partnerships alive in the scale up of HIV/AIDS prevention: Critical reflections on the roll-out of DEBI (Diffusion of Effective Behavioral Interventions). Am J Commun Psychol 2008;42:51–59.

18. Frieden TR. A framework for public health action: The health impact pyramid. Am J Public Health 2010;100(4):590–595.

19. Organista KC, Carillo H, Ayala G. HIV prevention with Mexican migrants: Review, critique, and recommendations. J Acquir Immune Defic Syndr 2004;37:S227–239.

20. Organista K. Towards a structural-environmental model of risk for HIV and problem drinking in Latino labor migrants: The case of day laborers. J Ethn Culture Diversity Social Work. 2007;16:95–125.

21. Díaz RM, Ayala G. Social discrimination and health: The case of Latino gay men and HIV risk. New York: Policy Institute of the National Gay and Lesbian Task Force; 2001.

22. Gonzalez JS, Hendriksen ES, Collins EM, Durán RE, Safren SA. Latinos and HIV/AIDS: Examining factors related to disparity and identifying opportunities for psychosocial intervention research. AIDS Behav. 2009;13(3):582–602.

23. Marin DV. HIV prevention in the Hispanic community: Sex, culture and empowerment. J Transcult Nurs. 2003;14:186–192.

24. Marin G. AIDS prevention among Hispanics: Needs, risk behaviors and cultural values. Pub Hlth Reports. 1989;104:411–415.

25. Triandis HC, Marin G, Lisansky J, Betancourt H. Simpatia as a cultural script for Hispanics. J Pers Soc Psychol 1985;47:1363–1375.

26. Sabogal F, et al. Hispanic familialism and acculturation: What changes and what doesn't? Hispanic J Behav Sci 1987;9:397–412.

27. Meyer M, Champion J. Protective factors for HIV infection among Mexican American men who have sex with men. J Assoc Nurses AIDS Care 2010;21:53–62.

28. Pulerwitz J, Amaro H, De Jong W, Gortmaker SL, Rudd R. Relationship power, condom use and HIV risk among women in the USA. AIDS Care 2002;14:789–800.

29. Bonomi AE, Anderson ML, Cannon EA, Slesnick N, Rodriguez MA. Intimate partner violence in Latina and non-Latina women. Am J Prev Med 2009;36:43–48.

30. Weidel JJ, Provencio-Vasquez E, Watson SD, Gonzalez-Guarda R. Cultural considerations for intimate partner violence and HIV risk in Hispanics. J Assoc Nurses AIDS Care 2008;19:247–251.

31. Gonzalez-Guarda R, M.,, Peragallo N, Urrutia MT, Vasquez EP, Mitrani VB. HIV risks, substance use, and intimate partner violence among Hispanic women and their intimate partners. J Assoc Nurses AIDS Care 2008;19(4):252–266.

32. Fernandez-Esquer ME, Atkinson J, Diamond P, Useche B, Mendiola R. Condom use self-efficacy among US- and foreign-born Latinos in Texas. J Sex Res 2004;41:390–399.

33. Díaz RM. Latino gay men and HIV: Culture, sexuality and risk behavior. New Yort: Routledge Press; 1998.

34. Bauermeister JA, Morales MM, González-Rivera M, Seda G. Sexual prejudice among Puerto Rican young adults. J Homosex. 2007;53:135–156.

35. Herek GM, Gonzalez-Rivera M. Attitudes toward homosexulaity among U.S. residents of Mexican descent. J Sex Res 2006;43:122–135.

36. Balan I, Carballo-Diéguez A, Ventuneac A, Remien RH. Intentional condomless anal intercourse among Latino MSM who meet sexual partners on the Internet. AIDS Educ Prev 2009;21:14–25.

37. Bauermeister JA. It's all about "connecting": Reasons for drug use among Latino gay men living in the San Francisco Bay Area. J Ethn Subst Abuse 2007;6:109–129.

38. Bauermeister JA. Latino gay men's drug functionality: The role of social networks and social support. J Ethn Subst Abuse 2008;7:41–65.

39. Ramirez-Valles J, Garcia D, Campbell RT, Diaz RM, Heckathorn DD. HIV infection, sexual risk behavior, and substance use among Latino gay and bisexual men and transgender persons. Am J Public Health 2008,98(6):1036–1042.

40. Hirsch JS, Munoz-Laboy M, Nyhus CM, Yount KM, Bauermeister JA. They "miss more than anything their normal life back home": Masculinity and extramarital sex among Mexican migrants in Atlanta. Perspect Sex Reprod Health 2009;41:23–32.

41. Bauermeister JA, Tross S, Ehrhardt AA. A review of HIV/AIDS system-level interventions. AIDS Behav 2009;13:430–448.

42. Guillamo-Ramos V, Bouris A, Jaccard J, Lesesne C, Ballan M. Familial and cultural influences on sexual risk behaviors among Mexicans, Puerto Rican and Dominican Youth. AIDS Educ Prev 2009;21(Suppl. 2):67–79.

43. Herbst JH, Kay LS, Passin WF, Lyles CM, Crepaz N, Marin BV. A systematic review and meta-analysis of behavioral interventions to reduce HIV risk behaviors of Hispanics in the United States and Puerto Rico. AIDS Behav 2007;11:25–47.

44. Rhodes SD, Foley KL, Zometa CS, Bloom FR. Lay health advisor interventions among Hispanics/Latinos: A qualitative systematic review. Am J Prev Med 2007;33(5):418–427.

45. Carballo-Diéguez A, Dolezal C, Leu CS, et al. A randomized controlled trial to test an HIV-prevention intervention for Latino gay and bisexual men: Lessons learned. AIDS Care 2005;17:314–328.

46. Díaz R. Hermanos de luna y sol: A model for HIV prevention with Latino gay men. In: Díaz RM, ed. Latino gay men and HIV: Culture, sexuality and risk behavior. New York: Routledge; 1998:151–175.

47. Somerville GG, Diaz S, Davis S, Coleman KD, Tavaras S. Adapting the popular opinion leader intervention for Latino young migrant men who have sex with men. AIDS Educ Prev 2006;18 (Suppl. A):137–148.

48. Toro-Alfonso J, Varas-Diaz N, Andujar-Bello I. Evaluation of an HIV/AIDS prevention intervention targeting Latino gay men and men who have sex with men in Puerto Rico. AIDS Educ Prev 2002;14:445–456.

49. Birkel RC, Golaszewski T, Koman JJI, Singh BK, Catan V, Souply K. Findings from the Horizontes Acquired Immune Deficiency Syndrome Education Project: The impact of indigenous outreach workers as change agents for injection drug users. Health Educ Quarterly 1993;20:523–538.

50. Colón IIM, Robles RR, Freeman D, Matos T. Effects of a HIV risk reduction education program among injection drug users in Puerto Rico. P R Health Sci J 1993;12:27–34.

51. González GM, Muñoz RF, Pérez-Arce P, Batki SL. Depression and HIV disease in injection drug users: A Spanish language feasibility study. J Counsel Psychol 1993;47:116–128.

52. Grella CE, Annon JJ, Anglin MD. Ethnic differences in HIV risk behaviors, self-perceptions and treatment outcomes among women in methadone maintenance treatment. J Psychoactive Drugs 1995;27:421–433.

53. Castro FG, Tafoya-Barraza HM. Treatment issues with Latinos addicted to cocaine and heroin. In Garcia JG, Zea MC, eds. Psychological interventions and research with Latino populations. Boston, MA: Allyn and Bacon; 1997:191–216.

54. Robles RR, Reyes JC, Colon HM, et al. Effects of combined counseling and case management to reduce HIV risk behaviors among Hispanic drug injectors in Puerto Rico: A randomized controlled study. J Subst Use Treat 2004;27:145–152.

55. Nyamathi AM, Flaskerud J, Bennett C, Leake B, Lewis C. Evaluation of two AIDS education programs for impoverished Latina women. AIDS Educ Prev 1994;6:296–309.

56. Flaskerud JH, Nyamathi AM, Uman GC. Longitudinal effects of an HIV testing and counseling programme for low-income Latina women. Ethn Health 1997;2:89–103.

57. Shain RN, Piper JM, Newton ER, et al. A randomized controlled trial of a behavioral intervention to prevent sexually transmitted disease among minority women. N Engl J Med 1999;340:93–100.

58. Suarez-Al-Adam M, Raffaelli M, O'Leary A. Influence of abuse and partner hypermasculinity on the sexual behavior of Latinas. AIDS Educ Prev 2000;12:263–274.

59. Raj A, Amaro H, Cranston K, et al. Is a general women's health promotion program as effective as an HIV-intensive prevention program in reducing HIV risk among Hispanic women? Pub Hlth Reports 2001;116:599–607.

60. Harvey SM, Henderson JT, Thorburn S, et al. A randomized study of a pregnancy and disease prevention intervention for Hispanic couples. Perspect Sex Reprod Health 2004;36:162–169.

61. Shain RN, Piper JM, Holden AE, et al. Prevention of gonorrhea and chlamydia through behavioral intervention: Results of a two-year controlled randomized trial in minority women. Sex Trans Dis 2004;31:401–408.

62. Peragallo N, DeForge D, O'Campo P, et al. A randomized clinical trial of an HIV-risk-reduction intervention among low-income Latina women. Nurs Res 2005;54:108–118.

63. Mishra SI, Conner RF. Evaluation of an HIV prevention program among Latino farmworkers. In: Mishra SI, Conner RF, Magana JR, eds. Crossing borders: The spread of HIV among migrant Latinos. Boulder, CO: Westview Press; 1996:157–181.

64. Rhodes SD, Hergenrather KC, Bloom FR, Leichliter JS, Montano J. Outcomes from a community-based, participatory lay health advisor HIV/STD prevention intervention for recently arrived immigrant Latino men in rural North Carolina. AIDS Educ Prev 2009;21 (Suppl. B):103–108.

65. Villarruel AM, Jemmott JB, III,, Jemmott LS. A randomized controlled trial testing an HIV prevention intervention for Latino youth. Arch Ped Adol Med 2006;160:772–777.

66. Pantin H, Prado G, Lopez B, et al. A randomized controlled trial of Familias Unidas for Hispanic adolescents with behavior problems. Psychosom Med 2009;71:987–995.

67. Prado G, Pantin H, Briones E, et al. A randomized controlled trial of a parent-centered intervention in preventing substance use and HIV risk behaviors in Hispanic adolescents. J Consult Clin Psychol 2007;75:914–926.

68. Sellers DE, McGraw SA, McKinlay JB. Does the promotion and distribution of condoms increase teen sexual activity? Evidence from an HIV prevention program for Latino youth. Am J Public Health 1994;84:1952–1959.

69. Harper GW, Bangi AK, Sanchez B, Doll M, Pedraza A. A quasi-experimental evaluation of a community-based HIV prevention intervention for Mexican-American female adolescents: the SHERO's program. AIDS Educ Prev 2009;21 (Suppl. B):109–123.

70. Lesser J, Koniak-Griffin D, Huang R, Takayanagi S, Cumberland WG. Parental protectiveness and unprotected sexual activity among Latino adolescent mothers and fathers. AIDS Educ Prev 2009;21(Suppl. 2):88–103.

71. Centers for Disease Control and Prevention. Compendium of Evidence-Based HIV Prevention Interventions; 2009. Accessed February 26, 2010 at, www.cdc.gov/hiv/topics/research/prs/evidence-based-interventions.htm.

72. Stallworth JM, Andia JF, Burgess R, Alvarez ME, Collins C. Diffusion of effective behavioral interventions and Hispanic/Latino populations. AIDS Educ Prev 2009;21 (Suppl. B):152–163.

73. Van Servellen G, Nyamathi A, Carpio F, et al. Effects of a treatment adherence enhancement program on health literacy, patient-provider relationships, and adherence to HAART among low-income HIV-positive Spanish-speaking Latinos. AIDS Patient Care STDs 2005;19:745–759.

74. Cohen MS, Kashuba AD. Antiretroviral therapy for prevention of HIV infection: New clues from an animal model. PLoS Med 2008;5(2):e30.

75. Feldblum PJ, Adeiga A, Bakare R, et al. SAVVY vaginal gel (C31G) for prevention of HIV infection: a randomized controlled trial in Nigeria. PLoS One 2008;3(1):e1474.

76. Ramjee G, Govinden R, Morar NS, Mbewu A. South Africa's experience of the closure of the cellulose sulphate microbicide trial. PLoS Med 2007;4(7):e235.

77. Rohan LC, Moncla BJ, Kunjara Na Ayudhya RP, et al. In vitro and ex vivo testing of tenofovir shows it is effective as an HIV-1 microbicide. PLoS One. 2010;5(2):e9310.

78. Carballo-Diéguez A, Stein Z, Sáez H, Dolezal C, Nieves-Rosa L, Díaz F. Frequent use of lubricants for anal sex among men who have sex with men: the HIV prevention potential of a microbicidal gel. Am J Public Health. 2000;90:1117–1121.

79. Flynn NM, Forthal DN, Harro CD, et al. Placebo-controlled phase 3 trial of a recombinant glycoprotein 120 vaccine to prevent HIV-1 infection. J Infect Dis 2005;191:654–665.

80. Newman PA, Lee SJ, Duan N, et al. Preventive HIV vaccine acceptability and behavioral risk compensation among a random sample of high-risk adults in Los Angeles (LA VOICES). Health Serv Res 2009;E-published 24 September 2009.

81. Millett GA, Ding H, Lauby J, al. e. Circumcision status and HIV infection among black and Latino men who have sex with men in 3 US cities. J Acquir Immune Defic Syndr 2007;46(5):643–650.

82. Xu F, Markowitz LE, Sternberg MR, Aral SO. Prevalence of circumcision and herpes simplex virus type 2 infection in men in the United States: the National Health and Nutrition Examination Survey (NHANES), 1999-2004. Sex Trans Dis 2007;34(7):479–484.

83. Reisen CA, Zea MC, Poppen PJ, Bianchi FT. Male circumcision and HIV status among Latino immigrant MSM in New York City. J LGBT Health Res 2008;15:29–36.

84. Dearing JW, Rogers EM, Meyer G, et al. Social marketing and diffusion-based strategies for communicating with unique populations: HIV prevention in San Francisco. J Health Commun 1996;1:343–363.

85. Conner RF, Takahasi L, Ortiz E, Archuleta E, Muniz J, Rodriguez J. The Solaar HIV prevention program for gay and bisexual Latino men: using social marketing to build capacity for service provision and evaluation. AIDS Educ Prev 2005;17:361–374.

86. Olshefsky AM, Zive MM, Scolari R, Zuñiga M. Promoting HIV risk awareness and testing in Latinos living on the U.S.-Mexico border: the Tú No Me Conoces social marketing campaign. AIDS Educ Prev 2007;19:422–435.

87. Martínez-Donate AP, Zellner JA, Fernández-Cerdeño A, et al. Hombres Sanos: exposure and response to a social marketing HIV prevention campaign targeting heterosexually identified Latino men who have sex with men and women. AIDS Educ Prev 2009;21 (Suppl. B):124–136.

88. Centers for Disease Control and Prevention. Act Against AIDS. 2009; Accessed February 26, 2010 at, http://www2c.cdc.gov/podcasts/media/pdf/ActAgainstAIDS.pdf.

89. Ramos RL, Hernandez A, Ferreira-Pinto JB, Ortiz M, Somerville GG. Promovisión: Designing a capacity-building program to strengthen and expand the role of promotores in HIV prevention. Health Promotion Practice 2006;7:444-449.

90. Painter TM. Connecting the dots: When the risks of HIV/STD infection appear high but the burden of infection is not known—The case of male Latino migrants in the Southern United States. AIDS Behav 2008;12:213–226.

91. Rotheram-Borus MJ, Swendeman D, Chovnick G. The past, present, and future of HIV prevention: integrating behavioral, biomedical and structural intervention strategies for the next generation of HIV prevention. Annu Rev Clin Psychol 2009;5:143–167.

92. Gindi RM, Erbelding EJ, Page KR. Sexually transmitted infection prevalence and behavioral risk factors among Latino and Non-Latino patients attending the Baltimore City STD clinics. Sex Transm Dis 2009;E-published 11 November 2009.

93. Varas-Diaz N, Marzán-Rodríguez M. The emotional aspect of AIDS stigma among health professionals in Puerto Rico. AIDS Care 2007;19:1247 1257.

94. González-Rivera M, Bauermeister JA. Children's attitudes toward persons with AIDS in Puerto Rico: A qualitative exploration of stigma through drawings and stories. Qual Health Res 2007;17:250–263.

95. Larios SE, Davis JN, Gallo LC, Heinrich J, Talavara G. Concerns about stigma, social support and quality of life in low-income HIV-positive Hispanics. Ethn Dis 2009;19:65–70.

96. Ramirez-Valles J, Fergus S, Reisen CA, Poppen PJ, Zea MC. Confronting stigma: Community involvement and psychological well-being among HIV-positive Latino gay men. Hispanic J Behav Sci 2005;27:101–119.

97. Kinsler JJ, Lee SJ, Sayles JN, Newman PA, Diamont A, Cunningham W. The impact of acculturation on utilization of HIV prevention services and access to care among an at-risk Hispanic population. J Health Care Poor Underserved 2009;20:996–1011.

98. Alvarez ME, Jakhmola P, Painter TM, et al. Summary of comments and recommendations from the CDC consultation on the HIV/AIDS epidemic and prevention in the Hispanic/Latino community. AIDS Educ Prev 2009;21 (Suppl. B):7–18.

99. Bernal G, Ortiz-Torres B. Barriers to research and capacity building at Hispanic-serving institutions: The case of HIV/AIDS research at the University of Puerto Rico. Am J Public Health 2009;99(Suppl. 1):S60–S65.

100. Ramos RL, Green NL, Shulman LC. Pasa la Voz: Using peer driven interventions to increase Latinas' access to and utilization of HIV prevention and testing services. J Health Care Poor Underserved 2009;20:29–35.

101. Lescano CM, Brown LK, Raffaelli M, Lima LA. Cultural factors and family-based HIV prevention intervention for Latino youth. J Ped Psychol 2009;34(10):1041–1052.

102. Korte JE, Shain R, Holden AE, et al. Reduction in sexual risk behaviors and infection rates among African Americans and Mexican Americans. Sex Trans Dis 2004;31:166–173.

Chapter 30 HIV/AIDS in Lesbian, Gay, Bisexual, and Transgender Communities*

GORDON MANSERGH AND DARREL HIGA

When it began turning up in children and transfusion recipients, that was a turning point... until then it was entirely a gay epidemic, and it was easy for the average person to say "So what?".

—HAROLD JAFFE, MD,
U.S. Centers for Disease Control and Prevention

Introduction

HIV/AIDS has tragically impacted populations of gay and bisexual men in the United States and around the world over the past 3 decades. Indeed, men who have sex with men (MSM)—a definition used in research that encapsulates behaviorally homosexual and bisexual men—were the first cases of HIV/AIDS identified in the epidemic.[1] MSM continue to be dramatically overrepresented in HIV incident and prevalent cases in the U.S.

Less research has been conducted on other lesbian, gay, bisexual, and transgender (LGBT) populations compared to MSM. Women who have sex only with other women are not generally seen as being at heightened risk for HIV infection.[2] Some behaviorally bisexual women may be at greater risk for HIV, although largely due to other factors and not based on sex with women.[3]

Transgender populations may be at especially high risk for HIV infection—primarily transgender individuals who have sex with men, and are generally (although not exclusively) male-to-female transitioned or transitioning persons.[4] However, relatively little research has been done with these communities, and this is a neglected and important area for future research.

In this chapter, we will address the HIV/AIDS epidemic among MSM and most of the existing HIV literature for LGBT populations. Given the historic import of MSM in the U.S. epidemic, we present a contextual picture of MSM behavior based on research and the environment in which that behavior exists for four periods of the epidemic: Emergence of an Epidemic (1981–1985); Understanding Behavior and Change (1986–1995); Management of a "Chronic Disease" (1996–2009); Now and Moving Forward (2010–and beyond).

The topic of HIV in lesbian, gay, bisexual, and transgender communities is vast, with a rich scientific, political, and sociocultural history over nearly 30 years. Limited space does not allow for full representation of that history here. We focus on summarizing behavioral research within the social context for gay and bisexual men.

Disclaimer: The findings and conclusions in this chapter are those of the authors and do not necessarily represent the views of the U.S. Centers for Disease Control and Prevention.

Emergence of an Epidemic (1981–1985)

In 1981, rare infections were observed among previously healthy young men in California and New York: five cases of *Pneumocystis carinii* pneumonia in Los Angeles,[1] and eight cases of Kaposi's sarcoma in New York City;[5] others soon followed.[6] Cofactors included a history of sexually transmitted diseases (STDs), substance use (commonly, amyl nitrites, known as "poppers", and other stimulants), and sex with other men.[6] Some circles began referring to the unknown illness as "gay cancer" or GRID—gay-related immune deficiency.[7,8] In the following year, cases were identified in nongay populations, including hemophiliacs[9] and Haitians,[10] and, later, injection drug users and children of infected mothers. A more accurate name, acquired immunodeficiency syndrome (AIDS), was officially adopted in 1982.[6] The prejudice and stigma associated with the disease based on early cases was well established by then, however, and the tone was set for a challenged public health and scientific response.

The political environment in the early years of AIDS made it particularly difficult to garner adequate support for a strong and rapid national response.[7,8,11] Although the U.S. Surgeon General, Dr. C. Everett Koop, disseminated HIV information to every U.S. household several years later,[12] President Reagan and his administration lacked direction and consensus on the issue during this period.[7,8,11] Pockets of funding were pieced together by committed scientists and agency administrators.[8,13] Traditional "shoe leather" epidemiology was undertaken by dedicated public health staff to better understand transmission and infection. Nonetheless, the early years of AIDS research and response were largely characterized by lack of an empowered, coordinated federal government response because of an absence of executive leadership and conflict with a socially conservative agenda.[8,11]

In contrast, LGBT communities quickly mobilized against AIDS. Living room meetings and grass roots activism led to programs of community outreach and advocacy for prevention and care. AIDS infiltrated communities in an era when gay men were beginning to live more visible lives in urban settings. The Stonewall uprising (a community response to police raids of a New York City gay bar in June 1969) had occurred a decade earlier, an historic event that symbolized the beginning of the modern gay equality movement and precipitated annual gay pride events around the country each June.[14,15] Harvey Milk was elected a San Francisco City Supervisor in 1977 as one of the first visible gay politicians in the United States; he and Mayor Moscone were assassinated by another politician a year later.[16] Several cities had passed antidiscrimination laws based on sexual orientation, and the first state (Wisconsin) did so in 1982.[17] Gay communities were building presence, and AIDS provided an unfortunate focal point around which to coalesce and mobilize. Agencies such as AIDS Project Los Angeles, the Gay Men's Health Crisis in New York City, and the San Francisco AIDS Foundation emerged. Now acting as institutions, these early LGBT grass roots organizations have diversified and now serve broader populations and address more health issues than HIV/AIDS.[18,19]

Observing and Acting

As HIV/AIDS emerged in the early 1980s, clinicians and scientists worked to better understand the new disease, particularly as it affected the hardest hit communities of MSM. Clinical and behavioral observation and documentation were the foundation of this process.[20] In a matter of months, and certainly within a few years, public health officials knew how HIV was and was not transmitted.[21–23] Given the devastation of the epidemic in gay communities, local prevention began early and continued to evolve based on information available at the time. This level of community investment and action was perhaps unprecedented in modern history, and particularly unique in that—and possibly because—it occurred in a small minority group that was highly stigmatized and marginalized in society.[11,24]

Public health researchers were lucky early on. A cohort study of MSM in San Francisco had begun in 1978, focusing on hepatitis B transmission,[25] which helped in understanding transmission and infection of the emerging disease.[26] Other cohort studies were soon under way outside of the U.S.[27,28] Through the San Francisco study, blood samples and behavioral data were retrospectively available for a large group of MSM; the cohort was already enrolled when AIDS first came to the attention of health officials. This allowed for in-depth examination of transmission factors for MSM regarding data collected prior to the first symptomatic cases of AIDS. The study cohort also allowed for assessment of participants over time, to better understand HIV seroconversion and infection progression.[29]

Cohort studies and other assessments of MSM[30–35] in the first critical years of the epidemic provided a basic understanding of HIV disease transmission and symptoms; the findings provided an empiric basis for which research on other populations followed.[36] Shortly after this period of the epidemic, the collective knowledge was distributed to every household in the U.S.[12] Thus, important progress was made by both LGBT and public health communities in the early years of AIDS, despite the sociopolitical environment.

Understanding Behavior and Change (1986–1995)

The next 10 years were marked by gradual progress in AIDS care due to developing effective drug therapy.[37] This period was also characterized by the proliferation of behavioral and psychosocial research that began to address significant changes that MSM were experiencing because of HIV/AIDS. As LGBT communities and grass roots AIDS organizations were responding to the epidemic with growing guidance and support from the federal government, researchers identified behavioral risk factors for acquiring HIV, examined how MSM were coping and living with AIDS from both individual and community perspectives, explored the impact of HIV testing on risk behavior, and investigated how HIV/AIDS was affecting diverse populations across the nation. In addition to these content areas, HIV prevention researchers sought greater involvement of MSM in the research process and began randomized control intervention studies.[38,39]

Identifying Behavioral Risk Factors Among MSM

The field of sexual behavior assessment and understanding grew immensely during this period of the epidemic. Researchers and practitioners gained an appreciation for the complexity of intimate behaviors as well as related perceptions and motivations, and started to identify critical factors of MSM risk behavior.

Unprotected Anal Sex. Early in the epidemic, unprotected anal sex was identified as a major HIV risk factor for MSM. Studies with larger samples of gay men confirmed findings from smaller studies[30] that receptive anal sex with multiple partners was associated with HIV infection.[40–44] Predictors of unprotected anal sex were also determined, including younger age,[45,46] more sexual partners,[45] preference for anal sex over other sexual activities,[46] low self-efficacy for sexual behavior change,[46,47] higher perceived peer norms for unsafe sex, and less knowledge of AIDS and its prevention.[46]

Number, Types, and Networks of Sex Partners. Several studies cited a strong correlation between the number of sexual partners and HIV infection.[40,43,44,48] In one study,[40] the odds ratio (and 95% confidence interval) of HIV seroconversion increased from OR=2.4 (95% CI, 1.2–4.7) when men had 1 or 2 partners per month to OR=3.2 (95% CI, 1.8–5.9) when they had 5 or more partners per month. Another study[43] found that the risk for HIV doubled with every increase of 30–40 sexual partners when HIV-positive study participants were compared with HIV-negative controls. Similarly, for a cohort of nonpartnered MSM in San Francisco,[44] HIV seropositivity was 17.6% for MSM with no sexual partners in the prior 2 years compared to 70.8% for MSM who had more than 50 partners within the same time period. Medical and public health experts strongly recommended that gay men limit the number of sex partners and avoid anonymous sex altogether.[49]

Despite the link between number of partners and HIV infection—and a great decline in risk behavior among MSM overall during this period of the epidemic—some MSM continued to have multiple partners.[45] Several hypotheses for this have been offered,[50] including prior sexual history and an expression of gay identification.[51] Although these motivations may seem in conflict with avoiding HIV infection, they represent the historical context and complex psychosocial-behavioral factors that may have contributed to HIV transmission, at least early in the epidemic.

Types of sexual partner relationships, such as primary or casual partners, were also thought to play a role in HIV transmission for MSM. Being single and having casual and anonymous sex was thought to confer higher risk for HIV infection compared to having sex with a primary or steady partner.[49] However, later studies found that partnered men were engaging in more unprotected anal sex than were nonpartnered men[52]; men often underestimated the risk associated with unprotected anal sex with primary partners, particularly when they did not know their partner's HIV status.[53,54] Other factors, such as wanting to experience intimacy, being in a longer-term relationship, and avoiding talking about HIV, may have facilitated unprotected sex for MSM in HIV-discordant primary relationships.[55]

As noted above, the HIV status of sexual partners may also be linked to HIV risk behavior. Studies conducted in this era and more recently have found that unprotected sex decreased with serodiscordant partners, but increased with seroconcordant partners,[56–58] foreshadowing a greater attention to seroadaptive strategies in the next era of the HIV epidemic.

Finally, sexual networks and selecting of partners based on demographic characteristics (e.g., age) may have facilitated HIV transmission for MSM. For example, sexual mixing patterns (e.g., having unprotected sex with at least one older sexual partner) may have contributed to HIV seroconversion for some men.[59,60] More recently, sexual networks, especially in relation to racial mixing patterns, would be considered a potentially important HIV risk factor for certain racial/ethnic groups, such as black MSM.[61,62]

Substance Use and Sexual Risk. Substance use, including alcohol use, was found to be associated with risk behavior and HIV infection[63,64] during this time period, specifically unprotected anal sex.[65] HIV infection was associated with heavy alcohol use, moderate to heavy drug use, and being younger;[63] heavy drinkers were more likely to have had receptive anal intercourse with more partners, had more anonymous sex, and were less likely to use condoms during anal sex. Frequent use of substances was associated with unprotected anal sex and "fisting" (insertion of the hand into the rectum)[65]; and men with a history of both unprotected receptive anal sex and use of "poppers" (amyl nitrite) were OR=5.5 (95% CI, 2.8–11.1) times more likely to be HIV-positive.[64]

Demographic Factors Associated With Risk for HIV Infection. During this period, demographic factors such as age, education, and geographic location were identified as risk factors for HIV/AIDS. Gay men recruited from three small cities in the South engaged in higher rates of risky sexual behaviors compared to gay men living in large metropolitan areas.[66] The authors hypothesized that gay men in smaller cities may have had fewer supports for making behavior change, and perhaps perceived that AIDS was a more distant threat to them relative to the threat faced by their urban peers. Younger age was generally associated with a heightened risk for HIV infection among U.S. MSM during this period of the epidemic,[67] including HIV seroconversion[68] and unprotected anal sex.[45] Potential contributing factors to the younger age-risk link were thought to be behavioral, biobehavioral, psychosocial, or methodologic (e.g., sampling bias) in nature.[67] Finally, having less education was also found to be associated with sexual risk behavior and HIV infection.[69,70]

Psychosocial Factors Associated With Risk for HIV Infection. During this decade of the HIV/AIDS epidemic, various psychosocial factors emerged as risk cofactors in HIV infection or unprotected sex. For example, childhood abuse was suspected early on as being linked to increased risk for HIV infection. One study found that 65% of a sample of mostly HIV-infected gay men had experienced some form of physical or sexual abuse as children.[71] Sexual compulsivity and sexual sensation seeking were also found to contribute to high-risk sexual behavior,[72–78] including prolonged sexual activity.[79] During this era of the epidemic, it was thought that negative affective states such as depression and anxiety may be linked to risky sex,[71] but a more recent review found little evidence of this.[80]

Community Adjustment: Living With AIDS and An Epidemic

Community Behavior Change. HIV prevention research studies from this time period focused largely on HIV risk factors, including the unprecedented, profound changes in sexual behavior in community samples of MSM.[81] One of the first studies to document these changes[82] found an early trend of nonmonogamous MSM engaging in fewer high-risk sexual behaviors, despite methodologic limitations.[83] Data from the AIDS Behavioral Research Project,[46,84] a longitudinal cohort study, suggested that gay men significantly decreased unprotected anal sex acts and increased using condoms. The San Francisco Men's Health Study[45] found that gay men in their sample drastically reduced unprotected anal sex over time, and the majority maintained these changes for at least 1 year prior to their last assessment. Research on gay men in New York City used retrospective designs to find that most men had reduced their sexual risk behavior by 70%[85]; condom use increased from 1.5% to 20% of the sample.[86] Further, 82.9% had abstained from receptive anal sex or consistently used a condom for anal sex for 1 year.[41] The Chicago Multicenter AIDS Cohort Study[87] reported significant reductions in unprotected receptive anal sex during the mid 1980s, but this effect was less dramatic a few years later. Altogether, these findings indicate that many gay men in large U.S. cities had substantially changed their sexual behavior in a short period of time.

Although evidence indicated that gay men and other MSM were reducing their behavioral risk for HIV transmission, concerns about "relapse" or reverting back to risky sexual behavior emerged during this time.[88–90] Longitudinal data on MSM from the Chicago Multicenter AIDS Cohort Study (MACS) indicated that 47% had a sexual risk relapse at least once over the span of 2 years[88]; another analysis of the same cohort found that 45% of the men were "lapsers" (i.e.,

sexually transmitted infections (STIs) were more likely to engage in unprotected anal sex. Others[119] found that childhood sexual abuse was associated with unprotected receptive anal sex in a sample of Puerto Rican MSM living in New York City.

Among Asian and Pacific Islander (A/PI) MSM, one of the earliest studies[120] suggested that A/PI MSM were more likely to engage in unprotected sex with white MSM than with men of other races/ethnicities; in addition, substance use was associated with sexual risk behavior in this sample. Research on American Indian and Native Alaskan MSM populations was scarce early in the epidemic, with the exception of surveillance data.[121] Only recently have researchers begun to examine HIV risk behaviors of Native Americans.[122]

Early Behavioral Interventions for MSM. During this period, there were many important advances in HIV behavioral prevention research, such as the establishment of national AIDS research centers and the requirement of community advisory boards to be an integral part of research and programs.[38] One of these notable advancements was the development and testing of individual- or small-group–level interventions for affected populations, including MSM.[123–125] These early interventions consisted of multiple components, including increasing knowledge of HIV and safer-sex practices, building skills such as using condoms or sexual assertiveness, promoting self-pride and responsibility toward others, and developing a socially supportive network. The interventions were often conducted at the individual or small-group level, and the findings generally indicated increases in condom use for anal sex or decreases in unprotected anal sex that were sustained over a few months. Being first-generation interventions, their efficacy was not always assessed thoroughly[126]; nevertheless, these studies were groundbreaking for starting to accumulate knowledge regarding evidence-based HIV prevention interventions for MSM.

Besides individual- and group-level interventions, community-level interventions that targeted gay men were also initiated during this period.[127,128] Based on diffusion of innovation theory,[129] one intervention involved identifying and training popular opinion leaders within the gay community of a small city to talk to their friends and acquaintances about HIV and safer sex. In one study, in comparison to men in two cities not receiving the intervention, men in the experimental city decreased unprotected anal sex by 25%, and increased condom use by 16% within a 2-month period[127]; there was also an 18% decrease in the percentage of men reporting multiple partners. The other study used the same procedures as the first study, but implemented the intervention at 6-month intervals in three different small cities; these researchers found reductions in unprotected anal sex.[128] These findings highlighted the importance of community-level interventions as an important complement to individual- and group-level interventions to reduce HIV risk for MSM.

In sum, a growing foundation of behavioral research of MSM was established during this period of the HIV/AIDS epidemic. Paralleling this growth, historic reductions in sexual risk behavior were documented among gay and bisexual men.[45,46,81–82,84] Demographic and psychosocial factors associated with HIV transmission were first identified and served as potential mediators and moderators for the development and testing of interventions to further reduce risk. Science was attempting to catch up with the Community.

Managing a "Chronic Disease" (1996–2009)

The introduction of antiretroviral therapy (ART) ushered in a new era for HIV/AIDS.[130] What was previously an AIDS epidemic was now becoming an HIV epidemic.[131] The prognosis and perception of an HIV-positive diagnosis transitioned from a life-threatening disease to a potentially manageable illness for many MSM. ART created a more hopeful trajectory for persons with HIV, but also raised concerns about complacency regarding sexual risk reduction, given "treatment optimism."[132,133] The issue of "barebacking," or intentional unprotected anal sex with nonprimary partners, also became more prominent in the research literature after ART.[134,135] Unprotected anal sex among MSM, particularly intentional unprotected anal sex, was very concerning because increasing STI rates at the time could foreshadow a resurgence of HIV incidence.[136] Within this section, we discuss these and other important issues of the period from 1996 to 2009.

Antiretroviral Therapy (ART)

Heightened HIV viral load reflects disease progression, particularly at two points: immediately after infection and near the end of life.[137,138] Protease inhibitors, in combination with other medications, became available in the mid-1990s, and were effective treatments that reduced viral load and disease progression for HIV-infected individuals. However, availability and implementation of these treatments introduced new challenges for HIV prevention.

Medication Adherence. Good adherence to HIV medications understandably contributes to the health-enhancing effects of treatment for HIV-positive people.[139,140] Beyond that, however, medication adherence is a concern due to the development and transmission of drug-resistant strains of HIV.[141] Thus, HIV prevention had begun to address adherence as a means to decrease HIV infectivity in MSM populations,[142,143] also referred to as community viral load. In a study on ART adherence among MSM,[144] 51% reported missing at least one day of medication. Moreover, an avoidant style of coping, alcohol use, and difficulty in discussing HIV with sex partners were associated with missed doses.[144] Cognitive-behavioral stress management techniques, combined with training on adherence to medications, have yielded some preliminary evidence of increasing medication adherence for MSM.[145,146]

Impact of ART on Sexual Risk. Besides hopeful expectations that ART would result in fewer AIDS cases,[147] concerns arose during this period that ART would lead to complacency in safer-sex practices for both HIV-positive and -negative MSM. However, findings from an early meta-analysis of studies conducted between 1996 and 2003 indicated that there were no differences in levels of unprotected sex between persons with HIV who were taking ART (largely MSM) and those who were not.[148] In addition, no differences were found in unprotected sex between persons with undetectable viral loads and those with detectable levels. Beliefs that persons taking ART or who had undetectable viral loads are less infectious were significantly associated with increased unprotected sex, regardless of HIV status. Findings from a more recent meta-analysis indicated that being on ART, having an undetectable viral load, and being more than 90% treatment-adherent were not associated with unprotected anal sex.[149] Summarizing recent longitudinal studies looking at the relationship between ART and unprotected sex,[150] researchers concluded that the association is still unclear and more research is needed.

Barebacking. Unprotected anal sex was, understandably, a primary focus of HIV prevention for MSM beginning early in the epidemic. It was during the present period of the epidemic, however, that the term "barebacking" emerged as sociocultural term referring to intentional unprotected anal sex.[131,132] Primary motivations for barebacking were enhanced emotional connection and physical stimulation,[131] among others. For some MSM, although not for others, barebacking included a label of self-identification.[151] According to a recent review,[152] the overall percentage of MSM who engage in barebacking is unknown, although self-identified barebackers appear to be among a minority of MSM. Factors associated with barebacking include: supportive sexual norms; a need to feel connected; HIV concordance with the partner, especially for HIV-positive men; and using the Internet to find sex partners.[152]

Seroadaptive Strategies Based on Accurate HIV Status and Disclosure. Unprotected anal sex under certain circumstances may be one of several community-generated, adaptive strategies that could reduce HIV risk.[153] In recent years, such community-generated strategies have been referred to as "seroadaptive" practices.[154,155] Seroadaptive behaviors are generally based on mutual HIV disclosure and recent testing, and behavioral adjustment to avoid condom use. Specific behaviors include HIV serosorting, negotiated safety, and strategic positioning (described below). These strategies are not necessarily endorsed by health officials, although they are sometimes practiced among MSM.[155] A critical element for all of the strategies is HIV status disclosure.

HIV Disclosure. Accurate knowledge and disclosure of HIV status to sex partners is strongly encouraged because it is assumed that risk behavior will be less if sex partners know they have a different serostatus from each another.[156] Two key elements of accurate HIV status disclosure are recent and ongoing testing over time, and honest disclosure and continued communication of HIV status to partners. HIV disclosure plays a critical role in serosorting behavior and other seroadapative strategies for managing transmission risk. However, HIV-positive MSM are more likely to disclose their status to primary partners and close friends than to casual sex partners.[157,158] The real-world interplay of disclosure and risky sex is complex and not fully understood yet.[159] Nonetheless, inconsistent disclosure has been linked to increased sexual risk, compared to consistent disclosure or nondisclosure of HIV status to partners.[157,160] Recent interventions centered on HIV status disclosure have demonstrated enhanced disclosure behavior,[161,162] which may reduce unprotected anal sex,[162] although more research is needed. Most studies on disclosure have focused on HIV-positive MSM; few studies have examined the experiences of HIV-negative MSM or men who do not know their HIV status.[158] This may change as HIV-status-based strategies become increasingly addressed in the research literature and MSM community.

As HIV diagnostic tests (such as viral load tests) have become more sophisticated, HIV-positive disclosure has become more nuanced and is a factor for sexual decision-making for many MSM.[160] In short, although HIV status disclosure has historically been a part of the HIV prevention for MSM, its practice and relation to unprotected sex is complex, is not fully understood, and will likely change as medical science develops further.

HIV Serosorting. "Serosorting" is a practice that refers to having unprotected sex with persons who are HIV seroconcordant and selectively using condoms with HIV-serodiscordant partners.[163–165] HIV serosorting may be considered controversial as a means for reducing HIV transmission and its potential effectiveness may differ for HIV-positive and HIV-negative MSM.[166] For HIV-positive MSM, transmission can be reduced if both partners discuss their current HIV status, but there is a potential for transmission of other STIs and, potentially, for HIV superinfection[164] (detection of HIV "superinfection" is difficult to assess[167] and has been minimally detected so far[168]). For truly HIV-negative MSM in mutually monogamous relationships, unprotected anal sex poses no risk of HIV transmission. However, the effectiveness of serosorting becomes limited for those who have multiple and concurrent sexual partners because of critical elements of knowing one's HIV status[164,165]—for example, how recent the HIV test was, the window of undetectable infection, and risk behavior since the last test[169]—and the percentage of MSM with undiagnosed HIV is high.[170]

Negotiated Safety. Whereas HIV serosorting can occur for both HIV-positive and -negative MSM, negotiated safety applies to HIV-negative men only. Specifically, "negotiated safety" refers to primary relationships where both partners are HIV-negative, and the partners have a clear agreement and ongoing communication about having only safe sex outside of their relationship.[171] As with barebacking, the overall prevalence of negotiated safety among MSM is unknown. Studies of MSM who use this strategy suggest that some men adhere to their rules, although ongoing testing and open communication are often difficult to maintain over time.[169,171,172] Although one study[173] reported that negotiated safety was not associated with HIV incidence, some MSM do break agreements and do not disclose unsafe sexual encounters with other partners to their primary partner,[169,172] thereby increasing the potential for HIV transmission. Further, there is speculation that most new infections among MSM occur within primary relationships.[174] More work is needed to better understand the complexity of personal interactions, including verbal and nonverbal communication, with primary as well as nonprimary partners.

Strategic Positioning. "Strategic positioning" refers to engaging in relatively lesser sexual risk behavior based on one's HIV status, in order to reduce risk for HIV transmission.[175] Specifically, HIV-positive MSM assume a receptive position in anal sex, and HIV-negative MSM assume an insertive position; this is often in the context of knowing or assuming HIV serodiscordance between partners.

The practice of strategic positioning as a risk reduction practice has been documented in many studies.[154,155,160,173,175] Some researchers have cautiously suggested that strategic positioning may contribute to decreasing HIV transmission rather than increasing it,[154,168] although others have questioned the behavior as an effective risk-reduction strategy.[176]

As a whole, HIV-seroadaptive strategies—namely, serosorting, negotiated safety, and strategic positioning—remain controversial because of understandable difficulties in effectively evaluating, implementing, and sustaining them over time by many people. Nevertheless, these community-generated practices are population-level adjustments to a 30-year epidemic. These approaches represent behavioral applications of HIV transmission information in the context of meeting other important human needs, such as emotional intimacy.[134]

Venues for Social and Sexual Connection

Social and sexual venues for MSM are opportune locales for risk-reduction efforts. During this period of the epidemic, venues such as bars, bathhouses, circuit parties, and the Internet became more of a focus of research for understanding MSM behavior and change.

Bars. Historically, bars were one of the few identifiable venues through which MSM could meet other MSM and delve into the MSM world.[177,178] Gay bars had a long existence before HIV/AIDS, and are discussed in more detail elsewhere.[177,179] Given that, substance use has played a key role and has been a central ingredient in socialization and sexuality development for many MSM.[179]

Bathhouses and Sex Clubs. Like bars, gay bathhouses and sex clubs existed well before HIV/AIDS and are considered a part of MSM sexual culture.[180] Gay bathhouses were first established in large cities in the 1950s and provided relatively safe and private places to meet other men for sex where homophobic violence and police interference were largely absent.[181] Bathhouses offer private rooms as well as common areas, and patrons wear a towel.[182]

Given the potential for anonymous sex and multiple partners in these environments, much controversy surrounded bathhouses early in the HIV epidemic, and many bathhouses were closed down for "public health" reasons when AIDS arrived.[183] Today, these venues are still largely perceived as high-risk for STIs and HIV, although recent studies have indicated that unprotected anal sex in these milieux is relatively uncommon,[182,184] and a majority of men engage in safer sex in these environments,[185] Additionally, bathhouses and sex clubs have provided community services such as HIV prevention outreach and STI/HIV testing and counseling.[180]

Circuit Parties and Other Events. Since the late 1980s, circuit parties have been popular affirming events for some MSM.[186,187] In an era when AIDS destroyed communities, circuit parties helped build them up—at least, symbolically.[187] Circuit parties, largely nonexistent today, were weekend-long events that often centered on music, dancing, other entertainment, and on themes. At large parties, such as the Palm Springs[188,189] and Miami[190] White Parties—which emphasize wearing white to the events—thousands of men would travel to the location and stay in host hotels for a long weekend.[186,187] Studies have found that substance use and sexual risk behavior were common in these environs[186,191,192] and were heightened during circuit party weekends compared to behavior during other weekends among the same individuals[193]— particularly circuit party weekends away from one's home town. Others have found similar results during trips to gay vacation destinations,[194] all opportune locales for risk-reduction interventions.[195]

Internet. Starting in the mid 1990s, MSM increasingly used the Internet to meet sexual partners, which raised questions about HIV transmission by meeting partners through this medium.[196] Although meeting sex partners online may prevent some unsafe HIV-discordant sex because disclosure of HIV status is common on site profiles, the Internet may also increase the efficiency of meeting sexual partners and thereby make it a risky sex environment.[197,198] In fact, one study found that a syphilis outbreak among MSM could be traced to a chat room network[199]; others have reported an association between STI/HIV risk factors (e.g., previous STI history, unprotected anal sex) and using the Internet to find sexual partners for MSM.[196,200,201]

According to a recent meta-analysis conducted with 14 studies published between 1988 and 2005, approximately 40% of American and European MSM recruited in studies offline used the Internet to look for sexual partners, with approximately 30% actually having sex with an partner who was met through an online site.[202] They found that unprotected anal sex was more common among MSM who used the Internet to find sexual partners than among those who did not. Despite the growing body of evidence that suggests using the Internet for sexual liaisons may be related to increased STI risk and unprotected sex, more research is needed to determine its relationship to HIV transmission risk.[150,197] Future research may continue to use the Internet and other technological tools for HIV prevention among MSM,[197,203] including social media venues. Texting interventions are being developed and tested among high-risk MSM.[204] Prevention efforts are needed for even newer technologies (e.g., GPS technology for partner acquisition).

Substance Use and Sexual Risk

Mentioned earlier, substance use has historically been a key element present in MSM communities and gay culture, and it continues to be so. A number of reviews or summaries have been written on substance use and sexual risk among MSM in this period of the HIV/AIDS epidemic.[205–207] The reviews point to somewhat differential results due to heterogeneous measurement and analytic approaches to the association of substance use and sexual risk behavior, including:

- Varying windows of behavioral recall (e.g., past 1 month, 12 months, lifetime)
- Varying specificity of the substance use–sex connection (e.g., both occurred independently or together during broad windows of assessment; both occurred together at sexual event-level analysis)
- Varying specificity of sexual risk behavior (e.g., "sex" in general; unprotected anal sex; unprotected anal sex with a partner of different HIV status than the respondent)
- Varying specificity of substance use (e.g., individual drug list; combined substances, such as "club drugs")
- Varying sophistication of analysis (e.g., bivariate analysis; multivariate analysis; covariates included in multivariate analysis).

Generally speaking, three types of research approaches have been undertaken to assess the association of substance use and sex risk behavior among MSM: global—that is, overall substance use and sexual risk behavior over the same assessment period (e.g., past 3 months), but not necessarily linked to each other; situational—that is, substance use during sex in general (e.g., past 3 months); and event-level—substance use and sexual behavior during a specific sexual episode—assessment.[206] These are important distinctions because different results may be found based on the particular approach taken. In recent years, sexual event-level research has become the preferred approach, given adequate sample size and statistical power, because of the contextual richness the approach offers in assessment. A recent review of event-level analyses for MSM[208] found that methamphetamine use and binge-alcohol drinking (5 or more drinks on one occasion) were the two substance-related practices consistently found to be associated with unprotected anal sex in a recent sexual encounter with another male. Other substance use, including alcohol (undefined or nonbinge), marijuana, cocaine, crack, ecstasy, ketamine, GHB, amyl nitrites, erectile dysfunction medications, and other substances, were either not consistently associated with sexual risk behavior or have not yet been adequately researched—particularly amyl nitrites (poppers), which are used by some MSM during sex.[209]

Methamphetamine Use. Methamphetamine use among MSM has received particular attention within gay communities and by public health and service agencies alike[210–212]; the issue has been discussed extensively elsewhere.[206,213] In short, a sociosexual culture has emerged among some MSM which involves sex while under the influence of methamphetamine because the substance can increase the sense of physical sensation and emotional connection, and its effects can last for hours and even days.[214] "Party and Play" (also known as P-n-P) is a commonly used term by MSM for getting high on methamphetamine and having sex—particularly when searching for sex partners on the Internet.[215,216]

STI/HIV prevention and substance abuse treatment agencies have worked together with MSM community activists to build awareness about the negative impact of methamphetamine use among MSM, and substance use assessment and counseling are increasingly integrated with HIV testing and risk-reduction programs.[214,217] Behavioral interventions have been developed for methamphetamine-using MSM in drug treatment[217]—also linked to HIV risk reduction— and not in drug treatment.[204,218-220] There are early indicators that methamphetamine use may be declining among MSM,[221] but assessment is still needed to monitor changes in use of meth-amphetamine and other substances among MSM over time.

Key Subgroups

HIV-Positive MSM. Given the growing population of HIV-positive MSM who are living longer and continuing to be sexually active, prevention efforts during this period of the epidemic have gradually shifted from focusing on noninfected MSM to increased emphasis on prevention for HIV-positive MSM.[136,222] Although a recent meta-analysis of studies focusing on HIV-positive MSM in the U.S. found that the majority reported safer sex practices that included using seroadaptive strategies, the prevalence of unprotected anal sex with HIV-negative or unknown-status partners was 26%.[149] Other investigators[223] found that unprotected anal sex was associated with substance use, lower expectations for condom use, negotiation of safer sex, and having a steady partner among MSM not on combination therapy. Reviewing 61 studies from 1980 to 2001,[224] researchers noted that a few psychosocial and interpersonal factors were related to unprotected anal sex for HIV-positive MSM, including sex with anonymous partners, having an attractive partner, having a sexual partner who was willing to engage in risky sex, and a having had a greater number of previous partners. Men who blamed others for becoming HIV-infected were also more likely to engage in unprotected anal sex with partners who were believed to be HIV-negative or unknown status. These findings reflect the complexity of issues facing HIV-positive MSM and the need for comprehensive interventions.

Young MSM. Since the late 1980s, younger MSM have had higher reported rates of sexual risk behavior compared to older MSM.[225] The Young Men's Survey[226] assessed HIV prevalence and risk behaviors of MSM between 15 and 22 years of age in six major cities and found a 7.2% HIV prevalence. Black and Latino MSM were found to have a higher HIV prevalence compared to whites and Asian/Pacific Islanders. Research also indicates that many young MSM are unaware of being infected.[226–228] Several correlates of HIV infection have been consistently identified for young MSM, including being of a man of color,[226,227,229] prior STI history,[227,230] a greater number of sexual partners,[227,230] and substance use.[227,229-231] Factors associated with unprotected sex in samples of young MSM in the U.S. include more perceived difficulty controlling sexual risk behavior,[232] sex with older partners,[56] sex with a greater number of partners,[232] having sex in commercial sex environments such as bathhouses,[232] less self-acceptance of being gay or bisexual,[220,233] and substance use or dependency.[230,232,233] Overall, these studies suggest that multiple issues contribute to increased HIV vulnerability for young MSM, and specific age-appropriate interventions may be necessary to reduce HIV risk in this population.[234,235]

MSM of Color. Although white MSM comprise a plurality of U.S. HIV/AIDS cases, **black MSM** comprise the group most disproportionately affected by HIV.[236] Recent systematic reviews and meta-analyses attempting to explain these disparities in HIV rates have concluded that behavioral risk factors alone cannot fully explain the high rates of HIV infection among black MSM.[61,237] According to these studies, black MSM have similar rates of unprotected anal sex as white MSM; have fewer lifetime, current, and casual sex partners; and report less substance use, in general and with sex, compared to white MSM. However, black MSM have higher rates of STIs that increase their vulnerability to HIV. Further, previous high rates of unprotected anal sex early in the epidemic may have contributed to current HIV incidence and prevalence rates for black MSM.[237] Given relatively tight-knit sexual networks among black MSM,[238] the chance of having sex with someone who may be experiencing a recent, acute HIV infection could be heightened. Factors such as undiagnosed HIV infection and lower rates of black MSM on ART[237] may increase the community's viral load[142] and potential for HIV transmission. Given these findings, interventions that facilitate early detection and treatment for STIs and HIV, and improved access to health care and medication may be the most effective interventions for the black MSM community as a whole. Additionally, despite great advances in culturally specific interventions[239] and successes of these interventions for black MSM,[240,241] more work is needed to address structural factors such as poverty, racism, and homophobia that may contribute to HIV vulnerability, particularly for black MSM. (See Chapter 33 for a more detailed discussion of HIV/AIDS among African Americans and blacks.)

Latino MSM are also disproportionately affected by HIV compared to white MSM.[236] Recent research has examined situational factors such as the sex partner's drug use, less communication about condom use, attractiveness of sex partners,[242,243] structural factors such as social discrimination,[244,245] and cultural factors such as *familismo* (or the importance of family) and *machismo* (or the importance of masculinity), which may contribute to sexual risk behaviors for Latino MSM.[246] Randomized, controlled intervention trials targeting Latino MSM are sparse.[247] Although baseline data indicated that men may be resilient in the face of social oppression, the intervention did not have an effect on levels of unprotected anal sex.[248] Thus, efficacious interventions specifically targeting Latino MSM have yet to be identified, although programs do exist in various communities. (See Chapter 34 for a more detailed discussion of HIV/AIDS among Latinos and Hispanics.)

Other race/ethnicities (including Asians, Pacific Islanders, American Indians, and Alaskan Native) among MSM have not been adequately studied, although surveillance data suggest that some of these groups have fewer cases compared to other MSM,[249] although their risk behavior actually may be high.[250] More research is needed to address the overrepresentation of HIV/AIDS in MSM of all race/ethnicities compared to what has been reported for the general heterosexual population in the U.S.

Behavioral Interventions for MSM

Behavioral intervention approaches continue to be an important component of efforts to curb the U.S. HIV epidemic. A number of HIV prevention intervention studies have been conducted with domestic and international MSM populations, and meta-analyses of these studies[251–254] have generally concluded that behavioral interventions are effective in reducing unprotected anal sex for MSM, although the average risk reduction at postintervention follow-up is approximately 27% and thus limited.[251,253] Interventions tended to be more effective if they were theory-based, addressed interpersonal skills, applied several delivery methods, and were given over multiple sessions.[251] Group-level interventions were found to be highly successful and cost-effective, especially if they included multiple sessions, used MSM interventionists, and emphasized skill building.[252, 255] MSM community-level interventions show evidence of efficacy and may be cost-advantageous.[252] However, current numbers of evidence-based interventions for MSM are insufficient due to multiple risk issues for and diversity of MSM communities.[256] Clearly, more behavioral interventions for MSM must be developed, tested, disseminated, and effectively adapted for MSM subgroups.

Now and Moving Forward (2010–on)

Current State of the Epidemic

MSM have dominated the HIV/AIDS epidemic in the U.S. MSM were the first cases identified and continue to be the largest group affected. CDC HIV/AIDS surveillance data illustrate this well.[257]

AIDS Case Trends. **Figure 30–1** presents both the annual estimated number of U.S. AIDS cases for adolescent and adult MSM and the percent of annual U.S. AIDS cases attributed to MSM, from 1985–2007;[257] 2007 is the most recent year data are available. Clearly, the number of annual AIDS cases increased from 1985 to 1992, and declined from 1993 (the first year in which the new CDC AIDS case definition was used) to 1999, after which time the annual number has been relatively stable. At the same time, the proportion of annual U.S. AIDS cases accounted for by MSM declined from approximately 2/3 in 1985 to slightly less than 1/2 in 2007. Given that MSM may account for an estimated 2% of the overall U.S. population 13 years of age and older and for an estimated 4% of the total U.S. male population,[258] MSM continue to be dramatically overrepresented in the U.S. epidemic. **Figure 30–2** shows how the increase and decrease in number of AIDS cases for MSM from 1985 to 1992 is reflected a few years later by a common curve for AIDS deaths. AIDS deaths for MSM peaked at roughly 40,000 in 1995, followed by a dramatic 2- to 3-year decline that parallels increasing access to and uptake of ART medications.[257]

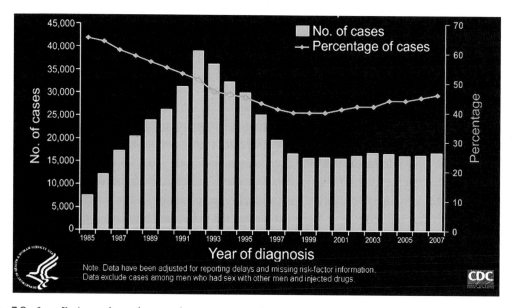

Figure 30–1. *Estimated numbers and percentages of AIDS cases among adult and adolescent MSM, 1985–2007—United States and dependent areas. Source: CDC.*

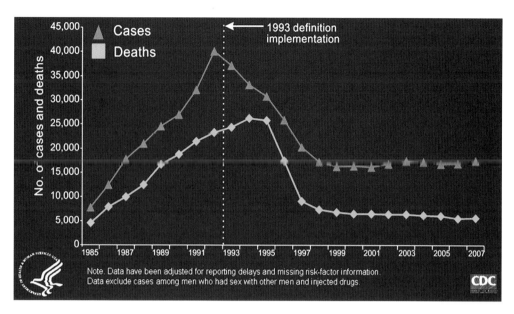

Figure 30–2. *Estimated numbers of AIDS cases and deaths among MSM, 1985–2007—United States and dependent areas. Source: CDC.*

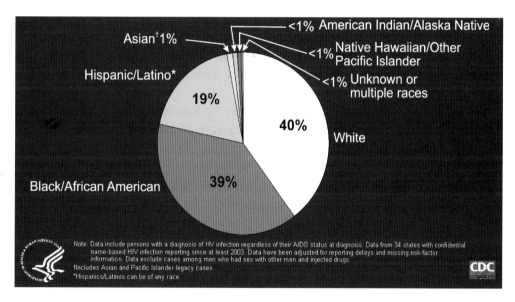

Figure 30–3. *Percentages of estimated HIV/AIDS cases among adult and adolescent MSM by race/ethnicity, 2007—34 states. Source: CDC.*

2007 HIV/AIDS Cases. In 2007, 34 states had well-established confidential name reporting for HIV infection.[257] **Figure 30–3** combines MSM having a diagnosis of AIDS for all states and HIV infection for the 34 states with confidential reporting in 2007 by race/ethnicity. Nearly as many MSM identified as black or African American (39%) as identified as white or Caucasian (40%), followed by Latino or Hispanic (19%). Given national race/ethnicity population estimates of 12.8% for blacks and 15.4% for Latinos,[258] these groups are overrepresented in HIV/AIDS cases among MSM today; this is particularly true for black MSM. The proportion of MSM with HIV/AIDS identified as white has steadily declined since U.S. surveillance data have been available (**Figure 30–4**), while black and Latino cases have increased.

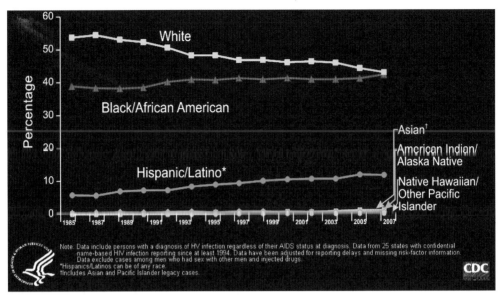

Figure 30–4. *Percentages of estimated HIV/AIDS cases among adult and adolescent MSM by race/ethnicity, 1985–2007—25 states. Source: CDC.*

Nearly 30 years into the epidemic, we still do not collect surveillance data specifically for the high-risk population of transgender persons.[4] More HIV epidemiologic and intervention research—as well as surveillance—is needed for these individuals.

HIV Risk Behavior. The U.S. National HIV Behavioral Surveillance System (NHBS) is a unique system established to monitor risk behavior; the system assesses behavior of three populations at risk for HIV infection—MSM, injection drug users, and high-risk heterosexuals—every 3 years. The first cycle of data collection for MSM occurred from November 2003 to April 2005, in 15 metropolitan statistical areas (MSAs) throughout the U.S. (**Figure 30–5**). An MSM venue-based procedure was used to systematically screen and assess adult males.[259] Among the 10,030 men who reported having sex with another male in the prior year, 5,912 (59%) reported having a main partner and 5,516 (55%) reported having a casual partner in the prior year (**Figure 30–6**). Among the men who had these partners types, 58% (3,429/5,912) and 36% (1,999/5,516), respectively, reported having unprotected anal sex at least once with that partner type within the year[259]; these data demonstrate that this risk behavior does continue among MSM. For years, an ongoing chorus has called for new and innovative approaches to reduce risk for HIV transmission among MSM.[114,131,187] The authors acknowledge that call and suggest specific directions in the next section.

Consistent with a systematic review,[237] black MSM do not demonstrate more unprotected anal sex with main or casual partners compared to other MSM (**Figure 30–6**). This is curious, given that black MSM have much higher HIV incidence than do white and other MSM.[256] Reasons for these somewhat incongruous circumstances are discussed by others,[61] and include several possibilities: black men may be more genetically susceptible to HIV infection, may be infectious for a longer period of time, or their sexual networks are more likely to be HIV-infected or infectious. More research is needed to allow a better understanding of the potentially complex dynamics of why black MSM have greater HIV incidence compared to other MSM in the U.S., and to inform the development of targeted behavioral and biomedical interventions.

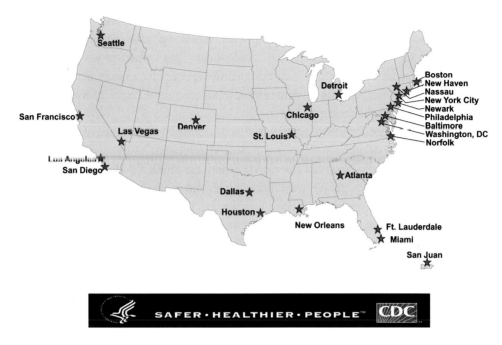

Figure 30–5. *National HIV Behavioral Surveillance System (NHBS) sites, 2006.*

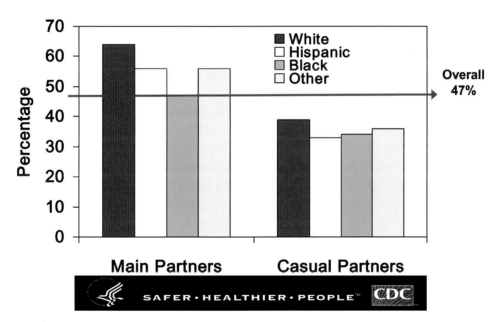

Figure 30–6. *Unprotected anal sex with male partners in the preceding 12 months, by MSM participant race/ethnicity, NHBS 2006 (n=10,030). Source: CDC.*

Future Scientific Directions

The future of HIV in gay and bisexual populations is dependent on behavioral and biomedical developments. Let us consider some potential directions.

New Directions for Behavior Change: Holistic Health. Early in the epidemic, behavioral deconstruction was necessary in order to identify modes of transmission and to prevent further infections. An entire field of epidemiologic and intervention research and related policy has, understandably, been developed based on risk-reduction approaches. Many behavioral interventions—particularly individual and small-group programs that are cognitive/behavior-based[260–262]—are designed to specifically change behaviors or alter potential mediators of risk behavior. Community-level interventions typically work to change behavior and norms affecting behavior.[127,128,263]

Behavioral deconstruction approaches were necessary and effective early in the epidemic, when the threat of death from AIDS was fresh and imminent. As was mentioned earlier, dramatic behavior changes were observed among MSM into the 1990s.[264] However, when effective treatments became available, people were living longer and the face of AIDS as death changed to one of HIV and life. Advertisements for antiretroviral treatments in gay media outlets presented attractive and athletic men who happened to be HIV-positive, and LGBT communities expressed concern about falsely glamorizing HIV/AIDS.[265,266] Fatigue in maintaining one-dimensional behavioral risk reduction,[267] combined with treatment optimism,[132,133] could help fuel increases in risky behavior. Cognitive/behavioral interventions focused on risk reduction that were tested during an era of antiretroviral therapy often had little or no differential effects versus control groups.[260–262,268,269]

Since the mid-1990s, there has been a growing movement toward broader approaches than HIV risk behavior deconstruction. Some researchers have called for attention to "syndemic" epidemics, such as HIV infection, substance abuse, and negative affect among MSM.[270] Others have encouraged broader wellness or holistic health approaches,[114,131,136,187,271] and still others have emphasized sexual health promotion, specifically.[272,273] Although the various approaches may have unique angles, a common element is that they effectively work to address HIV risk behavior in a framework broader than a single-issue behavioral deconstruction approach— namely, a broader holistic health framework.

In general, holistic health addresses the individual as having multiple needs and motivations, and not simply as a concern to reduce risk for HIV transmission. Such approaches can be presented at the individual, group, community, or policy level; however, a key distinction from a behavioral deconstructionist intervention at all levels is that a holistic constructionist intervention impacts multiple or broader issues beyond HIV risk reduction. These approaches tend to treat the individual as a complex organism with potentially competing physical, emotional, mental, and even spiritual health needs. For example, needs for emotional intimacy and physical connection may compete with and supersede the need to prevent HIV infection,[134] as with other emotional and mental health needs.[131,136,187] When effective interventions are determined, dissemination and adaptation are critical steps to implementing programs for behavior change in communities.

Biomedical Developments. In the future, there will be highly anticipated biomedical approaches to prevent HIV transmission, including the possibilities of vaccines, antiretroviral prophylaxis through oral or sexually-applied products, and other biomedical interventions. Regardless of the approach, however, first-generation biomedical interventions are likely to have "partial efficacy" and be less effective than the penile condom,[274] which is estimated to be approximately 90% to 95% effective when used correctly.[275] Thus, researchers must develop effective complex or hierarchical risk-reduction messages in the context of multiple biomedical options and various product characteristics, including a range of likely effectiveness.[276] For high-risk populations, such as MSM, effective multi-intervention messages will be critical for achieving a preferential epidemiologic impact.

As the biomedical intervention standard, condoms will continue to be central to HIV prevention. Condoms raise a complex range of attitudes, emotions, and symbolism for people, particularly MSM.[277–279] Research has demonstrated that although MSM have used condoms over the decades since HIV emerged, a notable decline in condom use has occurred since the inception of antiretroviral treatment in the mid-1990s (as mentioned earlier). Consistent use of condoms is difficult for a variety of reasons, including condom fatigue,[267,280] physical side effects,[281] and obstruction of intimacy.[134]

Microbicides are being developed for vaginal and rectal application. MSM in the US have reported that they would be willing to reduce their preferred microbicide efficacy level to prevent HIV transmission in order to use a rectal microbicide instead of a condom.[276] MSM have and will use a sexual lubricant product for reducing disease transmission,[282] and they have preferences that may help with product development and marketing of effective products.[277,279,283]

Clinical trials for pre-exposure prophylaxis (PrEP) use are under way, and promising results of one study among MSM were recently released.[284] It may be the case that PrEP is soon offered as an efficacious option for particularly high-risk MSM. Related laboratory research on monkey models is promising,[285,286] as is the well-established area of HIV transmission prophylaxis from mother-to-child.[287] Approximately 2% of MSM are already using ART for HIV pre-exposure prophylaxis, even before the results of efficacy trials are available.[288] MSM will be an obvious target for pre-exposure prophylaxis when it is recommended and available for use. Behavioral research is needed to prepare for targeted communications and interventions to maximize recommended usage.

Vaccine development and behavioral implications are discussed elsewhere in this text (see Chapter 41). Behavioral uptake and adherence—in the context of given vaccine efficacy and side effects—are critical concerns as generations of vaccines become available and accessible to MSM.

Human Rights

United States and Other Wealthy Nations. Rights and recognition of gay people will continue in the developed world. Gay marriage will provide legitimacy and societal support to same-sex unions; legal rights and responsibilities of marriage will eventually become a norm for LGBT individuals, as it is with heterosexual persons. Such policy changes could have a psycho-sociologic impact on sexual risk behavior, particularly on behavior outside of a recognized marriage.[289–291] Behavioral norms could move in the direction of reinforcing that social unit, also contributing to a decline in extramarital sex and, thus, the opportunity for HIV transmission. Legal rights and acceptance of gay adoption will further support building of the family unit for gay couples. Other laws defining health and legal rights of LGBT individuals and couples should serve to recognize and protect essential human rights[292,293] and ultimately affect health and potentially decrease HIV transmission in doing so.

Low- and Middle-Income Nations. MSM in developing country settings around the world are at disproportional risk for HIV infection, as are MSM in wealthier nations.[294] Based on pooled scientific findings,[295] MSM in low-income nations were approximately 7.8 times (95% CI, 7.2–8.4) more likely to be HIV-infected than the general population of their country. MSM in middle-income nations were 23.4 times more likely to be infected than their general population rate (95% CI, 22.8–24.0). LGBT populations in developing countries are generally at

39. Ross M, Kelly J. Interventions to reduce HIV transmission in homosexual men. In Peterson J, DiClemente R (Eds.): Handbook of HIV Prevention. New York: Springer; 2000 (pp. 201–214).

40. Darrow W, Echenberg D, Jaffe H et al. Risk factors for Human Immunodeficiency Virus (HIV) infections in homosexual men. Am J Public Health 1987;77:479–483.

41. Martin J, Garcia M, Beatrice S. Sexual behavior changes and HIV antibody in a cohort of New York City gay men. Am J Public Health 1989;79:501–503.

42. McCusker J, Stoddard A, Mayer K, Cowan D, Groopman J. Behavioral risk factors for HIV infection among homosexual men at a Boston Community Health Center. Am J Public Health 1988;78:68–71.

43. Moss AR, Osmond D, Bacchetti P, Chermann J, Barre-Sinoussi F, Carlson J. Risk factors for AIDS and HIV seropositivity in homosexual men. Amer J Epi 1987;125:1035–1047.

44. Winkelstein W, Lyman D, Padian N et al. Sexual practices and risk of infection by the Human Immunodeficiency Virus: The San Francisco Men's Health Study. JAMA 1987;257:321–325.

45. Ekstrand M, Coates T. Maintenance of safer sexual behaviors and predictors of risky sex: the San Francisco Men's Health Study. Am J Public Health 1990;80:973–977.

46. McKusick L, Coates T, Morin S, Pollack L, Hoff C. Longitudinal predictors of reductions in unprotected anal intercourse among gay men in San Francisco: the AIDS behavioral research project. Am J Public Health 1990;80:978–983.

47. Joseph J, Montgomery S, Emmons C et al. Perceived risk of AIDS: assessing the behavioral and psychosocial consequences in a cohort of gay men. J Appl Social Psych 1987;17:231–250.

48. Samuel M, Hessol N, Shiboski S, Engel R, Speed T, Winkelstein W. Factors associated with human immunodeficiency virus seroconversion in homosexual men in three San Francisco cohort studies, 1984-1989. J Acquir Immune Defic Syndr 1993;6:303–312.

49. McKusick L, Conant M, Coates T. The AIDS epidemic: A model for developing intervention strategies for reducing high-risk behavior in gay men. Sexually Transmitted Diseases 1985;12:229–234.

50. Aspinwall L, Taylor S, Shneider S, Dudley J. Psychosocial predictors of gay men's AIDS risk reduction behavior. Health Psych 1991;10:432–444.

51. Moore P. Beyond shame: reclaiming the abandoned history of radical gay sexuality. Boston: Beacon Press; 2004.

52. Hoff C, Coates T, Barrett D, Collette L, Ekstrand M. Differences between gay men in primary relationships and single men: implications for prevention. AIDS Educ Prev 1996;8:546–559.

53. Bosga M, De Wit J, de Vroome E, Houweling H, Schop W, Sandfort T. Differences in perception of risk for HIV infection with steady and non-steady partners among homosexual men. AIDS Educ Prev 1995;7:103–115.

54. McLean J, Boulton M, Brookes M et al. Regular partners and risky behavior: why do gay men have unprotected intercourse? AIDS Care 1994;6:331–341.

55. Remien R, Carballo-Dieguez A, Wagner G. Intimacy and sexual risk behavior in serodiscordant male couples. AIDS Care 1995;7429–438.

56. Dawson J, Fitzpatrick R, Reeves G et al. Awareness of sexual partners' HIV status as an influence upon high-risk sexual behavior among gay men. AIDS, 1994; 8:837–841.

57. Hoff C, Stall R, Paul J et al. Differences in sexual behavior among HIV discordant and concordant gay men in primary relationships. J Acquir Immune Defic Syndr Hum Retrovirol. 1997; 14:72–78.

58. Marks G, Crepaz N. HIV positive men's sexual practices in the context of self-disclosure of HIV status. J Acquir Immune Defic Syndr. 2001; 27:79–85.

59. Morris M, Zavisca, Dean L. Social and sexual networks: their role in the spread of HIV/AIDS among young gay men. AIDS EducPrev 1995;7: Suppl 24-35.

60. Service S, Blower S. HIV transmission in sexual networks: an empirical analysis. Proc Royal Society 1995;260:237–244.

61. Millett G, Peterson J, Wolitski R, Stall R. Greater risk for HIV infection of Black men who have sex with men: a critical literature review. Am J Public Health 2006;96:1007–1019.

62. Raymond H, McFarland W. Racial mixing and HIV risk among men who have sex with men. AIDS and Behav 2009;13:630–637.

63. Penkower L, Dew M, Kingsley L et al. Behavioral, health, and psychosocial factors and risk for HIV infection among sexually active homosexual men: the multicenter AIDS cohort study. Am J Public Health 1991;81:194–196.

64. Seage G, Mayer K, Horsburgh CR, Holmberg S, Moon M, Lamb G. The relation between nitrite inhalants, unprotected receptive anal intercourse, and the risk of human immunodeficiency virus infection. Amer J Epidem 1992;135:1–11.

65. Stall R, McKusick L, Wiley J, Coates T, Ostrow D. Alcohol and drug use during sexual activity and compliance with safe sex guidelines for AIDS: The AIDS Behavioral Research Project. Health Educ Quart 1986;13:359–371.

66. Kelly J, St. Lawrence J, Brasfield T, Stevenson Y, Diaz Y, Hauth A. AIDS risk behavior patterns among gay men in small southern cities. Am J Public Health 1990;80:416–418.

67. Mansergh G, Marks G. Age and risk of HIV infection in men who have sex with men. AIDS 1998;12:1119–1128.

68. Kingsley L, Zhou S, Bacellar H et al. Temporal trends in human immunodeficiency virus type 1 seroconversion, 1984-1989. Amer J Epidem 1991;135:331–339.

69. Easterbrook P, Chmiel J, Hoover D et al. Racial and ethnic differences in human immunodeficiency virus type 1 (HIV-1) seroprevalence among homosexual and bisexual men. The Multicenter AIDS Cohort Study. Amer J Epidem 1993;138:415–429;

70. Osmond D, Page K, Wiley J et al. HIV infection in homosexual and bisexual men 18 to 29 years of age: the San Francisco Young Men's Health Study. Am J Public Health 1994;84:1933–1937.

71. Allers C, Benjack K. Connections between childhood abuse and HIV infection. J Counseling Deve 1991;70:309–313.

72. Kalichman S, Rompa D. Sensation seeking and sexual compulsivity scales – reliability, validity, and predicting high risk behavior. J Pers Assess 1995;65:586–601.

73. Kalichman S, Johnson J, Adair V et al. Sexual sensation seeking—scale development and predicting AIDS risk behavior among homosexually active men. J Pers Assess 1994;62:385–397.

74. Kalichman S, Heckman T Kelly J. Sensation seeking as an explanation for the association between substance use and HIV-related risky sexual behavior. Arch Sexual Behav 1996;25:141–154.

75. Benotsch E, Kalichman S, Kelly J. Sexual compulsivity and substance use in HIV-seropositive men who have sex with men: prevalence and predictors of high-risk behaviors. Addic Behav 1990;24:857–868.

76. Chng C, Geliga-Vargas J. Ethnic identity, gay identity, sexual sensation seeking, and HIV risk taking among multiethnic men who have sex with men. AIDS Educ Prev 2000;12:326–339.

77. Parsons J, Halkitis P, Wolitiski R, Gomex C, The Seropositive Urban Men's Study Team. Correlates of sexual risk behaviors among HIV-positive men who have sex with men. AIDS Educ Prev 2003;15:383–400.

78. Semple S, Zians J, Grant I, Patterson T. Sexual compulsivity in a sample of HIV-positive methamphetamine-using gay and bisexual men. AIDS Beha 2006;10:587–598.

79. Semple S, Zians J, Strathdee S, Patterson T. Sexual marathons and methamphetamine use among HIV-positive men who have sex with men. Arch Sex Behav 2009;38:583–590.

80. Crepaz N, Marks G. Are negative affective states associated with HIV risk sexual behaviors? A meta-analytic review. Health Psych 2001;20:291–299.

81. Stall R, Coates T, Hoff C. Behavioral risk reduction for HIV infection among gay and bisexual men. Amer Psychologist 1988;43:8–885.

82. McKusick L, Horstman W, Coates T. AIDS and sexual behavior reported by gay men in San Francisco. Am J Public Health 1985;75:493-496.

83. Handsfield H. AIDS and sexual behavior in gay men. Am J Public Health 1985;7:1449.

84. Catania J, Coates T, Stall R et al. Changes in condom use among homosexual men in San Francisco. Health Psych 1991;10:190-199.

85. Martin J. The impact of AIDS on gay male sexual behavior patterns in New York City. Am J Public Health 1987;77:576–581.

86. Martin J, Dean L, Garcia M, Hall W. The impact of AIDS on a gay community: Changes in sexual behavior, substance use, and mental health. Amer J Community Psych 1987;17:269–293.

87. Ostrow D, Beltran E, Joseph J. Sexual behavior research on a cohort of gay men, 1984–1990: can we predict how men will respond to interventions? Arch Sex Behav 1994;23:531–551.

88. Adib S, Joseph J, Ostrow D, Tal M, Schwartz S. Relapse in sexual behavior among homosexual men: a 2-year follow-up from the Chicago MACS/CCS. AIDS 1996;5:S757–S760.

89. Kelly J, Kalichman S, Kauth M et al. Situational factors associated with AIDS risk behavior lapses and coping strategies used by gay men who successfully avoid lapses. Am J Public Health 1991;81:1335–1338.

90. Stall R, Ekstrand M, Pollack L, McKusick L, Coates T. Relapse from safer sex: The next challenge for AIDS prevention efforts. J Acquire Immune Defic Syndr 1990;3:1181–1187.

91. Emmons C, Joseph J, Kessler R, Wortman C, Montogomery S, Ostrow D. Psychosocial predictors of reported behavior change in homosexual men at risk for AIDS. Health Educ Quart 1986;13:331–345.

92. Centers for Disease Control and Prevention. Twenty-five years of HIV/AIDS—United States, 1981–2006. MMWR 2006;55:586–620.

93. Lyter D, Valdiserri R, Kinglsey L, Amoroso W, Rinaldo C. The HIV antibody test: why gay men and bisexual men want or do not want to know their results. Public Health Rep 1987;102:468–474.

94. Siegel K , Levine M, Brooks C, Kern R. The motives of gay men for taking or not taking the HIV antibody test. Social Problems 1989;36:368–383.

95. Higgins D, Galvotti C, O'Reilly K et al. Evidence for the effects of HIV antibody counseling and testing on risk behaviors. JAMA 1991;266:2419–2429.

96. Coates T, Stall R, Kegeles S, Lo B, Morin S, McKusick L. AIDS antibody testing. Amer Psychologist, 1988;43:859–864.

97. Marks G, Crepaz N, Senterfitt JD, Janssen R. Meta-analysis of high-risk sexual behavior in persons aware and unaware they are infected with HIV in the United States: implications for HIV prevention programs. J Acquir Immune Defic Syndr 2005;39:446–453.

98. Marks G, Crepaz N, Janssen RS. Estimating sexual transmission of HIV from persons aware and unaware that they are infected with the virus in the USA. AIDS 2006;20:1447–1450.

99. Morin S. AIDS: the challenge to psychology. Amer Psychologist 1988;43:838–842.

100. Coates T, Temoshok L, Mandel J. Psychosocial research is essential to understanding and treating AIDS. Amer Psychologist 1984:39:1309–1314.

101. Dilley J, Ochitill H, Perl M, Volderding P. Findings in psychiatric consultations with patients with acquired immune deficiency syndrome. Amer J Psychiatry 1985;142:82-85.

102. Morin S, Charles K, Malyon A. The psychological impact of AIDS on gay men. Amer Psychologist 1984;39:1288–1293.

103. Kelly J, Murphy D. Psychological interventions with AIDS and HIV: prevention and treatment. J Cons Clin Psych 1992;60:576–585.

104. Martin J, Dean L. Effects of AIDS-related bereavement and HIV-related illness on psychological distress among gay men: a 7-year longitudinal study, 1985-1991. J Consult Clin Psychol 1993;61:94–103.

105. Marzuk P, Tierney, H, Tardiff K et al. Increased risk of suicide in persons with AIDS. JAMA 1988;259:1333–1337.

106. Martin J. Psychological consequences of of AIDS-related bereavement among gay men. J Consult Clin Psychol 1988;56:856–862.

107. Neugebauer R, Rabkin J, Williams J, Remien R, Goetz R, Gorman J. Bereavement reactions among homosexual men experiencing multiple losses in the AIDS epidemic. Amer J Psychiatry 1992;149:1374–1379.

108. Joseph J, Montgomery S, Emmons C et al. Perceived risk of AIDS: assessing the behavioral and psychosocial consequences in a cohort of gay men. J Appl Social Psych 1987; 17:231–250.

109. Martin J, Dean L, Garcia M, Hall W. The impact of AIDS on a gay community: Changes in sexual behavior, substance use, and mental health. Amer J Community Psychol 1989;17:269–293.

110. Hays R, Turner H, Coates T. Social support, AIDS-related symptoms, and depression among gay men. J Consult Clin Psych 1992;60:463–469.

111. Lennon M, Martin J, Dean L. The influence of social support on AIDS-related grief reaction among gay men. Social Science Med 1990;31:477–484.

112. Taylor S, Kemeny M, Aspinwall L et al. Optimism, coping, psychological distress, and high-risk sexual behavior among men at risk for acquired immunodeficiency syndrome (AIDS). J Pers Social Psych 1992;63:460–473.

113. Turner H, Hays R, Coates T. Determinants of social support among gay men: the context of AIDS. J Health Social Beh 1993;34:37–53.

114. Rofes E. Reviving the Tribe: Regenerating Gay Men's Sexuality and Culture in the Ongoing Epidemic. New York: Harrington Park Press; 1996.

115. Valdiserri RO, Robinson, C, Lin LS, West GR, Holtgrave DR. Determining allocations for HIV-prevention interventions:assessing a change in federal funding policy. AIDS Public Policy J 1997;12:138–148.

116. Peterson J, Coates T, Catania J, Middleton L, Hilliard B, Hearst N. High-risk sexual behavior and condom use among gay and bisexual African-American men. Am J Public Health 1992;82:1490–1494.

117. Morales E. HIV infection and Hispanic gay and bisexual men. Hisp J Behav Stud 1990;12:212–222.

118. Ramirez J, Suarez E, de la Rosa G, Castro M, Zimmerman M. AIDS knowledge and sexual behavior among Mexican gay and bisexual men. AIDS Educ Prev 1994;6: 163–174.

119. Carballo-Dieguez A, Dolezal C. Association between history of childhood sexual abuse and adult HIV-risk sexual behavior in Puerto Rican men who have sex with men. Child Abuse Neg 1995;19:595–605.

120. Choi K, Coates T, Catania J, Lew S, Chow P. High HIV risk among gay and Asian and Pacific Islander men in San Francisco. AIDS 1995;9:306–308.

121. Metler R, Conway G, Stehr-Green J. AIDS surveillance among American Indians and Alaska Natives. Am J Public Health 1991;81:1469–1471.

122. Simoni J, Walters K, Balsam K, Meyers S. Victimization, substance use, and HIV risk behaviors among gay/bisexual/two-spirit and heterosexual American Indian men in New York City. Am J Public Health 2006; 96:2240–2245.

123. Valdiserri R, Lyter D, Leviton L, Callahan C, Kingsley L, Rinaldo C. AIDS prevention in homosexual and bisexual men: results of a randomized trial evaluating two risk reduction interventions. AIDS 1989;3:21–26.

124. Kelly J, St. Lawrence J, Hood H, Brasfield T. Behavioral intervention to reduce AIDS risk activities. J Consult Clin Psych 1989;57:60–67.

125. Kelly J, St Lawrence J, Betts R, Brasfield T, Hood H. A skills-training group intervention model to assist persons in reducing risk behaviors for HIV infection. AIDS Educ Prev 1990;2:24–35.

126. Lyles C, Crepaz N, Herbst J, Kay L. Evidence-based HIV behavioral prevention from the perspective of the CDC's HIV/AIDS prevention research synthesis team. AIDS Educ Prev 2006;18:21–31 (Suppl A).

127. Kelly J, St Lawrence J, Diaz et al. HIV risk behavior reduction following intervention with key opinion leaders of population: an experimental analysis. Am J Public Health 1991;81:168–171.

128. Kelly J, St Lawrence J, Stevenson LY et al. Community AIDS/HIV risk reduction: the effects of endorsements by popular people in three cities. Am J Public Health 1992;82:1483–1489.

129. Rogers EM. Diffusion of innovations. New York: Free Press; 1983.

130. Lemp GF, Porco TC, Hirozawa AM et al. Projected incidence of AIDS in San Francisco: the peak and decline of the epidemic. J Acquir Immune Defic Syndr Hum Retrovirol 1997;16:182–189.

131. Mansergh G. Paradigm shift for HIV prevention in the United States. AIDScience 2002;2:1–6. Access May 25, 2010, at www.aidscience.org/Articles/AIDScience021.asp.

132. Murphy S, Miller LC, Appleby PR, Marks G, Mansergh G. Antiretroviral drugs and sexual behavior in gay and bisexual men: When optimism enhances risk. XII International Conference on AIDS. Geneva, Switzerland: July 1998 [Abstract 14137].

133. Sullivan PS, Drake AJ, Sanchez TH. Prevalence of treatment optimism-related risk behavior andassociated factors among men who have sex with men in 11 states, 2000–2001. AIDS Behav 2007;11:123–129.

134. Mansergh G, Marks G, Colfax, GN, Guzman, R, Rader M, Buchbinder S. 'Barebacking' in a diverse sample of men who have sex with men. AIDS 2002;16:653–659.

135. Halkitis PN, Parsons JT. Barebacking among gay and bisexual men in New York City: explanations for the emergence of intentional unsafe behavior. Arch Sex Behav 2003;32:351–357.

136. Wolitski R, Valdiserri R, Denning P, Levine W. Are we headed for a resurgence of the HIV epidemic among men who have sex with men? Am J Public Health 2001;91:883–888.

137. Mellors J, Rinaldo C, Gupta P et al. Prognosis in HIV-1 infection predicted by the quantity of virus in plasma. Science 1996;272:1167–1170.

138. Schacker T, Hughes J, Shea T et al. Biological and virological characteristics of primary HIV infection. Annals Inter Med 1998;128:613–621.

139. Patterson DL, Swindells S, Mohr J, et al. Adherence to protease inhibitor therapy and outcomes in patients with HIV infection. Annals Intern Med 2000;133:21–30.

140. Mannheimer S, Kitchen S, Dubin JA, Gottlieb MS. Initial virological and immunological response to highly active antiretroviral therapy predicts long-term clinical outcome. Clin Infect Dis 2001;33:466–472.

141. Ross L, Lim M, Liao Q et al. Prevalence of antiretroviral drug resistance and resistance-associated mutations in antiretroviral therapy-naïve HIV-infected individuals from 40 United States cities. HIV Clin Trials 2007;8:1–8.

142. Stall R, Herrick A, Guadamuz T, Friedman M. Updating HIV prevention with gay men: current challenges and opportunities to advance health among gay men. In: Mayer K & Pizer H, ed. HIV prevention: a comprehensive approach. London: Academic Press; 2009 (pp. 169–202).

143. Porco T, Martin J, Page-Shafer K et al. Decline in HIV infectivity following the introduction of highly active antiretroviral therapy. AIDS 2004;18:81–88.

144. Halkitis P, Parsons, J, Wolitski R, Remien R. Characteristics of HIV antiretroviral treatments, access and adherence in an ethnically diverse sample of men who have sex with men. AIDS Care 2003;15:89–102.

145. Safren S, Otto, M, Worth J et al. Two strategies to increase adherence to HIV antiretroviral medication: Life-steps and medication monitoring. Behav Res Therapy 2001;39:1151–1162.

146. Antoni M, Carrico A, Duran R et al. Randomized clinical trial of cognitive behavioral stress management on human immunodeficiency virus viral load in gay men treated with highly active antiretroviral therapy. Psychol Med 2006;68:143–151.

147. Blower S, Gershengorn H, Grant R. A tale of two futures: HIV and antiretroviral therapy in San Francisco. Science 2000;287:650–654.

148. Crepaz N, Hart T, Marks G. Highly active antiretroviral therapy and sexual risk behavior: a meta-analytic review. JAMA 2004;292:224–236.

149. Crepaz N, Marks G, Liau A et al. Prevalence of unprotected anal intercourse among HIV-diagnosed MSM in the United States: a meta-analysis. AIDS 2009;23:1–13.

150. Elford J. Changing patterns of sexual behavior in the era of highly active antiretroviral therapy. Curr Opin Infect Dis 2006;19:26–32.

151. Parsons J, Bimbi D. Intentional unprotected anal intercourse among sex who have sex with men: barebacking – from behavior to identity. AIDS Behav 2007;11:277–287.

152. Berg R. Barebacking: a review of the literature. Arch Sex Behav 2009;38:754–764.

153. Xia Q, Molitor F, Osmond DH, Tholandi M, Pollack LM, Ruiz JD, Catania JA. Knowledge of sexual partner's HIV serostatus and serosorting practices in a California population-based sample of men who have sex with men. AIDS 2006 24;20:2081–2089.

154. McConnell J, Bragg L, Shiboski S, Grant R. 2010 Sexual seroadaptation: lessons for prevention and sex research from a cohort of HIV-positive men who have sex with men. 2010; PLoS ONE S (1): e8831. doi:10.1371/journal.pone.0008831.

155. Snowden J, Raymond H, McFarland W. Prevalence of seroadaptive behaviors of men who have sex with men, San Francisco, 2004. Sex Trans Infect 2009;85:469–476.

156. Pinkerton S, Galletly C. Reducing HIV transmission risk by increasing serostatus disclosure: a mathematical modeling analysis. AIDS Behav 2007;11:698–705.

157. Hart T, Wolitski R, Purcell D, Parsons J, Gomez C, Seropositve Urban Men's Study Team. Partner awareness of the serostatus of HIV-positive men who have sex with men: impact on unprotected sexual behavior. AIDS Behav 2005;9:155–166.

158. Wolitski RJ, Rietmeijer C, Goldbaum GM, Wilson RM. HIV serostatus disclosure among gay and bisexual men in four American cities: general patterns and relation to sexual practices. AIDS Care 1998;10:599–610.

159. Rosser BR, Horvath KJ, Hatfield LA, Peterson JL, Jacoby S, Stately A. Predictors of HIV disclosure to secondary partners and sexual risk behavior among a high-risk sample of HIV-positive MSM: results from six epicenters in the US. AIDS Care 2008;20:925–930.

160. Parsons J, Schrimshaw E, Wolitski R et al. Sexual harm reduction practices of HIV-sero-positive gay and bisexual men: serosorting, strategic positioning, and withdrawal before ejaculation. AIDS 2005;19:S13–S25 (Suppl 1).

161. Serovich J, Reed S, Grafsky E, Andrist D. An intervention study on men who have sex with men disclose their serostatus to casual sex partners: results from a pilot study. AIDS Educ Prev 2009;21:207–219.

162. Chiasson M, Shaw F, Humberstone M, Hirshfield S, Hartel D. Increased HIV disclosure three months after an online video intervention for men who have sex with men (MSM). AIDS Care 2009;21:1081–1089.

163. Zablotska I, Imrie J, Prestage G et al. Gay men's current practice of HIV seroconcordant unprotected anal intercourse: serosorting or seroguessing? AIDS Care 2009;21:501–510.

164. Truong HM, Kellogg T, Klausner JD et al. Increases in sexually transmitted infections and sexual risk behaviour without a concurrent increase in HIV incidence among men who have sex with men in San Francisco: a suggestion of HIV serosorting? Sex Transm Infect 2006;82:461–466.

165. Eaton L, Kalichman S, O'Connell D, Karchner W. A strategy for selecting sexual partners believed to pose little/no risks for HIV; serosorting and its implications for HIV transmission. AIDS Care 2009;21:1279–1288.

166. Golden M, Stekler J, Hughes J, Wood R. HIV serosorting in men who have sex with men: is it safe? JAIDS 2008;49:212–218.

167. Blackard JT, Mayer KH. HIV superinfection in the era of increased sexual risk-taking. Sex Transm Dis 2004;31:201–204.

168. Sidat MM, Mijch AM, Lewin SR, Hoy JF, Hocking J, Fairley CK. Incidence of putative HIV superinfection and sexual practices among HIV-infected men who have sex with men. Sex Health 2008;5:61–67.

169. Guzman R, Colfax G, Wheeler S, et al. Negotiated safety relationships and sexual behavior among a diverse sample of HIV-negative men who have sex with men. JAIDS 2005;38:82–86.

170. Wilson D, Regan D, Heymer K, Jin F, Prestage G, Grulich A. Serosorting may increase the risk of HIV acquisition among men who have sex with men. Sex Transm Dis 2010;37:13–17.

171. Kippax S, Noble J, Prestage, G et al. Sexual negotiation in the AIDS era: negotiated safety revisited. AIDS 1997;11:191–197.

172. Hoff C, Chajkravarty D, Beougher S et al. Serostatus differences and agreements about sex with outside partners among gay male couples. AIDS Educ Prev 2009;21:25–38.

173. Jin F, Crawford J, Prestage G et al. Unprotected anal intercourse, risk reduction behaviors, and subsequent HIV infection in a cohort of homosexual men. AIDS 2009;23: 243–252.

174. Sullivan PS, Salazar L Buchbinder S, Sanchez TH. Estimating the proportion of HIV transmissions from main sex partners among men who have sex with men in five US cities. AIDS 2009;23:1153–1162.

175. Van de Ven P, Kippax S, Crawford J et al. In a minority of gay men, sexual risk practice indicates strategic positioning for perceived risk reduction rather than unbridled sex. AIDS Care 2002;14:471–480.

176. Halkitis P, Moeller R, Pollack J. Sexual practices of gay, bisexual, and other non-identified MSM attending New York City gyms: patterns of serosorting, strategic positioning, and context selection. J Sex Res 2008;45:253–261.

177. Reitzes D, Diver J. Gay bars as deviant community organizations: the management of interactions with outsiders. Dev Behav 1982;4:1–18.

178. McKirnan, D, Peterson P. Psychosocial and cultural factors in alcohol and drug abuse: an analysis of a homosexual community. Addict Behav 1989;14:555–563.

179. Isarelstam S, Lambert S. Gay bars. J Drug Issues 1984;14:637–653.

180. Berube A. The history of gay bathhouses. In Colter E, Hoffman W, Pendleton E, Redick, A, Serlin D Eds): Policing public sex: queer politics and the future of AIDS activism. Boston, MA: South End Press; 1996 (pp. 187–220).

181. Chauncey G. Gay New York. New York: Basic Books; 1994.

182. Reidy W, Spielberg F, Wood R, Binson D, Woods W, Goldbaum G. HIV risk associated with gay bathhouses and sex clubs: findings from 2 Seattle surveys of factors related to HIV and sexually transmitted infections. Am J Public Health 2009;99: S165–S172.

183. Woods W, Binson D, Gay bathhouses and public health policy. New York: Harrington Park Press; 2003.

184. Beneden C, O'Brien K, Modeitt S, Yusem S, Rose A, Fleming D. Sexual behaviors in an urban bathhouse 15 years into the HIV epidemic. JAIDS 2002;30:522–526.

185. Binson, D, Woods W, Pollack L, Paul J, Stall R, Catania J. Differential HIV risk in bathhouses and public cruising areas. Am J Public Health 2001;91:1482–1486.

186. Mansergh G., Colfax, GN, Marks, G, Rader, M, Guzman, R, Buchbinder, S. The Circuit Party Men's Health Survey: Findings and Implications for Gay and Bisexual Men. Am J Public Health 2001;91:953–958.

187. Rofes E. Dry Bones Breath. New York: Harrington Park Press; 1998.

188. Palm Springs White Party. Accessed May 21, 2010, at: http://www.jeffrey.sanker.com.

189. Patel P, Taylor MM, Montoya JA, Hamburger ME, Kerndt PR, Holmberg SD. Circuit parties: sexual behaviors and HIV disclosure practices among men who have sex with men at the White Party, Palm Springs, California, 2003. AIDS Care 2006;18:1046–1049.

190. Miami White Party. Accessed May 21, 2010, at: http://www.careresource.org/white party/.

191. Mathison A, Ross M, Wolfson T, Franklin D, HNRC Group. Circuit party attendance, club drug use, and unsafe sex in gay men. J Subst Abuse 2001;13:119–126.

192. Lee SJ, Galanter M, Dermatis H, McDowell D. Circuit parties and patterns of drug use in a subset of gay men. J Addict Dis 2003;22:47–60.

193. Colfax GN. Mansergh G, Guzman R, Vittinghoff E, Marks G, Rader M, Buchbinder S. Drug use and sexual risk behavior among gay and bisexual men who attend circuit parties: a venue-based comparison. JAIDS 2001;28:373–379.

194. Kaufman M, Fuhrel-Forbis A, Kalichman S et al. On holiday: a risk behavior profile for men who have vacationed at gay resorts. J Homosex 2009;56,1134–1144.

195. Weidel JJ, Provencio-Vasquez E, Grossman J. Sex and drugs: high-risk behaviors at circuit parties. Amer J Mens Health 2008;2:344–352

196. McFarlane M, Bull S, Rietmeijer C. The internet as a newly emerging risk environment for sexually transmitted diseases. JAMA 2000;284:443–446.

197. Bull, S. McFarlane M. Soliciting sex on the Internet: what are the risks for sexually transmitted diseases and HIV? Sex Transm Dis 2000;27:545–550.

198. Rosser, BR, Miner M, Bockting W,et al. HIV risk and the Internet: Results of the men's INTernet sex (MINTS) study. AIDS Behav 2009;13:746–756.

199. Klausner J, Wolf W, Fischer-Ponce L, Zolt I, Katz M. Tracing a syphilis outbreak through cyberspace. JAMA 2000;284:447–449.

200. Benostsch E, Kalichman S, Cage M. Men who have met sex partners via the Internet: prevalence, predictors, and implications for HIV prevention. Arch Sex Behav, 2002;31:177–183.

201. Berry M, Raymond HF, Kellogg T, McFarland W, The Internet, HIV serosorting and transmission risk among men who have sex with men, San Francisco. AIDS 2008;22 :787–789.

202. Liau A, Millet G, Marks G. Meta-analytic examination of online sex-seeking and sexual risk behavior among men who have sex with men. Sex Transm Dis 2006;33:576–584.

203. Rhodes S, Hergenrather K, Duncan J et al. A pilot intervention utilizing Internet chat rooms to prevent HIV risk behaviors among men who have sex with men. Public Health Rep 2010;125:29–37 (Suppl 1).

204. Reback C, Ling D, Shoptaw S, Rohde J. Developing a Text Messaging Risk Reduction Intervention for Methamphetamine-Using MSM [Research Note]. The Open AIDS Journal 2010;4:116–122.

205. Leigh B, Stall R. Substance use and risky sexual behavior for exposure to HIV: Issues in methodology, interpretation, and prevention. Amer Psychol 1993;48:1035–1045.

206. Stall R, Purcell DW. Intertwining epidemics: A review of research on substance use among MSM and its connection to the HIV epidemic. AIDS Behav 2000;4:181–192.

207. Shoptaw S, Reback CJ. Methamphetamine use and infectious disease-related behaviors in MSM: Implications for interventions. Addiction 2007;102:103–135 (Suppl).

208. Vosburgh W, Mansergh G, Sullivan PS, Purcell DW. A review of the literature on event-level sexual risk behavior and substance use among men who have sex with men (under review).

209. Wilson H. The poppers--HIV connection. Focus 1999;14:5–6.

210. Halkitis PN, Parsons JT, Stirratt MJ. A double epidemic: crystal methamphetamine drug use in relation to HIV transmission among gay men. J Homosex 2001;41:17–35

211. Mansergh G, Purcell DW, Stall R et al. CDC consultation on methamphetamine use and sexual risk behavior for HIV/STD infection: Summary and suggestions. Public Health Rep 2006;121:127–132.

212. Mansergh G, Charania M, Purcell D. Developing innovative intervention approaches for methamphetamine-using MSM not currently in drug treatment [Editorial]. The Open AIDS Jour 2010;4:103–104.

213. Colfax G, Shoptaw S. The methamphetamine epidemic: implications for HIV prevention and treatment. Current HIV/AIDS Report 2005;2:194–199.

214. Peck J, Shoptaw S, Rotheram-Fuller E, Reback C, Bierman B. HIV-associated medical, behavioral, & psychiatric characteristics of treatment-seeking, methamphetamine-dependent men who have sex with men. J Addictive Disorders 2005;24:115–132.

215. Hirshfield S, Remien R, Walavalkar I et al. Crystal methamphetamine use predicts incident STD infection among men who have sex with men recruited online: a nested case-control study. J Med Internet Res 2004;6:42–49

216. Mimiaga M, Fair A, Mayer K et al. Experiences and sexual behaviors of HIV-infected MSM who acquired HIV in the context of crystal methamphetamine use. AIDS Educ Prev 2008;20:30–41.

217. Shoptaw S, Reback C, Peck J. Behavioral treatment approaches for methamphetamine dependence and HIV-related sexual risk behaviors among gay and bisexual men. Drug Alcoh Depend 2005;78:125–134.

218. Wu E, El-Bassel N, McVinney LD, Fontaine YM, Hess L. Adaptation of a couple-based HIV intervention for methamphetamine involved African American MSM. The Open AIDS Jour 2010;4:123–131.

219. Garfein R, Metzner M, Cuevas J, Bousman CA, Patterson T. Formative assessment of ARM-U: A modular intervention for decreasing risk behaviors among HIV-positive and HIV-negative methamphetamine-using MSM. The Open AIDS Jour 2010;4:105–115.

220. Zule W, Coomes CM, Karg R, Harris JL, Orr A, Wechsberg WM. Using a modified intervention mapping approach to develop and refine a single-session motivational intervention for methamphetamine-using MSM. The Open AIDS Jour 2010;4:132–140.

221. Stall R. Mental health, resiliency, and healthy development. The Sexual Health of Gay Men and Other MSM: HIV/STD Prevention Plus Conference. Boston, MA: The Fenway Institute, April 26, 2010.

222. Janssen R, Valdiserri R. HIV prevention in the United States: increasing emphasis on working with those living with HIV. JA IDS 2004;37: S119–S121 (Suppl 2).

223. Semple SL, Patterson TL, Grant I. HIV-positive gay and bisexual men: predictors of unsafe sex. AIDS Care 2003;15:3–15.

224. Crepaz N, Marks, G. Towards an understanding of sexual risk behavior in people living with HIV: a review of social, psychological, and medical findings. AIDS 2002;16:135–149.

225. Hays R, Kegeles S, Coates T. High HIV risk-taking among young gay men. AIDS 1990;4:901–907.

226. Valleroy L, MacKellar D, Karon J et al. HIV prevalence and associated risks in young men who have sex with men. JAMA 2000;284:198–204.

227. Lemp G, Hirozawa A, Givertz D, et al. Seroprevalence of HIV and risk behaviors among young homosexual and bisexual men: the San Francisco/Berkeley Young Men's Survey. JAMA 1994;272:449–454.

228. MacKellar D, Valleroy L, Secura G et al. Unrecognized HIV infection, risk behaviors, and perceptions of risk among young men who have sex with men. J Acquir Immune Defic Syndr 2005;38:603–614.

229. Osmond D, Page K, Wiley J et al. HIV infection in homosexual and bisexual men 18 to 29 years of age: the San Francisco Young Men's Health Study. Am J Public Health 1994;84:1933–1937.

230. Seage G, Mayer K, Lenderking W et al. HIV and Hepatitis B infection and risk behavior in young gay men and bisexual men. Public Health Rep 1997;112:158–167.

231. Harawa N, Greenland S, Bingham T, et al. Associations of race/ethnicity with HIV prevalence and HIV-related behaviors among young men who have sex with men in 7 urban centers in the United States. J Acquir Immune Defic Syndr 2004;35526–536.

232. Ekstrand M, Stall R, Paul J, Osmond D, Coates T. Gay men report high rates of unprotected anal sex with partners of unknown or discordant HIV status. AIDS 1999;13:1525–1533.

233. Waldo C, McFarland W, Katz M, MacKellar D, Valleroy L. Very young men gay and bisexual men are at risk for HIV infection: the San Francisco bay area young men's survey II. J Acquir Immune Defic Syndr 2000;24:168–174.

234. Kegeles S, Hays R, Coates T. The Mpowerment project: a community level HIV prevention intervention for young gay men. Am J Public Health 1996;86:1129–1136.

235. Rotheram-Borus M, Lee M, Murphy D et al. Efficacy of a preventive intervention for youths living with HIV. Am J Public Health 2001;91:400–405

236. Centers for Disease Control and Prevention. HIV and AIDS among gay and bisexual men (fact sheet, 2010). Accessed May 14, 2010 at, http://www/cdc/gov/nchhstp/newsroom/docsFastFacts-MSM-final508Comp.pdf

237. Millett G. Flores S, Peterson J, Bakeman R. Explaining disparities in HIV infection among black and white men who have sex with men: a meta-analysis of HIV risk behaviors. AIDS 2007;21:2083–2091.

238. Raymond H, McFarland W. Racial mixing and HIV risk among men who have sex with men. AIDS Behav 2009;1: 630–637.

239. Myrick R. In the life: culture-specific HIV communication programs designed for African American men who have sex with men. J Sex Res 1999;36:159–170.

240. Peterson J, Coates T, Catania J et al. Evaluation of an HIV risk reduction intervention among African-American homosexual and bisexual men. AIDS 1996;10: 319–325.

241. Wilton L, Herbst J, Coury-Doniger C et al. Efficacy of an HIV/STI prevention intervention for Black men who have sex with men: findings from the Many Men, Many Voices (3MV) project. AIDS Behav 2009;13:532–544.

242. Marks G, Millett G, Bingham T et al. Understanding differences in HIV sexual transmission among Latino and Black men who have sex with men: the Brothers y Hermanos study. AIDS Beh 2009;13:682–690.

243. Wilson P, Diaz R, Yoshikawa H, Shrout P. Drug use, interpersonal attraction, and communication: situational factors as predictors of episodes of unprotected anal intercourse among Latino gay men. AIDS Behav 2009;13:691–699.

244. Arreola S, Neilands T, Diaz R. Childhood sexual abuse and the sociocultural context of sexual risk among adult Latino gay and bisexual men. Am J Public Health 2009;99:S432–S438 (Suppl 2).

245. Diaz R, Ayala G, Bein E. Sexual risk as an outcome of social oppression: data from a probability sample of Latino gay men in three US cities. Cultural Diversity Ethnic Minority Psych, 2004; 10(3): 255–267.

246. Jarama SL, Kennamer JD, Poppen PJ, Hendricks M, Bradford J. Psychosocial, behavioral, and cultural predictors of sexual risk for HIV infection among Latino men who have sex with men. AIDS Behav 2005;9:513–523.

247. Carballo-Dieguez A, Dolezal C, Leu C et al. A randomized controlled trial to test an HIV-prevention intervention for Latino gay and bisexual men: lessons learned. AIDS Care 2005;17:314–328.

248. Herbst J, Kay L, Passin W et al. A systematic review and meta-analysis of behavioral interventions to reduce HIV risk behaviors of Hispanics in the United States and Puerto Rico. AIDS Behav 2006;11:25–47.

249. Centers for Disease Control and Prevention HIV/AIDS among Asians and Pacific Islanders [fact sheet, 2008]. Accessed June 1, 2010 at, http://www.cdc.gov/hiv/resources/factsheets/PDF/API.pdf.

250. Han CS. A qualitative exploration of the relationship between racism and unsafe sex among Asian Pacific Islander gay men. Arch Sex Behav 2008;37:827–837.

251. Herbst J, Sherba R, Crepaz N et al. A meta-analytic review of HIV behavioral interventions for reducing sexual risk behavior of men who have sex with men. J Acquir Immune Defic Syndr 2005;39:228–241.

252. Herbst J, Beeker C, Mathew A et al. The effectiveness of individual-, group-, and community-level HIV behavioral risk-reduction interventions for adult men who have sex with men. Amer J Preventive Med 2007;32:S38–S67.

253. Johnson W, Hedges L, Ramirez G et al. HIV prevention research for men who have sex with men: a systematic review and meta-analysis. J Acquir Immune Defic Syndr 2002;30:S118–S133 (Suppll 1).

254. Johnson W, Holtgrave D, McClellan W, Flanders W, Hill A, Goodman M. HIV intervention research for men who have sex with men: a 7-year update. AIDS Educ Prev 2005;17:568–589.

255. Task Force on Community Preventive Services. Recommendations for use of behavioral interventions to reduce the risk of sexual transmission of HIV among men who have sex with men. Amer J Prev Med 2007;32:S36–S37.

256. Sullivan P, Wolitski R. HIV infection among gay and bisexual men. In: Wolitski R, Stall R, Valdiserri R (Eds): Unequal opportunity: health disparities affecting gay and bisexual men in the United States. Oxford, UK: Oxford University Press; 2008 (pp. 220–247).

257. Centers for Disease Control and Prevention. CDC analysis provides new look at disproportionate impact of HIV and syphilis among U.S. gay and bisexual men (press release, 2010). Accessed May 24, 2010 at, http://www.cdc.gov/nchhstp/Newsroom/msmpressrelease.html.

258. U.S. Census Bureau. USA quick facts. Accessed May 24, 2010, at: http://quickfacts.census.gov/qfd/states/00000.html

259. Centers for Disease Control and Prevention. HIV risk, prevention, and testing behaviors – United States, NHBS: MSM, November 2003–April 2005. MMWR 2006;55:1–16.

260. Koblin B, Chesney M, Coates T. Effects of a behavioural intervention to reduce acquisition of HIV infection among men who have sex with men: The EXPLORE randomised controlled study. Lancet 2004;364:41–50.

261. Purcell DW, Metsch LR, Latka M et al. Interventions for seropositive injectors-research and evaluation: an integrated behavioral intervention with HIV-positive injection drug users to address medical care, adherence, and risk reduction. J Acquir Immune Defic Syndr 2004;37:S110–S118.

262. Mansergh GM, Koblin BA, McKirnan DJ et al. An intervention to reduce HIV risk of substance-using men who have sex with men: A two-group randomized trial with a non-randomized third group. PLoS-Med 2010;7(8):e1000329.

263. Kegeles SM, Hays RB, Pollack LM, Coates TJ. Mobilizing young gay and bisexual men for HIV prevention: a two-community study. AIDS 1999;13:1753–1762.

264. Ekstrand ML. Safer sex maintenance among gay men: are we making any progress? AIDS 1992;6:861–868.

265. Elliott S. Advertising: A Campaign for AIDS Drug Adds Warning. New York Times (Business Section); May 10, 2001.

266. Ritter J. Ads linked to rise in rate of HIV infections: City considers ban on drug billboards. USA Today (A04); April 6, 2001. Adapated by The Body; accessed May 23, 2010 at, http://www.thebody.com/content/art22690.html.

267. Ostrow DG, Silverberg MJ, Cook RL, et al. Prospective study of attitudinal and relationship predictors of sexual risk in the multicenter AIDS cohort study. AIDS Behav 2008;12:127–138.

268. Wolitski RJ, Gomez CA, Parsons JT. Effects of a peer-led behavioral intervention to reduce HIV transmission and promote serostatus disclosure among HIV-seropositive gay and bisexual men. AIDS 2005;19:S99–S109.

269. Garfein RS, Golub ET, Greenberg AE et al. A peer-education intervention to reduce injection risk behaviors for HIV and hepatitis C virus infection in young injection drug users. AIDS 2007;21:1923–1932.

270. Stall R, Mills TC, Williamson J et al. Association of co-occurring psychosocial health problems and increased vulnerability to HIV/AIDS among urban men who have sex with men. Am J Public Health 2003;93:939–942.

271. Heredia C. Serving body and soul. With music, games and art, Magnet adds a touch of fun to health checkups. San Francisco Chronicle; Sept 28, 2003. Accessed May 24, 2010 at, http://articles.sfgate.com/2003-09-28/living/17508465_1_gay-men-men-s-health-eric-rofes.

272. Van Kersteren NM, Kok G, Hospers HJ, Schippers J, De WIldt W. Systematic development of a self-help and motivational enhancement intervention to promote sexual health in HIV-positive MSM. AIDS Patient Care STDs 2006;20:858–875.

273. Mamary E, McCright J, Roe K. Our lives: an examination of sexual health issues using photovoice by non-gay identified African American men who have sex with men. Cult Health Sex 2007;9:359–370.

274. Forbes A. Microbicides: When, How and Why Care Now? The Body 2005 (Nov/Dec). Accessible May 25, 2010 at, http://www.thebody.com/content/art956.html.

275. Silverman BG, Gross TP. Use and effectiveness of condoms during anal sex: A review. Sex Transm Dis 1997;24:11–17.

276. Marks G, Mansergh G, Crepaz N, Murphy S, Miller LC, Appleby PR. Future HIV prevention options for men who have sex with men: Intention to use a potential microbicide during anal intercourse. AIDS Behav 2000;4:279–287.

277. Rader M, Marks G, Mansergh G et al. Preferences about the characteristics of future HIV prevention products among men who have sex with men. AIDS Educ Prev 2001;13:149–159.

278. Scott-Sheldon LA, Marsh KL, Johnson BT, Glasford DE. Condoms + pleasure = safer sex? A missing addend in the safer sex message. AIDS Care 2006;18:750–754.

279. Nodin N, Carballo-Dieguez A, Ventuneac AM, Balan IC, Remien R. Knowledge and acceptability of alternative HIV prevention biomedical products among MSM who bareback. AIDS Care 2008;20:106–115.

280. Adam BD, Husbands W, Murray J, Maxwell J. AIDS optimism, condom fatigue, or self-esteem? Explaining unsafe sex among gay and bisexual men. J Sex Res 2005;42:238–248.

281. Staff. Latex allergy and contraception. Contracept Rep March 1997;8:1–2 (Suppl 1).

282. Mansergh G, Marks G, Rader M, Colfax GN, Buchbinder S. Rectal use of nonoxynol-9 among men who have sex with men. AIDS 2003;17:905–909.

283. Carballo-Diéguez A, O'Sullivan LF, Lin P, Dolezal C, Pollack L, Catania J. Awareness and attitudes regarding microbicides and Nonoxynol-9 use in a probability sample of gay men. AIDS Behav 2007;11:271–276.

284. Grant RM, Lama JR, Anderson PL, McMahan V, Liu AY, Vargas L, Goicochea P, Casapía M, Guanira-Carranza JV, Ramirez-Cardich ME, Montoya-Herrera O, Fernández T, Veloso VG, Buchbinder SP, Chariyalertsak S, Schechter M, Bekker LG, Mayer KH, Kallás EG, Amico KR, Mulligan K, Bushman LR, Hance RJ, Ganoza C, Defechercux P, Postle B, Wang F, McConnell JJ, Zheng JH, Lee J, Rooney JF, Jaffe HS, Martinez AI, Burns DN, Glidden DV; iPrEx Study Team. Preexposure chemoprophylaxis for HIV prevention in men who have sex with men. N Engl J Med 2010 Dec 30;363(27):2587–2599.

285. Garcia-Lerma JG, Otten RA, Qari SH et al. Prevention of rectal SHIV transmission in macaques by daily or intermittent prophylaxis with emtricitabine and tenofovir. PLoS Med 2008;5:e28.

286. Garcia-Lerma JG, Paxton L, Kilmarx PH, Heneine W. Oral pre-exposure prophylaxis from HIV prevention. Trends Pharmacol Sci 2010;31:74–81.

287. Sturt AS, Dokubo EK, Sint TT. Antiretroviral therapy (ART) for treating HIV infection in ART-eligible pregnant women. Cochrane Database Syst Rev 2010;3:CD008440.

288. Mansergh GM, Koblin B, Colfax GN, McKirnan D, Flores SA, Hudson SM. Pre-efficacy use and sharing of antiretroviral medications to prevent sexually-transmitted HIV infection among U.S. men who have sex with men. JAIDS 2010;55:e14–e16.

289. Klausner JD, Pollack LM, Wong W, Katz MH. Same-sex domestic partnerships and lower-risk behaviors for STDs, including HIV infection. J Homosex 2006;51:137–144.

290. Kline TM, Martz G, Lesperance CJ, Waldo MC. Defining life partnerships: does sexual orientation matter? J Homosex 2008;55:606–618.

291. Marks G, Burris S, Peterman TA. Reducing sexual transmission of HIV from those who know they are infected: the need for personal and collective responsibility. AIDS 1999;13:297–306.

292. Human Rights Campaign. Marriage and Relationship Recognition (fact sheet, 2010). Accessed May 25, 2010 at, http://www.hrc.org/issues/5517.htm.

293. Wolitski R, Valdiserri, RO, Stall R. Health disparities affecting gay and bisexual men in the United States: An introduction. In Wolitski R, Stall R, Valdiserri, RO (Eds): Unequal Opportunity. New York: Oxford University Press; 2008 (pp. 3–32).

294. van Griensven F, de Lind van Wijngaarden JW, Baral S, Grulich A. (2009) The global epidemic of HIV infection among men who have sex with men. Curr Opinion HIV AIDS 2009;4:300–307.

295. Baral S, Sifakis F, Cleghorn F, Beyrer C. Elevated risk for HIV infection among men who have sex with men in low- and middle-income countries 2000–2006: A systematic review. PLoS Med 2007;4:e339.

296. Global Forum on MSM and HIV. Reaching MSM in a global HIV and AIDS epidemic: A policy brief; 2010. Accessed May 24, 2010, at http://www.msmandhiv.org/documents/MSMGF_ReachingMSMlowres.pdf.

297. Global Foum on MSM and HIV. Social discrimination against MSM: Implications for policy and programs; 2010. Accessed May 25, 2010 at, http://www.msmandhiv.org/documents/MSMGF_Social_Discrimination_Policy_Brief.pdf.

298. Northcraft GB, Neale MA. Organizational behavior: A management challenge. Chicago: Dryden Press, 1990.

299. Gibson JL, Ivancevich JM, Donnelly JH Jr. Organizations: Behavior, structure, processes (8th Ed). Boston: Irwin Inc, 1994.

300. Peters JW. Celebrities come out, without fanfare. New York Times (Fashion & Style Section); May 23, 2010. Accessed May 24, 2010 at, http://www.nytimes.com/2010/05/23/fashion/23outing.html?scp=3&sq=gay&st=cse.

Chapter 31 AIDS and Aging: A Living Experience

ELOISE RATHBONE-McCUAN, ERIN BOYCE,
AND SHARE DECOIX BANE

*They call me an "AIDS survivor" because I am living much longer than
the predicted longevity categorically assigned to me when first
diagnosed. Experimental drugs were quickly prescribed and my
eventual compliance with the HAART therapy regime dominated daily
living. Far too long I bought into the stigmatized stereotype of feeling
guilty, marking days off my extended life calendar and watching AIDS
deaths throughout my community network. As I kept living, mere survival
became insufficient, requiring me to reframe my understanding of what it
means to live more than less fully one day at a time.*

—PATRICK DeVeney

Introduction

In 1986, a 57-year-old man was autopsied to substantiate the presence of
Alzheimer's disease, with results suggesting the dementia was associated
with the human immunodeficiency virus (HIV). This diagnostic conclusion
was a case precedent of the virus in someone over 50 years age which supported observation that the virus might be associated with a progressive
dementia.[1] The following year, a second case study was published for a man
even older who was infected with HIV.[2] Prior to these case reports, little or
no medical practitioner interest had been shown for the possibility that
patients 50 years of age and older might be at risk for HIV infection. These
cases have provided the initial alert to geriatric physicians that HIV/AIDS
could occur undetected in older patients.[3] To this point, HIV/AIDS had been
portrayed as a virus almost exclusively contracted by younger, homosexual
men.

Over the past several decades, we have witnessed a significant increase
in the prevalence and incidence of HIV/AIDS among older Americans. During this time, there has also been a specific advocacy movement started in the
United States to raise awareness about HIV/AIDS risks among older people.
One goal was to challenge existing myths that older persons are sexually
inactive and, thus, not vulnerable to risks through sexual transmission. Significant progress has been made to understand the importance of providing
older people with prevention education as well as prompt access to HIV testing and treatment. Outreach is expanding, and more health and social services are being offered in communities where there are well developed
HIV/AIDS care networks and progressive comprehensive systems of elder

care. There is an expanding dialog between researchers and their funding agencies. Non-governmental organizations are beginning to cooperate and draw attention to how the HIV/AIDS pandemic threatens the global aging population.

Older Age-Related U.S. Reporting

Surveillance data have allowed us to understand the growing HIV/AIDS pandemic, quantify its magnitude, track the spatial distribution, and characterize disease progression.[4] Beginning in 1982 the U.S. Centers for Disease Control and Prevention (CDC) has collected and tracked incidence and prevalence rates of HIV/AIDS.[5] Initially, these rates were tracked under three age groups: under 25 years, 25–44 years, and over 44 years. Between 1983 and 1987, the CDC utilized an additional age category of over 49 years of age, and in 1988, again extended age categories to include 50–54 years, 60–64 years, and 65 and older, with further refinement added for 70 years and beyond.[6] The gradual extension of the chronological age variable was required because individuals were contracting the virus later in life and living longer as a result of effective highly-active antiretroviral therapy (HAART).

As of December 2001, the cumulative number of AIDS cases reported by the CDC was 816,149. Of that total, 90,513 (11%) were individuals 50 years of age and older when diagnosed. Of those diagnosed at 50 years of age and older, 47% were 50–54 years of age, 26% were 55–59, 14% were 60–64, and 13% were 65 years of age and older.[7] Between 1990 and 1999, the number of diagnosed AIDS cases increased and were most evident for older African American women, increasing from 24% to 53% for those 60 to 64 years of age and from 13% to 43% for those 65 years of age and older. This same age/gender trend was identified, to a lesser extent, among Hispanic women between 50 and 64 years of age. During this time, interval men 50 years of age and older who were diagnosed as HIV-positive through heterosexual contact increased 94%, and for older women, heterosexual transmission showed a 106% increase.[8] The public health implications were clear: older minority women and men were being infected with HIV through heterosexual transmission and were being diagnosed with AIDS at later life stages. Also, men who have sex with men showed an age increase at the time of their infection and diagnosis.

Beginning in 2001, the CDC provided the following data on the number of cases diagnosed each year by age group: between 2001 and 2007, the average number of new cases of HIV infection for adults ages 50–54 was 2,735; for those 55–59 years, 1482; for those 60–64 years, 754; and for those 65 years and older, 655.[9] In 2005, the CDC made available the first brief statistical overview of persons 50 years of age and older with HIV/AIDS: individuals 50 years of age and older accounted for 15% of new HIV/AIDS cases diagnosed. In 2001, 17% of persons living with HIV/AIDS were 50 years of age and older, and within 4 years it had increased to 24%. Older persons account for 19% of all AIDS cases and 35% of all deaths. The CDC profile further confirms the increasing racial and ethnic disparities in HIV/AIDS diagnoses among older persons. Rates were 12 times higher among African Americans (51.7/100,000) and 5 times higher for Hispanics (21.4/100,000) compared to whites (4.2/100,000). The position taken by the CDC makes clear that HIV/AIDS must be included as part of the ongoing national effort to reduce all types of health disparities for older minorities. Specific public health challenges must be addressed to enhance prevention, improve detection, and develop more appropriate service provision.

International HIV/AIDS data collection efforts do not offer age-refined categories for persons older than 49 years of age. Prevalence and incidence data collected by the World Health

Organization (WHO), the United Nations (UNAIDS), and Global AIDS generated from several hundreds nations does not afford a global picture of HIV/AIDS cases within the older population. This limits the ability to accurately estimate HIV/AIDS rates in the highest-impact nations. The number of HIV-infected older persons, if chronologically defined as 50 or older, is increasing as lives are extended by HAART therapy availability.

Advocacy for Older Americans

Advocacy is a process whereby individuals sharing a human need speak for themselves and others, often through personal effort and formal organizations taking action on their behalf. Federal funding agencies, specialized academic research units, professional organizations, local service provider agency coalitions, and individual campaigners have all been variously engaged in multifaceted HIV/AIDS elder advocacy for more than 20 years. Their efforts began with questions of how HIV/AIDS could be affecting the aging population, especially within the older gay community. Mental health risks such as depression, potential suicide risk, and drug addiction were important to identify. Health care needs based on potential disease comorbidity and drug toxicity suggested greater health risks for those with AIDS at an older age. Social service providers were questioning how to reduce social isolation, better coordinate service access, and offer educational programs to increase community awareness.

In 1988, the National Institute on Aging organized a workshop entitled *Aids in An Aging Society: What We Need to Know*. Some of these working papers and session summaries were then published in an issue of *Generations*, under the auspices of the Western Gerontological Society (now the American Society on Aging). The thematic consistency of the journal issue was for geriatric and gerontologic practitioners to recognize HIV/AIDS as a potential risk among older persons.[10] In 1989, SAGE (the acronym, at that time, for Senior Action in a Gay Environment, and now Services & Advocacy for GLBT Elders), a New York City social agency established 10 years prior to address the needs of aging lesbians, gays, bisexuals, and transgendered persons (LGBT), started the AIDS and Elderly Program. It was the first HIV/AIDS service program offered to LGBT elderly in the country.[11] Formation of the New York AIDS and Aging Task Force in 1990, then affiliated with the Brookdale Center on Aging of Hunter College, City University of New York, and the New York City Department of Aging, initiated small demonstration social service projects. For example, the task force helped organize volunteers to make home visits to isolated older AIDS patients and organized support groups for grandmothers caring for children of parents with HIV/AIDS. The staff from the Brookdale Center began to offer community education about emerging care needs for older ill patients and discuss an array of risk behaviors too often minimized in older groups. In 1991, the AIDS Community Research Initiative of America (ACRIA) was created and conducted the first community survey addressing AIDS within the older New York City population.[12]

The American Association of Retired Persons (AARP), the oldest and largest U.S. senior citizen advocacy organization, in 1993 incorporated issues of aging and HIV/AIDS into the agenda of its older women's educational initiative. Motivated by the importance for further education, AARP was a primary sponsor of a 1995 conference held in Washington, D.C. At this conference, topics such as the complexity of HIV transmission, AIDS treatment approaches, and lifestyle sexual activities issues experienced by midlife and older women were discussed.[13] A national AARP publication served to inform millions in the general older American population about general issues of HIV/AIDS applicable to those in later years.

Serv

Also in 1995, the first national targeted HIV/AIDS and aging conference was convened and, as a result, the New York Association of HIV Over Fifty (NAHOF) was created. The conference functioned as a small national idea exchange among professionals and consumers to share information and gain knowledge about the barriers to care faced by older persons with HIV/AIDS. The conference content was synthesized into an edited volume and published the following year. It provided a needed text for an expanding professional audience.[14] The purpose of NAHOF was to influence agencies within the city and state working with senior citizens to establish innovations linkages with HIV/AIDS service providers. Following the conference, Jane Fowler, a founding member of NAHOF, wanted to advocate for older women with HIV/AIDS. She recruited other older women with HIV/AIDS concerns and established a consumer community education effort. Their program was entitled HIV Wisdom for Older Women. Jane Fowler continues to be very active in older women's education.[15]

Several institutes of the National Institutes of Health (NIH) collaborated to sponsor a 2002 invitational workshop on mental health issues associated with HIV/AIDS. Exploratory attention was given to neurocognitive alterations such as immunosenesence, an area of particular interest to geriatric psychiatrists and neuropsychologists. In 2003, the *Journal of Acquired Immune Deficiency Syndromes (AIDS)* devoted an issue to AIDS and aging. The following year, a supplemental issue of *AIDS* was published, addressing new directions for HIV and aging mental health research and discussing evidence-based interventions for cognitive impairment.

In 2006 ACRIA began a survey of 1,000 persons throughout metropolitan New York area, gathering more information about effective services for those persons 50 years and older with recent HIV detection, those living in the community who were entering late midlife with long standing AIDS, and older patients with AIDS receiving long-term nursing care. The survey report recommendations were released in 2008 and are being used as guidelines for further service development.[16] Two international conferences on aging and AIDS were supported by the National Institute on Aging. The first was convened in November 2007 by the Institute of Behavioral Science at the University of Colorado in Boulder, and the second in November 2008 at the University of Michigan Population Studies Center. Both research meetings included papers addressing the patterns of HIV/AIDS infection among community elders and the roles and functions of older family caregivers in sub-Saharan and Asian countries with the highest rates of HIV/AIDS.

More recently, the First Annual National HIV/AIDS and Aging Awareness Day was held on September 18, 2009, advocating for greater national recognition of current and expanding needs of older persons with lives affected by HIV/AIDS.[17] At the November 2009 meeting of the NIH Office on AIDS Research Advisory Council (OARAC), the agenda was devoted to intensifying interdisciplinary aging and AIDS research interest and funding. Some topics of emerging importance are: the impact of HIV/AIDS on premature menopause, pre-HIV health conditions, and age-related, long-term HAART tolerance and its effect on brain function.[18] In 2010, the U.S. Department of Health and Human Services, Administration on Aging (DHHS/AoA) awarded a 5-year grant to SAGE to establish an LGBT National Technical Assistance Center to collect, analyze, and distribute research and practice material nationwide.[19] One of the Center's primary functions will be distribution of updated prevention and intervention information that targets the older MSM subgroup. The January 2010 issue of *Research on Aging (ROA)*, a supplemental issue of research papers, addressed the contributions of elderly HIV/AIDS family caregivers in Cambodia, Kenyan, South Africa, and Thailand.

The probability of more rigorous investigation on topics of aging and HIV/AIDS will undoubtedly provide timely, critical information concerning the impact of HIV/AIDS and the

H

13. American Association of Retired Persons. Midlife and older women and HIV/AIDS. Report on the Seminar. Washington DC:1994.

14. Zablotsky D, Kennedy M. Assessing the progress and promise of research on midlife and older adults with HIV/AIDS. In: Emlet CA, ed. HIV/AIDS and the Older Adult Challenges for individuals, families, and communities. New York NY: Springer: 2004;21–25.

15. Fowler JP. Aging with HIV: One woman's story. J AIDS 2003;33:S166–S168.

16. Karpiak SE, Shippy RA. Research on Older Adults with HIV. ACRIA. New York, NY;2008 Accessed October 8, 2009 at, http://www.acria.org.

17. Fauci AS, Hodes RJ, Whitescarver, J. Statement on National HIV/AIDS and Aging. National Institute on Aging, Rockhill, MD. September 2009. Accessed March 12, 2010 at, http://www.nia.nih.gov/News.

18. National Institutes of Health. Twenty-ninth meeting Office of AIDS Research Advisory Council. Rockhill MD: November 2009. Accessed January 12, 2010 at, http://www.oar.nih.gov/oarac/minutes110509.asp.

19. Services and Advocacy for Gay Lesbian and Transgender Elders National Resource Center on LGBT Aging. New York, NY.2009. Accessed January 20, 2010 at, http://www.sageusa.org/index.cfm.

20. Wetten K, Reif S, Whetten R, et al. Trauma, mental health, distrust and stigma among HIV-positive persons: Implications for effective care. Psychosomatic Med 2008;70:531–538.

21. Foster PP, Gaskins SW. Older African American's management of HIV/AIDS stigma. AIDS Care 2009;21:1306–1312.

22. Hardy DJ, Vance, DE. The neuropsychology of HIV/AIDS in older adults. Neurpsychol Rev 2009;19:263–272.

23. Aletha A, Bernstein L, Doyle, J et al. Factors associated with lack of interest in HIV testing in older at risk women. J Women's Health 2007;16:842–858.

24. Centers for Disease Control and Prevention. HIV testing recommendations 2009. Accessed March 31, 2010 at, http://www.aids.about.com/od/testing/a/testrec.htm.

25. Simone MJ, Applebaum J. HIV in older adults. Geriatrics 2008;63:6–12.

26. Sreenivas K, Beebe TJ, Merry SP, et al. The preferences of adult outpatients in medical or dental care settings for giving saliva, urine or blood for clinical testing. J Am Dent Assoc 2008;139:735-740.

27. Cherry-Peepers G, Daniels CO, Meeks V et al. Oral manifestations in the era of HAART. J Natl Med Assoc 2003;95:S21–S32.

28. Health Resources and Services Administration. Ryan White HIV/AIDS Federal Appropriations 2006-2009. Accessed March 10, 2010 at, http://www.hrsa.gov/reports/funding.htm.

29. Henry Kaiser Family Foundation. HIV Medicaid Policy Fact Sheet. Accessed February 2, 2010 at, http://www.kff.org/hivaids/7172.cfm.

30. Henry Kaiser Family Foundation. HIV Medicare Policy Fact Sheet. Accessed February 2, 1010 at, http://www.kff.org/hivaids/7171.cfm.

31. Sangho M, Shin J. Health care utilization among Medicare-Medicaid dual eligible: a count analysis. BMC. Public Health 2006;6:88.

32. Emlet CA, Gerkin A. The graying of HIV/AIDS: preparedness and needs of the aging network in a changing epidemic. J Gerontol Soc Work 2009;52:803-814.

33. HelpAge International. Mind the Gap: HIV and AIDS and older people in Africa. London 2008. Accessed December 10, 2009 at, http://www.helpage/briefing.

34. Zimmer Z. Household composition among elderly in sub-Saharan Africa in the context of HIV/AIDS. J Marriage and Family 2009;71:1086–1099.

35. Ice GH, Yogo J, Heh V, et al. The impact of care giving on the health and well being of Kenyan Lou grandparents. Res Aging 2010;32:40–68.

36. Kondel J, Saengtienchai C, Im-em W et al. AIDS and older people: An international perspective. Res Aging 2003;23:S153–S165.

37. Rathbone-McCuan E. Field study at Mezam Clinic and Shisong Hospital in Bamenda Cameroon. 2005. Unpublished.

Part VII

AIDS AND SOCIETY

16. Jia Y, Sun J, Fan L, et al. Estimates of HIV prevalence in a highly endemic area of China: Dehong Prefecture, Yunnan Province. Int J Epidemiol 2008;37:1287–1296.

17. Duan S, Guo H, Pang L, et al. Analysis of the epidemiologic patterns of HIV transmission in Dehong prefecture, Yunnan province. Zhonghua Yu Fang Yi Xue Za Zhi 2008;42:866–869.

18. Lu L, Jia M, Ma Y, et al. The changing face of HIV in China. Nature 2008;455:609–611.

19. Beyrer C, Razak MH, Lisam K, et al. Overland heroin trafficking routes and HIV-1 spread in South and Southeast Asia. AIDS 2000;17(1):75–83.

20. Stimson GV, Adelekan ML, Rhodes T. The diffusion of drug injection in developing countries. Int J Drug Policy 1996;7(4):245–255.

21. Des Jarlais DC, Choopanya K, Wenston J, et al. Risk reduction and stabilization of HIV seroprevalence among drug injectors in New York City and Bangkok, Thailand. In: Rossi GB, Beth-Giraldo E, Chieco-Bianchi L, Dianzani F, Giraldo G, Verani P, eds. Science Challenging AIDS Switzerland: S. Karger, Basel; 1992:207–213.

22. Wawer M, Gray R, Sewankambo N, et al. Rates of HIV-1 transmission per coital act, by stage of HIV-1 infection, in Rakai, Uganda. J Infect Dis 2005;191(9):1403–1409.

23. Des Jarlais DC, Friedman SR, Hopkins W. Risk reduction for the acquired immunodeficiency syndrome among intravenous drug users. Ann Intern Med 1985;103:755–759.

24. Friedman SR, Des Jarlais DC, Sotheran JL, et al. AIDS and self-organization among intravenous drug users. Int J Addict 1987;22:201–219.

25. Selwyn P, Feiner C, Cox C, et al. Knowledge about AIDS and high-risk behavior among intravenous drug abusers in New York City. AIDS 1987;1:247–254.

26. Des Jarlais DC, Hopkins W. "Free" needles for intravenous drug users at risk for AIDS: current developments in New York City. N Engl J Med 1985;313(23):1476.

27. Des Jarlais DC, Friedman SR. AIDS prevention programs for injecting drug users. In: Wormser GP, ed. AIDS and Other Manifestations of HIV Infection. Second ed. New York: Raven Press; 1992:645–658.

28. Jackson J, Rotkiewicz L. A coupon program: AIDS education and drug treatment. Paper presented at: III International Conference on AIDS,, 1987; Washington, D.C.

29. Watters JK, Estilo MJ, Clark GL, Lorvick J. Syringe and needle exchange as HIV/AIDS prevention for injection drug users. JAMA 1994;271(2):115–120.

30. Needle R, Burrows D, Friedman S, et al. Effectiveness of community-based outreach in preventing HIV/AIDS among injecting drug users. Int J Drug Policy 2005;16S:S45–S57.

31. Semaan S, Kay L, Strouse D, et al. A profile of U.S.-based trials of behavioral and social interventions for HIV risk-reduction. J Acquir Immune Defic Syndr 2002;30(Suppl 1):S30–S50.

32. Becker MH, Joseph JG. AIDS and Behavioral Change to Reduce Risk: a review. Am J Public Health 1988;78(4):394–410.

33. Bandura A. Social Learning Theory. Englewood, NJ: Prentice-Hall; 1977.

34. Fishbein M, Ajzen I. Belief, Attitude, Intention and Behavior: An Introduction to Theory and Research. Boston: Addison-Wesley; 1975.

35. Brown BS, Beschner GM, eds. Handbook on Risk of AIDS: Injection Drug Users and Sexual Partners. Westport, CT: Greenwood Press; 1993.

36. Stephens RC, Simpson DD, Coyle SL, McCoy C, National AIDS Research Consortium. Comparative effectiveness of NADR interventions. In: Brown BS, Beschner GM, eds. Handbook on risk of AIDS. Westport, CT: Greenwood Press; 1993.

37. Meader N, Li R, Des Jarlais D, Pilling S. Psychosocial interventions for reducing injection and sexual risk behaviour for preventing HIV in drug users (Review). New York: Cochrane Collaboration; 2010.

38. Semaan S, Des Jarlais DC, Sogolow E, et al. A meta-analysis of the effect of HIV prevention interventions on the sex behaviors of drug users in the United States. J Acqui Immune Defic Syndr 2002;30(suppl 1):S73–S93.

39. Des Jarlais DC, Friedman SR, Sotheran JL, et al. Continuity and change within an HIV epidemic: injecting drug users in New York City, 1984 through 1992. JAMA 1994;271(2):121–127.

40. Latkin C, W. M, Vlahov D, Oziemkowska M, Celentano D. People and places: behavioral settings and personal network characteristics as correlates of needle sharing. J Acquir Immune Defic Syndr 1996;30:273–280.

41. Neaigus A, Friedman SR, Curtis R, et al. The relevance of drug injectors' social and risk networks for understanding and preventing HIV infection. Soc Sci Med 1994;38(1):67–78.

42. Des Jarlais DC, Choopanya K, Frischer M, et al. Cross-cultural similarities in AIDS risk reduction among injecting drug users. Paper presented at: IX International Conference on AIDS, 1993; Berlin.

43. Wiebel W, Jimenez A, Johnson W, et al. Risk Behavior and HIV seroincidence among out-of-treatment IDUs: four-year prospective study. J Acquir Immune Defic Synd 1996;12(3):282–289.

44. Wiebel W. The indigenous leader outreach model: intervention manual. Rockville: National Institute on Drug Abuse; 1993.

45. Friedman SR, de Jong W, Wodak A. Community development as a response to HIV among drug injectors. AIDS 1993;S263–S269.

46. Friedman SR, Des Jarlais DC, Neaigus A, et al. Organizing drug injectors against AIDS: preliminary data on behavioral outcomes. Psychol Addict Behav 1992;6(2):100–106.

47. Broadhead RS, Heckathorn DD, Weakliem DL, et al. Harnessing peer networks as an instrument for AIDS prevention: results from a peer driven intervention. Public Health Rep 1998;113 Suppl 1:42–57.

48. Costenbader F, Astone N, Latkin C. The dynamics of injection drug users' personal networks and HIV risk behaviors. Addiction 2006;101:1003–1013.

49. Friedman SR, Bolyard M, Maslow C, et al. Harnessing the power of social networks to reduce HIV risk. Focus 2005;20(1):5–6.

50. Broadhead RS, Heckathorn DD, Altice FL, et al. Increasing drug users' adherence to HIV treatment: results of a peer-driven intervention feasibility study. Soc Sci Med 2002;55(2):235–246.

51. Latkin C, Hua W, Davey M. Factors associated with peer HIV prevention outreach in drug-using communities. AIDS Educ Prev 2004;16(6):499–508.

52. McKnight C, Des Jarlais D, Bramson H, et al. Respondent-driven sampling in a study of drug users in New York City: notes from the field. J Urban Health 2006;83(7):i54–i59.

53. Blankenship K, Bray S, Merson M. Structural interventions in public health. AIDS 2000;14(Suppl 1):S11–S21.

54. Des Jarlais DC. Structural interventions to reduce HIV transmission among injecting drug users. AIDS 2000;14(1):S41–S46.

55. Sumartojo E, Laga Me. Structural factors in HIV prevention. AIDS 2000;14(Suppl 1):S1–S73.

56. Rhodes T. Risk environments and drug harms: a social science for harm reduction approach. Int J Drug Policy 2009;20:193–201.

57. Buning EC, van Brussel GHA, van Santen G. Amsterdam's Drug Policy and its Implications for Controlling Needle Sharing. In: Battjes RJ, Pickens RW, eds. Needle Sharing Among Intravenous Drug Abusers: National and International Drug Perspectives. Research Monograph 80. Rockville, MD: National Institute on Drug Abuse; 1988:59–74.

58. Stimson GV, Alldritt LJ, Dolan KA, Donoghoe MS, Lart RA. Injecting Equipment Exchange Schemes: Final Report. London: London: Monitoring Research Group, Goldsmith's College; 1988.

59. Espinoza P, Bouchard I, Ballian P, et al. Has the open sale of syringes modified the syringe exchanging habits of drug addicts? Paper presented at: IV International Conference on AIDS, 1988; Stockholm, Sweden.

60. Ingold FR, Ingold S. The effects of the liberalization of syringe sales on the behavior of intravenous drug users in France. Bull Narcotics 1989;41:67–81.

61. Wodak A. Needle exchange and bleach distribution programmes: the Australian experience. Int J Drug Policy 1995;6(1):46–56.

62. Lurie P, Reingold AL, eds. The Public-Health Impact of Needle-Exchange Programs in the United States and Abroad: Summary, Conclusions, and Recommendations. San Francisco, CA: University of California, San Francisco, Institute for Health Policy Studies; 1993.

63. Normand J, Vlahov D, Moses LE, eds. Preventing HIV Transmission: The Role of Sterile Needles and Bleach. Washington, D.C.: National Academy Press/National Research Council/ Institute of Medicine; 1995.

64. Des Jarlais DC, Friedman SR. AIDS and legal access to sterile drug injection equipment. Ann Am Acad Political Soc Sci 1992;521:42–65.

65. Gostin L. The legal environment impeding access to sterile syringes and needles: the conflict between law enforcement and public health. J Aquir Immune Defic Syndr 1998;18(1):S60–S70.

66. Anderson W. The New York needle trial: the politics of public health in the age of AIDS. Am J Public Health 1991; 81:1506–1517.

67. McKnight C, Des Jarlais D, Perlis T, et al. Syringe exchange programs—United States, 2005. MMWR 2007;56(44):1164–1167.

68. Hagan H, Des Jarlais DC, Purchase D, et al. The Tacoma syringe exchange. J Addict Dis 1991;10(4): 81–88.

69. Ljungberg B, Christensson B, Tunving K, et al. HIV prevention among injecting drug users: three years of experience from a syringe exchange program in Sweden. J Acquir Immune Defic Syndr 1991;4:890–895.

70. Frischer M, Des Jarlais DC, Green S, et al. Modeling AIDS awareness and behavior change among IDUs in Glasgow and New York. Paper presented at: 9th International Conference on AIDS, 1993; Berlin.

71. Stimson GV, Keene J, Parry-Langdon N. Evaluation of the syringe exchange programme Wales, 1990–91. Final Report to the Welsh Office: The Centre for Research on Drugs and Health Behavior, University of London; 1991.

Although in many countries the highest rates of sexual violence have been reported for rape by intimate partners, in South Africa, men are more likely to report having raped a woman who is not an intimate partner.[4] In South Africa, 28% of men report having raped, and 21% of these disclosed having raped a non-intimate partner.[4] The WHO Multi-Country Study reported the prevalence of rape victimization by an intimate partner varied from 6% in Japan and Serbia and Montenegro to 59% in rural Ethiopia. Rape by a man who was not a partner varied from less than 1% in rural Ethiopia and Bangladesh to more than 10% in Peru, Samoa and urban Tanzania.[3]

Gender-Based Violence and HIV: Making the Connections

A discussion of the connections between gender-based violence and HIV must be prefaced by clarification of what is meant by "gender." The word is often used synonymously with "sex," but this is incorrect as sex differences are rooted in biology, whereas gender differences stem from sexual socialization. This encompasses differences in ways men and women learn to position themselves socially and act as social and sexual beings. Thus, gender refers to the socially learned ways of being a man or woman, and the power and possibilities so entailed.

Research from South Africa has shown that women who experience highly controlling practices from their male partner and intimate partner violence, in both respects, have a 50% greater HIV incidence. Calculation of the Population Attributable Fractions indicates that HIV incident infections in women could be reduced by 13.9% and 11.9%, respectively, if women were not exposed to the most highly controlling practices and partner violence.[1] Furthermore, it has also shown that women who experience sexual abuse in childhood have a 66% higher HIV incidence.[5] These findings support a body of evidence from both low- and high-prevalence settings, which has shown associations between gender-based violence and male controlling practices experienced by women and their HIV serostatus.[6–9]

Evidence suggests that these connections arise through multiple pathways (**Figure 33–1**). Gender power inequities and violence are integrally linked, with violence both a consequence of the former, at both a societal and relationship level, and an act that serves to reproduce power inequities.[10] At their heart, the intersections of HIV/AIDS, gender inequity and gender-based violence stem from the patriarchal nature of society, and ideals of masculinity that are predicated on control of women and valorize male strength and toughness.[10,11] These ideals readily translate into sexually risky behaviors, sexual predation, and other acts of violence against women.[10] They also translate into an expectation that men have an unquestionable right to have multiple partners and to control both their sexual encounters and women whom they partner. Evidence from South Africa and India shows that men who perpetrate violence are more likely to be HIV infected.[4,9] While individual women may resist male power, women are largely expected by society to accept such male behavior. Particularly in developing countries, acquiescent femininities are normative. Abuse enhances the likelihood that women will relinquish attempts at influencing the timing and circumstances of sex, resulting in more frequent sex and less condom use.[12–15]

As suggested by **Figure 33–1**, rape is a potential cause of direct infection with HIV. Intimate partner violence and gender inequity impact on HIV risk through longer-acting indirect risk pathways, which are the most important sources of HIV risk from a population perspective. These involve both chronically abusive relationships where women are repeatedly exposed to the same individual, as well as women who have had prior, but not necessarily ongoing, exposure to violence (in childhood or as adults) and controlling practices.

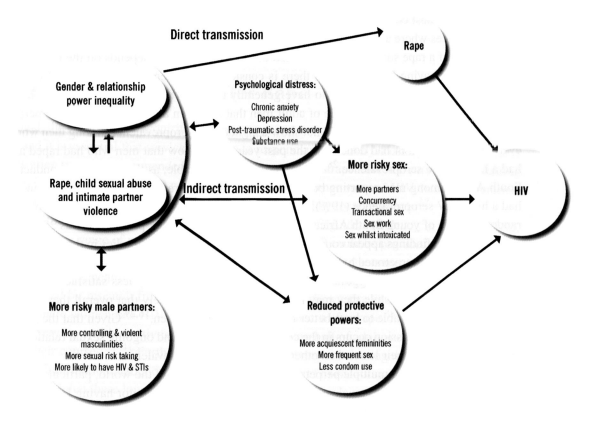

Figure 33–1. *Conceptual model showing pathways through which gender-based violence and gender and relationship power inequity place woman at risk of HIV. Source: Jewkes et al.*[1]

Exposure to gender-based violence, including controlling behavior of a partner, is seen from developing and developed countries to be associated with high-risk sexual behavior, including multiple and concurrent sexual partnerships, increased numbers of overall partners, lower levels of condom use, increased substance use and sex while intoxicated, and increased participation in transactional sex as well as commercial sex work.[2,6,16–22] This is partly due to the psychological impact of violence, which can last many years after the violent acts.[23] Women may be more willing to engage in risky sex, and less able to refuse unwanted advances, when drunk, drugged, dissociating, or desperately seeking affection, or otherwise unable to resist controlling partners.[21–23] Thus, the abuse feeds a vicious cycle, enhancing risk of HIV infection as well as risk of further abuse.

Rape and HIV Risks

Since HIV is sexually transmissible, there is a potent concern about transmission occurring through rape. This compounds the trauma and violation of rape, irrespective of the specific risks involved, and appropriate counselling and provision of postexposure antiretroviral prophylaxis are essential features of high-quality postrape care. The risks of HIV acquisition during rape are highly context dependent. Clearly, they are much higher if the perpetrator is known to be HIV-infected and not on treatment than, for example, a college student date rape in a low-prevalence

101. Bandura A. (1994). Social cognitive theory and exercise of control over HIV infection. In DiClemente RJ, Peterson JL (Eds): Preventing AIDS: Theories and methods of behavioral interventions. New York, NY, US: Plenum Press; 1994 (pp. 25–59).

102. Rotheram-Borus MJ, Lee MB, Gwadz M, Draimin B. An intervention for parents with AIDS and their adolescent children. Am J Public Health 2001;91:1294–1302.

103. Abel E, Rew L, Gortner EM, Delvill CL. Cognitive reorganization and stigmatization among persons with HIV. J Adv Nurs 2004;47:510 25.

104. Eigo J, Harrington M, McCarthy M, Spinella S, SugdenR. FDA action handbook. New York City: ACT UP Archives; 1988. Accessed December 23, 2008, at http://www.actupny.org/documents/FDAhandbook1.html.

105. Hadijpateras A. Unraveling the dynamics of HIV-AIDS related stigma and discrimination: The role of community based research. London: ACORN/ASAP Publication; 2004.

106. International Planned Parenthood Federation Civil society declaration on the UN high level meeting on AIDS. London: International Planned Parenthood Federation; 2008. Accessed December 23, 2008, at http://www.ippf.org/en/Resources/Statements/Civil+Society+Declaration+on+the+UN+High+Level+Meeting+on+AIDS.htm.

107. Pryor JB, Beadle de Palomo F, Little SE, Engle NM, Ahmed M, Anderson G, Campos P, Sheoran B, Stupplebeen D, Schroeder K, Candelario N, Koll G, Roque F, Curry L, Clear A, McQuie H, Raymond D, Rios-Ellis B, Arroyo L, Diaz G. Reducing HIV-related stigma in diverse communities in the United States. Unpublished manuscript, Illinois State University; 2010.

108. Harm Reduction Coalition. Accessed on December 15, 2010 at http://www.harmreduction.org/index.php.

109. Lyles CM, Kay LS, Crepaz N, Herbst JH, Passin WF, Kim AS, Rama SM, Thadiparthi S, DeLuca JB, Mullins MM. Best-Evidence Interventions: Findings From a Systematic Review of HIV Behavioral Interventions for US Populations at High Risk, 2000–2004. Am J Public Health 2007;97:133–143.

110. Maughan-Brown B. Stigma rises despite antiretroviral roll-out: A longitudinal analysis in South Africa. Soc Sci Med 2010;70:368–374.

111. Pulerwitz J, Michaelis A, Weiss E, Brown L, Mahendr V. Reducing HIV-related stigma: Lessons learned from Horizons research and programs. Public Health Rep 2010;125;272–281.

112. Herek GM, Glunt EK. An epidemic of stigma: public reactions to AIDS. Am Psychol 1988;43:886–891.

Part VIII

AIDS IN SPECIFIC GEOGRAPHIC REGIONS

Chapter 35 AIDS IN AFRICA

JOEP M.A. LANGE, ELLY KATABIRA, AND
ANDREW KAMBUGU

*Even in London or New York or Paris, Africans do not easily lose the
habit of catching your eye as you pass. Raise an eyebrow in greeting
and a flicker of a smile starts in their eyes. A small thing? No. It is the
prize that Africa offers the rest of the world: humanity.*

—RICHARD DOWDEN, Africa: Altered States,
Ordinary Miracles. Portobello Books, London, 2008.

*Why is it that we are always talking about the problem of drug
distribution when there is virtually no place in Africa where one cannot
get a cold beer or a cold Coca Cola?*

—JOEP LANGE, International AIDS Conference, July 2004,
Barcelona, Catalunya, Spain

Introduction

The HIV epidemic originated in sub-Saharan Africa[1] and of a global total of
approximately 33 million people living with HIV/AIDS, this region currently
is home to two-thirds of that number. All seven countries with an adult HIV
prevalence of greater than 15% are located in southern Africa. Although there
are concentrated epidemics in other regions of the world, overall adult HIV
prevalence in sub-Saharan Africa generally dwarfs that seen elsewhere.[2] In
no other region has HIV created such devastation or has had such a visible
impact on public life.

Yet, when AIDS first emerged in the early 1980s in young gay men from
the East and West Coast of the United States (U.S.), there was not the slight-
est notion about what was going on in Africa.[3,4] Although it sounds paradoxical, this may be considered fortunate—if HIV/AIDS had first emerged
where it originated, rather than affecting the vocal communities in the U.S.
where substantial market incentives also existed, the breathtaking history of
HIV drug development[5] might not have occurred. Instead the pace would
more likely have resembled that for tuberculosis or malaria treatments, which
has been exceedingly slow.

Origins and Epidemiology of HIV

For details on the epidemiology of HIV and its spread in sub-Saharan Africa,
we refer to the chapter on epidemiology in this book. Although HIV comprises several related viruses that have crossed into the human population on
multiple occasions from nonhuman primate reservoir species in Africa, when

we speak about HIV in this chapter we refer to HIV-1, group M (for "main" or "major"), unless we state otherwise. Only the HIV-1 group M lineage has reached pandemic proportions: it has a global distribution and accounts for more than 99% of the HIV infections.[1] Chimpanzees and gorillas are the only nonhuman primates known to harbor viruses closely related to HIV-1 (SIVcpz and SIVgor, respectively). Phylogenetic analyses showed that gorillas acquired SIV from chimpanzees, and that viruses from the SIVcpz/SIVgor lineage have been transmitted to humans (in central Africa) on at least four occasions, leading to HIV-1 groups M, N ("new"), O ("outlier") and the newly discovered group P. The natural reservoir of HIV-1 pandemic group M and nonpandemic group N is the chimpanzee (*Pan troglodytes troglodytes*), and that of nonpandemic groups O and P is the gorilla.[6–9] HIV-2 is the result of at least eight distinct cross-species transmissions of SIV from sooty mangabeys (SIVsmm) in west Africa, corresponding to HIV-2 groups A through H.[1,7,10] HIV-2 is less transmissible than HIV-1, both heterosexually and vertically.[11–13] HIV-2 infection also progresses more slowly than does HIV-1 infection.[11,14]

The term *subtype* (A to D, F to H, J, K) is used within HIV-1 group M. Different subtypes dominate in different regions. Subtype B accounts for most infections in the United States and Europe; subtype C predominates in southern Africa and in India; and subtype D is common in eastern Africa. However, matters are even more complicated by the fact that recombination plays a large role in the evolution of both SIV and HIV. The existence of clear recombinants, with genomes that are mosaics of distinct lineages, has led to the introduction of a formal system for recognizing them.[15] These *circulating recombinant forms* (CRFs) represent virus populations that have diversified from a single, ancestral strain generated by recombination between two or more of the recognized M group subtypes.[15] The "missing" subtypes, E and I, have been reclassified as CRFs after detailed analysis of their genomes revealed that they had recombinant origins. Some CRFs are the dominant HIV-1 group M strain in some locales (e.g., CRF01_AE in Thailand, CRF02_AG in Nigeria).[1,15,16] There is also abundant evidence of recombination among the SIVs of different primate species, and even between groups M and O.[17] The progenitor of HIV-1, SIVcpz, has been determined to be a recombinant between the SIVs of red-capped mangabeys and greater spot-nosed monkeys, two prey species of chimpanzees.[18] All strains of HIV are, thus, ultimately recombinant in origin, their genomes a mosaic of two monkey viruses, trafficked through an ape intermediary. As Michael Worobey summarizes it: "The virus that first appeared on the medical world's radar in high-risk populations in the U.S.A. made an extraordinary journey there: from African monkeys, then to the apes that preyed upon them, then on to human beings in central Africa and beyond."[1]

This may not be the end of the story. Since human beings in sub-Saharan Africa continue to be exposed to a plethora of primate lentiviruses through hunting and handling of primate bushmeat, additional zoonotic transfers of primate lentiviruses must be considered.[7]

Although AIDS only emerged or was recognized in 1981, the estimate is that HIV-1 group M had been introduced in humans in 1931 (1915–1930).[1,19] For the two main HIV-2 groups A and B these estimates are 1940 (1924–1956) and 1945 (1931–1959), respectively. The HIV epidemic could take off in Africa because of urbanization and mobility of people and subsequently spread to the rest of the world, where it was first recognized, through international travel.[20,21]

By the time HIV was recognized, it had already become endemic in central and east Africa.[22,23] One can conclude that, given the lack of awareness about this new infection, its long incubation period to disease development, and the preponderance of confounding diseases in settings with limited diagnostic possibilities, the spread of the virus to these levels could not have been prevented. The story is very different for southern Africa. Here, the epidemic took off in the early 1990s, after we already knew much about this horrific disease, about the virus, and about the way it was transmitted. This represents a huge failure of both national governments—in particular, the South African government, which espoused AIDS denialism[24,25]—and the international HIV prevention community. Fortunately, epidemic trends in many sub-Saharan African countries have improved, although the annual number of new infections is no reason for complacency.[26] There is increasing recognition of high infection rates in men who have sex with men (MSM), who, due to stigmatization and criminalization, are often not openly gay and may spread the virus to other groups in the population.[27,28]

Disease Manifestations

The spectrum of HIV and AIDS-related disease manifestations in sub-Saharan Africa differs from that in the developed world. In African adults, tuberculosis (TB) is the most frequent cause of death, whereas *Pneumocystis jirovecii* pneumonia is relatively uncommon. Bacterial pneumonias also play an important role in mortality. In children, especially infants, *Pneumocystis jirovecii* pneumonia does appear to be an important contributor to mortality.[29–36] A particular challenge in sub-Saharan Africa is that in many settings there is a limited ability to make a correct laboratory diagnosis of an opportunistic disease.

HIV and tuberculosis form a deadly liaison. Not only is tuberculosis a leading cause of death in people with HIV infection, but conversely HIV has exacerbated the tuberculosis epidemic globally and especially in Africa. In some sub-Saharan African countries up to 70% of people with tuberculosis are also HIV positive.[37] HIV is also an important driver of the spread of multidrug-resistant (MDR) tuberculosis, including extensively drug resistant (XDR) tuberculosis.[38] Yet, integration of HIV and TB services has been exceedingly slow. Between 1995 and 2008, the directly observed therapy, short course (DOTS) strategy enabled treatment of 43 million patients with tuberculosis, but until 2004 this strategy did not explicitly include HIV interventions. Most HIV services still do not include specific activities for tuberculosis care and prevention. Many lives must have been lost due to this negligence. Rapid scale-up of effective and integrated services for tuberculosis and HIV is mandatory.[37] New tools to diagnose tuberculosis and drug resistance within hours,[39] if used widely, could make a major difference.[40] Although isoniazid preventive therapy in HIV-positive individuals has long been known to be efficacious,[41–44] its use has been limited.[37,45] Likewise, cotrimoxazole preventive therapy—another life-saving intervention that may prevent *Pneumocystis jirovecii*, *Toxoplasma gondii*, *Isospora belli*, and bacterial infections,[42,46–50] and which also has antimalarial activity[51]—is often not provided.[52]

There is no more effective way to break the deadly connection between HIV and tuberculosis than to initiate highly active antiretroviral therapy (HAART) in a timely manner.[53,54] This is just one of the many benefits of early HAART initiation, which we will discuss later.

African patients with HIV infection, like those from elsewhere, often suffer from dermatologic afflictions. A very common problem, largely limited to tropical environments, is papular pruritic eruption, which probably reflects a hypersensitivity to insect bites.[55] Because of the endemic nature of human herpesvirus type 8 (HHV-8) or Kaposi's sarcoma-associated herpesvirus (KSHV) in certain African countries, Kaposi's sarcoma (KS) is very common in HIV-infected persons in the region. The demographics are very different from those in the developed world, where KS is primarily a disease of MSM. In sub-Saharan Africa men, women and children are all commonly affected.[56,57]

While no data on global prevalence exist, HIV-associated nephropathy (HIVAN) is likely to be highest in sub-Saharan Africa.[58–60] HAART slows down HIVAN progression.[61,62]

Concomitant infections of HIV and either hepatitis B virus (HBV) or hepatitis C virus (HCV) (or both) are not uncommon. HIV co-infection leads to considerably higher rates of liver disease progression in both HBV[63] and HCV infected individuals.[64,65] Timely initiation of HAART will slow down progression of liver disease.[66,67] In the case of HBV coinfection, it is fortunate that a tenofovir-based HAART regimen has dual activity against HIV and HBV. Moreover, such a regimen virtually always contains either lamivudine (3TC) or emtricitabine (FTC), agents that also have anti-HBV activity[68,69].

Uptake of currently available treatment for HCV infection—peginterferon-α plus ribavirin[70,71]—in sub-Saharan Africa has been limited because of its complexity, poor tolerability, and cost plus the fact that patients' HCV status is often not known. However, clinical trials are underway for multiple anti-HCV compounds with novel mechanisms of action and oral curative therapy may eventually be feasible. It is hoped that this will lead to expanded testing and treatment of HCV infections worldwide, similar to what has happened with HIV and HAART.[72]

With increased access to effective treatment, and while new infections continue to occur,[26] the HIV-infected population in sub-Saharan Africa is aging. It has been estimated that in 2007 approximately 3 million HIV-infected adults over 50 years of age were living in this region.[73] This will increase the burden of chronic or aging diseases, which are exacerbated by HIV.[74]

Prevention of HIV Infection

The 2010 UNAIDS report on the Global AIDS Epidemic brought good news. New infections in sub-Saharan Africa have fallen by nearly 20% in the last 10 years, and AIDS-related deaths are down by nearly 20% in the last 5 years. Yet, in 2009 an estimated 2.6 (2.3–2.9) million people became newly infected, 69% of those living in sub-Saharan Africa. For every person starting HIV treatment, two new infections occur.[26] There is, thus, no reason for complacency with regard to HIV prevention.

Some individual countries exempted, the HIV prevention response in sub-Saharan Africa overall may be characterized as "too little, too late," with the AIDS denialism embraced by the former South African government being particularly shameful.[24,25]

It has become clear that, in the absence of an effective preventive HIV vaccine, no single HIV prevention intervention will be sufficient.[75] Apart from increasing knowledge about and access to "classic" HIV prevention tools such as behavior modification, condom use, and harm reduction strategies for people who are injecting-drug users (IDUs), it is necessary for structural interventions to occur simultaneously to decrease gender inequality and stigma associated with particular lifestyles and for new HIV prevention tools to be rolled out in a synergistic manner. It is also crucial for HIV prevention efforts to be based on thorough knowledge of regional, national, and local epidemics and targeted accordingly.[2,76]

The ideal HIV prevention tool would be an HIV vaccine with activity against virtually all HIV strains. Although one clinical trial in Thailand, utilizing a recombinant canarypox vector vaccine with booster injections of a recombinant gp120 subunit protein vaccine, has shown some effect in preventing new HIV infections in a low-risk population,[77] the ideal vaccine is still out of reach. Nevertheless, the Thai trial results, passive protection studies with broad neutralizing antibodies in nonhuman primates, a new yield of broad neutralizing antibodies, and new targets for vaccine design have generated renewed hope that a clinically useful preventive HIV vaccine can be developed.[78]

Findings from nonrandomized studies have already made it highly likely that male circumcision has significantly reduced risk of HIV infection among men in sub-Saharan Africa.[79] This was finally confirmed in three large, randomized, controlled clinical trials, conducted in, respectively, South Africa, Kenya, and Uganda, which showed a reduction in female-to-male transmission of 51% to 61%.[56,80–82] Unfortunately, circumcision of HIV-infected men does not seem to directly reduce HIV risk for their female partners; nevertheless, women will benefit from male circumcision programs in the long term.[83,84] However, the roll-out of male circumcision is lagging behind in many countries: Kenya having made the most progress.[26]

There is a great and longstanding need for female-controlled HIV prevention methods, such a female condoms and vaginal microbicides.[85,86] Although female condoms have been available for about two decades, their uptake has been disappointing. In 2008, while 2.4 billion male condoms were distributed, the figure for female condoms was only 18.2 million (Sipple S, Center for Health and Gender Equity, Washington DC). In 2009 a new version, made of softer material for quieter use and less costly to produce, was licensed by the FDA, but marketing efforts are falling short.

The cervical diaphragm is another potential female-controlled HIV prevention method. Unfortunately, a large, open-label controlled trial, conducted in Southern Africa, comparing an intensive HIV prevention regimen (control arm) with that regimen plus a cervical diaphragm and lubricant gel (intervention arm), failed to show an additional effect of the intervention on HIV incidence. However, this does not represent conclusive evidence of the lack of effect of such a cervical barrier: self-reported condom use at last intercourse was substantially higher in the controls (85%) than in the intervention group (54%). Self-reported use of the diaphragm and gel was only about 73% and might have further compromised the power of this study.[87]

Until recently, the quest to find an effective vaginal microbicide focused on nonantiretroviral-based products showed dismal results.[88–93] A new era seems to be heralded by the successful outcome of the CAPRISA 004 trial, conducted in sexually active HIV-uninfected women in KwaZulu-Natal, which found that a 1% vaginal gel formulation of the nucleotide analogue reverse transcriptase inhibitor tenofovir reduced HIV incidence by 54% in high adherers[94]. Such HIV-specific microbicides could fill an important HIV prevention gap, especially for women unable to negotiate monogamy or condom use[94]. It would also be desirable to develop rectally applied microbicides given the frequency of rectal intercourse not only among MSM, but also among heterosexual men and women[95]. The biological plausibility of rectal microbicides has not been established, however.

Antiretrovirals may also be used systemically to prevent HIV acquisition (pre-exposure prophylaxis, [PrEP]). A recent large, randomized, controlled clinical trial conducted in Peru, Ecuador, South Africa, Brazil, Thailand, and the United States, comparing once-daily tenofovir disoproxil fumarate and emtricitabine (TDF/FTC) with placebo in MSM or transgender women having sex with men showed a 44% reduction in HIV incidence in the active arm. In post hoc analyses, pill use on 90% of days was recorded at 49% of visits on which efficacy was 73%.[96] This success evidently mirrors that of the CAPRISA trial, in which TDF was used locally. Other studies on systemic and local use of TDF or TDF/FTC to prevent HIV acquisition are ongoing.

It is also evident that successful antiretroviral treatment decreases HIV transmission probability to extremely low levels,[97,98] and the scaling up of antiretroviral therapy has been proposed as a strategy to curb the growth of the HIV epidemic.[99] A strategy of universal voluntary HIV testing of those 15 years and older and immediate antiretroviral therapy in those found to be positive, according to a mathematical model based on data from South Africa, could lead to rapid reductions of HIV prevalence and reduce this to less than 1% within 50 years.[100] Although this model has been criticized as being overly simplistic and optimistic,[101] and may be context-dependent,[102] it has generated an enormous interest in "test-and-treat" strategies as a valuable addition to the HIV prevention armamentarium.

A study in rural Tanzania demonstrated that improved treatment of curable STIs led to lower rates of HIV transmission,[103] but these results have not been shown in other studies and settings.[104–108] Likewise, three intervention trials looking at the effect of suppressive antiviral therapy for herpes simplex virus type 2 (HSV-2), on either HIV acquisition[109,110] or HIV transmission,[111] did not have a positive outcome. Yet, as Hayes et al. demonstrated in a recent review,[112] observational and biological data provide compelling evidence of the importance of STIs, including HSV-2, in HIV transmission. These authors conclude: "It is time for a new phase of exploration of how, when, and in whom to include STI control as a key component of HIV prevention, driven by basic research to elucidate the mechanisms by which STIs and vaginal infections facilitate HIV transmission. From a policy perspective, treatment of curable STIs is an essential part of primary health care and is a cheap, simple, and effective intervention when appropriately targeted and delivered. It should be promoted as an essential component of HIV control programs in communities in which the burden of STIs is substantial."[112]

Since a considerable proportion of HIV transmissions takes place in serodiscordant couples, couples voluntary counseling and testing (CVCT) has been proposed as an additional strategy to reduce sexual transmission of HIV.[113]

For thorough coverage of prevention of mother-to-child transmission of HIV (PMTCT), we refer to the chapter on that subject in this book. It is evident that HAART during pregnancy and breastfeeding is the way forward, although WHO guidelines still leave room for a suboptimal regimen in women "who do not need treatment for their own health."[114]

HIV Treatment and Treatment Access

When HAART was introduced in 1996 in the developed world there was great reluctance to also make it widely available in resource-poor settings. Although it was now, unlike in the days of mono- and dual therapy, hard to argue the clinical benefits of antiretroviral therapy, this treatment was considered far too expensive and complex for anything but sophisticated medical environments. It is our personal belief that the fact that the International AIDS Conference in 2000 was held for the first time in sub-Saharan Africa (Durban, South Africa), forced a breakthrough in scaling up access to HAART in resource-poor settings. Shortly before the Durban conference UNAIDS and five major pharmaceutical companies announced an agreement on significant price reductions of antiretrovirals for least-developed nations, especially in sub-Saharan Africa: the Accelerating Access Initiative.[115,116] This was followed by a United Nations General Assembly Special Session (UNGASS) on HIV/AIDS, firmly putting antiretroviral treatment in resource-poor settings on the agenda. The World Health Organization (WHO) subsequently included antiretrovirals in the Essential Medicines list and formulated guidelines for a public health approach to treatment of HIV. New and substantial funding mechanisms, such as the World Bank's Multi-country AIDS Program (MAP), the Global Fund to Fight AIDS, TB and Malaria (GFATM) and the U.S. President's Emergency Plan for AIDS Relief (PEPFAR), were established. Through its "3-by-5" initiative, WHO set a target of 3 million people in resource-poor settings on HAART by the end of 2005. In the meantime, prices of a number of antiretrovirals continued to fall; to a significant extent, this is the result of generic competition.[115] Although the "3-by-5" target was not met, progress has been remarkable. At the end of 2009, 5.2 million people in low- and middle-income countries were receiving HAART, and it is estimated that about 14.4 million life-years have been gained by providing antiretroviral therapy since 1996.[26] This is a striking example of what health gains can be made if the will and resources are there. Unfortunately, the current global economic crisis and policy changes threaten to level off funding for HIV/AIDS, which would undermine the tremendous progress that has been made and would be a grave mistake.[117–119] For the sake of sustainability, African countries themselves should also invest more in health and healthcare.

Notwithstanding the specter of decreased funding for HIV/AIDS, the newest WHO antiretroviral therapy guidelines call for earlier initiation of therapy,[69] in a move toward ending the double standard between HIV treatment guidelines for the developed and developing world. Initiating antiretrovirals early increases survival for those infected,[120–122] slows down HIV-related aging,[74] greatly reduces TB incidence,[53] and is also likely to reduce HIV incidence.[97–100] It will also greatly decrease the occurrence of immune reconstitution inflammatory syndrome (IRIS), [123,124] as well as early mortality during HAART.[125] Lastly, in settings where human resources for health are scarce, it will allow for task shifting.

For HAART to be successful, people must engage in HIV care and be adherent to therapy. It is estimated that in low- and middle-income countries, which have experienced a massive scale-up of antiretroviral therapy over the past few years, approximately 76% of patients who have started HAART are retained in care during the first year of follow-up[126]—not exactly a reassuring figure. Adherence and loss to follow-up may be negatively affected by factors such as food insecurity, lack of transportation, lack of money, and work and child care responsibilities.[127,128] Apart from addressing the aforementioned factors, a single-tablet regimen is likely to contribute to improving adherence.[129] Moreover, in a study conducted in Kenya, support by mobile phone short message service significantly improved HAART adherence and rates of viral suppression.[130]

With increasing coverage of antiretroviral therapy in sub-Saharan Africa, it is inevitable that drug resistance does occur, but until now the extent of this appears to be limited.[132,133] Patterns of drug resistance mutations may be HIV-1 subtype dependent.[133–136] Because of drug resistance, there is a need for affordable second- and third-line regimens in resource-poor settings, although replacing stavudine-based first-line regimens with safer ones remains a priority.[69]

HIV-2 infection poses a particular treatment challenge, since non-nucleoside reverse transcriptase inhibitors (NNRTI) are not active against it and some protease inhibitors, especially non-boosted ones, may also exhibit insufficient activity.[137]

Health Systems in Africa

Sub-Saharan Africa holds approximately 11% of the global population while it carries 40% of the global burden of communicable diseases, and utilizes only 1% of global health spending. Low income countries in sub-Saharan Africa on average annually spend only $17.30 per capita on health care.[138] Slogans like "Health for All" and "Universal Access" appear to pretend that it is possible to deliver decent health care for this amount of money, but this is a fallacy. Health systems in sub-Saharan Africa are to a large extent decrepit. Health care workers often have to work under abominable conditions and are underpaid. These conditions underlie a large brain drain, from rural to urban settings, from some African countries to others, and from African countries to other continents, which aggravates an already severe shortage of human resources for health.[139]

The premier problem is that not enough money is spent on health and health care, not by national governments themselves and not by the donor community. The second is that donor money is often not used in the most efficient manner. Most of it goes to the public sector. Yet a recent paper showed that development assistance for health to governments of developing countries had a negative and significant effect on government spending on health.[140] It is clear that business as usual will not do and that sub-Saharan Africa needs new models to finance health care.[141,142]

Conclusions

The introduction of HAART in the developed world has been one of the success stories of modern medicine. The antiretroviral roll out in resource-poor settings, especially in sub-Saharan Africa, has been another staggering accomplishment, yet its further expansion is under threat. Numbers of new infections are falling, but still far too large. Vaginal microbicides and PrEP will be valuable additions to the HIV prevention armamentarium and increase our chances to turn the tide of the HIV epidemic decisively, as will further roll out of antiretroviral therapy. AIDS exceptionalism has brought us to where we are and has taught us that what seemed impossible is possible. We now need to move on to health exceptionalism, providing access to quality medical care for all.

References

1. Worobey M. The origins and diversification of HIV. In: Volberding PA, Sande MA, Lange J, Greene WC, Gallant J, Eds. Global HIV/AIDS Medicine. Philadelphia: Saunders Elsevier 2008:13–21.
2. UNAIDS/WHO. AIDS epidemic update 2009. Geneva; 2009.
3. CentersforDiseaseControl. *Pneumocystis* pneumonia—Los Angeles. MMWR 1981;30:250–252.
4. CentersforDiseaseControl. Kaposi's sarcoma and *Pneumocystis* pneumonia among homosexual men - New York City and California. MMWR 1981;30(409–410).
5. Broder S. The development of antiretroviral therapy and its impact on the HIV-1/AIDS pandemic. Antiviral Res 2010 Jan;85(1):1–18.
6. Keele BF, Van Heuverswyn F, Li Y, Bailes E, Takehisa J, Santiago ML, et al. Chimpanzee reservoirs of pandemic and nonpandemic HIV-1. Science 2006 Jul 28;313(5786):523–526.
7. Van Heuverswyn F, Peeters M. The origins of HIV and implications for the global epidemic. Curr Infect Dis Rep 2007 Jul;9(4):338–346.
8. Neel C, Etienne L, Li Y, Takehisa J, Rudicell RS, Bass IN, et al. Molecular epidemiology of simian immunodeficiency virus infection in wild-living gorillas. J Virol Feb;84(3):1464–1476.
9. Plantier JC, Leoz M, Dickerson JE, De Oliveira F, Cordonnier F, Lemee V, et al. A new human immunodeficiency virus derived from gorillas. Nat Med 2009 Aug;15(8):871–872.
10. Hahn BH, Shaw GM, De Cock KM, Sharp PM. AIDS as a zoonosis: scientific and public health implications. Science 2000 Jan 28;287(5453):607–614.
11. Kanki P. Human immunodeficiency virus type 2 (HIV-2). AIDS Rev. 1999;1:101–108.
12. Kanki PJ, Travers KU, Mboup S, Hsieh CC, Marlink RG, Gueye NA, et al. Slower heterosexual spread of HIV-2 than HIV-1. Lancet 1994 Apr 16;343(8903):943–946.
13. Adjorlolo-Johnson G, De Cock KM, Ekpini E, Vetter KM, Sibailly T, Brattegaard K, et al. Prospective comparison of mother-to-child transmission of HIV-1 and HIV-2 in Abidjan, Ivory Coast. JAMA 1994 Aug 10;272(6):462–466.
14. Reeves JD, Doms RW. Human immunodeficiency virus type 2. J Gen Virol 2002 Jun;83(Pt 6):1253–265.
15. Robertson DL, Anderson JP, Bradac JA, Carr JK, Foley B, Funkhouser RK, et al. HIV-1 nomenclature proposal. Science 2000 Apr 7;288(5463):55–56.
16. Kijak GH, McCutchan FE. HIV diversity, molecular epidemiology, and the role of recombination. Curr Infect Dis Rep. 2005 Nov;7(6):480–488.

17. Takehisa J, Zekeng L, Ido E, Yamaguchi-Kabata Y, Mboudjeka I, Harada Y, et al. Human immunodeficiency virus type 1 intergroup (M/O) recombination in cameroon. J Virol 1999 Aug;73(8):6810–6820.

18. Bailes E, Gao F, Bibollet-Ruche F, Courgnaud V, Peeters M, Marx PA, et al. Hybrid origin of SIV in chimpanzees. Science 2003 Jun 13;300(5626):1713.

19. Korber B, Muldoon M, Theiler J, Gao F, Gupta R, Lapedes A, et al. Timing the ancestor of the HIV-1 pandemic strains. Science 2000 Jun 9;288(5472):1789–796.

20. Shilts R. And the Band Played On: Politics, people and the AIDS epidemic. New York: Viking Penguin 1987.

21. Engel J. The epidemic: a global history of aids. New York: Harper Collins 2006.

22. Serwadda D, Mugerwa RD, Sewankambo NK, Lwegaba A, Carswell JW, Kirya GB, et al. Slim disease: a new disease in Uganda and its association with HTLV-III infection. Lancet 1985 Oct 19;2(8460):849–852.

23. Quinn TC, Mann JM, Curran JW, Piot P. AIDS in Africa: an epidemiologic paradigm. Science. 1986 Nov 21;234(4779):955-63.

24. Geffen N. Justice after AIDS denialism: should there be prosecutions and compensation? J Acquir Immune Defic Syndr 2009 Aug 1;51(4):454–455.

25. Chigwedere P, Essex M. AIDS denialism and public health practice. AIDS Behav 2010 Apr;14(2):237–247.

26. UNAIDS. UNAIDS Report on the Global AIDS Epidemic. Geneva; 2010.

27. Sanders EJ, Graham SM, Okuku HS, van der Elst EM, Muhaari A, Davies A, et al. HIV-1 infection in high risk men who have sex with men in Mombasa, Kenya. AIDS 2007 Nov 30;21(18):2513–2520.

28. Smith AD, Tapsoba P, Peshu N, Sanders EJ, Jaffe HW. Men who have sex with men and HIV/AIDS in sub-Saharan Africa. Lancet 2009 Aug 1;374(9687):416–422.

29. Ansari NA, Kombe AH, Kenyon TA, Mazhani L, Binkin N, Tappero JW, et al. Pathology and causes of death in a series of human immunodeficiency virus-positive and -negative pediatric referral hospital admissions in Botswana. Pediatr Infect Dis J 2003 Jan;22(1):43–47.

30. Lucas S. The pathology of HIV infection. Lepr Rev 2002 Mar;73(1):64–71.

31. Ansari NA, Kombe AH, Kenyon TA, Hone NM, Tappero JW, Nyirenda ST, et al. Pathology and causes of death in a group of 128 predominantly HIV-positive patients in Botswana, 1997–1998. Int J Tuberc Lung Dis 2002 Jan;6(1):55–63.

32. Grant AD, Sidibe K, Domoua K, Bonard D, Sylla-Koko F, Dosso M, et al. Spectrum of disease among HIV-infected adults hospitalised in a respiratory medicine unit in Abidjan, Cote d'Ivoire. Int J Tuberc Lung Dis 1998 Nov;2(11):926–934.

33. Rana F, Hawken MP, Meme HK, Chakaya JM, Githui WA, Odhiambo JA, et al. Autopsy findings in HIV-1-infected adults in Kenya. J Acquir Immune Defic Syndr Hum Retrovirol 1997 Jan 1;14(1):83–85.

34. Lucas SB, Hounnou A, Koffi K, Beaumel A, Andoh J, De Cock KM. Pathology of paediatric human immunodeficiency virus infections in Cote d'Ivoire. East Afr Med J 1996 May;73(5 Suppl):S7–8.

35. Greenberg AE, Lucas S, Tossou O, Coulibaly IM, Coulibaly D, Kassim S, et al. Autopsy-proven causes of death in HIV-infected patients treated for tuberculosis in Abidjan, Cote d'Ivoire. AIDS 1995 Nov;9(11):1251–1254.

36. Lucas SB, Hounnou A, Peacock C, Beaumel A, Djomand G, N'Gbichi JM, et al. The mortality and pathology of HIV infection in a west African city. AIDS 1993 Dec;7(12):1569–1579.

37. Ghebreyesus TA, Kazatchkine M, Sidibe M, Nakatani H. Tuberculosis and HIV: time for an intensified response. Lancet 2010 May 22;375(9728):1757–78.

38. Nathanson E, Nunn P, Uplekar M, Floyd K, Jaramillo E, Lonnroth K, et al. MDR tuberculosis--critical steps for prevention and control. N Engl J Med 2010 Sep 9;363(11):1050–1058.

39. Boehme CC, Nabeta P, Hillemann D, Nicol MP, Shenai S, Krapp F, et al. Rapid molecular detection of tuberculosis and rifampin resistance. N Engl J Med 2010 Sep 9;363(11):1005–1015.

40. Small PM, Pai M. Tuberculosis diagnosis—time for a game change. N Engl J Med 2010 Sep 9;363(11):1070–1071.

41. Pape JW, Jean SS, Ho JL, Hafner A, Johnson WD, Jr. Effect of isoniazid prophylaxis on incidence of active tuberculosis and progression of HIV infection. Lancet 1993 Jul 31;342(8866):268–272.

42. Lange JM. HIV-related morbidity and mortality in sub-Saharan Africa: opportunities for prevention. AIDS 1993 Dec;7(12):1675–1676.

43. Eldred LJ, Churchyard G, Durovni B, Godfrey-Faussett P, Grant AD, Getahun H, et al. Isoniazid preventive therapy for HIV-infected people: evidence to support implementation. AIDS 2010 Nov;24 Suppl 5:S1–3.

44. Lawn SD, Wood R, De Cock KM, Kranzer K, Lewis JJ, Churchyard GJ. Antiretrovirals and isoniazid preventive therapy in the prevention of HIV-associated tuberculosis in settings with limited health-care resources. Lancet Infect Dis 2010 Jul;10(7):489–498.

45. Getahun H, Granich R, Sculier D, Gunneberg C, Blanc L, Nunn P, et al. Implementation of isoniazid preventive therapy for people living with HIV worldwide: barriers and solutions. AIDS 2010 Nov;24 Suppl 5:S57–65.

46. Wiktor SZ, Sassan-Morokro M, Grant AD, Abouya L, Karon JM, Maurice C, et al. Efficacy of trimethoprim-sulphamethoxazole prophylaxis to decrease morbidity and mortality in HIV-1-infected patients with tuberculosis in Abidjan, Cote d'Ivoire: a randomised controlled trial. Lancet 1999 May 1;353(9163):1469–1475.

47. Chintu C, Bhat GJ, Walker AS, Mulenga V, Sinyinza F, Lishimpi K, et al. Co-trimoxazole as prophylaxis against opportunistic infections in HIV-infected Zambian children (CHAP): a double-blind randomised placebo-controlled trial. Lancet 2004 Nov 20-26;364(9448):1865–1871.

48. Mermin J, Lule J, Ekwaru JP, Malamba S, Downing R, Ransom R, et al. Effect of co-trimoxazole prophylaxis on morbidity, mortality, CD4-cell count, and viral load in HIV infection in rural Uganda. Lancet 2004 Oct 16–22;364(9443):1428–1434.

49. Grimwade K, Sturm AW, Nunn AJ, Mbatha D, Zungu D, Gilks CF. Effectiveness of cotrimoxazole prophylaxis on mortality in adults with tuberculosis in rural South Africa. AIDS 2005 Jan 28;19(2):163–168.

50. Grimwade K, Swingler GH. Cotrimoxazole prophylaxis for opportunistic infections in children with HIV infection. Cochrane Database Syst Rev 2006(1):CD003508.

51. Bloland PB, Redd SC, Kazembe P, Tembenu R, Wirima JJ, Campbell CC. Co-trimoxazole for childhood febrile illness in malaria-endemic regions. Lancet 1991 Mar 2;337(8740):518–520.

52. Walker AS, Ford D, Gilks CF, Munderi P, Ssali F, Reid A, et al. Daily co-trimoxazole prophylaxis in severely immunosuppressed HIV-infected adults in Africa started on combination antiretroviral therapy: an observational analysis of the DART cohort. Lancet 2010 Apr 10;375(9722):1278–1286.

53. Lawn SD, Myer L, Edwards D, Bekker LG, Wood R. Short-term and long-term risk of tuberculosis associated with CD4 cell recovery during antiretroviral therapy in South Africa. AIDS 2009 Aug 24;23(13):1717–1725.

54. Harries AD, Zachariah R, Corbett EL, Lawn SD, Santos-Filho ET, Chimzizi R, et al. The HIV-associated tuberculosis epidemic--when will we act? Lancet 2010 May 29;375(9729):1906–1919.

55. Resneck JS, Jr., Van Beek M, Furmanski L, Oyugi J, LeBoit PE, Katabira E, et al. Etiology of pruritic papular eruption with HIV infection in Uganda. JAMA 2004 Dec 1;292(21):2614–2621.

56. Bayley AC. Occurrence, clinical behaviour and management of Kaposi's sarcoma in Zambia. Cancer Surv 1991;10:53–71.

57. Wabinga HR, Parkin DM, Wabwire-Mangen F, Mugerwa JW. Cancer in Kampala, Uganda, in 1989-91: changes in incidence in the era of AIDS. Int J Cancer 1993 Apr 22;54(1):26–36.

58. Okpechi I, Swanepoel C, Duffield M, Mahala B, Wearne N, Alagbe S, et al. Patterns of renal disease in Cape Town South Africa: a 10-year review of a single-centre renal biopsy database. Nephrol Dial Transplant 2010 Oct 27.

59. Eke FU, Anochie IC, Okpere AN, Eneh AU, Ugwu RN, Ejilemele AA, et al. Microalbuminuria in children with human immunodeficiency virus (HIV) infection in Port Harcourt, Nigeria. Niger J Med 2010 Jul–Sep;19(3):298–301.

60. Arendse CG, Wearne N, Okpechi IG, Swanepoel CR. The acute, the chronic and the news of HIV-related renal disease in Africa. Kidney Int 2010 Aug;78(3):239–245.

61. Szczech LA, Edwards LJ, Sanders LL, van der Horst C, Bartlett JA, Heald AE, et al. Protease inhibitors are associated with a slowed progression of HIV-related renal diseases. Clin Nephrol. 2002 May;57(5):336–341.

62. Kalayjian RC. The treatment of HIV-associated nephropathy. Adv Chronic Kidney Dis 2010 Jan;17(1):59–71.

63. Thio CL, Seaberg EC, Skolasky R, Jr., Phair J, Visscher B, Munoz A, et al. HIV-1, hepatitis B virus, and risk of liver-related mortality in the Multicenter Cohort Study (MACS). Lancet 2002 Dec 14;360(9349):1921–1926.

64. Benhamou Y, Bochet M, Di Martino V, Charlotte F, Azria F, Coutellier A, et al. Liver fibrosis progression in human immunodeficiency virus and hepatitis C virus coinfected patients. The Multivirc Group. Hepatology 1999 Oct;30(4):1054–1058.

65. Graham CS, Baden LR, Yu E, Mrus JM, Carnie J, Heeren T, et al. Influence of human immunodeficiency virus infection on the course of hepatitis C virus infection: a meta-analysis. Clin Infect Dis 2001 Aug 15;33(4):562–569.

66. Hoffmann CJ, Seaberg EC, Young S, Witt MD, D'Acunto K, Phair J, et al. Hepatitis B and long-term HIV outcomes in coinfected HAART recipients. AIDS 2009 Sep 10;23(14):1881–1889.

67. Qurishi N, Kreuzberg C, Luchters G, Effenberger W, Kupfer B, Sauerbruch T, et al. Effect of antiretroviral therapy on liver-related mortality in patients with HIV and hepatitis C virus coinfection. Lancet 2003 Nov 22;362(9397):1708–1713.

68. Matthews GV, Seaberg E, Dore GJ, Bowden S, Lewin SR, Sasadeusz J, et al. Combination HBV therapy is linked to greater HBV DNA suppression in a cohort of lamivudine-experienced HIV/HBV coinfected individuals. AIDS 2009 Aug 24;23(13):1707–715.

69. WHO. Antiretroviral Therapy for HIV Infection in Adults and Adolescents: Recommendations for a Public Health Approach: 2010 revision. Geneva: WHO 2010.

70. Torriani FJ, Rodriguez-Torres M, Rockstroh JK, Lissen E, Gonzalez-Garcia J, Lazzarin A, et al. Peginterferon Alfa-2a plus ribavirin for chronic hepatitis C virus infection in HIV-infected patients. N Engl J Med 2004 Jul 29;351(5):438–450.

71. Chung RT, Andersen J, Volberding P, Robbins GK, Liu T, Sherman KE, et al. Peginterferon Alfa-2a plus ribavirin versus interferon alfa-2a plus ribavirin for chronic hepatitis C in HIV-coinfected persons. N Engl J Med 2004 Jul 29;351(5):451–459.

72. Thomas DL. Curing hepatitis C with pills: a step toward global control. Lancet 2010 Oct 30;376(9751):1441–1442.

73. Negin J, Cumming RG. HIV infection in older adults in sub-Saharan Africa: extrapolating prevalence from existing data. Bull World Health Organ 2010 Nov 1;88(11):847–853.

74. Mills EJ, Rammohan A, Awofeso N. Ageing faster with AIDS in Africa. Lancet 2010;376:1441–1442.

75. Merson M, Padian N, Coates TJ, Gupta GR, Bertozzi SM, Piot P, et al. Combination HIV prevention. Lancet 2008 Nov 22;372(9652):1805–1806.

76. UNAIDS. UNAIDS Annual Report: Knowing your epidemic. Geneva; 2007.

77. Rerks-Ngarm S, Pitisuttithum P, Nitayaphan S, Kaewkungwal J, Chiu J, Paris R, et al. Vaccination with ALVAC and AIDSVAX to prevent HIV-1 infection in Thailand. N Engl J Med 2009 Dec 3;361(23):2209–2220.

78. Haynes BF, Liao HX, Tomaras GD. Is developing an HIV-1 vaccine possible? Curr Opin HIV AIDS 2010 Sep;5(5):362–367.

79. Weiss HA, Quigley MA, Hayes RJ. Male circumcision and risk of HIV infection in sub-Saharan Africa: a systematic review and meta-analysis. AIDS 2000 Oct 20;14(15):2361–2370.

80. Auvert B, Taljaard D, Lagarde E, Sobngwi-Tambekou J, Sitta R, Puren A. Randomized, controlled intervention trial of male circumcision for reduction of HIV infection risk: the ANRS 1265 Trial. PLoS Med. 2005 Nov;2(11):e298.

81. Bailey RC, Moses S, Parker CB, Agot K, Maclean I, Krieger JN, et al. Male circumcision for HIV prevention in young men in Kisumu, Kenya: a randomised controlled trial. Lancet 2007 Feb 24;369(9562):643–656.

82. Gray RH, Kigozi G, Serwadda D, Makumbi F, Watya S, Nalugoda F, et al. Male circumcision for HIV prevention in men in Rakai, Uganda: a randomised trial. Lancet 2007 Feb 24;369(9562):657–666.

83. Wawer MJ, Makumbi F, Kigozi G, Serwadda D, Watya S, Nalugoda F, et al. Circumcision in HIV-infected men and its effect on HIV transmission to female partners in Rakai, Uganda: a randomised controlled trial. Lancet. 2009 Jul 18;374(9685):229–237.

84. Baeten JM, Celum C, Coates TJ. Male circumcision and HIV risks and benefits for women. Lancet 2009 Jul 18;374(9685):182–184.

85. Cecil H; Perry MJ; Seal DW; Pinkerton S. The female condom: what have we learned thus far. AIDS and Behavior 1998;2:241–256.

86. Elias CJ, Heise LL. Challenges for the development of female-controlled vaginal microbicides. AIDS 1994 Jan;8(1):1–9.

87. Padian NS, van der Straten A, Ramjee G, Chipato T, de Bruyn G, Blanchard K, et al. Diaphragm and lubricant gel for prevention of HIV acquisition in southern African women: a randomised controlled trial. Lancet. 2007 Jul 21;370(9583):251–261.

88. Van Damme L, Govinden R, Mirembe FM, Guedou F, Solomon S, Becker ML, et al. Lack of effectiveness of cellulose sulfate gel for the prevention of vaginal HIV transmission. N Engl J Med 2008 Jul 31;359(5):463–472.

89. Kreiss J, Ngugi E, Holmes K, Ndinya-Achola J, Waiyaki P, Roberts PL, et al. Efficacy of nonoxynol 9 contraceptive sponge use in preventing heterosexual acquisition of HIV in Nairobi prostitutes. JAMA 1992 Jul 22-29;268(4):477–482.

90. Van Damme L, Ramjee G, Alary M, Vuylsteke B, Chandeying V, Rees H, et al. Effectiveness of COL-1492, a nonoxynol-9 vaginal gel, on HIV-1 transmission in female sex workers: a randomised controlled trial. Lancet 2002 Sep 28;360(9338):971–977.

91. Skoler-Karpoff S, Ramjee G, Ahmed K, Altini L, Plagianos MG, Friedland B, et al. Efficacy of Carraguard for prevention of HIV infection in women in South Africa: a randomised, double-blind, placebo-controlled trial. Lancet 2008 Dec 6;372(9654):1977–1987.

92. McCormack S, Ramjee G, Kamali A, Rees H, Crook AM, Gafos M, et al. PRO2000 vaginal gel for prevention of HIV-1 infection (Microbicides Development Programme 301): a phase 3, randomised, double-blind, parallel-group trial. Lancet 2010 Oct 16;376(9749):1329–1337.

93. Grant RM, Hamer D, Hope T, Johnston R, Lange J, Lederman MM, et al. Whither or wither microbicides? Science 2008 Jul 25;321(5888):532–534.

94. Abdool Karim Q, Abdool Karim SS, Frohlich JA, Grobler AC, Baxter C, Mansoor LE, et al. Effectiveness and safety of tenofovir gel, an antiretroviral microbicide, for the prevention of HIV infection in women. Science 2010 Sep 3;329(5996):1168–1174.

Chapter 36 AIDS in Eastern Europe and Central Asia

DMITRY LIOZNOV, KRISTI RUUTEL, ANNELI UUSKULA,

AND JACK A. DEHOVITZ

AIDS does not inevitably lead to death,
especially if you suppress the co-factors that support the disease.
It is very important to tell this to people who are infected.

—LUC MONTAGNIER

Introduction

A number of factors place the emerging democracies of Eastern Europe at high risk for HIV infection, other sexually transmitted infections (STIs), and tuberculosis (TB).[1]

First, political transition in the early 1990s led to dramatic declines in income, a significant increase in unemployment, and widened income inequities. This economic disarray also led to an expansion of informal and criminal economies.[2] Second, the highly structured public health system rooted in the Soviet tradition has been unable to effectively make the transition to meet post-Soviet challenges. The Soviet model was based on a highly centralized and hierarchical sanitary-epidemiologic system, which was characterized by a large labor force and minimal emphasis on technology. Thus, while surveillance was highly developed, health promotion efforts remained rudimentary.[3] These changes have been confounded by dramatic increases in injection drug use (IDU), the enormous production of opiates from the Central Asian state of Afghanistan, and consequent drug trafficking.[4]

The HIV epidemic in Eastern Europe is substantial and increasing rapidly. While HIV incidence rates vary across the region, certain trends are clear. An estimated 150,000 people were infected with HIV in 2007 bringing the total number of people living with HIV in Eastern Europe and Central Asia to 1.6 million, compared to 630,000 in 2001.[5] IDU remains the primary risk factor in Eastern Europe, although the proportion of HIV infected women (and subsequent vertical transmission to children) is increasing.[6]

Implementation of known interventions to reduce transmission in injecting-drug users (IDUs) has been impeded by challenges in scaling up opioid substitution therapy (OST) as well as other harm-reduction efforts (including needle exchange programs). In 2005, WHO added methadone and buprenorphine to the WHO model list of essential medicines for opioid addiction treatment. While OST has been shown to reduce HIV incidence in drug users,[7] it is variably and inadequately available in the region. Its use is proscribed in Russia, and while the Ministry of Health of Kazakhstan allowed the implementation of a pilot project, it remains generally unavailable there. Programs have been initiated in Ukraine, Estonia, and Georgia, but access to these services remains inadequate. For example it is estimated that there are over 400,000 IDUs in Ukraine, but there are less than 2,000 patients on OST in that country.[8]

The specific epidemiology and prevention efforts in the region are described below.

Central Europe

Central Europe: Czech Republic, Poland, and Hungary

With the exception of Poland, the burden of HIV in Central Europe has remained low.[9] Poland has the highest rate of new HIV infections in the region (~750/year), and approximately 7,500 of the estimated 25,000 people living with HIV are women. The epidemic in Poland is primarily driven by IDU. The high rate of new infections contrasts with both Hungary and the Czech Republic, which have fewer than 100 cases of HIV reported per year, mostly in men who have sex with men (MSM). A series of studies confirm the low rates of infection in these countries.[10–13] Fortunately, the government of Poland has responded forthrightly with model care and treatment programs. Antiretrovirals are universally available, a clinical trials infrastructure is in place, and AIDS Centers have been developed within infectious diseases hospitals in all major large cities.[14] Highly active antiretroviral therapy (HAART) is available free of charge for patients in all three countries.

HIV Epidemiology and Prevention in Baltic Countries, Belarus, and Ukraine

Epidemiology of HIV-Infection

Eastern European countries, especially Estonia and Ukraine, have experienced the fastest growing HIV-epidemics in the world in the last decade. Even though the first cases of HIV were diagnosed in late 1980s (1987 in Ukraine and Latvia, 1988 in Estonia and Lithuania), the major epidemics started in late 1990s and were driven by IDU. The majority of HIV cases have been diagnosed among males and people aged 20–34 years. However, in recent years the proportion of females and people older than 35 years of age has increased.[15–20]

In **Belarus** the peak of the epidemic was in 2002 when 915 HIV cases were diagnosed (9.2 per 100,000 population). The epidemic then appeared to wane, increasing again in 2007–2008 (10.2 and 9.1 new cases per 100,000 population, respectively).[20] The transmission pattern has changed since early 2000, with the proportion of new cases attributed to heterosexual transmission steadily increasing (27% of total new diagnoses in 2001, 74% in 2008).[20,21] More than 50% of all cases have been diagnosed among IDUs and approximately 40% have been heterosexual cases.[20]

In **Estonia** a rapid increase in new HIV infections was detected among IDUs in 2000 and 2001. In 2001 1,474 HIV cases were diagnosed (108 per 100,000). The number of new cases has decreased since 2002, down to 411 (306 per 100,000 population) in 2009.[16] Data on transmission routes is limited and based only on the data from AIDS counseling centers (where approximately one-third of all new cases have been diagnosed). Thus, IDUs accounted for 90% of new

HIV-cases in 2001, 66% in 2003, 54% in 2007, and 48% in 2009. At the same time, the absolute numbers of diagnosed HIV-infections among non-IDUs have not increased. (The increase in the non-IDU proportion is due to the decrease of absolute numbers of IDUs diagnosed with HIV).[22]

In **Latvia** an HIV outbreak among IDUs began at the end of 1997 and by 1998 almost 50% of all HIV cases were diagnosed among this subgroup.[23] By 2006 70% of all cases could be attributed to IDU. The epidemic peaked in 2001, when 807 new cases (34.3 per 100,000) were diagnosed. In general the number of newly diagnosed cases has been decreasing, although a small increase was observed during 2006–2008.[20] In 2009, 275 new cases (12.1 per 100,000) were detected.[17]

In **Lithuania** the majority of HIV cases in 1998–1996 were diagnosed among men who have sex with men (MSM) and heterosexuals (especially sailors). Between 1997 and 2003 the majority of new cases were diagnosed among IDUs (70% in 1997, 78% in 2001) and since 2004 the proportion of heterosexually transmitted cases has increased.[24] Following a decline in the annual number of new HIV diagnoses since 2003 the number of new cases in 2009 rose to 180 (5.3 per 100,000),[18] compared to 95 cases (2.8 per 100,000) diagnosed in 2008.[20]

The increase in injecting drug use in **Ukraine** began in the early 1990s.[25] An HIV outbreak among IDUs was first detected in 1995 and by 1997 at least one HIV case among IDUs was registered in each of the 27 administrative regions. Among those living with HIV at that time 84% were IDUs. Since 1999 more heterosexually transmitted cases have been diagnosed, primarily among women whose sexual partners have been IDUs. In 2004, on average 34 new cases of HIV, eight cases of AIDS and five AIDS deaths were registered daily.[26] The number of officially registered new HIV cases has risen from 1,490 in 1995 to 19,840 in 2009 (43 per 100,000). Within the same period the proportion of IDUs among new cases has decreased from 69% to 36%.[19]

Coinfections

Hepatitis C and B

In 1990s the rates of hepatitis B and C increased throughout the region. For example in Estonia between 1992 and 1998, there was a marked increase in the rates of hepatitis B (6 per 100,000 in 1992 and 34 per 100,000 in 1998) and hepatitis C (0.4 per 100,000 in 1992 and 25 per 100,000 in 1998). Since 2002, the incidence of both hepatitis B and C has decreased, to 3.3 and 2.7 cases per 100,000 inhabitants respectively (2007).[16] In Latvia an increase in hepatitis B and C incidence occurred until 2000–2001, both in the general population and among injecting drug users. Decreasing incidence has been observed since 2001.[27] Among HIV-positive people, there were reports of HCV prevalence of 20–40% in Belarus, more than 40% in Latvia, and more than 70% in Estonia, Lithuania, and Ukraine.[28]

Tuberculosis

The incidence rate of tuberculosis started to increase in the region in the 1990s. For example in Estonia the incidence increased rapidly from 21 per 100,000 in 1992 to 48 per 100,000 in 1998. In Latvia the incidence of TB was 29 per 100,000 in 1991 and 74 per 100,000 in 1998. In recent years substantial progress has been made in the management of this epidemic and TB incidence has begun to decrease in all three Baltic countries. Nonetheless they still have the highest proportion of MDR TB cases in European Union (Latvia, 17.1%; Lithuania, 21.3%; Estonia, 14.7%).[29,30]

In Ukraine the incidence of TB rose from 41.7 per 100 000 population in 1995 to 84.1 per 100,000 in 2005. In 2004, Ukraine had the highest HIV prevalence in adult incident TB cases (8.3%) in Europe, but other studies estimate this figure to be nearer to 9.4%. In Kiev the prevalence of HIV infection in TB patients has increased from 6.3% in 2004 to 10.1% in 2005.[31] In Donetsk Oblast in 2006 the prevalence of HIV among patients with TB was 15.5% in the civilian sector and 23.7% in the prison inmates.[32]

Mother-to-Child Transmission (MTCT) of HIV

The total number of MTCT cases by the end of 2008 was 138 in Belarus, 33 in Estonia, 33 in Latvia, 1 in Lithuania, and 601 in Ukraine. The proportion of MTCT cases among all newly diagnosed HIV cases has remained below 2%, except in Ukraine where it was 3% in 2008.[20] At the same time the MTCT rate in Ukraine has decreased from 15% in 2001 to 6.2% in 2007 and the proportion of women not receiving prophylaxis treatment has decreased from 18% in 2001 to 7% in 2007.[33] In Latvia, on average, around four cases of vertical HIV transmission are reported in Latvia every year, which amounts to 20 cases per 100,000 newborns. In addition, approximately 30 HIV positive pregnant women are detected annually.[17] In Estonia similar patterns have been observed.[16]

AIDS

The number of AIDS cases has increased steadily. At the end of 2008 a total of 724 AIDS cases were diagnosed in Latvia, 206 in Lithuania, 252 in Estonia, 1,328 in Belarus, and 19,427 in Ukraine. The rates per 1 million population in 2008 were 43.6 for Latvia, 16.3 for Lithuania, 45.5 for Estonia, 36.2 for Belarus, and 22.3 for Ukraine. Tuberculosis has been the main AIDS associated disease. Of importance is to note that while in Western Europe the most common AIDS-associated diseases in 2008 were pneumocystis pneumonia (22%), wasting syndrome due to HIV (9%), and tuberculosis (TB) (9%), in the East of the WHO European Region (including also Belarus, Estonia, Latvia, Lithuania, Ukraine) TB ranked first (32%), followed by HIV-related wasting syndrome and extrapulmonary TB.[20]

Risk Groups

Injecting Drug Users

The estimated number of IDUs is 60,000 in Belarus, 13,800 in Estonia, 12,000 in Latvia, 8,000 in Lithuania, and 375,000 in Ukraine.[28] There have been a number of new studies to estimate HIV prevalence among IDUs in these countries. The mean HIV prevalence among IDUs in Ukraine in studies conducted in 2008–2009 in 30 regions was 22.9%. There were major differences across different regions—HIV prevalence ranged from 3.4 to 55.2%.[19] An HIV prevalence rate of 55% has been described among IDUs in Estonia's capital city Tallinn, 22% in Riga, Latvia, and 8% in Vilnius, Lithuania.[34] Unfortunately, only limited data on HIV prevalence in IDUs for Belarus is available. Rapidly increasing HIV prevalence rates among IDUs were already detected in the 1990s—in Svetlogorsk (known as the state's drug capital) in 1996 HIV prevalence among 1,000 IDUs was 16% and in a study conducted in 1997—74%.[35,36] Existing

54. Emmanuelli J,Desenclos J. Harm reduction interventions, behaviours and associated health outcomes in France, 1996-2003. Addiction 2005;100:1690–1700.

55. Van Den Berg C, Smit C, Van Brussel G, et al. Full participation in harm reduction programmes is associated with decreased risk for human immunodeficiency virus and hepatitis C virus: evidence from the Amsterdam Cohort Studies among drug users. Addiction 2007;102:1454–1462.

56. Des Jarlais DC, Arasteh K, Gwadz M. Increasing HIV prevention and care for injecting drug users. Lancet 2010;20;375:961–963.

57. Burrows D. Advocacy and coverage of needle exchange programs: results of a comparative study of harm reduction programs in Brazil, Bangladesh, Belarus, Ukraine, Russian Federation, and China. Cad Saude Publica 2006;22:871–879.

58. Estonia: National Report on the Implementation of the Declaration of Commitment on HIV/AIDS. Reporting period: January 2009—December 2009. Tallinn 2010. Accessed at http://data.unaids.org/pub/Report/2010/estonia_2010_country_progress_report_en.pdf

59. Niccolai LM, Toussova OV, Verevochkin SV, et al. High HIV prevalence, suboptimal HIV testing, and low knowledge of HIV-positive serostatus among injection drug users in St. Petersburg, Russia. AIDS Behav 2008.

60. Caplinskas S, Likatavièius G. Recent sharp rise in registered HIV infections in Lithuania. Euro Surveill 2002;6(26):pii=1939.

61. Jürgens R. HIV/AIDS in prisons: recent developments. Canadian HIV/AIDS Policy & Law Review 2002;7(2/3):13–20.

62. Mounier-Jack S, Nielsen S, Coker RJ. HIV testing strategies across European countries. HIV Medicine 2008;9(Suppl. 2):13–19.

63. Lai T, Rätsep M, Rüütel K, et al. Modelling Estonia's concentrated HIV epidemic. A case study. WHO 2009. Available at, http://www.euro.who.int/document/E93235.pdf

64. UNAIDS, 2008. Report on the global AIDS epidemic. Geneva, UNAIDS.

65. Pokrovsky V. Nowhere HIV spreads as soon as in Russia. November 26, 2009. Argumenty i facty. Zdorovi'e. p.11–12.

66. Pokrovskiy VV, Yankina ZK, Pokrovskiy VI. Epidemiological Investigation of the First Case of the Acquired Immunodeficiency Syndrome (AIDS) Detected in the USSR. Zhurnal Mikrobiologii 1987;12:6–10.

67. Bobkov A, Garaev MM, Rzhnaninova A, et al. Molecular epidemiology of HIV-1 in the former Soviet Union: analysis of env V3 sequences and their correlation with epidemiologic data. AIDS 1994;8:619-624.

68. Euro HIV (2003) HIV/AIDS Surveillance in Europe. Mid-year report. Saint-Maurice, Institut de Veille Sanitaire.

69. Information on Officially Registered HIV Cases in Russian Federation by October 31, 2009. Russian Federal AIDS Center. http://www.hivrussia.ru/stat/2009/10.shtml

70. Reference on HIV-infection in Russian Federation in 2009. Russian Federal AIDS Center. 2009.

71. Selivanov Ye.A., Danilova T.N. Degtereve I.N., Grigorian M.Sh. Measures to Ensure the Infections Safety of Blood Transfusion in the Russian Federation. HIV-infection and Immunosuppressive Conditions. 2009;1(1):62–67.

72. Frolova O., Shikareva I., Novoselova O. Epidemiological Situation on TB with HIV in Russian Federation. 3rd All Russian scientific conference MDR-TB in HIV-infected patients; May 12–13, 2009; Moscow, Russia. p.56-57. http://hivpolicy.ru/upload/File/RelatedFiles/news/3449/bulletin_7_2009.pdf

73. Smolskaya T, Liitsola K, Zetterberg V, Golovanova E, Kevlova N, Konovalova N, Sevastianova K, Brummer-Korvenkontio H, Salminen M. HIV epidemiology in the Northwestern Federal District of Russia: dominance of HIV type 1 subtype A. AIDS Res Hum Retroviruses. 2006 Nov;22(11):1074–1080.

74. Khanina TA, Selimova LM, Kazennikova EV, Bobkov AF, Bobkova MR, Pokrovsky VV, Zverev SIa, Braganza R, Nicolson K, Weber D. Biological properties of HIV-1 variants circulating among drug users in Russia. Vopr Virusol. 2005 Jul–Aug;50(4):24-8. [Article in Russian]

75. Bobkov AF, Kazennova EV, Selimova LM, Khanina TA, Ryabov GS, Bobkova MR, Sukhanova AL, Kravchenko AV, Ladnaya NN, Weber JN, Pokrovsky VV. Temporal trends in the HIV-1 epidemic in Russia: predominance of subtype A. J Med Virol. 2004 Oct;74(2):191–196.

76. Khaldeeva, N., Hillis, S.D., Vinogradova, E., Voronin, E., Rakhmanova, A., Yakovlev, A., Jamieson, D.J., Ryder, R.W. HIV-1 seroprevalence rates in women and relinquishment of infants to the state in St. Petersburg, Russia, 2002. Lancet 2003;362:1981–1982.

77. Hillis SD, Phd EK, Akatova N, Kissin DM, Vinogradova EN, Rakhmanova AG, Stepanova E, Jamieson DJ, Robinson J, Vitek C, Miller WC. Antiretroviral Prophylaxis to Prevent Perinatal HIV Transmission in St. Petersburg, Russia: Too Little, Too Late. J Acquir Immune Defic Syndr. 2010 Feb 3. [Epub ahead of print]

78. Kissin DM et al. Rapid HIV testing and prevention of perinatal HIV transmission in high-risk maternity hospitals in St. Petersburg, Russia. Am J Obstet Gynecol 2008;198(2):183–183.

79. Zabina H, Kissin D, Pervysheva E, Mytil A, Dudchenko O, Jamieson D, Hillis S. Abandonment of infants by HIV-positive women in Russia and prevention measures. Reprod Health Matters. 2009 May;17(33):162–170.

80. Fomina M Yu, Voronin EE. Neurological aspects at children with a perinatal HIV-infection. Zn Infectologii 2010;1(2):18–27. [Article in Russian]

81. State of the narcological service and the main trends of registered morbidity in the Russian Federation in 2006, National Scientific Addiction Centre of the Federal State Agency for Health and Social Development, Statistical Reports, Moscow, 2006

82. Platt L., Sutton A. J., Vickerman P., Koshkina E., Maximova S., Latishevskaya N., Hickman M., Bonell C., Parry J., Rhodes T. Measuring risk of HIV and HCV among injecting drug users in the Russian Federation. Eur J Public Health, Aug 2009; 19: 428 – 433.

83. Niccolai LM, Shcherbakova IS, Toussova OV, Kozlov AP, Heimer R. The Potential for Bridging of HIV Transmission in the Russian Federation: Sex Risk Behaviors and HIV Prevalence among Drug Users (DUs) and their Non-DU Sex Partners. J Urban Health. 2009 Jun 9. [Epub ahead of print] (Vol. 86, No. 1:131–143.)

84. RHRN Annual Report 2007. Russian Harm Reduction Network. Russia. Accessed at http://www.harmreduction.ru/files/otchet_vssv_2007.pdf)

85. Gyarmathy VA, Li N, Tobin KE, Hoffman IF, Sokolov N, Levchenko J, Batluk J, Kozlov AA, Kozlov AP, Latkin CA. Correlates of Unsafe Equipment Sharing among Injecting Drug Users in St. Petersburg, Russia. Eur Addict Res. 2009 Jun 5;15(3):163–170. [Epub ahead of print]

86. Country Progress Report of the Russian Federation on the Implementation of the Declaration of Commitment on HIV/AIDS. Reporting period: January 2006–December 2007. www.unaids.ru/files/documents/en350.pdf

87. Moshkovich GF et al. Prevention of HIV infection and other blood borne infections amongst injecting drug users in Nizhny Novgorod associated with harm reduction. Journal of Microbiology, Epidemiology and Immunobiology. 2000;(4):78–82 [Original in Russian].

88. Rhodes T et al. HIV transmission and HIV prevention associated with injecting drug use in the Russian Federation. Inter J Drug Policy, 2004;15:1–16.

89. Niccolai LM, Shcherbakova IS, Toussova OV, Kozlov AP, Heimer R. The Potential for Bridging of HIV Transmission in the Russian Federation: Sex Risk Behaviors and HIV Prevalence among Drug Users (DUs) and their Non-DU Sex Partners. J Urban Health. 2009 Jun 9. [Epub ahead of print]

90. Russia (2008): HIV/AIDS TRaC Study of Risk, Health-seeking Behaviors, and Their Determinants, Among Men Who Have Sex with Men in Eight Regions of the Russian Federation. Second Round. PSI, 2009.

91. Benotsch EG, Somlai AM, Pinkerton SD, Kelly JA, Ostrovski D, Gore-Felton C, Kozlov AP. Drug use and sexual risk behaviours among female Russian IDUs who exchange sex for money or drugs. Inter J STD AIDS, 2004;15:343–347.

92. Kozlov, A., Shaboltas, A., Toussova, O. HIV incidence and factors associated with HIV acquisition among injections drug users in St. Petersburg, Russia. AIDS 2006;20;901–906.

93. Harm reduction Developments 2008. Countries with Injection-Driven HIV Epidemics. OSI. 2008.

94. Open Health Institute (2006) Harm Reduction Programs in the Civilian and Prison Sectors of the Russian Federation: Assessment of Best Practices. Washington, DC: The World Bank.

95. Lioznov D, Nikolaenko S Gutova L. Stigmatization in HIV-infected patients. International Conference Urbanization and Health. April 7–8, 2010. Kiev, Ukraine.

96. HIV in prison in low-income and middle-income countries. K. Dolan, B. Kite, E. Black, C. Aceijas, G.V. Stimson. Lancet Infect Dis 2007; 7: 32–41

97. Kononec A., Sidorova S. Tuberculosis and HIV in Institutions of Penitentiary System of Russia. 3rd All Russian scientific conference MDR-TB in HIV-infected patients; May 12–13, 2009; Moscow, Russia. p.52-53 http://hivpolicy.ru/upload/File/RelatedFiles/news/3449/bulletin_7_2009.pdf)

98. Morozov A, Fridman AN. HIV testing, prevalence, and risk behaviours among prisoners incarcerated in St. Petersburg, Russia. Proceedings of the XIII International AIDS Conference; July 9–14, 2000; Durban, South Africa. Abstract MoPpC1103)

99. Nikolayev Y. Immunodeficiency virus outbreak registered in Nizhnekamsk colony. April 13 2001; Asian Harm Reduction Network. Accessed February 16, 2009, at: http://www.ahrn.net/index.php?option=content&task=view&id=1308&Itemid=2

100. Transatlantic Partners Against AIDS. On Russian Federation State Financing of Measures to Prevent and Fight HIV/AIDS, 2007–2010. Accessed February 16, 2009 at, http://www.hivpolicy.net/topics/?id=40&page=138.

101. Onischenko G.G. HIV-infection: a Challenge to Humanity. HIV-infection and Immunosuppressive Conditions 2009;1(1):5–9.

102. UNAIDS, 2009. Report on the global AIDS epidemic. Geneva, UNAIDS.

103. Yurin O.G., Kraevsky A.A., Afonina L.Yu., Balaganin V.A. and others. Phosphazid—New Russian-made anti-viral medicine. Epidemiol Infect Dis 2001;1:43–45. [Article in Russian]

104. Galegov GA. Nikavir (phosphazide)—an antiretroviral agent: anti-HIV activity, toxicology, pharmacokinetics and some perspectives of its clinical use. Antibiot Khimioter 2004;49(7):3,5-8. [Article in Russian]

105. UNDP, 2005. Central Asia Human Development Report. Bringing down barriers: Regional cooperation for human development and human security.

106. Turkmenistan: Public Health Remains in Critical Condition. EURASIA INSIGHT, 1/08/10. Accessed April 20, 2010, at http://www.eurasianet.org/departments/insightb/articles/eav010810.shtml.

107. WHO, 2003. European Observatory on Health Care Systems. Health Care in Central Asia, Policy Brief. Accessed April 20, 2010 at, http://www.euro.who.int/document/obs/carbrief120202.pdf.

108. World Bank, 2004. Epidemiologic Surveillance Systems in Eastern Europe and Central Asia: An Overview.

109. Marquez PV, et al., Communicable Diseases: A Perpetual Challenge in Central Asia, Strategy Note. Washington, DC: World Bank, 2006.

110. World Bank, 2004. HIV/AIDS and Tuberculosis in Central Asia. Country Profiles.

111. AIDS Prevention Republic Center. Epidemiological situation for HIV/AIDS in Kazakhstan for December 2009 and by January 1, 2010. Accessed April 20, 2010 at, http://depzdrav.gov.kz/hospitalnews/502190110.

112. Epidemiological Situation in Kyrgyzstan. Accessed February 2, 2010 at, http://www.aids.gov.kg/ru/news/.

113. Lukyanov N.B., Ruziev M.M., Soliev A.A. Epidemiological characteristics of HIV infection in Tadzhikistan. The 3rd Eastern Europe and Central Asia AIDS Conference; October 28–30, 2009; Moscow, Russia. Vol. 1 (pp. 169–170).

114. Central Asia AIDS Control Project, 2009. Regional Strategy on HIV Control in Central Asia for 2009–2015. Accessed April 20, 2010 at, www.caap.info/.

115. World Bank, 2008. Blood Services in Central Asian Health Systems: A Clear and Present Danger of Spreading HIV/AIDS and Other Infectious Diseases.

116. Bayizbekova DA. Monitoring and Estimation of measures on PMTCT and counteraction to HIV/AIDS among children. The 3rd Eastern Europe and Central Asia AIDS Conference; October 28–30, 2009; Moscow, Russia. Vol 1(pp. 53–54).

117. Zkusopov BS, Dooronbekova AZh. Estimation of Coverage and Quality of HIV Testing of IDUs, SW,Prisoners and TB-patients in Central Asian countries. The 3rd Eastern Europe and Central Asia AIDS.Conference; October 28–30, 2009; Moscow, Russia. Vol. 1 (pp. 324–325).

118. IHRA, 2008. The Global State of Harm Reduction 2008. Mapping the response to drug-related HIV and hepatitis C epidemics.

119. HIV Outbreak is Under Control, 12/14/07. Accessed April 20, 2010 at, http://www.shymkent.com/news/detail/1573.

120. Lillis J. Government in Kazakhstan Addresses HIV-infection Scandal. EURASIA INSIGHT, 10/25/06 , Accessed April 20, 2010, at http://www.eurasianet.org/departments/insight/articles/eav102506.shtml.

121. Program of Counteraction to HIV/AIDS in Kazakhstan in 2006–2010. Accessed April 20, 2010 at, http://ru.government.kz/docs/p061216~1.htm.

122. Osh's Physician brings HIV. Accessed April 20, 2010, at http://www.medicall.ru/news/22354.html.

123. Dozen jailed in Uzbekistan in HIV scandal: report. 04/02/10. Accessed April 20, 2010 at, http://www.euronews.net/2010/04/02/dozen-jailed-in-uzbekistan-in-hiv-scandal-report/.

124. Bekieva M. Chimkent Tragedy or About Mass HIV Infected Children in Kazakhstan. 01.11.06. Accessed April 20, 2010 at, http://www.ferghana.ru/article.php?id=4679.

125. Lillis J. Government in Kazakhstan Addresses HIV-infection Scandal. EURASIA INSIGHT, 10/25/06. Accessed April 20, 2010 at, http://www.eurasianet.org/departments/insight/articles/eav102506.shtml.

126. Country Coordinating Mechanism, Republic of Uzbekistan, Proposal Form—Round 7: The Global Fund to Fight AIDS, TB, and Malaria (2007). Accessed March 1, 2007 at, http://www.theglobalfund.org/en/files/apply/call7/notapproved/7UZBH_1601_0_full.pdf .

127. World Bank, 2004. Reversing the Tide: Priorities for HIV/ AIDS Prevention in Central Asia.

128. Dzhalbieva ID, Bozgunchiev M, Esenamanova AT, Akumatova D.I. Estimation of Substitution Therapy on the Mental Health of HIV-infected IDUs in Prisons. The 3rd Eastern Europe and Central Asia AIDS Conference; October 28–30, 2009; Moscow, Russia. Vol. 1 (pp. 133–134).

129. Petrenko II, Mosunova NA, Davletgalieva TI, Surtaeva SK. Implementation of Pilot Opioid-Substitute Therapy Program in Kazakhstan. The 3rd Eastern Europe and Central Asia AIDS Conference; October 28–30, 2009; Moscow, Russia. Vol. 1 (pp. 139–140).

130. Najibullah F. Tajik Mullahs Enlisted To Battle HIV/AIDS. 10/18/08 Accessed April 20, 2010 at, http://www.rferl.org/content/Tajik_Mullahs_Battle_HIV_AIDS/1330898.html.

131. Niaytbekov Sh., Meymanaliev T.S., Seytalieva Ch.T. The Role of Islam in forming cultural wealth and involving religion leadersof Central Asia in counteraction to HIV/AIDS The 3rd Eastern Europe and Central Asia AIDS Conference; October 28–30, 2009; Moscow, Russia. Vol. 1 (p. 344).

Chapter 37 AIDS IN ASIA AND THE PACIFIC

YING-RU LO,* THI THANH THUY NGUYEN,*

PADMINI SRIKANTIAH, JEAN-LOUIS EXCLER,

MASSIMO GHIDINELLI,* AND JAI P. NARAIN*

Your beliefs become your thoughts.
Your thoughts become your words.
Your words become your actions.
Your actions become your habits.
Your habits become your values.
Your values become your destiny.

—MAHATMA GANDHI

Introduction

The first AIDS cases in Asia and the Pacific were reported from Thailand and China in 1984 and 1985, respectively.[1-3] Twenty-five years into the global HIV epidemic, the Asia–Pacific region with an estimated 4.6 million persons living with HIV/AIDS in 2008, bears the second-highest burden in the world.[4] More than 95% of HIV infections are found in nine countries: Cambodia, China, India, Indonesia, Myanmar, Nepal, Papua New Guinea, Thailand, and Vietnam. The overall HIV prevalence in Asia and the Pacific remains low, at 0.1% to 0.3% in the South-East Asia and Western Pacific Regions compared with sub-Saharan Africa, where the prevalence is 4.9% in adults above the age of 15 years.[4] However, due to the large population in Asia and the Pacific (India and China account for 62% of the total population of 4.166 billion in Asia and the Pacific in 2010[5]), even a low HIV prevalence translates into a large number of people living with HIV.

The HIV epidemic in this densely populated region is characterized by wide variations in epidemiologic pattern, both by geographic area and subpopulation. Several factors contribute to the wide variation in pattern, but four of the most important ones are: (1) variations in behavioral factors, (2) differences in biological factors, (3) the timing of introduction of HIV into populations with high-risk behavior, and (4) the level of response targeting those populations.[1,6]

In most countries, cross-sectional and sentinel surveillance data suggest that the predominant modes of HIV transmission are through unprotected sex and through needle-sharing among injecting drug users (IDUs) (**Figure 37–1**). HIV prevalence remains highest among populations most at risk for acquiring

---

The author is a staff member of the World Health Organization. The author alone is responsible for the views expressed in this publication and they do not necessarily represent the decisions or policies of the World Health Orcanization.

Abbreviations Used

- ART—antiretroviral therapy
- ARV—antiretroviral
- EWI—early warning indicator
- Global Fund—Global Fund to fight AIDS, Tuberculosis and Malaria
- HIV-DR—HIV drug resistance
- IDU—injecting-drug user
- MSM—men who have sex with men
- NGO—nongovernmental organization
- OST—opioid substitution therapy
- PITC—provider-initiated testing and counseling
- PMTCT—prevention of mother-to-child transmission (of HIV)
- STI—sexually transmitted infection
- TB—tuberculosis
- UNAIDS—Joint United Nations Programme on HIV/AIDS
- UNODC—United Nations Office on Drugs and Crime
- WHO—World Health Organization

HIV, such as people who inject drugs, female sex workers and their clients and, increasingly, men who have sex with men (MSM), male sex workers and transgender people.

Overall, the HIV epidemic in Asia and the Pacific is still rampant, and several countries including Indonesia, Papua New Guinea, and the Philippines, have recently recorded growing HIV epidemics.[1,7–9] In a number of countries, such as Indonesia and Thailand, HIV has spread to lower-risk populations.[1,7,10] However, in Asia, it is unlikely that the HIV epidemic will be sustained in the general population, as is the case in a number of countries in sub-Saharan Africa.[11]

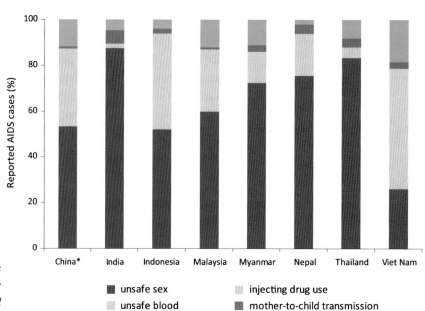

Figure 37–1. *Distribution of reported AIDS cases by mode of transmission in selected Asian countries in 2008.*

Epidemiology of HIV in Asia and the Pacific

History of the HIV Epidemic

The patterns of the HIV epidemics in the Asia–Pacific region are diverse and are evolving over time, although the pattern of transmission has been similar. In most countries, MSM and IDUs were the first populations infected with HIV, followed by spread among female sex workers and transmission to their male clients.[1,6] In Thailand, injecting drug use and commercial sex work contributed to the largest proportion of new infections, and then gradually increased among MSM (**Figure 37–2**).[12] In Asia, most women with HIV were infected by their sexual partner. The HIV epidemic in children reflects HIV infection in women as the final link in the chain of transmission.

The HIV epidemic in Papua New Guinea is emerging and, in 2008, the HIV prevalence was 1.5% among the general population.[8,13,14] This is of great concern in the Pacific region. Among the smaller island nations of the Pacific, the vast majority of HIV infections are found in New Caledonia, Fiji, French Polynesia, and Guam.[4,8]

Populations Most at Risk for Acquiring HIV

The features of the HIV epidemic in most-at-risk populations are complex, reflecting the socio-cultural environment from which they originate. As the behaviors of these populations are highly stigmatized and illegal, periodic and regular surveys may be biased and usually underestimate the HIV prevalence. In addition, the definitions for these different populations and means to

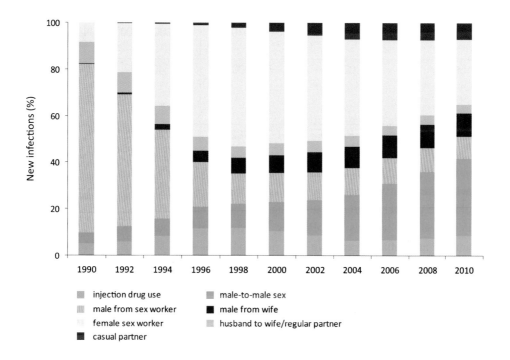

Figure 37–2. *Estimated new HIV infections by mode of transmission, Thailand, 1990–2010.*

TABLE 37–1	Estimated Size of High-Risk Populations in Selected Countries, Asia, and the Pacific (2003–2008)			
Country	Number of female sex workers (range or point estimate)	Number of men who have sex with men (range or point estimate)	Number of injecting drug users (range or point estimate)	[a,b,c]Data sources (year)
Bangladesh	60 000–90 000	40 000–150 000	20 000–40 000	Ministry of Health (2004)
Cambodia	34,000[a]	1,400–8,300[b]	2,000[c]	[a]Ministry of Health (2009) [b]Family Health International (2008) [c]National Authority for Drug Control (2008)
China	2 800,000–4,500,000[a]	1,070,000[b]	1,800,000–2,900,000[a]	[a]Ministry of Health (2005) [b]UN Theme group (2007)
India	800,000–1,200,000	2,500,000	106,000–223,000	National AIDS Control Programme (2006)
Indonesia	221,000	766,000	220,000	Ministry of Health, Indonesia (2008)
Malaysia	40,000–60,000[a]	5,000[b]	104,000–135,000[a]	[a]Ministry of Health (2008) [b]Malaysian AIDS Council (2008)
Myanmar	60,000	240,000	75,000	Ministry of Health (2008)
Nepal	31,000	135,000	28,000	Ministry of Health and Population (2007)
Philippines	128,000–156,000	203,000–610,000	7,000–14,000	National AIDS Council (2007)
Thailand	145,000	560,000	40,000	The Asian Epidemic Model Projections for HIV/AIDS in Thailand, 2005–2025 (2008)
Vietnam	29,000–87,000	161,000–482,000	111,000–274,000	Ministry of Health (2009)

reach representative samples differ among countries. In contrast, data on the extent of spread within the general population are easier to obtain, although this is insufficient in settings where HIV prevalence remains concentrated in most-at-risk populations. Nevertheless, several Asian countries are gathering reliable data on population size estimates (**Table 37–1**), prevalence of HIV, and risk behaviors among most-at-risk populations.[1,6]

Female Sex Workers. Sex work in Asia is classified as *direct* (open, formal), or *indirect* (hidden, informal).[15] Direct sex work is brothel- and street-based, whereas indirect sex work takes place mostly in entertainment establishments such as karaoke bars and massage parlors. The size of female sex worker populations (15–49 years of age) varies within and across countries (**Table 37–1**), from 0.2% to 2.6%.[16] Within countries, the proportion and number of female sex workers is generally higher in areas with a high demand for sexual services, such as major urban areas, ports, and mining and border areas.[1] The duration of sex work is 2 years or less in surveyed Thai female sex workers, and 3 to 5 years among female sex workers in selected sites in Myanmar.[17,18] The median age of female sex workers ranges from the mid-20s and 30 years: Thailand, 30 years[17]; Nepal, 26.5 years[19]; Myanmar (Yangon) 24 years and Myanmar (Mandalay), 23 years.[18] In Cambodia, 55% of female sex workers surveyed were 15–24 years of age[20] and in Vietnam, 48% of street-based sex workers and 64% of sex workers in karaoke bars were less than 30 years of age.[21]

The highest HIV prevalence is reported from Myanmar where all five sentinel HIV surveillance sites reported an HIV prevalence of more than 15%.[22] In India, out of 125 sites, 55 had an HIV prevalence of less than 1% and, in 17 sites, it was above 10%. Large cities such as Mumbai and Pune have recorded an HIV prevalence of more than 30%.[23] HIV prevalence among female sex workers varies widely, and is generally higher among direct sex workers than among indirect sex workers. For example, in Indonesia, HIV prevalence varied from 6% to 16% in direct sex workers, whereas it ranged from 1.6% to 9% in indirect sex workers.[7] In Vietnam, more than 10% of sex workers were HIV-infected in five out of seven provinces. However, the highest HIV prevalence was among indirect sex workers in Can Tho (29%) and Hanoi (23%), coupled with high levels of injecting drug use.[24] In Thailand, HIV prevalence among female sex workers has declined dramatically over the years (**Figure 37–3**).[10] Similar trends have been documented in Cambodia[25] and in the southern states of India.[23] In contrast, HIV prevalence among female sex workers is increasing in some countries. Sentinel surveillance data from China show that HIV

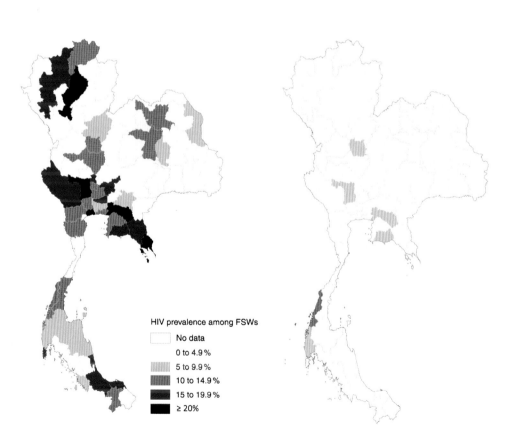

Figure 37–3. *Comparison of HIV prevalence among female sex workers, by district, Thailand (1998 vs 2008).*

prevalence among female sex workers increased from 0.02% in 1995 to 0.3% in 2007.[26] In most of the provinces, HIV prevalence remains 1% or less, but in a few settings in severely affected provinces, the prevalence has exceeded 3%.

A high turnover of sex workers is associated with an increased risk of HIV and other sexually transmitted infections (STIs). For example, in Cambodia, 60% of the sex workers surveyed were new to sex work (≤12 months).[20] The constant renewal of the population of female sex workers, who are at highest risk for acquiring and transmitting HIV to their sexual partners, highlights the importance of sustained targeted prevention programs.[1]

Injecting-Drug Users (IDUs). Historically, HIV prevalence among IDUs in Asia has been among the highest in the world.[27] HIV prevalence among IDUs remains uncontrolled in most countries. In Asia, HIV prevalence among IDUs varies widely, from 0% in the Maldives to more than 50% in Indonesia.[1] Countries in Asia with the highest concentration of IDUs include Cambodia, China, most states of India, Indonesia, Malaysia, Myanmar, Nepal, Thailand, and Vietnam.[3,26,27] China and India have the largest estimated populations of IDUs in Asia (**Table 37–1**).[1,3,27,28] Wide variations in HIV prevalence are observed within countries; this is particularly pronounced in large countries such as China, Indonesia, and India. For example, in India, HIV prevalence ranged from 0% to 30% in 50 sentinel sites across 23 states; it varies between 0.01% among adult males in the south to around 4% in the northeast region bordering Myanmar and China.[27,29] In China, the largest concentration of IDUs is found in the southern provinces.[3,26] Similar geographic variations are reported in smaller countries such as Myanmar, where HIV prevalence among IDUs ranged from 13% in Taunggyi to 55% in Myitkyina.[27]

In Asia, a high proportion of people who inject drugs share injecting equipment (**Figure 37–4**). In Bangladesh, more than 70% of IDUs share injecting equipment.[30] China, India, Indonesia, Myanmar, the Philippines, and Vietnam also report a high proportion of needle–syringe sharing[3,27] with variations within countries (**Figure 37–4**). In Bangladesh, HIV prevalence among IDUs was relatively low, at 7.1% in 2007, despite high levels of sharing of injecting

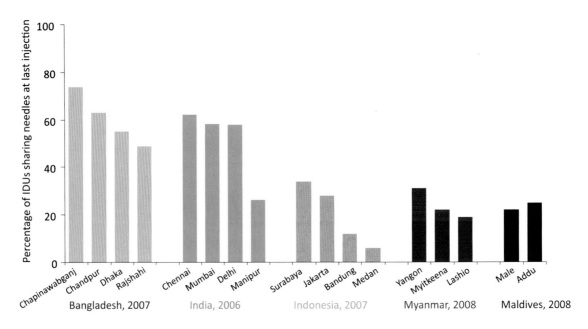

Figure 37–4. *Percentage of injecting drug users sharing injecting equipment at last injection, selected cities, 2006–2008*

equipment.[31] Several factors may have contributed to this observation, including limited sexual transmission due to the high prevalence of male circumcision, declining rates of syphilis, small size of sharing networks, and patterns of drug use that limit HIV transmission.[1] In Kathmandu, Nepal, sharing of injecting equipment decreased from 46% to 7%[19] and in Manipur from 55% to 26%,[23] largely due to early implementation of large-scale harm-reduction programs, including provision of clean injecting equipment.

The overlap between networks of drug users and sex workers is less well studied. In Vietnam, HIV infection among sex workers was highly correlated with injecting drug use; injecting sex workers were 3.5 to 31 times more likely to be HIV infected than are noninjectors. Among street-based sex workers in Hai Phong, only 3% of sex workers without a history of injecting were HIV infected compared with 55% of those who ever injected.[24] Data from 2006 to 2008 from selected cities in Asia show that large numbers of IDUs buy sex and that most of them do not use condoms (**Figure 37–5**).[1] The proportion of IDUs who bought sex during the past year from a female sex worker varied within and across countries.[1] In Bangladesh, the proportion of IDUs who visited a female sex worker varied from 46% to 66%, and only 14% to 43% used a condom.[30]

Amphetamine-Type Stimulants. Amphetamine and polydrug use are on the rise in several countries in Asia and is increasingly being linked to the risk for HIV transmission.[32] Methamphetamine and amphetamine are reportedly the most common amphetamine-type stimulants used globally. The crystalline formulation can be injected. HIV prevalence among injectors of amphetamine-type stimulants is poorly documented, and data are lacking to determine an association between high-risk sexual behavior among users of amphetamine-type stimulants and increased risk for HIV infection.[32]

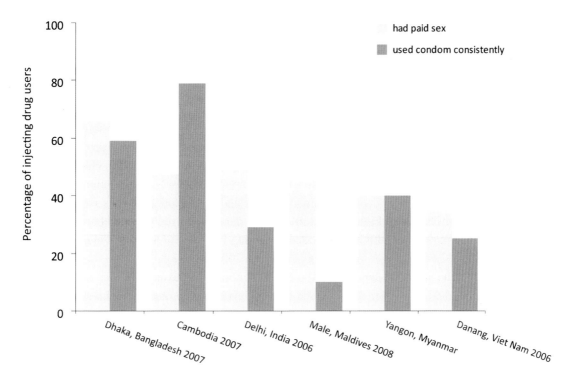

Figure 37–5. *Percentage of injecting drug users engaging in unsafe sexual behaviors in the past year, selected cities, 2006–2008*

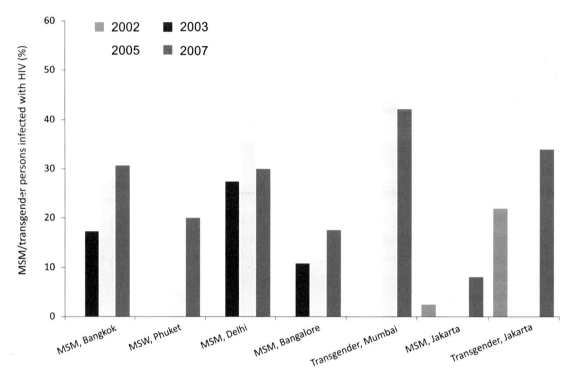

Figure 37–6. *Trends in HIV prevalence among men who have sex with men and transgender persons in selected cities in Asia (2002–2007)*

Men Who Have Sex With Men (MSM) and Transgender Populations. The estimated population size of MSM varies considerably between countries (**Table 37–1**). The estimated prevalence of male-to-male sex in Southeast Asia is 4%, and in South Asia, 7%–8%.[33] An increasing number of studies report that a significant proportion of MSM have heterosexual sex and are married. In Southeast Asia, lifetime prevalence of heterosexual sex among MSM ranged between 25% and 61%; between 3% and 13% were married.[34]

Between 2000 and 2009, the number of countries reporting data on HIV infection and other STIs among these populations has increased. These include Bangladesh,[31] Cambodia,[35] China,[26,35] India,[23] Indonesia,[36] Japan,[37] Lao PDR,[38] Myanmar,[22] Nepal,[1] Philippines,[37] Singapore,[37] Republic of Korea,[37] Thailand,[39–41] and Vietnam.[1,24,42] Four countries recorded an HIV prevalence of more than 20% among MSM and transgender persons (India, Indonesia, Myanmar, and Thailand) (**Figure 37–6**). In-country data show wide variation between sites, populations, and over time, with HIV prevalence ranging from 0% to 5.8% in China between 2001 and 2006 and 2.6% to 14.4% in Cambodia between 2000 and 2005.[37]

In Asia, the high prevalence of HIV infection within male sexual networks and among transgender individuals is further compounded by high levels of unprotected anal sex, large numbers of sexual partners, buying and selling sex, and significant levels of sexual contact with females. These constitute ideal conditions for accelerating the spread of HIV and other STIs, both within populations of MSM and to the general population.[1]

Limited data are available on HIV incidence among MSM. A 6-month prospective cohort study in Nanjing, China showed an HIV incidence of 5.12 per 100 person-years (PY) among MSM. Risk factors predictive of HIV acquisition were male sex >20 years, recruiting male sex partners mostly at saunas, positive diagnosis of syphilis at baseline, and having multiple male sex partners during the past six months.[43] In Thailand, the HIV incidence was 5.7/100 PY in a cohort of MSM in Bangkok, and 2.7/100 PY among MSM attending an HIV testing and counseling clinic.[39,41]

Survey reports indicate that HIV prevalence is higher among transgender populations than among MSM. Alarmingly high levels of 42% were reported from Mumbai in 2007, six times higher than among MSM (8.4%).[25] In Indonesia, HIV infection among transgender populations was four to seven times higher than among MSM: 14% and 2% in Bandung, 25% and 5.6% in Surabaya; 34% and 8.1% in Jakarta, respectively.[7] Available data indicate a high prevalence of bacterial and viral STIs among MSM and transgender populations, which are important cofactors for HIV transmission.[1]

HIV in Prison and Other Closed Settings. Prisoners are particularly vulnerable to HIV infection.[44] As HIV is often concentrated in prisons and other closed settings, incarcerated populations may also play an important role in the dynamics of HIV epidemics. Upon release, the majority of prisoners return to the cities and towns they came from. Resumption of risk behaviors such as unprotected sex and drug injecting shortly after release from prison is common. HIV-infected prisoners who are unaware of their HIV status can transmit HIV to their sexual partners and those with whom they share injecting equipment.[44]

Data from India, Indonesia, and Thailand illustrate that HIV prevalence in prison is between 2 and 15 times higher than that in the general population, suggesting that HIV may be transmitted in prison.[44] HIV risk behaviors, such as injecting drug use, having sex, and tattooing, are common in prisons. About 30%–50% of all inmates with a history of injecting drug use continue to inject in prison. Data on other risk behaviors in prison in the region are limited. It is known that both consensual and coerced homosexual or heterosexual activity occurs in prisons. Tattooing and penile modification are reportedly common in Indonesia and Thailand.[44]

HIV in Women and Children

Globally, women account for 50% of the total number of people living with HIV. The proportion of women living with HIV in Asia is much lower but has been steadily increasing, from 19% in 2000 to 35% in 2008.[4] In Thailand, the proportion of women among reported cumulative AIDS cases increased from 14% in 1990 to 39% in 2008.[45] In China, in 2008, nearly 30% of adults living with HIV were women. An increasing proportion of new HIV infections in Thailand is being observed among low-risk women infected by their husbands or regular male partners. Similar trends are observed in China and Indonesia (17%).[1,26] In 2008, an estimated 161,000 children (range 87,000–243,000, <15 years of age) were living with HIV in Asia and the Pacific.[4]

Tuberculosis/HIV Coinfection

The World Health Organization (WHO) estimates that of the 9.4 million incident tuberculosis (TB) cases globally, an estimated 1.2–1.6 million are HIV infected. Of these, 13% are in Southeast Asia alone. Overall, five countries in Asia with the highest HIV burden also have a high HIV prevalence among new TB cases: Thailand (17%), Cambodia (15%), Myanmar (11%), India (6.7%), and Vietnam (3.7%).[46] The mortality among HIV-positive active TB cases is high.[47] HIV prevalence trends among TB patients mirrors trends in the general population. In Cambodia, HIV prevalence among the general population fell to an estimated 0.8% among the adult

countries in the Pacific do not consider same-sex behavior as a criminal offence (personal communication Shivananda Khan, APCOM; Dominique Ricard, WHO Lao; Narantuya Jadambaa, WHO Mongolia; Pengfei Zao, WHO Vietnam). In India, the Delhi High Court in 2009 ruled that sex between two consenting same-sex adults should not be considered criminal behavior.[1,66,67] In 2008, Nepal issued a bill recognizing transgender persons as a *third* gender.[1,68]

In most countries, interventions for MSM and transgender persons are implemented through NGOs. The key interventions are peer outreach, promotion and distribution of condoms and water-based lubricants, and referral to HIV testing and STI screening and treatment.[69] Major progress has been made in India where comprehensive operational guidelines have been developed for implementing HIV prevention interventions among MSM. As of March 2009, 129 targeted interventions were in place exclusively for MSM, of which 37 are managed by community-based organizations.[1,69] Most countries in Asia have implemented some interventions but coverage remains low.[1]

HIV Testing and Counseling

In Asia and the Pacific, limited data are available on population-based coverage of HIV testing. A few surveys indicate that the proportion of the adult population who have been tested and counseled is low. However, this does not indicate what proportion of people most in need of testing is actually receiving this service.[1]

HIV testing and counseling for pregnant women is the single and only entry point to interventions for PMTCT of HIV. Yet, WHO guidance for provider-initiated HIV testing and counseling (PITC) during antenatal care, labor and delivery, and postpartum remains ambiguous for countries with low and concentrated HIV epidemics.[70] With the exception of Malaysia and Thailand, where policies for routine recommendation of HIV testing have been implemented in antenatal care services, access of pregnant women to PMTCT in Asia and Pacific has historically been very low.[1] Reported rates of HIV testing among pregnant women increased from 4% in 2004 to 8% in 2007, which are among the lowest in the world.[1,65] An increase was reported in 2008 in Southeast Asia, with coverage of up to 13% of pregnant women attending antenatal care services, and this could be due to adoption of the PITC approach in addition to the classical client-initiated approach.[1]

WHO recommends provider-initiated HIV testing for all new active TB cases and the administration of ART for those who test HIV positive.[71,72] HIV testing and counseling is the single and only gateway for HIV-positive new TB cases to access ART early to reduce the current high death rates among HIV-positive TB patients.[47,73] Cambodia, India, and Thailand have made progress in scaling up PITC for active TB cases. In Cambodia, 39% of notified TB cases had been tested for HIV; of those tested, 21% were HIV-positive, but fewer than 20% of them received ART.[48] Based on reports received from nine states in India in 2009, the proportion of TB patients with known HIV status increased from 34% to 62%.[74] Of those tested for HIV, 12% had an HIV-positive test result. In Thailand, HIV testing and counseling among TB patients had increased from 52% in 2006 to 79% in 2008.[1,75]

In all countries of Asia and the Pacific, policy guidelines mention that HIV testing and counseling should be targeted at high-risk populations as part of a comprehensive package of interventions for the prevention and treatment of HIV and other STIs. Overall, the proportion of sex workers, IDUs, and MSM receiving an HIV test in the past 12 months was 30%, 28%, and 23%, respectively, with few intercountry variations. Data on the proportion of people who tested HIV-positive and accessed HIV care, support, and treatment services are not available.[1]

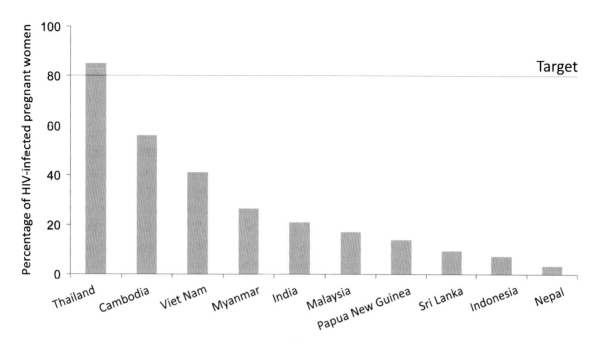

Figure 37–9. *Percentage of pregnant women with access to antiretroviral prophylaxis, Asia, 2008.*

Prevention of Mother-to-Child Transmission of HIV

Prevention of mother-to-child transmission of HIV is one of the most powerful HIV prevention measures. It combines prevention with care and treatment for both the mother and the child. Clinical trials and additional data suggest that treating pregnant women with a CD4 count at or below 350 cells/mm^3 could prevent at least 75% of all mother-to-child transmission, while also providing the best available treatment for the mother's health.[76] A growing number of countries have now developed and implemented national PMTCT plans. However, the overall progress in implementing comprehensive interventions for PMTCT in Asia–Pacific has been slow and constrained by several factors, including limited coverage of antenatal care and delay in introduction of PITC. Antenatal and postpartum care services are often not equipped and trained to provide HIV treatment and care and, hence, fail to test all pregnant women and infants for HIV, stage their disease when HIV infected, and provide prophylactic ARVs or ART.[65] In addition, infrastructural issues, such as lack of access to clean water, limit infant-feeding options for many women.[77]

Although the provision of any ARV for HIV-infected pregnant women has increased over the past few years, only 25% of all cases in East and Southeast Asia could be reached and benefit from ARVs in 2008.[65] Regional statistics indicate that single-dose ARV regimens continue to be the most commonly used in Asia–Pacific, although country-by-country disaggregated data are limited. Coverage with ARV prophylaxis of infants born to mothers living with HIV in East and Southeast Asia increased from 16% in 2007 to 25% in 2008, falling below the average coverage rate of 32% for all low- and middle-income countries worldwide.[65] Wide variations in coverage are observed between countries (**Figure 37–9**). In Thailand in 2008, almost 100% of the 781,898 pregnant women who delivered in the public sector received HIV testing and counseling and 95% of the 6,085 with a positive HIV test result received ARVs.[1] However, larger countries face major challenges. Notable progress has been recorded in India, which bears the highest number of pregnant women needing ARVs in Asia. In 2008, 4.2 million pregnant women were tested at 4,817 government facilities. However, only 51% of mother–baby pairs of pregnant women who tested positive for HIV received any ARV prophylaxis, indicating a high loss to follow-up after HIV testing.[1] In 2010, the National AIDS Control Organization plans to move to more effective multidrug ARV prophylaxis, as recommended by WHO in 2009.[1]

In many countries, use of ANC services remains suboptimal, especially among marginalized population groups. These populations have high rates of deliveries at home, making the full implementation of PMTCT services rather problematic. Key challenges in implementing ARV prophylaxis include developing strategies to test pregnant women for HIV in ares with low and concentrated epidemics, identifying mechanisms to reduce losses to follow-up between HIV testing and counseling, and care during the antenatal, labor/delivery, and postpartum periods. These difficulties are further complicated by the vertical nature of most public health programs, including those for HIV and maternal and child health, whereby referrals for and follow-up of pregnant mothers and newborns across different services become challenging, often resulting in high dropout rates.[1]

WHO's new recommendations released in November 2009 on the use of ARVs for treating HIV-infected pregnant women and preventing HIV infection in infants emphasize the scale-up of quality programs globally, including in countries with limited resources. These new recommendations have great potential for improving the mother's own health and reducing the risk of MTCT to 5% or lower, from a background transmission risk of 35% (in the absence of any interventions and with continued breastfeeding). This would allow countries to eliminate pediatric HIV. Combined with improved infant feeding practices, the recommendations can help to reduce both child mortality and new HIV infections.[78] Implementation of the new guidelines will require a paradigm shift in promoting the continuity of services for mother and child across services for maternal, newborn, and child health, and for HIV treatment.

Antiretroviral Therapy

Thailand was among the first countries in Asia to start ART in public health facilities. Cambodia and China started soon after, but the majority of treatment scale-up in Asia–Pacific countries has taken place since 2004. From 2003 to 2008, the number of people receiving ART increased from an estimated 67,000 HIV-infected persons across the nine countries with the highest HIV burden in the Asia–Pacific region to over 500,000 (**Figure 37–10**).[65,79] This expansion in treatment access has been accompanied by significant improvements in survival and decreases in morbidity among persons accessing care.[80–82] Analyses of national program data from six countries indicate an overall 12-month survival rate of 79% (65%–82%), which is similar to the rates of survival in other resource-limited settings.[65]

The extent of coverage with ART varies widely across Asian countries. Cambodia and Thailand are approaching universal access, and nearly 80% of persons who require therapy currently receive it. In Cambodia, ART services are now available at 91% of the 56 district referral hospitals.[65] Since 2006, ART services in Thailand have been integrated into the government's universal healthcare coverage scheme, and ART is now available at 95% of the 1,066 hospitals designated for the provision of ART across Thailand's 1,057 districts. An estimated 179,557 HIV-infected persons were receiving treatment, representing 71% of those in need as of 2008.[1] In other countries, ART programs continue to expand, with treatment coverage ranging from 13% to 40% of those in need of it.[1,65]

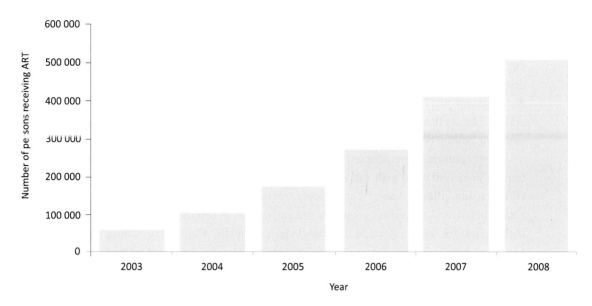

Figure 37–10. *Scale up of antiretroviral therapy in the Asia–Pacific Region, 2003–2008.*

The success of ART programs in Asia–Pacific have largely been the result of strong national efforts coupled with high commitment from the government, civil society and advocacy groups, NGOs and donor agencies, and the global WHO 3 by 5 Initiative. Key challenges to scaling up remain and need to be addressed, including: identifying and linking HIV-infected persons to care earlier in the course of disease to prevent early mortality; access to treatment for difficult-to-reach and most-at-risk population groups; implementing appropriate measures to support treatment adherence and preventing loss to follow up; and strengthening health systems to monitor program progress and support the effective long-term decentralization of HIV treatment services. Continued advocacy and research for affordable and better tolerated drugs, as well low-cost strategies to monitor treatment response, are also essential elements to ensure the long-term success of ART in Asia and the Pacific.[1,65]

Strategic Information

Strategic information is the data and knowledge required to inform policy-making, program development, and adjustment. This information is of critical importance for advocacy and resource mobilization, targeting interventions at the most affected populations and areas, monitoring progress toward planned program objectives, as well as measuring the impact of interventions, and accountability to donors, policy makers, and the civil society. The key components of HIV strategic information include the following:

- Surveillance for HIV, STIs, and risk behaviors
- Surveillance for HIV drug resistance (HIV-DR)
- Program monitoring and evaluation
- Research.

Surveillance for HIV, STIs, and Risk Behaviors

Systematic collection of data on biological and behavioral indicators is the basis for estimating the burden of HIV/AIDS and for monitoring the impact of the national response to the epidemic.[83–87] Facility-based sentinel surveillance surveys among different population groups are the mainstay of HIV serologic data collection, while community-based surveys are needed to collect data on risk behaviors. In "concentrated" epidemics, it is most important to conduct surveillance among populations engaging in high-risk behaviors.[1,88]

Most countries have adopted and implemented the WHO/UNAIDS-initiated second generation HIV surveillance, with variations in terms of periodicity, methodology, and sustainability. HIV serosurveillance surveys are widely conducted. Repeat rounds of HIV serosurveillance and/or behavioral surveillance surveys are carried out at sentinel sites in selected populations at higher risk for HIV infection in Bangladesh, Bhutan, Cambodia, China, India, Indonesia, Maldives, Mongolia, Myanmar, Nepal, the Philippines, Sri Lanka, Thailand, Timor-Leste, and Vietnam. Cambodia, India, Myanmar, Papua New Guinea, and Thailand also have introduced HIV serosurveillance surveys among pregnant women attending antenatal care services, male military recruits, and youth.[1] India, Indonesia, Malaysia, Nepal, the Philippines, and Vietnam have conducted integrated biological and behavioral surveys. Sampling methodologies, such as respondent-driven sampling, have been successfully used to reach high-risk populations in some countries.[1] Unfortunately, routine reporting of HIV/AIDS and STI cases is generally poor or nonexistent in most countries, with the notable exception of China, Maldives, Malaysia, Sri Lanka, and Thailand. Issues of quality have been raised, such as incompleteness, inaccuracy, and duplication of data. Information on HIV incidence is generally lacking. Thailand is the only country that conducts regular, laboratory-based surveillance for HIV incidence among female sex workers and pregnant women attending antenatal care services.[1]

Several countries have proceeded with estimation and projections of HIV population size. The lack of availability of a reliable size of high-risk populations remains a major data gap, and a barrier to effective planning and delivery of services for these populations. National AIDS programs are taking greater ownership of the process and producing national estimates of people living with HIV including of various most-at-risk populations. In recent years, capacity has increased at the national level for using HIV estimate and projection tools published by WHO and UNAIDS.[1,89] In Cambodia, Indonesia, and Thailand, HIV estimates and projections were made using the Asian Epidemic model.[90]

Implementation of Surveillance and Prevention Activities for HIV Drug Resistance

Because of the occurrence of mutations during HIV replication, the chronic nature of HIV infection, and the need for lifelong treatment, the development of HIV-DR is inevitable in populations receiving ART. Several Asian countries have adapted the WHO global strategy for HIV-DR to their local context.[91] Key elements of this strategy include the implementation of systematic surveys to assess the prevalence of transmitted and acquired HIV-DR, and the collection and analysis of program-based "early warning indicators" (EWIs) that provide information on preventable HIV-DR.

Surveillance and monitoring protocols for HIV-DR have been developed in selected countries, including Cambodia, China, India, Indonesia, Malaysia, Myanmar, Papua New Guinea, Thailand, and Vietnam.[92] Surveys to evaluate transmitted HIV-DR among recently infected individuals have been implemented in selected populations in several countries, including blood donors in Thailand, clients attending HIV testing and counseling services in Vietnam and India, and IDUs in Indonesia. In surveyed Asia–Pacific countries, the detected prevalence of transmitted HIV-DR is below 5%.[91] Surveys to assess the development of acquired HIV-DR among persons receiving first-line ART have been implemented in India and Indonesia; analysis of the results is under way. At present, nine national reference laboratories are accredited by WHO for HIV-DR testing in the Asia–Pacific region, which support the implementation of surveillance activities. Finally, the collection and analyses of EWIs has been piloted in several countries, including China, Cambodia, Papua New Guinea, Vietnam, and Indonesia, and will be expanded to India and Myanmar in 2010. In each setting, these indicators, which include prescribing practices, appointment-keeping, and continuity of drug supply, reflect the quality of first-line HIV treatment services. Evaluation of these factors at both the site and national levels can serve to guide the development of program-based interventions to improve treatment services to prevent HIV-DR, and maximize the benefits of affordable first-line ART to those in need.

Program Monitoring and Evaluation

An efficient monitoring and evaluation system is the cornerstone of measuring a country's progress in providing universal access to prevention, care, and treatment services, and achieving the Millennium Development Goals (that is, to "halt and reverse the spread of HIV" by 2015). An increasing number of countries are annually reporting progress on the health sector response toward the global goal of universal access to prevention, treatment, and care.[1,65] Monitoring of interventions focuses on priority health sector interventions, such as HIV testing and counseling, PMTCT, prevention and treatment of HIV and other STIs for most-at-risk populations, health care, and ART. However, linking monitoring and evaluation to the planning and implementation of program interventions at the country level remains suboptimal.[1]

Research

Identifying and conducting priority translational and operational research to improve public health programs and practices should be an integral part of any HIV/AIDS control program. The results of research should be disseminated as quickly as possible and used to improve local programs and policies. Many Asian countries benefit from sophisticated infrastructures and strong capacity to conduct HIV research on molecular epidemiology, epidemiologic and behavioral studies in different populations, ART, microbicides, pre-exposure prophylaxis with ARVs, HIV-DR, and more sophisticated research such as HIV vaccines. For example, Thailand has been a pioneer in this area, with several studies demonstrating the effectiveness of ARVs for PMTCT, leading to the revision of global WHO recommendations on the use of ARVs for PMTCT in low- and middle-income countries.[93–96] Thailand, India, China, Australia, and Japan are actively involved in the clinical development of an HIV vaccine.[97–102] Several countries (Malaysia, Thailand, Indonesia) have conducted research studies on OST for drug users.[64,103,104] Major epidemiologic and behavioral studies are being conducted among MSM, flagging the need to target the growing and often hidden epidemic among this group.[42] Research collaborations and networks, such as the HIV Netherlands Australia Thailand Research Collaboration founded in 1996 in Bangkok, were among the first to build local research capacity in low- and middle-income countries in Asia, and in conducting HIV prevention and treatment research. TREAT Asia (Therapeutics Research, Education, and AIDS Training in Asia), a network of clinics, hospitals, and research institutions working with civil society to ensure the safe and effective delivery of treatment for HIV throughout Asia and the Pacific, was launched in 2001. TREAT Asia seeks to strengthen capacity for HIV research through education and training programs developed by experts in the region. Such support provides a unique opportunity for countries to develop their research infrastructure and expertise, while undertaking studies that are relevant to the country and the region. Similarly, AVAN (AIDS Vaccine Asian Network) is a regional collaborative network for AIDS vaccine development.[105] Long-term investments combined with a collaborative spirit between groups and countries have strengthened the capacity of research institutions and trained a new generation of young researchers at the national and regional levels to undertake high-quality research.

National Strategic Planning and Resource Allocation

Over the past decade, most countries in Asia have prepared national strategic plans for a multisectoral response to the HIV epidemic. The development of such plans, usually for a duration of 5 years, as well as the monitoring and reporting of their implementation, fall under the responsibility of an overarching national authority on AIDS, or a national AIDS council/commission with representatives from various ministries, civil society, and development partners. In most Asian countries, the Ministry of Health chairs this multisectoral body, highlighting the paramount role that the health sector continues to play in national responses to the HIV epidemic.[106–108] In line with the overall strategic plan, each sector would develop specific plans, including that of the National AIDS Program of the Ministry of Health.[1,109]

National strategic plans on HIV/AIDS, as part of the national health plans, have become increasingly ambitious in their goals and targets. Scaling-up of interventions has thus far been supported by substantive allocation of resources, mainly from development partners, but also from national budgets. However, regional investments in the health sector—HIV being no exception—as a percentage of gross domestic product is lower for Asia than for any other region in the world. In low- and middle-income countries across the region, the Global Fund to fight AIDS, TB and Malaria (Global Fund) has emerged as the main financing mechanism throughout the nine rounds of grant proposal and funding implemented since the its establishment in 2002. Between 2002 and December 2009, 23 low- and middle-income countries in Asia have received more than $1 billion USD to support HIV interventions, of which one-third was in 2009 alone.[110] Asia is second to Sub-Saharan Africa in terms of investments for HIV responses. The heavy reliance on external funding is documented by the proportion of patients receiving ART through Global Fund resources, which, on a regional average, is about two-thirds, but reaches almost 100% in some low-income countries.[110] However, similar proportions are applicable, with little variation, to virtually all HIV-related activities, including prevention efforts, especially those for population groups at high risk for HIV infection. Although external funding has been critical in providing the economic backbone of public health efforts to curb the HIV epidemic in Asia and in enhancing the participation of civil society, increased commitment of public resources is clearly needed to address the issue of long-term sustainability.

Conclusion

The HIV epidemic in Asia and the Pacific is characterized by wide variation in epidemiologic patterns, both by geographic area and subpopulation, coupled with evolving modes of transmission. Typically, HIV prevalence remains highest among populations most at risk for acquisition of HIV, such as people who inject drugs, sex workers and their clients and, increasingly, MSM. Even in areas with declining HIV epidemics, pockets of high transmission remain and new epidemics are arising among new population groups even before existing epidemics have been controlled. Countries that have shown commitment at the highest level of the Ministry of Health and the government to issuing policies towards universal coverage of interventions—such as the 100% condom program approach, PITC, PMTCT, and ART—have been successful in averting new HIV infections and decreasing morbidity and mortality due to HIV. However, because of limited coverage, interventions for IDUs, MSM, and transgender persons have not been as successful. Early recognition of the importance of linking prevention, care, and treatment, promoting a continuum of care for people living with HIV, early engagement of civil society, and strengthening strategic information systems in many countries are key factors for successful HIV control in the Asia–Pacific region.

Acknowledgments

This chapter is based on the publication *HIV/AIDS in the South-East Asia Region*, New Delhi, India, World Health Organization Regional Office for South-East Asia (2009) available at http://www.searo.who.int/LinkFiles/Publications_HIV_AIDS_Report2009.pdf. We thank the WHO Regional Offices for South-East Asia and Western Pacific Regions for providing the latest HIV surveillance and programme data from Member States. We acknowledge Renu Garg, MD, MPH, for providing the data, figures and references from the publication *HIV/AIDS in the South-East Asia Region* (2009), Thi Thanh Thuy Nguyen MD, MSc, for providing the data and figures from the Western Pacific Region (2009), and Bandana Malhotra, DVD, for editing the chapter.

References

1. WHO. HIV/AIDS in the South-East Asia Region. New Delhi, India: World Health Organization Regional Office for South-East Asia; 2009. Accessed 19 March 2010 at, http://www.searo.who.int/LinkFiles/Publications_HIV_AIDS_Report2009.pdf

2. Phanuphak P, Locharernkul C, Panmuong W, Wilde H. A report of three cases of AIDS in Thailand. Asian Pac J Allergy Immunol 1985;3:195–199.

3. Mesquita F, Jacka D, Ricard D, et al. Accelerating harm reduction interventions to confront the HIV epidemic in the Western Pacific and Asia: the role of WHO (WPRO). Harm Reduct J 2008;5:26. Accessed 23 April 2010 at, http://www.harmreductionjournal.com/content/5/1/26.

4. UNAIDS, WHO. AIDS epidemic update 2009. Geneva, Switzerland: UNAIDS; 2009. Accessed 23 April 2010 at, http://data.unaids.org/pub/Report/2009/JC1700_Epi_Update_2009_en.pdf.

5. United Nations, Department of Economic and Social Affairs, Population Division (2008). World Population Prospects: The 2008 revision. Accessed 19 March 2010 a,t http://esa.un.org/unpp/index.asp?panel=2

6. Ruxrungtham K, Brown T, Phanuphak P, Ruxrungtham K, Brown T, Phanuphak P. HIV/AIDS in Asia. Lancet 2004;364:69–82.

7. Department of Health (DepKes), Statistics Indonesia (BPS), US Agency for International Development (USAID), National AIDS Commission (KPA), Family Health International – Aksi Stop AIDS (ASA). Integrated biological–behavioral surveillance (IBBS) among most-at-risk groups (MARG), Indonesia. Surveillance highlights: Female sex workers. Jakarta, Indonesia: Ministry of Health Indonesia; 2007. Accessed 30 March 2010 at, http://www.aidsindonesia.or.id/wp-content/plugins/downloads-manager/upload/IBBSHighlightsFSW2007-eng.pdf.

8. Commission on AIDS in the Pacific. Turning the tide: an open strategy for a response to AIDS in the Pacific: report of the Commission on AIDS in the Pacific—Suva, Fiji UNAIDS Pacific Region. Bangkok, Thailand: Commission on AIDS in the Pacific; 2009. Accessed 30 March 2010 at, http://data.unaids.org/pub/Report/2009/20091202_pacificcommission_en.pdf.

9. UNAIDS, WHO, UNICEF. Country profile Philippines. Accessed 19 March 2010 at, http://www.aidsdatahub.org/files/country_reviews/philippines_country_review.pdf.

10. HIV sentinel surveillance. Thailand: Ministry of Health; 2008.

11. De Cock KM, De Lay P. HIV/AIDS estimates and the quest for universal access. Lancet 2008;371:2068–70.

12. Family Health International and Bureau of AIDS, TB and STIs. The Asian Epidemic Model. Projections for HIV/AIDS in Thailand: 2005–2025. Bangkok, Thailand: Ministry of Public Health Thailand; 2008.

13. UNAIDS, WHO, UNICEF. Epidemiological Fact Sheet on HIV and AIDS: Papua New Guinea. Geneva, Switzerland: UNAIDS; 2008 update.

14. Sladden T. Twenty years of HIV surveillance in the Pacific—what do the data tell us and what do we still need to know? Pac Health Dialog 2005;12:23–37.

15. WHO. Toolkit for monitoring and evaluation of interventions for sex workers. New Delhi, India: World Health Organization Regional Offices for South-East Asia and the Western Pacific; 2009. Accessed on 16 November 2010 at, http://www.searo.who.int/LinkFiles/Publications ToolKitMandE.pdf.

16. Vandepitte J, Lyerla R, Dallabetta G, et al. Estimates of the number of female sex workers in different regions of the world. Sex Transm Infect 2006;82 (Suppl 3):iii18–25.

17. Bureau of Epidemiology, Ministry of Public Health Thailand. Behavior surveillance survey 2008. Bangkok, Thailand: Ministry of Health Thailand, 2008.

18. National AIDS Programme. Behavioral surveillance survey: injecting drug users and female sex workers. Naypidaw, Myanmar: Department of Health, Ministry of Health Myanmar; 2008. Accessed 30 March 2010, at, http://www.whomyanmar.org/LinkFiles/HIVAIDS_IDU_and_FSW.pdf

19. FHI. Integrated biological and behavioral surveillance survey (IBBS) among injecting drug users in Kathmandu. Kathmandu, Nepal: Family Health International; 2009.

20. Sopheab H, Morineau G, Neal JJ, Saphonn V, Fylkesnes K. Sustained high prevalence of sexually transmitted infections among female sex workers in Cambodia: high turnover seriously challenges the 100% Condom Use Programme. BMC Infect Dis 2008;8:167.

21. WHO. Targeted HIV prevention for injecting drug users and sex workers. Viet Nam's first large-scale national harm reduction initiative. Hanoi, Vietnam: WHO; 2009.

22. National AIDS Programme. Report of the HIV sentinel sero-surveillance survey. Naypyidaw, Myanmar: Ministry of Health; 2009.

23. National AIDS Control Organization. HIV sentinel surveillance report. New Delhi, India: Ministry of Health and Family Welfare; 2008.

24. Results from the HIV/STI integrated biological and behavioral surveillance (IBBS) in Vietnam, 2005–2006. Vietnam: Ministry of Health; 2007. Accessed 19 March 2010 at, http://www.fhi.org/nr/rdonlyres/etpiez3jktbiyvwcnx6upuefj7kqefygm4b5h5dplftlbyrgxhfnsakq24y3aymclczypl4cdn6cxj/vietnamibbs2006englishhv.pdf.

25. National Center for HIV/AIDS, Dermatology and STD Cambodia. Report of a consensus workshop. HIV estimates and projections for Cambodia 2006–2012. Phnom Penh, Cambodia: National Center for HIV/AIDS, Dermatology and STD, Ministry of Health Cambodia; 2007.

26. State Council AIDS Working Committee Office and UN theme group on AIDS. A joint assessment of HIV/AIDS prevention, treatment and care in China (2007). Accessed 19 March 2010 at, http://www.unaids.org.cn/uploadfiles/20080725151739.pdf.

27. Sharma M, Oppenheimer E, Saidel T, Loo V, Garg R. A situation update on HIV epidemics among people who inject drugs and national responses in South-East Asia Region. AIDS 2009;23:1405–13.

28. Mathers BM, Degenhardt L, Phillips B, et al.; 2007 Reference Group to the UN on HIV and Injecting Drug Use. Global epidemiology of injecting drug use and HIV among people who inject drugs: a systematic review. Lancet 2008;372:1733–45.

29. National AIDS Control Organization. Report of the Expert Group on size estimation of populations with high-risk behaviour for NACP-III Planning. The National AIDS Control Programme-Phase III (2006–2011). New Delhi, India: Ministry of Health and Family Welfare; 2006.

30. National AIDS/STD Programme. Behavioural surveillance survey: technical report 2006–2007. Dhaka, Bangladesh: Directorate General of Health Services, Ministry of Health and Family Welfare; 2008.

31. National AIDS/STD Programme. Sentinel surveillance, 2007. Dhaka, Bangladesh: Ministry of Health; 2007.

32. Degenhardt L, Mathers B, Guarinieri M, et al.; the Reference Group to the United Nations on HIV and Injecting Drug Use. Meth/amphetamine use and associated HIV: Implications for global policy and public health. Int J Drug Policy 2010 Sep;21:347–358.

33. Cáceres C, Konda K, Pecheny M, Chatterjee A, Lyerla R. Estimating the number of men who have sex with men in low and middle income countries. Sex Transm Infect 2006; 82 (Suppl 3):iii3–9.

34. Cáceres CF, Konda K, Segura ER, Lyerla R. Epidemiology of male same-sex behaviour and associated sexual health indicators in low- and middle-income countries: 2003-2007 estimates. Sex Transm Infect 2008;84 (Suppl 1):i49–i56.

35. de Lind van Wijngaarden JW, Brown T, Girault P, Sarkar S, van Griensven F. The epidemiology of human immunodeficiency virus infection, sexually transmitted infections, and associated risk behaviors among men who have sex with men in the Mekong Subregion and China: implications for policy and programming. Sex Transm Dis 2009;36:319–24.

36. Integrated biological-behavioral surveillance (IBBS) among most-at-risk-groups (MARG), Indonesia. Surveillance highlights: Female sex workers. Jakarta, Indonesia: Ministry of Health; 2007.

37. WHO. Health sector response to HIV/AIDS among men who have sex with men. Report of a consultation. Manila, Philippines. WHO Regional Office for the Western Pacific Region; 2009. Accessed 30 March at, http://www.wpro.who.int/internet/resources.ashx/HSI/report/MSM+Report+_HOK_Feb2009_for+web.pdf

38. Sheridan S, Phimphachanh C, Chanlivong N, et al. HIV prevalence and risk behaviour among men who have sex with men in Vientiane Capital, Lao People's Democratic Republic, 2007. AIDS 2009;23:409–14.

39. van Griensven F, Thanprasertsuk S, Jammaroeng R, et al. Evidence of a previously undocumented epidemic of HIV infection among men who have sex with men in Bangkok, Thailand. AIDS 2005;19:521–6.

40. van Griensven F, Varangrat A, Wimonsate W, et al. Trends in HIV prevalence, estimated hiv incidence, and risk behavior among men who have sex with men in Bangkok, Thailand, 2003–2007. J Acquir Immune Defic Syndr 2010;53:234–239

41. Ananworanich J, Phanuphak N, South East Asia Research Collaboration with Hawaii 004 Protocol Team, et al. Incidence and characterization of acute HIV-1 infection in a high-risk Thai population. J AIDS 2008;49:151–5.

42. van Griensven F, de Lind van Wijngaarden JW, Baral S, Grulich A. The global epidemic of HIV infection among men who have sex with men. Curr Opin HIV AIDS 2009;4:300–7.

43. Yang H, Hao C, Huan X, et al. HIV incidence and associated factors in a cohort of men who have sex with men in Nanjing, China. Sex Transm Dis 2010 Feb 23. [Epub ahead of print] Accessed 30 March 2010 at, http://www.ncbi.nlm.nih.gov/pubmed/20182406

44. WHO. HIV prevention, care and treatment in prisons in South-East Asia. New Delhi, India: World Health Organization, Regional Office for South-East Asia; 2007.

45. Bureau of Epidemiology, Ministry of Public Health Thailand. Annual AIDS case reporting 2008. Bangkok, Thailand: Ministry of Health Thailand, 2008.

46. WHO. Global tuberculosis control: a short update to the 2009 report. Geneva, Switzerland: World Health Organization; 2009. Accessed on 19 March at, http://whqlibdoc.who.int/publications/2009/9789241598866_eng.pdf

47. Atun RA, Lebcir RM, Drobniewski F, McKee M, Coker RJ. High coverage with HAART is required to substantially reduce the number of deaths from tuberculosis: system dynamics simulation. Int J STD AIDS 2007;18:267–273.

48. WHO. Tuberculosis control in the Western Pacific Region: 2009 report. Manila, Philippines: World Health Organization, Regional Office for the Western Pacific; 2009.

49. Raizada N, Chauhan LS, Khera A, et al. HIV seroprevalence among tuberculosis patients in India, 2006–2007. PLoS One 2008;3:e2970.

50. WHO. Priority interventions: HIV/AIDS prevention, treatment and care in the health sector. Geneva, Switzerland: World Health Organization; 2009.

51. De Cock KM, Fowler MG, Mercier L, et al. Prevention of mother-to-child HIV transmission in resource-poor countries: translating research into policy and practice. JAMA 2000;283:1175–1182.

52. WHO. Essential prevention and care interventions for adults and adolescents living with HIV in resource-limited settings. Geneva, Switzerland: World Health Organization; 2008.

53. Commission on AIDS in Asia. Redefining AIDS in Asia, 2008. Delhi, India: Oxford University Press; 2008.

54. Hanenberg RS, Rojanapithayakorn W, Kunasol P, et al. Impact of Thailand's HIV-control programme as indicated by the decline of sexually transmitted diseases. Lancet 1994;344:243–245.

55. WHO. Joint UNFPA/WHO meeting on 100% condom use programme. Manila, Philippines: WHO Regional Office for the Western Pacific; 2006. Accessed 19 March 2010 and available at http://www.wpro.who.int/internet/resources.ashx/HSI/report/MtgRep_UNFPA_WHO_100CUP.pdf.

56. National AIDS Programme. National strategic plan for HIV & AIDS in Myanmar: Progress report. Myanmar: Ministry of Health; 2008.

57. Gangopadhyay DN, Chanda M, Sarkar K, et al. Evaluation of sexually transmitted diseases/human immunodeficiency virus intervention programs for sex workers in Calcutta, India. Sex Transm Dis 2005;32:680–684.

58. Verma R, Shekhar A, Khobragade S, et al. Scale-up and coverage of Avahan: a large-scale HIV-prevention programme among female sex workers and men who have sex with men in four Indian states. Sex Transm Infect 2010;86 (Suppl 1):i76–82. doi:10.1136/sti.2009.039115.

59. Mogasale V, Wi TC, Das A, et al. Quality assurance and quality improvement using supportive supervision in a large-scale STI intervention with sex workers, men who have sex with men/transgenders and injecting-drug users in India. Sex Transm Infect 2010b;86 (Suppl 1):i83–88.doi:10.1136/sti.2009.038364.

showed a prevalence of 7.5%.[23] (The Garífuna is an ethnic group of mixed ancestry who live primarily in Central America, along the Caribbean Coast in Belize, Guatemala, St. Vincent, Nicaragua, and Honduras including the mainland, and on the island of Roatán. There are also diaspora communities of Garinagu in the U.S., particularly in Los Angeles, Miami, New York, and other major cities). Individuals from border areas and mobile populations have a higher risk of acquiring and/or transmitting HIV. In borders cities, the frequent high population growth, intense commerce, drug trafficking, sex tourism, and bidirectional mobility increase the risk of acquiring and transmitting HIV. In Mexico, for example, Tijuana has the highest incidence of HIV after Mexico City. Nearly 50% of MSM in Tijuana and 75% of MSM in San Diego, California, report having male sex partners from across the border.[24] In Paraguay, regions bordering Brazil and Argentina (Alto Paraná, Amambay, and Itapúa), present a higher HIV prevalence after Asunción.[25] Prevalence among incarcerated people was reported as 12% to 17% in different populations in Brazil and 37% in Buenos Aires, Argentina.[26]

Caribbean

At the end of 2008, it was estimated that 240,000 (220,000–260,000) individuals were living with HIV in the Caribbean; of these, 20,000 (16,000–24,000) had new infections. Although these numbers represent a relatively small proportion of the global epidemic, the Caribbean is the most affected region after Sub-Saharan Africa, with an adult HIV prevalence of 1.0% (0.9–1.1%). Three-quarters of the people living with HIV/AIDS (PLWHA) in the Caribbean reside in Haiti and the Dominican Republic.[27] The 2007 estimated HIV prevalence for the 15- to 49-year-old population ranged from 3.3% in the Bahamas, to 2.2% in Haiti, and 1.6% in Jamaica. Cuba has a completely opposite picture, having the lowest HIV prevalence in the Americas (including the U.S. and Canada).[28] The highly questioned isolation policy implemented in Cuba in the first years of the epidemic changed to a comprehensive policy that allowed a successful containment of the epidemic. The policy includes an active promotion of testing (with 6 million inhabitants between 14 and 49 years of age, 1.6 million tests are performed annually), reinforced by systematic investigation of partners (which constitutes the source of 25% of all reported cases), a strong health promotion strategy (including a 6-week educational course for all new patients), and universal coverage for antiretroviral therapy.[29]

The HIV data in the Caribbean should be considered with caution, as HIV surveillance is limited and both HIV prevalence and AIDS cases are thought to be widely underestimated. Most of the local information comes through the Caribbean Epidemiological Center (CAREC), which collects HIV and AIDS data from 11 countries (but not from Haiti). A considerable share (17%) of AIDS cases reported in the Caribbean have no assigned risk category, perhaps because they are reported after death or because of insufficient information about sexual preferences.[30] The primary mode of HIV transmission in CAREC member countries is sexual, with a male-to-female ratio close to 1:1. There is a shift of the epidemic to younger populations, in particular, young females. Available data show that the 20- to 49-year-old group is the most affected by HIV/AIDS, accounting for more than 65% of cases annually. In Haiti, a survey of 10,000 individuals showed HIV prevalence ranging from 1.1% to 3.8% in different districts, with higher prevalence associated with increased age and number of sexual partners (**Figures 38–1 and 38–2**).[31] Here, too, the HIV epidemic is shifting to younger populations, in particular, young women. Norms that tolerate males having multiple concurrent sexual partners, and young women maintaining relationships with older men, are among the factors underlying these findings.

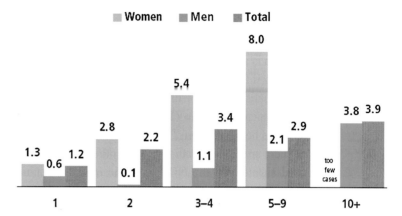

Figure 38–1. *HIV prevalence in Haiti, 2005–2006, by number of lifetime sexual partners.*

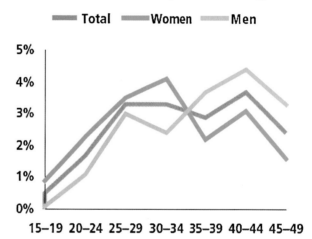

Figure 38–2. *HIV prevalence in Haiti, 2005–2006, by sex and age.*

Compared with previous years, the number of new infections seems to have stabilized and even decreased in countries such as the Dominican Republic and Haiti. It is challenging to determine the exact cause of the reduction in new HIV infections, as behavioral data in the region are scarce. The efficacy of preventive interventions reported by the Dominican Republic, such as increased condom use and a reduction in the number of sexual partners among men, could have an impact on the decrease in HIV prevalence.[32] In Haiti, the HIV rate among pregnant women declined from 6.0% in 1996 and 5.1% in 2000 to 3.4% in 2004. In the Bahamas, HIV rates among pregnant women declined from 4.8% in 1993 to 3.0% in 2002.[33] However, recent surveys among vulnerable populations indicate HIV infection rates continue to be disturbingly high in female sex workers, but also in MSM and drug users. It is uncertain how the recent natural catastrophe in Haiti will affect the overall health care system and, in particular, the already weak HIV program, but it seems that GHESKIO, the main program providing care for PLWHA, is coping with the situation.[34]

HIV rates among commercial sex workers in Jamaica remained stable between 1997 and 2005, at 9%; in the Dominican Republic, HIV rates in 2000 ranged from 4.5% to 12.4%,[35] while surveys carried out in Guyana in 2000[36] and in Surinam in 2004[37] showed HIV prevalence rates as high as 30.6% and 21%, respectively. Sexual work in the Caribbean has had a significant role in HIV transmission in the context of high poverty and unemployment, where young women are particularly at risk. Concurrent drug use worsens the HIV risk due to higher prevalence of unprotected sexual activity with multiple partners, violent victimization, and migration between high and low HIV prevalence areas. Thus, more integral and effective means must be found to reduce HIV infection rates among female sex workers.

There is a paucity of epidemiologic data on HIV among MSM, attributed largely to frequent underreporting as a consequence of the illegality, stigmatization, and discrimination surrounding homosexuality in the Caribbean, but HIV prevalence as high as 33% in Jamaica (2000), 11% in the Dominican Republic (1998), 6.7% in Surinam (2005), and 20.4% in Trinidad and Tobago (2005) has been reported.[38]

There are limited data regarding other populations at high risk. Although crack/cocaine use caused an increase the HIV epidemic in the Bahamas in the 1990s, injection drug use is, at present, rare in most Caribbean countries, with the exception of Bermuda and Puerto Rico. HIV prevalence in patients hospitalized for drug rehabilitation in Jamaica between 1991 and 2003 was 4.6%.[39]

Data from prison inmates shows HIV rates of 6.7% in Jamaica, 4.9% in Trinidad and Tobago, and 25.8% in Cuba.[40] Another study in Belize showed a prevalence of 4%.[41] In 118 homeless individuals from Jamaica, St. Lucia, and Trinidad and Tobago, the self-reported HIV rates were 7%, 12%, and 34%, respectively.[42]

Caribbean life consists of high levels of intraregional mobility and interdependence. Short- and long-term migration is often linked to economic factors and is a major determinant driving the HIV epidemic. Illegal migrants face limited access to health services and increased vulnerability. In the Dominican Republic, the bateyes population (workers on sugar plantations, usually Haitian migrants) is disproportionately affected by HIV.

Mother-to-Child HIV Transmission

With approximately 11 million pregnancies each year, Latin America and the Caribbean report an unacceptably high number of children affected by two highly preventable infections: HIV and syphilis.

As the approach for both infections is fairly similar, the Pan American Health Organization (PAHO) promotes an integrated approach to reduce mother-to-child transmission (MTCT) of HIV and the incidence of congenital syphilis. In collaboration with other UN agencies, PAHO launched in 2008 the Regional Initiative for the Elimination of Mother to Child Transmission of HIV and Congenital Syphilis. The ultimate goal of this initiative is the reduction of HIV to 2% and the reduction of congenital syphilis incidence to 0.5 cases per 1,000 live births by 2015. [43]

However, much work remains to be done. In spite of current preventive interventions available to prevent HIV MTCT, UNAIDS estimated that during 2008, 6,900 (4,200–9,700) and 2,300 (1,400–3,400) newly infected children were born in Latin America and the Caribbean, respectively.[44] During the same period, only 54% of pregnant women had access to HIV testing (19% in 2004) (**Figure 38–3**), and only five countries (Argentina, Belize, Costa Rica, Cuba, and Guyana) tested at least 80% of their pregnant women. Furthermore, among the 32,000 (24,000 to 41,000) mothers living with HIV, as estimated for 2008, 54% (36%–87%) received antiretroviral drugs during pregnancy, a little more than the global figure of 45% but quite far from the >95% reached in developed regions, with only few countries providing >80% of the ARV coverage of pregnant women in need.[45]

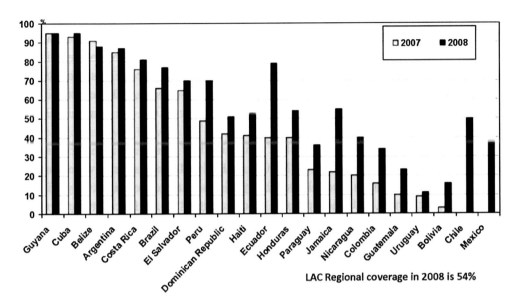

Figure 38–3. *Proportion of pregnant women tested for HIV in LAC, 2007–2008.*[46]

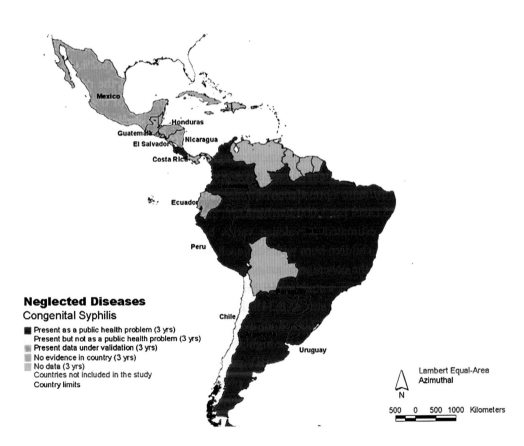

Figure 38–4. *Presence of Congenital Syphilis in the LAC region.*[49]

Part IX

THE FUTURE

the adult population and at very few instances of mother-to-child transmission as exceptions due to special circumstances.

A project named AIDS 2031 has been created to improve and sustain our activities during the coming years leading up to the 50th anniversary after the first report of AIDS (in 1981), to do better than what we have achieved so far. AIDS 2031 was established in 2007 by Peter Piot, executive director of UNAIDS at that time, for the purpose of bringing together experts in HIV/AIDS and related fields to examine the likely trajectory of the pandemic and the response required. We must focus on next generation, both because it is the young people who will bear the brunt as infected and affected by the epidemic they will inherit from us and as those who have to carry the burden of sustained prevention, care, and treatment, as well as the socioeconomic consequences of the pandemic. The recommendations are published in the AIDS 2031 report, *An Agenda for the Future*.

Young people are also carrying our hopes for the future regarding scientific advances. Today, we do not know for sure if it will be possible to develop an efficient vaccine or a cure, but some present-day school children might become the future scientists, succeeding to achieve those goals. In science, one should expect the unexpected.

Background

Epidemiologic Findings

It is difficult to learn the specific prevalence among young people, as the designation "young people" is not well-defined. In the present article, adolescence is defined as the period between childhood and adulthood, corresponding to 12 through 18 years of age.

Globally, young people between 15 and 24 years of age account for 45% of all new HIV infections, according to UNAIDS. However, the burden of adolescence is further increased by the fact that more than 10% are having first sex before age 15[1] and thereby are exposed to the risk of being HIV-infected. In addition, there are many children younger than 15 years of age, particularly in Asia and Eastern Europe, who acquire HIV infection through injecting drug use.

Generalized Epidemics

The burden of HIV infections is unevenly distributed among regions and countries, sub-Saharan Africa being home for 66% of the global total. Almost two-thirds of all young people with HIV live in Sub-Saharan Africa, where around 75% of all infections in young people between 15 and 24 years of age occur among women. The HIV prevalence among young people in southern Africa is considerably higher than in other parts of Africa. For instance, the prevalence among South African youths is two times greater than among Ugandan youth.[2] In 2007, The HIV prevalence among pregnant women in rural South Africa was 37.5% in the age group 20–24 years, and 13.7 among those under 20 years of age.

There is a great discrepancy between the HIV prevalence of boys and girls 15–24 years of age. Girls may have more than six times higher prevalence compared to same-age boys in the group 15–19 years old,[3] although the magnitude differs between years and locations; thus, three times higher is more often cited.[4,5] In general, women with male sexual partners 5 years older or more are several times more likely to become HIV-infected than are women with same-age partners.

A study from Tanzania showed that girls who became sexually active before the age of 16 have higher HIV prevalence (8%) than those who delayed sex until they were 20 years of age or older.[6] In South Africa, the proportion of girls having sex before 15 years of age rose fro 5.3 to 5.9%.[7] The same report found that the age of sexual partners 5 years older than themselves rose from 18.5% in 2005 to 27.6% in 2008. In Lesotho, the male partner was 5 years older or more in 53% and more than 10 years older in 19%.[8] The relationship between early coital debut (e.g., before age 15) and associated HIV risk factors, such as partner age differences, forced sex, and lack of condom use, were studied in South Africa.[9]

Recently, the percentage of HIV-infected young pregnant women (15–24 years of age) has been reported to decline in 14 of 17 African countries with adequate survey data.[10] From a scientific point of view, it is unclear if the decline is a result of interventions, spontaneous change of sexual behavior (linked, perhaps, to economic and social development), or due to the natural course of the epidemic; regardless, it is a hopeful sign.

Concentrated Epidemics

In contrast to the generalized epidemics with predominantly heterosexual transmission in the general public, young people in countries with concentrated epidemics are subject to other risks of HIV transmission, namely, through injecting drug use, sex work (including trafficking of young people), and other forms of sexual abuse (as in families and prisons, including pedophilic and pornographic abuse of minors).

A UNICEF study in Ukraine in 2008 revealed that most at-risk adolescents living with HIV were commercial sex workers, men who have sex with men, and injecting drug users. The adolescents were more exposed to HIV infection than were older representatives of such groups, due to lack of knowledge. The majority of teenage female sex workers had provided services for the first time when they were younger than 16 years (the average age was 14 years), for food, clothing, and protection. Many combined commercial sex and injecting drug use. Every tenth boy among those living on the streets has practiced anal sex with a male, often for a reward of money, clothes, or drugs.[11]

HIV infections in young people are reported also from Western countries. For instance, the U.S. Centers for Disease Control and Prevention (CDC) estimated that about 56,000 people 13–24 years of age were living with HIV in the U.S. in 2006, 60% of them being African-Americans.[12]

Behavior and Risk Factors

An analysis of the sexual behavior at the beginning of the 21st century from 59 countries revealed substantial differences in sexual behavior by region and gender.[13] No trend toward earlier debut was found, but a shift to later marriage causing an increase of premarital sex was seen. It is notable that the prevalence of premarital sex was higher in industrialized countries than in developing countries. The prevalence was higher in men than in women. Monogamy is the dominant pattern everywhere, but, having had more than one partner during the past year is more common in men than in women, and is more common in developed countries. Condom use has increased everywhere, but still remains low in many developing countries. The diversity between regions indicated mainly social and economic determinants.

In a multivariate logistic regression analysis of data from Zambia, the lifestyle among sexually active in-school adolescents was studied and the adjusted odds ratios were calculated.[14]

Chapter 40 — DEVELOPMENT OF ANTIVIRAL THERAPEUTICS FOR HIV-1 INFECTION AND AIDS

KENJI MAEDA, DEBANANDA DAS, AND HIROAKI MITSUYA

I believe that the struggle against death, the unconditional and self-willed determination to live, is the mode of power behind the lives and activities of all outstanding men.

—HERMANN HESSE

Introduction

Highly active antiretroviral therapy (HAART) refers to the utilization of a combination of antiretroviral drugs for treatment of HIV-1 infection, and it has made an immense impact on the quality of life and prognosis of HIV-1-inflicted individuals over the last ten years. Indeed, HAART significantly suppresses the replication of HIV-1 and substantially extends the life expectancy of HIV-1-infected individuals.[1–3] Recent analyses have revealed that life expectancy in HIV-1-infected individuals treated with HAART increased between 1996 and 2005, that mortality rates for HIV-1-infected persons have become much closer to general mortality rates since the introduction of HAART, and that first line HAART with boosted protease inhibitor (PI)-based regimens has resulted in less resistance within and across drug classes.[4] However, the ability to provide effective long-term antiretroviral therapy for HIV-1 infection has still remained a complex issue since those who initially achieved favorable viral suppression to undetectable levels have experienced treatment failure.[5–8] In addition, it is evident that, in general, even with the currently available antiretroviral drugs, only partial immunologic reconstitution is attained.

At present, we should say that in regard to the development of new anti-HIV-1 therapeutics, we have faced a variety of challenges different than those encountered during the design of first-line drugs.[9–18] The issue of the emergence of drug-resistant HIV-1 variants is one of the most formidable challenges in the era of HAART. Indeed, it is notable that the very features that contribute to their specificity and antiretroviral activity also provide the virus with a strategy to develop drug resistance[5,19–21]; it seems inevitable that this resistance issue will remain problematic for many years to come. However, a few recently developed PIs, such as darunavir (DRV) and tipranavir (TPV), have been relatively successful in treating individuals carrying multiple-PI-resistant HIV-1 variants.[22,23] Nevertheless, a number of recent studies indicate that cross-resistance is a major obstacle to therapy with all classes of antiretroviral agents.[20,24]

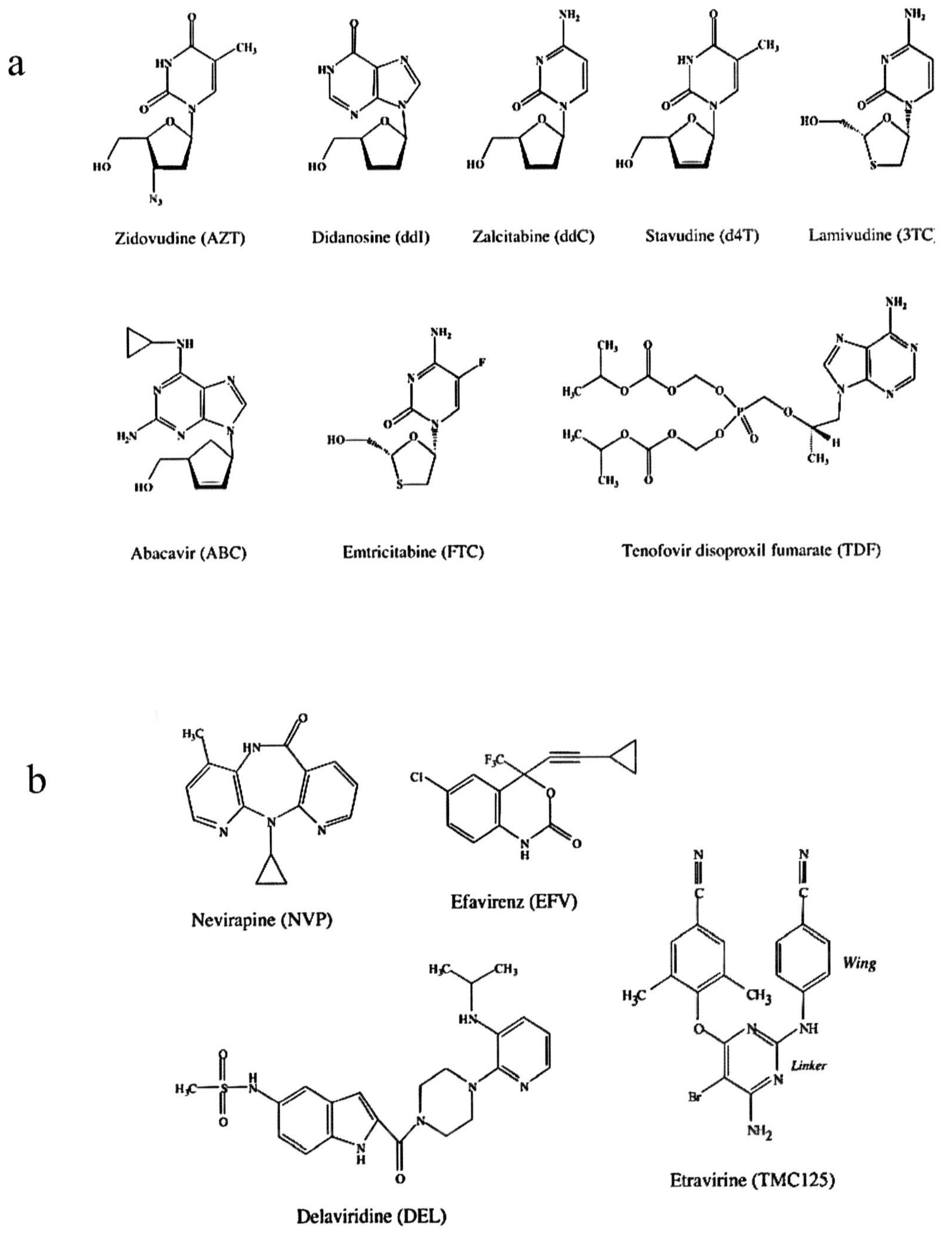

TABLE
40–1

Figure 40–1. *Clinically approved anti-HIV drugs.* (**a**) *nucleoside and nucleotide RT inhibitors;* (**b**) *non-nucleoside RT inhibitors;* (**c**) *protease inhibitors.*

It is notable that during treatment with HAART, inadequate drug concentrations can result from a number of factors, including nonadherence, pharmacokinetics, and lack of drug potency, among others. In addition, anatomic sanctuary sites may exist where drug concentrations do not achieve adequate levels despite apparent therapeutic plasma drug concentrations. HIV-1 replication can occur in such settings, and the selective pressure of antiretroviral therapy leads to the emergence of HIV-1-harboring, drug-resistant mutations. These drug-resistant variants can be generated de novo, but perhaps more commonly arise from the pool of integrated proviruses that

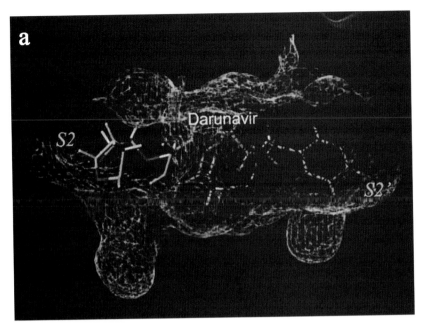

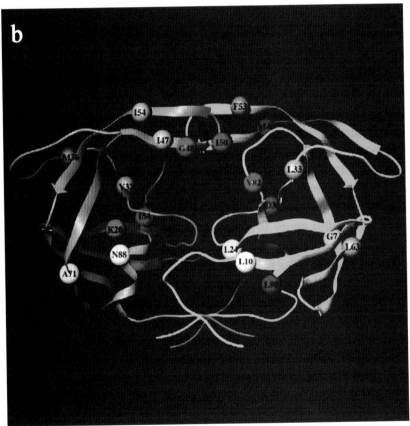

Figure 40–5. *HIV-1 protease.* (**a**) *The hydrophobic cavity within protease with darunavir docked (PDB ID 1S6G). The brown and green regions are lipophilic while the blue regions are hydrophilic (determined using MOLCAD). The S2 and S2' subsites are indicated. This figure was generated using Sybyl 7.0.* (**b**) *Structure of protease homodimer with positions of amino acid residues associated with clinical resistance to current PIs indicated. Primary and secondary mutations are indicated with red and white spheres, respectively. The protease monomers are shown in green and orange ribbons. Mutations are shown on only one monomer for clarity. This figure was generated using Maestro version 7.0.*

PIs may be chemically unique from each other, they occupy a similar space within the protease binding cavity, which explains how individual mutations may cause PI cross-resistance.

Structural analysis of primary mutations has formed the basis for our current understanding of PI resistance at the molecular level. One such mutation is V82A, originally described after selection with ritonavir or indinavir.[123–125] This mutation is capable of conferring HIV-1 resistance to a number of PIs, particularly early-generation compounds. Crystal structures of protease containing V82A complexed with either natural substrates or a PI were compared (these enzymes also contained D25N, a mutation that inactivated the enzyme to prevent cleavage of the substrate but did not appear to affect hydrogen bonding between protease and ligand).[126] V82A results in significant changes in the crystal structures of the protease complexed to PI including changes in the flap position and subsequent disruption of hydrogen bonding as well as the loss of van der Waals interactions between mutant protease and PI.

In contrast, crystal structures between natural substrate peptides complexed to either wild-type protease or V82A mutant protease have not demonstrated significant changes. Molecular interactions between protease and the longer natural substrates consists mainly of extensive backbone-backbone hydrogen bonds as well as more extensive van der Waals interactions.[110,111,126] This suggests that the side chain substitution V82A has little effects on substrate binding, but has a much greater detrimental effect on PI binding. Others have shown that multi-drug-resistant (MDR) protease with mutations at multiple positions (amino acids L10, M36, M46, I54, L63, A71, V82, I84, and L90) has an expanded active site cavity.[127] Again, the binding of PIs to this MDR protease was noticeably different than binding to wild-type protease. Although the crystal structure of this MDR protease with natural substrates was not assessed, this work provides further insight into the structural effects of multiple protease resistance mutations.

Development of Protease Inhibitors Active Against PI-Resistant Variants

To further understand the difference between substrate binding and PI binding to protease, an analysis of the structures of eight different inhibitors complexed to protease has been conducted. King and colleagues[128] demonstrated that, despite the chemical differences of the drugs, all compounds occupied a similar volume within the active site cavity that is termed the "inhibitor envelope". If the inhibitor envelope was compared to the "substrate envelope," the space within the protease that is occupied by a natural substrate, the inhibitors protrude from the substrate envelope in very distinct locations. At these positions, PIs may have van der Waals interactions with amino acid positions such as G48, I50, V82, and I84. It is known that mutations at these residues result in PI primary resistance (**Figure 40–5b**), and therefore these mutations likely disrupt PI and protease molecular associations.

On the other hand, these same mutations have little effects on natural substrates that do not make molecular interactions at these amino acid positions.[128] King et al. have also demonstrated that darunavir (DRV, Prezista®, TMC114) binds approximately 2 orders of magnitude more tightly to the wt enzyme ($Kd : 4.5 \times 10^{-12}$ M) than APV ($Kd : 3.9 \times 10^{-10}$ M). Thus, DRV's potency against multi-drug resistant HIV-1 variants may also be due to a combination of its high affinity and close fit within the substrate envelope.[129] The mutation profile for amprenavir is also different compared to that for other PIs, providing more evidence that PIs that have greater resemblance to natural substrates will be less affected by primary mutations selected by first generation PIs. However, mimicking the shape of protease substrates is only one element in designing effective PIs. Another key element that differentiates substrate binding and PI binding is the significant amount of hydrogen bonding between backbone atoms of substrate and protease that is mostly lacking in protease/PI binding. Because mutations of backbone atoms of proteases cannot occur, disruption of these bonds is more difficult compared to hydrogen bonds that many PIs form between amino acid side chains, which can be affected by substitution mutations. Further development of analogs of amprenavir has successfully exploited these elements and has resulted in certain PIs with significant activity against MDR HIV-1.

Amprenavir contains a tetrahydrofuranyl (THF) urethane moiety that interacts with the S2 region of the protease active site upon drug binding. Replacing THF of amprenavir with a *bis*-THF component led to the synthesis of two PIs, DRV and its prototype TMC126 (**Figure 40–6a**).[130–132] TMC126 differs slightly from amprenavir due to a replacement of 4-aminobenzene-sulfonamide with 4-methoxybenzenesulfonamide which interacts with protease at the S2′ subsite, while darunavir is identical to amprenavir with the exception of the *bis*-THF. Based on analysis of darunavir, the larger *bis*-THF rings of TMC126 and darunavir protrude slightly more from the substrate envelope compared to the THF ring of amprenavir.[129] Despite this, both drugs have increased activity against both wild-type as well as clinical isolates containing multi-PI-resistant mutations.[21,133,134] At least one explanation for this is the improved hydrogen bond stability with the protease backbone conferred by the *bis*-THF ring (**Figure 40–6b**), as mentioned above.[21,129,135] Although the THF ring of amprenavir is able to form hydrogen bonds with the backbone carboxylate oxygen of D30, *bis*-THF has an additional hydrogen bond with the main chain atoms of D29 in the S2 subsite of protease. This extra hydrogen bond may account for a 10-fold increase in activity of TMC126 and DRV against a panel of clinical isolates with various combinations of protease resistance mutations.[21,136] Attempts to design compounds capable of further exploiting these critical interactions with the main-chains of D29 and D30 in the S2 subsite are currently under way.[19,137–140]

It has been reported that, on the opposite side of these same inhibitor molecules, the P2′ substituents such as the 4-aminobenzenesulfonamide found on amprenavir and darunavir or the 4-methoxybenzenesulfonamide of TMC126 also introduce hydrogen bonding with the carboxyl backbone of D30′ in the S2′ subsite (**Figure 40–6b**).[136] Compounds designed to optimize this interaction have also demonstrated good in vitro activity against PI-resistant HIV-1 variants.[141] Maximization of hydrogen bond interactions between the protease backbone and TMC126 or darunavir results in highly favorable enthalpic contributions that drive inhibitor binding. This differs from first-generation PIs (i.e., nelfinavir, saquinavir, and indinavir), which have unfavorable enthalpic interactions with the protease. Binding of these PIs to the protease was entropically driven as a result of the burial of hydrophobic residues of these compounds. Thus, mimicking the backbone hydrogen bonding of natural substrates in at least two separate subsites of the protease has yielded more thermodynamically adaptable PIs capable of overcoming protease resistance conferred by amino acid substitutions.[129,142]

As mentioned above, amprenavir selects for a unique pattern of protease resistance mutations compared to first-generation PIs, and this holds true for the structurally similar TMC126 and darunavir. TMC126 resistance appears to be mediated by a novel mutation, A28S, along with subsequent acquisition of I50V.[133] Although I50V has been demonstrated to confer primary resistance on amprenavir in clinical isolates, A28S has not been described yet as a common protease resistance mutation, likely because of the effect this mutation has on the catalytic efficiency of the protease.[133,143] Computational modeling analysis does not indicate TMC126 has interactions with either the backbone or side group of A28, which suggests that the reduction in potency with TMC126 is due to either steric hindrance caused by the larger serine of A28S, or possibly

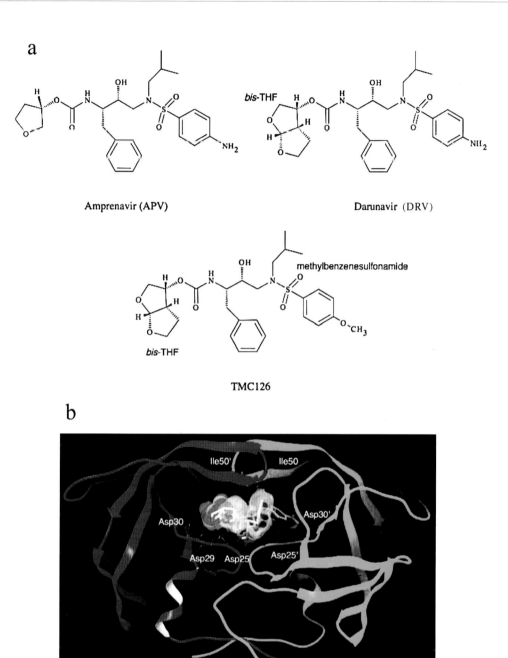

Figure 40–6. *Comparative structures of darunavir (DRV) and its related PIs and interactions with HIV-1 protease.* **(a)** *Structures of amprenavir (APV), DRV, and TMC126.* **(b)** *Structure of HIV-1 protease complexed with DRV. DRV is shown in sticks with the van der Waals force surface. Locations of amino acids (Asp25, Asp29, Asp30, and Ile50 and corresponding amino acids in the other subunit), which form strong hydrogen bond interactions, are also shown.*

due to unfavorable solvation energy effects during binding.[133] Although the pharmacokinetic properties of TMC126 were not suitable for further clinical development, the related compound DRV had significant activity against multi-PI-resistant HIV-1 from clinical isolates and favorable pharmacokinetics.[121,134,144] The FDA granted accelerated approval for DRV in June 2006. The Office of AIDS Research Advisory Council (OARAC), which develops guidelines for the use of antiretroviral agents in HIV-1-infected adults and adolescents, currently recommends DRV as a treatment option for treatment-naïve and treatment-experienced adults and adolescents. Phase III trials demonstrated that antiviral efficacy of DRV combined with RTV is superior to the LPV combined with RTV for first-line therapy.[144] It is noteworthy that DRV is the first drug that did not come with a price increase in the area of antiretroviral drug development.

Despite the chemical similarities of TMC126 and DRV, A28S has yet to be described after DRV selection (Koh and Mitsuya, unpublished data). The reasons for this are unclear at this point. Instead, clinical HIV-1 strains harboring R41T and K70E have been isolated.[134] Isolates harboring these two mutations were found to have eight-fold to ten-fold resistance to DRV, twenty-fold resistance to saquinavir, and six-fold resistance to lopinavir. Otherwise, resistance remained less than four-fold for all other first generation PIs. The molecular mechanisms that allow R41T and K70E to confer darunavir resistance is also currently unknown, as site-directed mutants carrying one or both of these mutations show no reduction in sensitivity to any PI tested.[134] Nonetheless, there appears to be a higher genetic barrier to the emergence of resistance to both TMC126 and darunavir, and both drugs have been shown to maintain potent antiviral activity against multi-PI–resistant strains, suggesting that their unique interactions with HIV-1 protease can provide the framework for developing subsequent generations of PIs.

Inhibition of HIV-1 Protease Dimerization as a New Modality of HIV-1 Intervention

Dimerization of HIV-1 protease subunits is an essential process for the acquisition of the proteolytic activity of HIV-1 protease, which plays a critical role in the maturation and replication of the virus.[145,146] Hence, inhibition of protease dimerization represents a unique target for potential intervention of HIV-1 infection. Two HIV-1 protease monomer subunits (each containing 99 amino acids) are connected by a four-stranded antiparallel beta-sheet involving the *N*- and *C*- termini of both monomer subunits (**Figure 40–7a,b,c**). Therefore, the catalytic activity of the dimerized protease is thought to be abolished by reagents that block protease dimerization. This strategy has been explored by several groups[147,148] who targeted the antiparallel beta-sheet that contributes close to 75% of the dimerization energy.[149]

Koh et al. have recently developed an intermolecular fluorescence resonance energy transfer (FRET)-based HIV-1-expression assay employing cyan and yellow fluorescent protein-tagged protease monomers (**Figure 40–7d**).[150] Using such an assay system, a group of nonpeptidyl small molecule inhibitors of HIV-1 protease dimerization have been identified. These inhibitors, including DRV and TMC-126, blocked protease dimerization at concentrations of as low as 0.01 µM and also blocked HIV-1 replication in vitro with IC_{50} values of 0.0002–0.48 µM. These agents also inhibited the proteolytic activity of mature HIV-1 protease. With the exception of tipranavir, a CCR5 inhibitor and a soluble $CD4^+$ inhibitor, other approved anti-HIV-1 agents failed to block the dimerization event. It is assumed that once protease monomers dimerize to become a mature protease, this dimerization inhibition mechanism does not cause dissociation of protease monomers, suggesting that these agents block dimerization at its nascent stage of protease maturation. The proteolytic activity of the mature protease that managed to undergo dimerization despite the presence of these agents is likely to be inhibited by the same agents acting as conventional PIs. Such a dual-inhibition mechanism should lead to highly potent inhibition of HIV-1 and contribute to the above-mentioned high genetic barrier of DRV against the emergence of resistant HIV-1 variants.

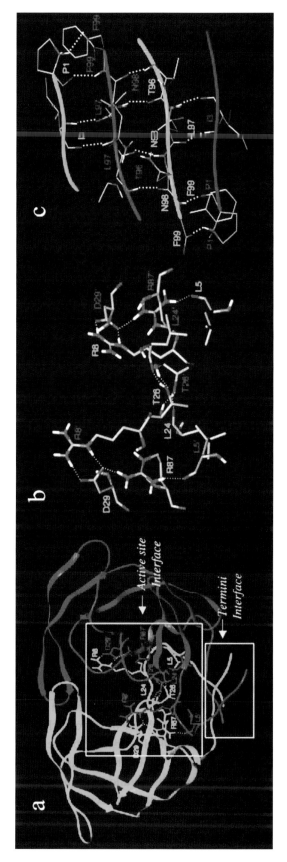

Figure 40–7. *Critical amino acid residues for protease dimerization and inhibition of the dimerization by DRV.* **(a)** *Two interfaces, active site and termini interfaces responsible for protease dimerization. The locations of two interfaces are shown. One monomer is shown in green ribbon while the other monomer in red ribbon.* **(b)** *Active site interface. The inter-molecular hydrogen bond interactions between protease monomers A and B are D29-R8'; R87-L5'; L24-T26'; L24-L5'; R8'-L5'; and T26-T26' are shown. The corresponding amino acids of monomer A also forms hydrogen bonds with monomer B (i.e., R8-D29' etc.). An intra-molecular hydrogen bond interaction between D29 and R87 is shown by white dotted lines. The residues forming critical intermolecular contacts between two monomer subunits are shown by atom color types (C:grey, N:blue, O:red, H:white). The residues of chain A are labeled green and those of chain B are labeled red.* **(c)** *Four stranded antiparallel beta-sheets involving the N- and C- termini of both monomer subunits. Two HIV-1 protease monomer subunits are connected by four stranded antiparallel beta-sheets involving the N- and C- termini of both subunits. Mature dimerized protease has as many as 12 hydrogen bonds in this N- and C-terminal region.* **(d)** *Inhibition of protease dimerization by DRV. COS7 cells were exposed to 1 μM of DRV and subsequently co-transfected with a plasmid encoding HIV-1 tagged with cyan or yellow fluorescent protein. After 72 hours, cultured cells were examined in the FRET-HIV-1 assay system where if CFP$^{A/B}$ ratios are <1.0, there is no FRET, indicating disruption of dimerization, using confocal microscopy Fluoview FV500 confocal laser scanning microscope, and CFP$^{A/B}$ ratios were determined and plotted. The CFP$^{A/B}$ ratio values for PR$_{WT}^{CFP}$/PR$_{WT}^{YFP}$ were 1.19 and 0.78 in the absence and presence of DRV, respectively.[150] Note that all the CFP$^{A/B}$ ratio values were greater than 1.0 except for those of DRV.*

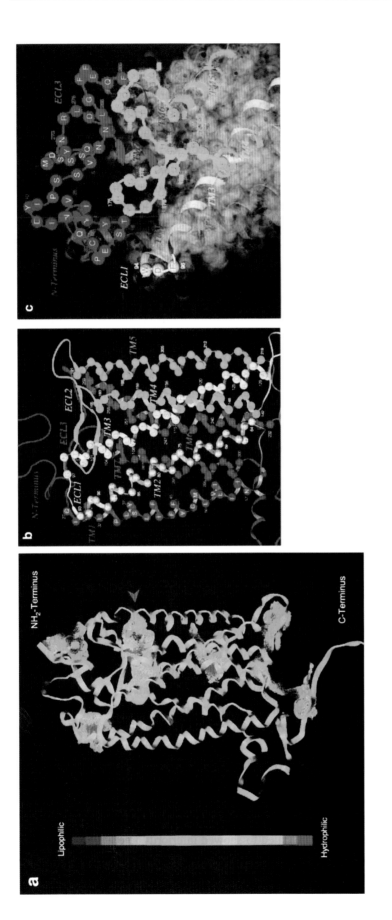

Figure 40–9. (a) *Hydrophobic cavities within CCR5. Six hydrophobic cavities are identified within human CCR5, defined using MOLCAD (Sybyl 7.0). Note the largest hydrophobic cavity (red arrow head) that is likely to accommodate a molecule of the size of reported CCR5 inhibitors[182].* **(b)** *A side-view of the TM domains of CCR5. TM2, TM3, and TM4 are above the plane of the paper, and TM6 and TM7 are below the plane.* **(c)** *A top-view of the extra-cellular loop regions of CCR5. The following assignments have been made for loops: N-terminus, 1 to 26; ECL1, residues 94 to 96; ECL2, residues 166 to 190; ECL3, residues 260 to 278.[183]* **(d)** *Structures of selected CCR5 inhibitors.*

achieved a viral load less than 50 copies/ml which was similar to the efavirenz arm.[191] Maraviroc was approved by the FDA in August 2007 for treatment-experienced people who have HIV-1 strains that are resistant to multiple antiretroviral drugs. It was also approved in November 2009 for individuals with drug-sensitive HIV-1 strains, who initiate HAART including MVC.

CXCR4 Inhibitors

Targeting another chemokine receptor, CXCR4, which HIV-1 exploits for its cellular entry, has proven to be highly challenging. Although proof of concept has been demonstrated in early phases of clinical trials, none of these compounds have proved suitable for chronic administration. AMD3100, which is a bicyclam analog, has potent activity against X4-tropic HIV-1 in vitro, while clinical development as an AIDS drug was abandoned because of the lack of obvious activity in the clinical trial.[192] However, it was found that the AMD3100 had the ability to increase the mobilization of CD34[+] stem cells into the peripheral circulation.[193] AMD3100 has been approved by the FDA as a hematopoietic stem cell mobilizer for transplantation. Another bicyclam analog, AMD070, is a newer CXCR4 inhibitor that is orally bioavailable, but development has been halted because histological abnormality of the liver was seen in the preclinical studies.

Conclusions

The development of antiretroviral therapy for HIV-1 infection and AIDS has witnessed one of the most dramatic progressions in the history of medicine, combining swift drug development, short-lived trends, unprecedented levels and volumes of clinical trial results, and continuous evolution. In 1987, just 4 years following the discovery of the culprit responsible for AIDS, the first antiretroviral drug, AZT, became clinically available. As of this writing, more than 30 drugs (if the combination agents incorporating two or three antiretrovirals are included) have been approved for the treatment of HIV-1 infection and AIDS. Now, every year, guidelines for therapy are revised multiple times by various organizations, including the U.S. Department of Health and Human Services (DHHS), the International AIDS Society–USA Panel, the British HIV Association, and so on. Such frequent and substantial revisions of treatment guidelines have not been seen in any areas of treatment of any other disease in history. Of note, such guidelines at one time asked patients and clinicians to "choose and combine" drugs listed in alphabetical order; however, as can be seen in the most recent *Guidelines for the Use of Antiretroviral Agents in HIV-1-Infected Adults and Adolescents*, released in December 2009, the DHHS Panel strongly recommends using "ready-to-administer mixtures" in far more specific ways.[194,195] For example, the DHHS Panel now classifies treatment regimens as "Preferred," "Alternative," "Acceptable," "Regimens that may be acceptable but more definitive data are needed," and "Regimens to be used with caution." One can say that, within a surprisingly rapid rate, the treatment practice for HIV-1 infection and AIDS has reached such a highly mature stage as the treatment practice of hypertension.

However, as has been the cases with RT and protease inhibitors we have seen over a period of more than 2 decades, we are to encounter a variety of formidable challenges that are different from those we faced in the development and clinical practice of the first antiretroviral drugs. A key element in future drug design strategies will be to generate novel agents—rather than "me-too" drugs—that would work against both wild-type and drug-resistant HIV-1 strains with a new

35. Sarafianos SG, Das K, Hughes SH, Arnold E. Taking aim at a moving target: designing drugs to inhibit drug-resistant HIV-1 reverse transcriptases. Curr Opin Struct Biol 2004;14:716–730.

36. Menéndez-Arias L. Mechanisms of resistance to nucleoside analogue inhibitors of HIV-1 reverse transcriptase. Virus Res 2008;134:124–146.

37. Richman DD. Antiviral drug resistance. Antiviral Res 2006;71:117–121.

38. Sarafianos SG, Marchand B, Das K, Himmel DM, Parniak MA, Hughes SH, Arnold E. Structure and function of HIV-1 reverse transcriptase: molecular mechanisms of polymerization and inhibition. J Mol Biol. 2009;385:693–713.

39. Yin PD, Das D, Mitsuya H. Overcoming HIV drug resistance through rational drug design based on molecular, biochemical, and structural profiles of HIV resistance. Cell Mol Life Sci. 2006;63:1706–1724.

40. Kohlstaedt LA, Wang J, Friedman JM, Rice PA, Steitz TA Crystal structure at 3.5 A resolution of HIV-1 reverse transcriptase complexed with an inhibitor. Science 1992;256:1783–1790.

41. Jacobo-Molina A, Ding J, Nanni RG, Clark Jr. AD, Lu X, Tantillo C, Williams RL, Kamer G, Ferris AL, Clark P, Hizi A, Hughes SH, Arnold E. Crystal structure of human immunodeficiency virus type 1 reverse transcriptase complexed with double-stranded DNA at 3.0 A resolution shows bent DNA. Proc Natl Acad Sci USA 1993;90;6320–6324.

42. Kati WM, Johnson KA, Jerva LF, Anderson KS. Mechanism and fidelity of HIV reverse transcriptase. J Biol Chem 1992;267:25988–25997.

43. Huang H, Chopra R, Verdine GL, Harrison SC. Structure of a covalently trapped catalytic complex of HIV-1 reverse transcriptase: implications for drug resistance. Science 1998;282;1669–1675.

44. Hsieh JC, Zinnen S, Modrich P. Kinetic mechanism of the DNA-dependent DNA polymerase activity of human immunodeficiency virus reverse transcriptase. J Biol Chem 1993;268:24607–24613.

45. Larder BA, Darby G, Richman DD. HIV with reduced sensitivity to zidovudine (AZT) isolated during prolonged therapy. Science 1989;243:1731–1734.

46. Rooke R, Tremblay M, Soudeyns H, DeStephano L, Yao XJ, Fanning M, Montaner JS, O'Shaughnessy M, Gelmon K, Tsoukas C, Gill J, Ruedy J, Wainberg MA, the Canadian Zidovudine Multi-Centre Study Group. Isolation of drug-resistant variants of HIV-1 from patients on long-term zidovudine therapy. Canadian Zidovudine Multi-Centre Study Group. AIDS 1989;3:411–415.

47. Arion D, Kaushik N, McCormick S, Borkow G, Parniak MA. Phenotypic mechanism of HIV-1 resistance to 3'-azido-3'-deoxythymidine (AZT): increased polymerization processivity and enhanced sensitivity to pyrophosphate of the mutant viral reverse transcriptase. Biochemistry 1998;37:15908–15917.

48. Meyer PR, Matsuura SE, So AG, Scott WA. Unblocking of chain-terminated primer by HIV-1 reverse transcriptase through a nucleotide-dependent mechanism. Proc Natl Acad Sci USA 1998;95:13471–13476.

49. Tuske S, Sarafianos SG, Clark Jr AD, Ding J, Naeger LK, White KL, Miller MD, Gibbs CS, Boyer PL, Clark, P, Wang G, Gaffney BL, Jones RA, Jerina DM, Hughes SH, Arnold E. Structures of HIV-1 RT-DNA complexes before and after incorporation of the anti-AIDS drug tenofovir. Nat Struct Mol Biol 2004;11:469–474.

50. Shafer RW, Kozal MJ, Winters MA, Iversen AK, Katzenstein DA, Ragni MV, Meyer 3rd WA, Gupta P, Rasheed S, Coombs R, Katzman M, Fiscus S, Merigan TC. Combination therapy with zidovudine and didanosine selects for drug-resistant human immunodeficiency virus type 1 strains with unique patterns of pol gene mutations. J Infect Dis 1994:169:722–729.

51. Shirasaka T, Yarchoan R, O'Brien MC, Husson RN, Anderson BD, Kojima E, Shimada T, Broder S, Mitsuya H. Changes in drug sensitivity of human immunodeficiency virus type 1 during therapy with azidothymidine, dideoxycytidine, and dideoxyinosine: an in vitro comparative study. Proc Natl Acad Sci USA 1993:90;562–566.

52. Shirasaka T, Kavlick MF, Ueno T, Gao WY, Kojima E, Alcaide ML, Chokekijchai S, Roy BM, Arnold E, Yarchoan R, Mitsuya H. Emergence of human immunodeficiency virus type 1 variants with resistance to multiple dideoxynucleosides in patients receiving therapy with dideoxynucleosides. Proc Natl Acad Sci USA 1995;92:2398–2402.

53. Maeda Y, Venzon DJ, Mitsuya H. Altered drug sensitivity, fitness, and evolution of human immunodeficiency virus type 1 with pol gene mutations conferring multi-dideoxynucleoside resistance. J Infect Dis 1998;177:1207–1213.

54. Ueno T, Shirasaka T, Mitsuya H. Enzymatic characterization of human immunodeficiency virus type 1 reverse transcriptase resistant to multiple 2',3'-dideoxynucleoside 5'-triphosphates. J Biol Chem 1995;270:23605–23611.

55. St Clair MH, Martin JL, Tudor-Williams G, Bach MC, Vavro CL, King DM, Kellam P, Kemp SD, Larder BA. Resistance to ddI and sensitivity to AZT induced by a mutation in HIV-1 reverse transcriptase. Science 1991;253:1557–1559.

56. Boyer PL, Tantillo C, Jacobo-Molina A, Nanni RG, Ding J, Arnold E, Hughes SH. Sensitivity of wild-type human immunodeficiency virus type 1 reverse transcriptase to dideoxynucleotides depends on template length, the sensitivity of drug-resistant mutants does not. Proc Natl Acad Sci USA 1994;91:4882–4886.

57. Harrigan PR, Stone C, Griffin P, Najera I, Bloor S, Kemp S, Tisdale M, Larder B. Resistance profile of the human immunodeficiency virus type 1 reverse transcriptase inhibitor abacavir (1592U89) after monotherapy and combination therapy. CNA2001 Investigative Group. J Infect Dis 2000;181, 912–920.

58. Winters MA, Shafer RW, Jellinger RA, Mamtora G, Gingeras T, Merigan TC. Human immunodeficiency virus type 1 reverse transcriptase genotype and drug susceptibility changes in infected individuals receiving dideoxyinosine monotherapy for 1 to 2 years. Antimicrob Agents Chemother 1997;41;757–762.

59. Schinazi RF, Lloyd Jr RM, Nguyen MH, Cannon DL, McMillan A, Ilksoy N, Chu CK, Liotta DC, Bazmi HZ, Mellors JW. Characterization of human immunodeficiency viruses resistant to oxathiolane-cytosine nucleosides. Antimicrob Agents Chemother 1993;37;875–881.

60. Schuurman R, Nijhuis M, van Leeuwen R, Schipper P, de Jong D, Collis P, Danner SA, Mulder J, Loveday C, Christopherson C, Kwok S, Sninsky J, Boucher CAB. Rapid changes in human immunodeficiency virus type 1 RNA load and appearance of drug-resistant virus populations in persons treated with lamivudine (3TC). J Infect Dis 1995;171;1411–1419.

61. Johnson MS, McClure MA, Feng DF, Gray J, Doolittle RF. Computer analysis of retroviral pol genes: assignment of enzymatic functions to specific sequences and homologies with nonviral enzymes. Proc Natl Acad Sci USA 1986;83;7648–7652.

62. Lacey SF, Reardon JE, Furfine ES, Kunkel TA, Bebenek K, Eckert KA, Kemp SD, Larder BA. Biochemical studies on the reverse transcriptase and RNase H activities from human immunodeficiency virus strains resistant to 3'-azido-3'-deoxythymidine. J Biol Chem 1992;267;15789–15794.

63. Boyer PL, Imamichi T, Sarafianos SG, Arnold E, Hughes SH. Effects of the Delta67 complex of mutations in human immunodeficiency virus type 1 reverse transcriptase on nucleoside analog excision. J Virol 2004;78:9987–9997.

64. Boyer PL, Sarafianos SG, Arnold E, Hughes SH. Selective excision of AZTMP by drug-resistant human immunodeficiency virus reverse transcriptase. J Virol 2001;75:4832–4842.

65. Sarafianos SG, Clark Jr AD, Das K, Tuske S, Birktoft JJ, Ilankumaran P, Ramesha AR, Sayer JM, Jerina DM, Boyer PL, Hughes SH, Arnold E. Structures of HIV-1 reverse transcriptase with pre- and post-translocation AZTMP-terminated DNA. Embo J 2002;21;6614–6624.

66. Larder BA, Bloor S, Kemp SD, Hertogs K, Desmet RL, Miller V, Sturmer M, Staszewski S, Ren J, Stammers DK, Stuart DI, Pauwels R. A family of insertion mutations between codons 67 and 70 of human immunodeficiency virus type 1 reverse transcriptase confer multinucleoside analog resistance. Antimicrob Agents Chemother 1999;43:s1961–1967.

67. Matamoros T, Franco S, Vazquez-Alvarez BM, Mas A, Martinez MA, Menendez-Arias L. Molecular determinants of multi-nucleoside analogue resistance in HIV-1 reverse transcriptases containing a dipeptide insertion in the fingers subdomain: effect of mutations D67N and T215Y on removal of thymidine nucleotide analogues from blocked DNA primers. J Biol Chem 2004;279;s24569–24577.

68. Boyer PL, Sarafianos SG, Arnold E, Hughes SH. Nucleoside analog resistance caused by insertions in the fingers of human immunodeficiency virus type 1 reverse transcriptase involves ATP-mediated excision. J Virol 2002;76;9143–9151.

69. Mas A, Parera M, Briones C, Soriano V, Martinez MA, Doming E, Menendez-Arias L. Role of a dipeptide insertion between codons 69 and 70 of HIV-1 reverse transcriptase in the mechanism of AZT resistance. Embo J 2000;19:5752–5761.

70. Meyer PR, Lennerstrand J, Matsuura SE, Larder BA, Scott WA. Effects of dipeptide insertions between codons 69 and 70 of human immunodeficiency virus type 1 reverse transcriptase on primer unblocking, deoxynucleoside triphosphate inhibition, and DNA chain elongation. J Virol 2003;77:3871–3877.

71. Julias JG, McWilliams MJ, Sarafianos SG, Alvord WG, Arnold E, Hughes SH. Mutation of amino acids in the connection domain of human immunodeficiency virus type 1 reverse transcriptase that contact the template-primer affects RNase H activity. J Virol 2003;77:8548–8554.

72. Julias JG, McWilliams MJ, Sarafianos SG, Arnold E, Hughes SH. Mutations in the RNase H domain of HIV-1 reverse transcriptase affect the initiation of DNA synthesis and the specificity of RNase H cleavage in vivo. Proc Natl Acad Sci USA 2002;99:9515–9520.

73. Shaw-Reid CA, Feuston B, Munshi V, Getty K, Krueger J, Hazuda DJ, Parniak MA, Miller MD, Lewis D. Dissecting the effects of DNA polymerase and ribonuclease H inhibitor combinations on HIV-1 reverse-transcriptase activities. Biochemistry 2005;44;1595–1606.

74. Petropoulos CJ, Parkin NT, Limoli KL, Lie YS, Wrin T, Huang W, Tian H, Smith D, Winslow GA, Capon DJ, Whitcomb JM. A novel phenotypic drug susceptibility assay for human immunodeficiency virus type 1. Antimicrob Agents Chemother 2000;44;920–928.

75. Shafer RW, Hertogs K, Zolopa AR, Warford A, Bloor S, Betts BJ, Merigan TC, Harrigan R, Larder BA. High degree of interlaboratory reproducibility of human immunodeficiency virus type 1 protease and reverse transcriptase sequencing of plasma samples from heavily treated patients. J Clin Microbiol 2001;39:1522–1529.

76. Nikolenko GN, Palmer S, Maldarelli F, Mellors JW, Coffin JM, Pathak VK. Mechanism for nucleoside analog-mediated abrogation of HIV-1 replication: balance between RNase H activity and nucleotide excision. Proc Natl Acad Sci USA 2005;102:2093–2098.

77. Klarmann GJ, Hawkins ME, Le Grice SF. Uncovering the complexities of retroviral ribonuclease H reveals its potential as a therapeutic target. AIDS Rev 2002;4:183–194.

78. Min BS, Miyashiro H, Hattori M. Inhibitory effects of quinones on RNase H activity associated with HIV-1 reverse transcriptase. Phytother Res 2002;16 (Suppl 1):S57–62.

79. Shaw-Reid CA, Munshi V, Graham P, Wolfe A, Witmer M, Danzeisen R, Olsen DB, Carrol SS, Embrey M, Wai JS, Miller MD, Cole JL, Hazuda DJ. Inhibition of HIV-1 ribonuclease H by a novel diketo acid, 4-[5-(benzoylamino)thien-2-yl]-2,4-dioxobutanoic acid. J Biol Chem 2003;278:2777–2780.

80. Sarafianos SG, Das K, Clark Jr AD, Ding J, Boyer PL, Hughes SH, Arnold E. Lamivudine (3TC) resistance in HIV-1 reverse transcriptase involves steric hindrance with beta-branched amino acids. Proc Natl Acad Sci USA 1999;96:10027–10032.

81. Margot NA, Isaacson E, McGowan I, Cheng AK, Schooley RT, Miller MD. Genotypic and phenotypic analyses of HIV-1 in antiretroviral-experienced patients treated with tenofovir DF. AIDS 2002;16;1227–1235.

82. Miller MD. K65R, TAMs and tenofovir. AIDS Rev 2004;6:22–33.

83. Hayakawa H, Kohgo S, Kitano K, Ashida N, Kodama E, Mitsuya H, Ohrui H. Potential of 4′-C-substituted nucleosides for the treatment of HIV-1. Antivir Chem Chemother 2004;15:169–187.

84. Kodama EI, Kohgo S, Kitano K, Machida H, Gatanaga H, Shigeta S, Matsuoka M, Ohrui H, Mitsuya H. 4′-Ethynyl nucleoside analogs: potent inhibitors of multidrug-resistant human immunodeficiency virus variants in vitro. Antimicrob Agents Chemother 2001;45:1539–1546.

85. Kohgo S, Mitsuya H, Ohrui H. Synthesis of the L-enantiomer of 4′-C-ethynyl-2′-deoxycytidine. Biosci Biotechnol Biochem 2001;65:1879–1882.

86. Nakata H, Amano M, Koh Y, Kodama E, Yang G, Bailey CM, Kohgo S, Hayakawa H, Matsuoka M, Anderson KS, Cheng YC, Mitsuya H. Activity against human immunodeficiency virus type 1, intracellular metabolism, and effects on human DNA polymerases of 4′-ethynyl-2-fluoro-2′-deoxyadenosine. Antimicrob Agents Chemother 2007;51:2701–2708.

87. Michailidis E, Bruno Marchand B, Ei-Ichi Kodama E-I, Kamlendra Singh K, Matsuoka M, Ashida N, Kirby K, Ryan EM, Sawani 1 AM, Eva Nagy E, Mitsuya H, Parniak MP, Sarafianos SG. Novel mechanism of inhibition of HIV-1 reverse transcriptase by 4′-ethynyl-2-fluoro-deoxyadenosine triphosphate, a translocation defective reverse transcriptase inhibitor. J. Biol. Chem. 2009;284:35681–35691.

88. de Béthune MP. Non-nucleoside reverse transcriptase inhibitors (NNRTIs), their discovery, development, and use in the treatment of HIV-1 infection: a review of the last 20 years (1989–2009). Antiviral Res 2010;85:75–90.

89. De Clercq E. Anti-HIV drugs: 25 compounds approved within 25 years after the discovery of HIV. Int J Antimicrob Agents 2009;33:307–320.

90. De Clercq E. The role of non-nucleoside reverse transcriptase inhibitors (NNRTIs) in the therapy of HIV-1 infection. Antiviral Res 1998;38:153–179.

91. Esnouf R, Ren J, Ross C, Jones Y, Stammers D, Stuart D. Mechanism of inhibition of HIV-1 reverse transcriptase by non-nucleoside inhibitors. Nat Struct Biol 1995;2:303–308.

92. Spence RA, Kati WM, Anderson KS, Johnson KA. Mechanism of inhibition of HIV-1 reverse transcriptase by nonnucleoside inhibitors. Science 1995;267:988–993.

93. Tantillo C, Ding J, Jacobo-Molina A, Nanni RG, Boyer PL, Hughes SH, Pauwels R, Andries K, Janssen PA, Arnold E. . Locations of anti-AIDS drug binding sites and resistance mutations in the three-dimensional structure of HIV-1 reverse transcriptase. Implications for mechanisms of drug inhibition and resistance. J Mol Biol 1994;243:369–387.

94. Buckheit Jr RW, Fliakas-Boltz V, Yeagy-Bargo S, Weislow O, Mayers DL, Boyer PL, Hughes SH, Pan BC, Chu SH, Bader JP. Resistance to 1-[(2-hydroxyethoxy)methyl]-6-(phenylthio)thymine derivatives is generated by mutations at multiple sites in the HIV-1 reverse transcriptase. Virology 1995;210:186–193.

95. Byrnes VW, Sardana VV, Schleif WA, Condra JH, Waterbury JA, Wolfgang JA, Long WJ, Schneider CL, Schlabach AJ, Wolanski BS, Graham DJ, Gotlib L, Rhodes A, Titus DL, Roth E, Blahy OM, Quintero JC, Staszewski S, Emini EA. Comprehensive mutant enzyme and viral variant assessment of human immunodeficiency virus type 1 reverse transcriptase resistance to nonnucleoside inhibitors. Antimicrob Agents Chemother 1993;37:1576–1579.

96. Ding J, Das K, Moereels H, Koymans L, Andries K, Janssen PA, Hughes SH, Arnold E. . Structure of HIV-1 RT/TIBO R 86183 complex reveals similarity in the binding of diverse nonnucleoside inhibitors. Nat Struct Biol 1995;2:407–415.

97. Das K, Lewi PJ, Hughes SH, Arnold E. Crystallography and the design of anti-AIDS drugs: conformational flexibility and positional adaptability are important in the design of non-nucleoside HIV-1 reverse transcriptase inhibitors. Prog Biophys Mol Biol 2005;88:209–231.

98. Smerdon SJ, Jager J, Wang J, Kohlstaedt LA, Chirino AJ, Friedman JM, Rice PA, Steitz TA. . Structure of the binding site for nonnucleoside inhibitors of the reverse transcriptase of human immunodeficiency virus type 1. Proc Natl Acad Sci USA 1994;91:3911–3915.

99. Hsiou Y, Ding J, Das K, Clark Jr AD, Boyer PL, Lewi P, Janssen PA, Kleim JP, Rosner M, Hughes SH, Arnold E. The Lys103Asn mutation of HIV-1 RT: a novel mechanism of drug resistance. J Mol Biol 2001;309:437–445.

100. Janssen PA, Lewi PJ, Arnold E, Daeyaert F, de Jonge M, Heeres J, Koymans L, Vinkers M, Guillemont J, Pasquier E, Kukla M, Ludovici D, Andries K, de Bethune MP, Pauwels R, Das K, Clark Jr AD, Frenkel YV, Hughes SH, Medaer B, De Knaep F, Bohets H, De Clerck F, Lampo A, Williams P, Stoffels P. In search of a novel anti-HIV drug: multidisciplinary coordination in the discovery of 4 [[1 [[4-[(1E)-2-cyanoethenyl]-2,6-dimethylphenyl]amino]-2-pyrimidinyl]amino]benzonitrile (R278474, rilpivirine). J Med Chem 2005;48:1901–1909.

101. Zhan P, Liu X, Li Z, Pannecouque C, De Clercq E. Design strategies of novel NNRTIs to overcome drug resistance. Curr Med Chem 2009;16:3903–3917.

102. Ludovici DW, Kukla MJ, Grous PG, Krishnan S, Andries K, de Bethune MP, Azijn H, Pauwels R, De Clercq E, Arnold E, Janssen PA. Evolution of anti-HIV drug candidates. Part 1: From alpha-anilinophenylacetamide (alpha-APA) to imidoyl thiourea (ITU). Bioorg Med Chem Lett 2001;11_2225–2228.

103. Ludovici DW, Kavash RW, Kukla MJ, Ho CY, Ye H, De Corte BL, Andries, K, de Bethune MP, Azijn H, Pauwels R, Moereel HE, Heeres J, Koymans LM, de Jonge MR, Van Aken KJ, Daeyaert FF, Lewi PJ, Das K, Arnold E, Janssen PA. Evolution of anti-HIV drug candidates. Part 2: Diaryltriazine (DATA) analogues. Bioorg Med Chem Lett 2001;11:2229–2234.

104. Das K, Clark Jr AD, Lewi PJ, Heeres J, De Jonge MR, Koymans LM, Vinkers HM, Daeyaert F, Ludovici DW, Kukla MJ, De Corte B, Kavash RW, Ho CY, Ye H, Lichtenstein MA, Andries K, Pauwels R, De Bethune MP, Boyer PL, Clark P, Hughes SH, Janssen PA, Arnold E. Roles of conformational and positional adaptability in structure-based design of TMC125-R165335 (etravirine) and related non-nucleoside reverse transcriptase inhibitors that are highly potent and effective against wild-type and drug-resistant HIV-1 variants. J Med Chem 2004;47:2550–2560.

105. Katlama C, Haubrich R, Lalezari J, Lazzarin A, Madruga JV, Molina JM, Schechter M, Peeters M, Picchio G, Vingerhoets J, Woodfall B, De Smedt G, DUET-1 and DUET-2 study groups. Efficacy and safety of etravirine in treatment-experienced, HIV-1 patients: pooled 48 week analysis of two randomized, controlled trials. AIDS 2009;23:2289–2300.

106. Pelemans H, Esnouf R, De Clercq E, Balzarini J. Mutational analysis of trp-229 of human immunodeficiency virus type 1 reverse transcriptase (RT) identifies this amino acid residue as a prime target for the rational design of new non-nucleoside RT inhibitors. Mol Pharmacol 2000;57:954–960.

107. Chou KC, Tomasselli AG, Reardon IM, Heinrikson RL. Predicting human immunodeficiency virus protease cleavage sites in proteins by a discriminant function method. Proteins 1996;24:51–72.

108. Kohl NE, Emini EA, Schleif WA, Davis LJ, Heimbach JC, Dixon RA, Scolnick EM, Sigal IS. Active human immunodeficiency virus protease is required for viral infectivity. Proc Natl Acad Sci USA 1988;85:4686–4690.

109. Pettit SC, Sheng N, Tritch R, Erickson-Viitanen S, Swanstrom R. The regulation of sequential processing of HIV-1 Gag by the viral protease. Adv Exp Med Biol 1998;436:15–25.

110. Prabu-Jeyabalan M, Nalivaika E, Schiffer CA. Substrate shape determines specificity of recognition for HIV-1 protease: analysis of crystal structures of six substrate complexes. Structure 2002;10:369–381.

111. Prabu-Jeyabalan M, Nalivaika E, Schiffer CA. How does a symmetric dimer recognize an asymmetric substrate? A substrate complex of HIV-1 protease. J Mol Biol 2000;301:1207–1220.

112. Louis JM, Weber IT, Tozser J, Clore GM, Gronenborn AM. HIV-1 protease: maturation, enzyme specificity, and drug resistance. Adv Pharmacol 2000;49:111–146.

113. Gatanaga H, Das D, Suzuki Y, Yeh DD, Hussain KA, Ghosh AK, Mitsuya H. Altered HIV-1 gag protein interactions with cyclophilin A (CypA) on the acquisition of H219Q and H219P substitutions in the CypA binding loop. J Biol Chem 2006;281:1241–1250.

114. Doyon L, Croteau G, Thibeault D, Poulin F, Pilote L, Lamarre D. Second locus involved in human immunodeficiency virus type 1 resistance to protease inhibitors. J Virol 1996;70:3763–3769.

115. Gatanaga H, Suzuki Y, Tsang H, Yoshimura K, Kavlick MF, Nagashima K, Gorelick RJ, Mardy S, Tang C, Summers MF, Mitsuya H. Amino acid substitutions in Gag protein at non-cleavage sites are indispensable for the development of a high multitude of HIV-1 resistance against protease inhibitors. J Biol Chem 2002;277:5952–5961.

116. Zhang YM, Imamichi H, Imamichi T, Lane HC, Falloon J, Vasudevachari MB, Salzman NP. Drug resistance during indinavir therapy is caused by mutations in the protease gene and in its Gag substrate cleavage sites. J Virol 1997;71:6662–6670.

117. Tamiya S, Mardy S, Kavlick MF, Yoshimura K, Mistuya H. Amino acid insertions near Gag cleavage sites restore the otherwise compromised replication of human immunodeficiency virus type 1 variants resistant to protease inhibitors. J Virol 2004;78:12030–12040.

118. Yusa K, Harada S. Acquisition of multi-PI (protease inhibitor) resistance in HIV-1 in vivo and in vitro. Curr Pharm Des 2004;10:4055–4064.

119. Tisdale M, Myers RE, Maschera B, Parry NR, Oliver NM, Blair ED. Cross-resistance analysis of human immunodeficiency virus type 1 variants individually selected for resistance to five different protease inhibitors. Antimicrob Agents Chemother 1995;39:1704–1710.

120. Watkins T, Resch W, Irlbeck D, Swanstrom R. Selection of high-level resistance to human immunodeficiency virus type 1 protease inhibitors. Antimicrob Agents Chemother 2003;47:759–769.

121. Hertogs K, Bloor S, Kemp SD, Van den Eynde C, Alcorn TM, Pauwels R, Van Houtte M, Staszewski S, Miller V, Larder BA. Phenotypic and genotypic analysis of clinical HIV-1 isolates reveals extensive protease inhibitor cross-resistance: a survey of over 6000 samples. AIDS 2000;14:1203–1210.

122. Kemper CA, Witt MD, Keiser PH, Dube MP, Forthal DN, Leibowitz M, Smith DS, Rigby A, Hellmann NS, Lie YS, Leedom J, Richman D, McCutchan JA, Haubrich R. Sequencing of protease inhibitor therapy: insights from an analysis of HIV phenotypic resistance in patients failing protease inhibitors. AIDS 2001;15:609–615.

123. Molla A, Korneyeva M, Gao Q, Vasavanonda S, Schipper PJ, Mo HM, Markowitz M, Chernyavskiy T, Niu P, Lyons N, Hsu A, Granneman GR, Ho DD, Boucher CA, Leonard JM, Norbeck DW, Kempf DJ. Ordered accumulation of mutations in HIV protease confers resistance to ritonavir. Nat Med 1996;2:760–766.

124. Condra JH, Schleif WA, Blahy OM, Gabryelski LJ, Graham DJ, Quintero JC, Rhodes A, Robbins HL, Roth E, Shivaprakash M, Titus D, Yang T, Tepplert H, Squires KE, Deutsch PJ, Emini EA. In vivo emergence of HIV-1 variants resistant to multiple protease inhibitors. Nature 1995;374:569–571.

125. Deeks SG, Grant RM, Beatty GW, Horton C, Detmer J, Eastman S. Activity of a ritonavir plus saquinavir-containing regimen in patients with virologic evidence of indinavir or ritonavir failure. AIDS 1998;12:F97–F102.

126. Prabu-Jeyabalan M, Nalivaika EA, King NM, Schiffer CA. Viability of a drug-resistant human immunodeficiency virus type 1 protease variant: structural insights for better antiviral therapy. J Virol 2003;77:1306–1315.

127. Logsdon BC, Vickrey JF, Martin P, Proteasa G, Koepke JI, Terlecky SR, Wawrzak Z, Winters MA, Merigan TC, Kovari LC. Crystal structures of a multidrug-resistant human immunodeficiency virus type 1 protease reveal an expanded active-site cavity. J Virol 2004;78:3123–3132.

128. King NM, Prabu-Jeyabalan M, Nalivaika EA, Schiffer CA. Combating susceptibility to drug resistance: lessons from HIV-1 protease. Chem Biol 2004;11:1333–1338.

129. King NM, Prabu-Jeyabalan M, Nalivaika EA, Wigerinck P, de Bethune MP, Schiffer CA. Structural and thermodynamic basis for the binding of TMC114, a next-generation human immunodeficiency virus type 1 protease inhibitor. J Virol 2004;78:12012–12021.

130. Ghosh AK, Kincaid JF, Walters DE, Chen Y, Chaudhuri NC, Thompson WJ, Culberson C, Fitzgerald PM, Lee HY, McKee SP, Munson PM, Duong TT, Darke PL, Zugay JA, Schleif WA, Axel MG, Lin J, Huff JR. Nonpeptidal P2 ligands for HIV protease inhibitors: structure-based design, synthesis, and biological evaluation. J Med Chem 1996;39:3278–3290.

131. Ghosh AK, Krishnan K, Walters DE, Cho W, Cho H, Koo Y, Trevino J, Holland L, Buthod J. Structure based design: novel spirocyclic ethers as nonpeptidal P2-ligands for HIV protease inhibitors. Bioorg Med Chem Lett 1998;8:979–982.

132. Ghosh AK, Thompson WJ, Fitzgerald PM, Culberson JC, Axel MG, McKee SP, Huff JR, Anderson PS. Structure-based design of HIV-1 protease inhibitors: replacement of two amides and a 10 pi-aromatic system by a fused bis-tetrahydrofuran. J Med Chem 1994;37:2506–2508.

133. Yoshimura K, Kato R, Kavlick MF, Nguyen A, Maroun V, Maeda K, Hussain KA, Ghosh AK, Gulnik SV, Erickson JW, Mitsuya H. A potent human immunodeficiency virus type 1 protease inhibitor, UIC-94003 (TMC-126), and selection of a novel (A28S) mutation in the protease active site. J Virol 2002;76:1349–1358.

134. De Meyer S, Azijn H, Surleraux D, Jochmans D, Tahri A, Pauwels R, Wigerinck P, de Bethune MP. TMC114, a novel human immunodeficiency virus type 1 protease inhibitor active against protease inhibitor-resistant viruses, including a broad range of clinical isolates. Antimicrob Agents Chemother 2005;49:2314–2321.

135. Tie Y, Boross PI, Wang YF, Gaddis L, Hussain AK, Leshchenko S, Ghosh AK, Louis JM, Harrison RW, Weber IT. High resolution crystal structures of HIV-1 protease with a potent non-peptide inhibitor (UIC-94017) active against multi-drug-resistant clinical strains. J Mol Biol 2004;338:341–352.

136. Surleraux DL, Tahri A, Verschueren WG, Pille GM, de Kock HA, Jonckers TH, Peeters A, De Meyer S, Azijn H, Pauwels R, de Bethune MP, King NM, Prabu-Jeyabalan M, Schiffer CA, Wigerinck PB. Discovery and selection of TMC114, a next generation HIV-1 protease inhibitor. J Med Chem 2005;48:1813–1822.

137. Ghosh AK, Sarang Kulkarni S, Anderson DD, Hong L, Baldridge A, Wang Y-F, Chumanevich AA, Kovalevsky AY, Tojo Y, Koh Y, Tang J, Weber IT, Mitsuya H. Design, synthesis, protein-ligand X-ray

structures and biological evaluation of a series of novel macrocyclic HIV-1 protease inhibitors to combat drug-resistance. J Med Chem 2009;52:7689–705.

138. Ghosh AK, Chapsal BD, Mitsuya H. Darunavir, a new PI with dual mechanism: from a novel drug design concept to new hope against drug-resistant HIV. In "Aspartic Acid Proteases as Therapeutic Targets: Ed. Ghosh, A.K.", Wiley-VCH GmbH & Co. KgaA, Weinheim. 2010: in press.

139. Mitsuya H, Ghosh AK. Development of HIV-1 protease inhibitors, antiretroviral resistance and current challenges of HIV/AIDS management. In "Aspartic Acid Proteases as Therapeutic Targets: Ed. Ghosh, A.K.", Wiley-VCH GmbH & Co. KgaA, Weinheim. 2010: in press.

140. Tojo Y, Koh Y, Amano M, Aoki M, Das D, Ghosh AK, Mitsuya H. Novel protease inhibitors (PIs) containing macrocyclic components and 3(R),3a(S),6a(R)-bis-Tetrahydrofuranylurethane (bis-THF) that are potent against multi-pi-resistant HIV-1 variants in vitro. Antimicrob. Agents Chemother 2010;54:3460–3470.

141. Surleraux DL, de Kock HA, Verschueren WG, Pille GM, Maes LJ, Peeters A, Vendeville S, De Meyer S, Azijn H, Pauwels R, de Bethune MP, King NM, Prabu-Jeyabalan M, Schiffer CA, Wigerinck PB. Design of HIV-1 protease inhibitors active on multidrug-resistant virus. J Med Chem 2005;48:1965–1973.

142. Ohtaka H, Freire E. Adaptive inhibitors of the HIV-1 protease. Prog Biophys Mol Biol 2005;88;193–208.

143. Hong L, Hartsuck JA, Foundling S, Ermolieff J, Tang J. Active-site mobility in human immunodeficiency virus, type 1, protease as demonstrated by crystal structure of A28S mutant. Protein Sci 1998;7:300–305.

144. Madruga JV, Berger D, McMurchie M, Suter F, Banhegyi D, Ruxrungtham K, Norris D, Lefebvre E, de Béthune MP, Tomaka F, De Pauw M, Vangeneugden T, Spinosa-Guzman S, TITAN study group. Efficacy and safety of darunavir-ritonavir compared with that of lopinavir-ritonavir at 48 weeks in treatment-experienced, HIV-infected patients in TITAN: a randomised controlled phase III trial. Lancet 2007;370:49–58.

145. Wlodawer A, Miller M, Jaskolski M, Sathyanarayana BK, Baldwin E, Weber IT, Selk LM, Clawson L, Schneider J, Kent SB. Conserved folding in retroviral proteases: crystal structure of a synthetic HIV-1 protease. Science 1989;245:616–621.

146. Navia MA, Fitzgerald PM, McKeever BM, Leu CT, Heimbach JC, Herber WK, Sigal IS, Darke PL, Springer JP. Three-dimensional structure of aspartyl protease from human immunodeficiency virus HIV-1. Nature 1989;337:615–620.

147. Bowman MJ, Byrne S, Chmielewski J. Switching between allosteric and dimerization inhibition of HIV-1 protease. Chem Biol 2005;12:439–444.

148. Frutos S, Rodriguez-Mias RA, Madurga S, Collinet B, Reboud-Ravaux M, Ludevid D, Giralt E. Disruption of the HIV-1 protease dimer with interface peptides: structural studies using NMR spectroscopy combined with [2-(13)C]-Trp selective labeling. Biopolymers 2007;88:164–173.

149. Levy Y, Caflisch A, Onuchic JN, Wolynes PG. The folding and dimerization of HIV-1 protease: evidence for a stable monomer from simulations. J Mol Biol 2004;340:67–79.

150. Koh Y, Matsumi S, Amano M, Das D, Davis D, Li J, Leshchenko S, Baldridge A, Shioda T, Yarchoan R, Ghosh AK, Mitsuya H. Potent inhibition of HIV-1 replication by non-peptidyl small molecule inhibitors of HIV-1 protease dimerization. J Biol Chem 2007;282:28709–28720.

151. Randolph JT, DeGoey DA. Peptidomimetic inhibitors of HIV protease. Curr Top Med Chem 2004;4:1079–1095.

152. Chrusciel RA, Strohbach JW. Non-peptidic HIV protease inhibitors. Curr Top Med Chem 2004;4:1097–1114.

153. Larder BA, Hertogs K, Bloor S, van den Eynde CH, DeCian W, Wang Y, Freimuth WW, Tarpley G. Tipranavir inhibits broadly protease inhibitor-resistant HIV-1 clinical samples. AIDS 2000;14:1943–1948.

154. Turner, SR, Strohbach JW, Tommasi RA, Aristoff PA, Johnson PD, Skulnick HI, Dolak LA, Seest EP, Tomich PK, Bohanon MJ, Horng MM, Lynn JC, Chong KT, Hinshaw RR, Watenpaugh KD, Janakiraman MN, Thaisrivongs S. Tipranavir (PNU-140690): a potent, orally bioavailable nonpeptidic HIV protease inhibitor of the 5,6-dihydro-4-hydroxy-2-pyrone sulfonamide class. J Med Chem 1998;41:3467–3476.

155. Back NK, van Wijk A, Remmerswaal D, van Monfort M, Nijhuis M, Schuurman R, Boucher CA. In-vitro tipranavir susceptibility of HIV-1 isolates with reduced susceptibility to other protease inhibitors. AIDS 2000;14:101–102.

156. Poppe SM, Slade DE, Chong KT, Hinshaw RR, Pagano PJ, Markowitz M, Ho DD, Mo H, Gorman 3rd RR, Dueweke TJ, Thaisrivongs S, Tarpley WG. Antiviral activity of the dihydropyrone PNU-140690, a new nonpeptidic human immunodeficiency virus protease inhibitor. Antimicrob Agents Chemother 1997;41:1058–1063.

157. Rusconi S, La Seta Catamancio S, Citterio P, Kurtagic S, Violin M, Balotta C, Moroni M, Galli M, d'Arminio-Monforte A. Susceptibility to PNU-140690 (Tipranavir) of human immunodeficiency virus type 1 isolates derived from patients with multidrug resistance to other protease inhibitors. Antimicrob Agents Chemother 2000;44:1328–1332.

158. Doyon L, Tremblay S, Bourgon L, Wardrop E, Cordingley MG. Selection and characterization of HIV-1 showing reduced susceptibility to the non-peptidic protease inhibitor tipranavir. Antiviral Res 2005;68:27–35.

159. Schake D. Molecular significance of tipranavir related codon 33 protease gene mutations. AIDS 2005;19:218–219.

160. Schake D. How flexible is tipranavir in complex with the HIV-1 protease active site? AIDS 2004;18:579–580.

161. Muzammil S, Kang LW, Armstrong AA, Jakalian A, Bonneau PR, Schmelmer V, Amzel LM, Freire E. Unique response of tipranavir to multi-drug resistant HIV-1 protease suggests new ways of combating drug resistance. In XIV International HIV Drug Resistance Workshop: Quebec Canada, 2005 [Abstract 63].

162. Ribera E, Curran A. Double-boosted protease inhibitor antiretroviral regimens: what role? Drugs 2008;68:2257–2267.

163. Mathias A, Lee M, Callebaut C, Xu L, Tsai L, Murray B, Liu H, Yale K, Warren D, Kearney B. sGS-9350: a Pharmaco-enhancer without anti-HIV activity. In: Program and abstracts of the 16th Conference on Retroviruses and Opportunistic Infections; February 8–11, 2009, Montréal, Canada. [Abstract 40].

164. Pommier Y, Johnson AA, Marchand C. Integrase inhibitors to treat HIV/AIDS. Nat Rev Drug Discov 2005;4:236–248.

165. Chiu TK, Davies DR. Structure and function of HIV-1 integrase. Curr Top Med Chem 2004;4:965–977.

166. Cushman M, Sherman P. Inhibition of HIV-1 integration protein by aurintricarboxylic acid monomers, monomer analogs, and polymer fractions. Biochem Biophys Res Commun 1992;185:85–90.

167. Fesen MR, Kohn KW, Leteurtre F, Pommier Y. Inhibitors of human immunodeficiency virus integrase. Proc. Natl Acad. Sci. USA 1993;90:2399–2403.

168. Goldgur Y, Craigie R, Cohen GH, Fujiwara T, Yoshinaga T, Fujishita T, Sugimoto H, Endo T, Murai H, Davies DR. Structure of the HIV-1 integrase catalytic domain complexed with an inhibitor: A platform for antiviral drug design. Proc. Natl Acad. Sci. USA 1999;96:13040–13043.

169. Hazuda DJ, Felock P, Witmer M, Wolfe A, Stillmock K, Grobler JA, Espeseth A, Gabryelski L, Schleif W, Blau C, Miller MD. Inhibitors of strand transfer that prevent integration and inhibit HIV-1 replication in cells. Science 2000;287:646–650.

170. Steigbigel RT, Cooper DA, Kumar PN, Eron JE, Schechter M, Markowitz M, Loutfy MR, Lennox JL, Gatell JM, Rockstroh JK, Katlama C, Yeni P, Lazzarin A, Clotet B, Zhao J, Chen J, Ryan DM, Rhodes RR, Killar JA, Gilde LR, Strohmaier KM, Meibohm AR, Miller MD, Hazuda DJ, Nessly ML, DiNubile MJ, Isaacs RD, Nguyen BY, Teppler H, BENCHMRK Study Teams. Raltegravir with optimized background therapy for resistant HIV-1 infection. N Engl J Med 2008;359:339–354.

171. Sato M, Motomura T, Aramaki H, Matsuda T, Yamashita M, Ito Y, Kawakami H, Matsuzaki Y, Watanabe W, Yamataka K, Ikeda S, Kodama E, Matsuoka M, Shinkai H. Novel HIV-1 integrase inhibitors derived from quinolone antibiotics. J Med Chem 2006;49:1506–1508.

172. DeJesus E, Berger D, Markowitz M, Cohen C, Hawkins T, Ruane P, Elion R, Farthing C, Zhong L, Cheng AK, McColl D, Kearney BP for the 183-0101 Study Team. Antiviral activity, pharmacokinetics, and dose response of the HIV-1 integrase inhibitor GS-9137 (JTK-303) in treatment-naive and treatment-experienced patients. J Acquir Immune Defic Syndr. 2006;43:1–5.

173. Shimura K, Kodama E, Sakagami Y, Matsuzaki Y, Watanabe W, Yamataka K, Watanabe Y, Ohata Y, Doi S, Sato M, Kano M, Ikeda S, Matsuoka M. Broad anti-retroviral activity and resistance profile of a novel human immunodeficiency virus integrase inhibitor, elvitegravir (JTK-303/GS-9137). J Virol 2007;82:764–774.

174. Vandeckerckhove L. GSK-1349572, a novel integrase inhibitor for the treatment of HIV infection. Curr Opin Investig Drugs 2010;11:203–212.

175. Min S, Song I, Borland J, Chen S, Lou Y, Fujiwara T, Piscitelli SC. Pharmacokinetics and safety of S/GSK1349572, a next-generation HIV integrase inhibitor, in healthy volunteers. Antimicrob Agents Chemother 2010;54:254–258.

176. Alkhatib G, Combadiere C, Broder CC, Feng Y, Kennedy PE, Murphy PM, Berger EA. CC CKR5: a RANTES, MIP-1alpha, MIP-1beta receptor as a fusion cofactor for macrophage-tropic HIV-1. Science 1996;272:1955–1958.

177. Deng H, Liu R, Ellmeier W, Choe S, Unutmaz D, Burkhart M, Di Marzio P, Marmon S, Sutton RE, Hill CM, Davis CB, Peiper SC, Schall TJ, Littman DR, Landau NR. Identification of a major co-receptor for primary isolates of HIV-1. Nature 1996;381:661–666.

178. Kuritzkes DR. HIV-1 entry inhibitors: an overview. Current Opinion in HIV and AIDS 2009;4:82–87.

179. Wild CT, Shugars DC, Greenwell TK, McDanal CB, Matthews TJ. Peptides corresponding to a predictive alpha-helical domain of human immunodeficiency virus type 1 gp41 are potent inhibitors of virus infection. Proc Natl Acad Sci USA 1994;91:9770–9774.

180. Hardy H, Skolnik PR. Enfuvirtide, a new fusion inhibitor for therapy of human immunodeficiency virus infection. Pharmacotherapy 2004;24:198–211

181. Kilby JM, Lalezari JP, Eron JJ, Carlson M, Cohen C, Arduino RC, Goodgame JC, Gallant JE, Volberding, P, Murphy RL, Valentine F, Saag MS, Nelson EL, Sista PR, Dusek A. The safety, plasma pharmacokinetics, and antiviral activity of subcutaneous enfuvirtide (T-20), a peptide inhibitor of gp41-mediated virus fusion, in HIV-infected adults. AIDS Re Hum Retroviruses 2002;18:685–693.

182. Maeda K, Das D, Ogata-Aoki H, Nakata H, Miyakawa T, Takaoka Y, Ding J, Arnold E, Mitsuya H. Structural and molecular interactions of CCR5 inhibitors with CCR5. J Biol Chem 2006;281:12688–12698.

183. Maeda K, Das D, Yin P, Tsuchiya K, Ogata-Aoki H, Nakata H, Norman K, Hackney L, Takaoka Y, Mitsuya H. Involvement of the second extracellular loop and transmembrane residues of CCR5 in inhibitor binding and HIV-1 fusion. Insights to mechanism of allosteric inhibition. J Mol Biol 2008;381:956–974

184. Dorr P, Westby M, Dobbs S, Griffin P, Irvine B, Macartney M, Mori J, Rickett G, Smith-Burchnell C, Napier C, Webster R, Armour D, Price D, Stammen B, Wood A, Perros M. Maraviroc (UK-427,857), a potent, orally bioavailable, and selective small-molecule inhibitor of chemokine receptor CCR5 with broad-spectrum antihuman immunodeficiency virus type 1 activity. Antimicrob Agents Chemother 2005;49:4721–4732.

185. Fätkenheuer G, Pozniak AL, Johnson MA, Plettenberg A, Staszewski S, Hoepelman AI, Saag MS, Goebel FD, Rockstroh JK, Dezube BJ, Jenkins TM, Medhurst C, Sullivan JF, Ridgway C, Abel S, James IT, Youle M, van der Ryst E. Efficacy of short-term monotherapy with maraviroc, a new CCR5 antagonist, in patients infected with HIV-1. Nat Med 2005;11:1170–1172.

186. Gulick RM, Lalezari J, Goodrich J, Clumeck N, DeJesus E, Horban A, Nadler J, Clotet B, Karlsson A, Wohlfeiler M, Montana JB, McHale M, Sullivan J, Ridgway C, Felstead S, Dunne MW, van der Ryst E, Mayer H, MOTIVATE Study Teams. Maraviroc for previously treated patients with R5 HIV-1 infection. N Engl J Med 2008;359:1429–1441.

187. Fätkenheuer G, Nelson M, Lazzarin A, Konourina I, Hoepelman AI, Lampiris H, Hirschel B, Tebas P, Raffi F, Trottier B, Bellos N, Saag M, Cooper DA, Westby M, Tawadrous M, Sullivan JF, Ridgway C, Dunne MW, Felstead S, Mayer H, van der Ryst E, MOTIVATE 1 and MOTIVATE 2 Study Teams.Subgroup analyses of maraviroc in previously treated R5 HIV-1 infection. N Engl J Med 2008;359:1442–1455.

188. Hardy D, Reynes J, Konourina I, Wheeler D, Moreno S, van der Ryst E, Towner W, Horban A, Mayer H, Goodrich J. Efficacy and safety of maraviroc plus optimized background therapy in treatment-experienced patients infected with CCR5-tropic HIV-1: 48-week combined analysis of the MOTIVATE studies. In: 15th Conference on Retroviruses and Opportunistic Infections; 3–6 February 2008, Boston, MA [abstract #792].

189. Hoepelman IM, Ayoub A, Heera J. The incidence of severe liver enzyme abnormalities and hepatic adverse events in the Maraviroc Clinical Development Programme. In: 11th European AIDS Conference/EACS; 24–27 October 2007, Madrid, Spain [poster LBP7.9/1].

190. Saag M, Ive P, Heera J, Tawadrous M, DeJesus E, Clumeck N, Cooper D, Horban A, Mohapi L, Mingrone H, Reyes-Teran G, Walmsley S, Hackman F, van der Ryst E, Mayer H. A multicenter, randomized, double-blind, comparative trial of a novel CCR5 antagonist, maraviroc versus efavirenz, both in combination with combivir (zidovudine [ZDV]/lamivudine [3TC]), for the treatment of antiretroviral naive subjects infected with R5 HIV-1: week 48 results of the MERIT study. In: 4th IAS conference; 22–25 July 2007, Sydney, Australia [abstract #WESS104].

191. Heera J, Saag M, Ive P, Whitcomb J, Lewis M, McFadyen L, Goodrich J, Mayer H, van der Ryst E, Westby M. Virological correlates associated with treatment failure at week 48 in the phase III study of maraviroc in treatment naïve patients. In: 15th Conference on Retroviruses and Opportunistic Infections; 3–6 February 2008, Boston, MA [abstract #40LB].

192. Hendrix CW, Collier AC, Lederman MM, Schols D, Pollard RB, Brown S, Jackson JB, Coombs RW, Glesby MJ, Flexner CW, Bridger GJ, Badel K, MacFarland RT, Henson GW, Calandra G. Safety, pharmacokinetics, and antiviral activity of AMD3100, a selective CXCR4 receptor inhibitor, in HIV-1 infection. J Acquir Immune Defic Syndr 2004;37:1253–1262.

193. Liles WC, Rodger E, Broxmeyer HE, Dehner C, Badel K, Calandra G, Christensen J, Wood B, Price TH, Dale DC. Augmented mobilization and collection of CD34+ hematopoietic cells from normal human volunteers stimulated with granulocyte-colony-stimulating factor by single-dose administration of AMD3100, a CXCR4 antagonist. Transfusion 2005;45:295–300.

194. The DHHS Panel on Antiretroviral Guidelines for Adultsand Adolescents—A Working Group of theOffice of AIDS Research Advisory Council (OARAC). (2009) Guidelines for the Use of Antiretroviral Agents in HIV-1-Infected Adults and Adolescents, released on December 1, 2009.

195. Thompson MA, Aberg JA, Cahn P, Montaner JSG, Rizzardini G, Telenti A, Gatell JM, Günthard HF, Hammer SM, Hirsch MS, Reiss P, Richman DD, Volberding PA, Yeni P, Schooley RT. Antiretroviral Treatment of Adult HIV Infection. 2010 Recommendations of the International AIDS Society–USA Panel. JAMA 2010;304:321–333.

Chapter 41 AN HIV VACCINE: IS IT POSSIBLE? ARE WE GETTING CLOSER?

JAMES F. STANFORD AND CAROL W. STANFORD

Some see a hopeless end, while others see an endless hope.

WORLD AIDS DAY QUOTES—ANONYMOUS

Introduction

As we close in on 3 decades since the discovery of the human immunodeficiency virus[1] (HIV) and the first descriptions of the acquired immunodeficiency syndrome[2,3] (AIDS) the recent declarations that we are entering a "renaissance" in HIV vaccine development[4] and that controlling and ultimately ending the HIV /AIDS pandemic is a "a feasible goal"[5] are being met with differing reactions. These have comprised the full range of possibilities—continued skepticism to cautious optimism and now include a true sense of excitement for the beginning of the era in which one of the world's greatest plagues might be brought under control.

The successes along the path to a preventative vaccine have repeatedly provided hope that something easier than lifelong medication and consistent sexual behavior change—namely, a one-time series of shots—will be a legitimate way to slow and ultimately end the pandemic. Setbacks and failures along the way have reinforced how truly difficult this endeavor is.

Interested and engaged followers of this effort—including patients, their families and advocates, investigators, funders, global vaccine workers, and public health leaders—all experienced disappointment as we learned the STEP trial,[6,7] a proof-of-concept phase IIB trial of replication-incompetent recombinant adenovirus 5 (rAd5) vector vaccine carrying HIV genes gag, pol, and nef, was unsuccessful. Not only did the trial demonstrate that the vaccine conferred no protection and no effect on a recipient's viral RNA levels, there was actually an increased acquisition of HIV in subgroups of vaccine recipients who were uncircumcised and who had higher pre-existing rAd5 antibody titers. Was this simply a failure of this specific vaccine? Or is it a sign that the entire viral vector and other primarily T-cell–directed vaccine strategies are flawed?[8–14]

Although some see the recently published RV 144 trial[15] as an early validation signal that we're on the right path and that vaccine protection against HIV transmission has finally been seen[4,5,16] others may fear that this vaccine strategy combining two previously failed concepts was ill-advised[17] and may not be real vaccine-induced protection but a chance event.[18] Especially given the fact that the modified intent-to-treat analysis reached statistical significance, whereas the as-treated analysis, which included only patients who received all of the planned vaccine injections, failed to do so.[15]

TABLE 41–1	Challenges in the Development of an HIV Vaccine[a]
	• Immune correlates of protection unclear
	• Numerous HIV variants with extensive viral clade and sequence diversity
	• HIV integrates into the cellular genome
	• Attenuated viruses unsafe for human use
	• Infected cells transmit the infection and cell-to-cell transfer of infection
	• Viral evasion of humoral and cellular immune responses
	• Early establishment of latent viral reservoirs and immune sanctuaries of the body (e.g., brain and testes)
	• Virus compromises immune function
	• Antibody responses are typically type specific
	• No method exists to elicit broadly reactive neutralizing antibodies
	• Autoimmune responses may be induced
	• Lack of a small animal model
	• Little pharmaceutical interest

[a]Adapted from: Barouch DH, *Nature.* 2008;455:614 and Levy JA (Ed). *HIV and the Pathogenesis of AIDS, 3rd ed.* Washington, DC: ASM Press;2007:397–428.

Very recently published rational design work utilizing advances in structural biology, high-throughput screening of sera, and reverse engineering has resulted in the discovery of exceptionally potent and broadly neutralizing antibodies as well as information regarding their mechanism(s) of action.[19,20,21,22] However, transforming this knowledge into vaccine immunogens that will be able to elicit similar antibodies that prove protective against HIV transmission will not be easy.

Advances in HIV/AIDS Immunopathogenesis Inform Vaccine Research

Developing an HIV preventative vaccine has proved challenging and elusive for a number of reasons[8,10,11,14,23] (**Table 41–1**).

HIV and the pathogenesis of both early acute and chronic HIV infection/AIDS differ in many respects from those of other viruses/associated diseases. Therefore, not all insights gained from studying these historic vaccines will necessarily be beneficial. Tremendous worldwide diversity exists with multiple clades/subtypes and recombinant viruses, and rapid development of HIV variants (quasi-species) due to an extremely error-prone reverse transcriptase enzyme. HIV integrates into the cellular genome, establishes reservoirs of latency, and infects immune system silent sanctuaries of the body (i.e., brain and testes).[23] With HIV, cell-to-cell transfer of infection takes place,[25] autoimmunity may be induced, and the virus itself infects and compromises CD4+ cells, which normally coordinate both B cell and T cell functions needed to respond to the invading threat.

Levy[23] has suggested that the ideal HIV vaccine would induce local immunity at all entry sites, induce both cellular and humoral immune responses against virus-infected cells, induce antibodies that neutralize and do not enhance infection,[66] induce responses in both innate and adaptive immune systems, include responses that recognize latently infected cells, be safe, be long-lasting, and not induce autoantibodies.

The field of HIV vaccine research has enjoyed steady gains stemming from advances in our understanding of basic pathobiology of acute and chronic HIV infection,[26–55] mechanisms of immune system evasion,[8,10,11,14,23,25,26,32-35,39,41,42,44,47,49,56–71] immune and genomic correlates of natural HIV control and /or resistance found in "long-term nonprogressors," "elite controllers,"[71–80] and "heavily exposed, persistently seronegative" (HEPS) individuals such as the Nairobi prostitute cohort.[81,81b,82]

Early transmission and the events that characterize early acute infection proceed quite rapidly and are extremely dynamic, but if completely understood may reveal some vulnerabilities that could be exploited as targets for an effective vaginal/rectal microbicide as well as an HIV preventative vaccine. Recent data from the SIV rhesus macaque model of female HIV-1 infection[87,99] reveals that only a very small number of virus particles (in fact, a single virus in 80% of cases and two to five viruses in the other 20%) cross mucous membranes within hours of their arrival at the mucous membrane. There they initially establish small transmitted/founder virus focuses[51,51b,67] before multiplying and disseminating. The virus that crosses[23,26,26b,42,87,99,101,183,184] appears to be primarily a free virus, utilizing only CCR5 as its coreceptor (regardless of the coreceptor tropism of the transmitter). This knowledge also reveals a "genetic bottleneck"[42] of sorts, in terms of the viral diversity story, and perhaps a vulnerability of HIV that could be used in the quest for an effective and safe vaccine.

Clarifying whether HIV traverses mucous membranes by transcytosis, movement between cells, or across tears in the mucosa is a high priority in that the answer to this question will determine how important it might be to generate mucosal immunity through vaccination.[42,47,47b]

The transmitted/founder virus(es) infect intraepithelial dendritic cells[101] and undergo a necessary local expansion during the first week to generate sufficient virus and infect cells to disseminate and establish a self-propagating systemic infection throughout lymphoid organs.[42,87,99,101] Replication explodes at the beginning of the second week of infection in the lymphatic system, where HIV finds many more target cells than at the founder focus. Extremely rapid and profound depletion of resting HIV-specific CD4+ memory cells[26–29,45] in the gut ensues as the virus levels in the blood and tissues peak at the end of the second week.[42,45] Immune system activation,[32-36,64] triggered—at least, in part—by bacterial translocation[36] across the gut mucosa, plays a key role in accelerating and perpetuating viral replication at basically all phases of infection and contributes to progression to chronic established HIV infection.

Adaptive immune responses, initially in the form of CD8+ cytotoxic lymphocytes, make their debut at about the beginning of the third week, and although they initially result in a dramatic 3- to 5-log drop in viral RNA blood levels by about four weeks this appears to be "too little too late"[30,42,47,56,60,65] as initially expanded HIV-specific CD8+ T-cell clones rapidly disappear later during primary infection[30] and are unable to prevent viral seeding of immune sanctuaries[23] (brain and testes) and infection of cells capable of latency.[23,72] Humoral adaptive responses—consisting initially of blocking antibodies and only later, neutralizing antibodies—appears to be quite ineffective[31,37] as the virus's ability to rapidly divide and mutate outpaces the host's ability to form neutralizing antibody responses.[10,25,58,60,68–70]

Because of concerns that adaptive immune responses from a vaccine-primed memory population of lymphocytes emerge too slowly to contain early spread after transmission attention is being focused on determining whether innate mechanisms contribute to HIV prevention, aborted, or controlled/attenuated infection. The role of innate immune responses[42,43,44,48,95,96] (including the roles of natural killer [NK] cells, dendritic cells, and non-neutralizing antibody responses such as antibody-dependent cellular cytotoxicity [ADCC]) at mucosal surfaces and in the tissues is being studied, but requires much greater emphasis. Newer assays that are less cumbersome, easier to interpret, and more relevant for ADCC and other immune responses may help spur interest and more research in some of these areas. Interestingly, resistance to simian immunodeficiency virus infection in sooty mangabeys (SIVsm) appears to relate to innate immune effector mechanisms with less gut damage and less immune system activation seen in this natural host infection.[95,96]

Our current understanding of these early transmission events calls for new vaccine concepts requiring pre-existing and/or constantly present innate and adaptive mucosal immune defense or extremely fast-acting amnestic responses to prevent established infection or control early infection before it can disseminate, establish a chronic state, and before devastating CD4 depletion[42,71] occurs.

Nonhuman Primates: Our Partners in Understanding, Treating, and Preventing HIV/AIDS

HIV passed from chimpanzees to humans around 1934 with obvious devastating consequences.[83] While much has been and will continue to be learned about HIV transmission, disease resistance, progression, and HIV prevention (via both microbicide candidates and vaccines), there are many peculiarities regarding natural lentiviral infections/diseases and susceptibility of nonhuman primates to HIV, simian immunodeficiency virus (SIV), and other lentiviruses. A thorough discussion of this interesting topic is beyond the scope of this chapter; the interested reader is referred to several excellent reviews and trusted sources.[23,48,68, 84–88]

The major limitation surrounding HIV study in animal models is that the virus does not replicate in most species tested, including rodents and nonhuman primates (the rare exceptions being gibbon apes and chimpanzees, in which HIV-1 does not typically cause an AIDS-like disease).[84] Although chimpanzees are the closest species in evolutionary terms to humans, they are endangered, costly to maintain, and their use can be of ethical concern. HIV viral surrogates, primarily simian immunodeficiency virus (SIV) and a chimeric HIV/SIV (SHIV) model of infection have been utilized.[23,48,68,84,85,89–94] Simian immunodeficiency virus is generally not pathogenic ("apathogenic") in its natural hosts, which are the African green monkey and sooty mangabeys.[48,84,86–88,95,96] However, experimental infection in non-natural hosts, such as the Asian rhesus macaques (*Macaca mulatta*) results in a disease (SIVmac) which is quite similar to AIDS in humans in many important respects.[48,84,85,89–94]

In light of the recent (2007) failure of the Merck rAD5 vaccine (the STEP trial) and other unsuccessful vaccine strategies that have failed to mirror nonhuman primate model protection (despite eliciting potent cytotoxic CD8+ T-cell responses in both rhesus macaques and humans), there has been an important re-evaluation of the use of nonhuman primate models for HIV vaccine preclinical development. Experts in the field recommend that nonhuman primate studies should no longer act as "clinical trial gatekeepers,"[84] but should instead be used for studying pathogenesis,[41] generating hypotheses, and as "immune gatekeepers,"[84] for progression to phase I clinical testing (**Figure 41–1**).

More pathogenic nonhuman primate models—for example, SIVmac—which utilize more stringent heterologous viral challenge[97,98] may be more predictive of successful human

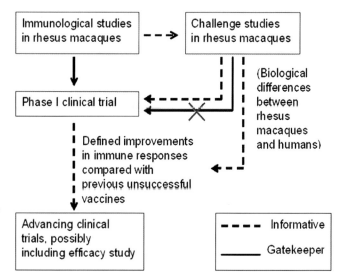

Figure 41–1. *SIV rhesus macaque model: immune versus clinical trials "gatekeeper." Source: Shedlock DJ, Silvestri G, Weiner DB. Monkeying around with HIV vaccines: using rhesus macaques to define "gatekeepers" for clinical trials. Nature Reviews Immunology 2009;9(10):717–728. Used by permission of the publisher.*

TABLE 41–2	Recommendations for Preclinical Challenge Studies of T-Cell–based Vaccines[a]
	• Use stringent challenge virus (SIVMAC$_{239}$, SIVMAC$_{251}$)
	• Design study with adequate power and follow-up time
	• Model clinical regimen with vaccine schedule and dose
	• Select rhesus monkeys that lack MHC alleles associated with efficient virologic control (Mamu-A*01, Mamu-B*17, Mamu
	• Avoid use of a homologous Env antigen
	• Assess promising vaccine concepts against both homologous and heterologous viral challenges.

[a]Source: Barouch DH. Challenges in the development of an HIV-1 vaccine. Nature 2008 Oct 2;455(7213):613–619. Used by permission of the publisher.

protection (**Table 41–2**). Use of these models, along with better measures of immune responses[84] (which are standardized, quantifiable, broad, potent, and relevant), are currently informing a new generation of clinical trials. Importantly, these animal model immune responses are benchmarked against immune responses seen with earlier human HIV vaccines which failed to lower viral set points and failed to protect humans from HIV infection.

Earlier nonhuman primate model studies utilized high-dose SIV or SHIV intravenous challenge to assure uniform infection of all control group animals.[48,84] As most of the world's HIV pandemic is the result of heterosexual transmission, information gleaned from the female sexual transmission SIVmac model[87,99] has been informative and enlightening. Important discoveries have been made regarding the pathogenesis of early, acute SIV infection of rhesus macaques[42,44,46,52,87,99-100] where the disease in SIVmac appears to mirror human pathology and pathogenesis quite well.[102] Additionally, the use of repeated, low-dose mucosal (vaginal, rectal, oral) challenge[87,99-106] is believed to be much more relevant to actual human sexual and perinatal transmission of HIV. All of these recent advances are no doubt moving the field forward in important and hopeful pathways of inquiry and discovery.

HIV Vaccine as Part of an Overall Prevention Strategy

As we continue to make progress toward the ultimate goal of a safe and effective vaccine, we must remain ever cognizant of our critical partnership with and obligations to our patients and clinical trial volunteers for ethically sound, just, transparent, and reasoned human testing of vaccine candidates. This is especially important to recognize when this testing occurs in the developing world[111–117,159] which bears more than 90% of the devastation. Strides are being made in rolling out life-saving and life-extending antiretroviral (ARV) treatment in the Third World,[118] where it is so desperately needed and where the concept of "treatment as prevention"[5,119] potentially could be realized. Twenty to forty percent of those who need antiretroviral treatments (40% of those with CD4 counts of <200 cells/mm^3 or 20% of those with <350 cells/mm^3) are now receiving such therapy.[18,118]

Although a strong evidence base for proven prevention interventions[5] now exists (male circumcision in various settings and populations, consistent condom use, education/counseling for behavior change, screening of blood supplies, needle exchange programs, ARV treatment to prevent vertical transmission, and prevention and treatment of drug and alcohol abuse) and we have begun to achieve the basic science underpinnings for successful vaginal/rectal microbicides,[42,46,120] it is indeed discouraging to realize that these interventions are accessible only to a minority of persons globally who need them.[5] The sobering fact remains that as of 2010, for every person who is receiving ARV treatment there are six others who become newly infected.[18]

Clearly, our best hope for turning the pandemic around lies in the concept of "combination prevention,"[5] the largest and most important components of which are ARV drugs and a safe and effective vaccine.[5]

Learning From Natural Infection/Natural Protection

Common wisdom among HIV vaccine experts is that natural protection and/or control of HIV infection (a low or undetectable viral set point and lack of progressive immune destruction and disease) occur rarely in infected humans and that very detailed correlates of protection from HIV infection are still poorly understood.[8,10,11,14,23,26,37,39,40,41,42,47,49,50,57,67,70] Therefore what to look for in a vaccine is similarly unclear. At the same time we have learned more about this virus in a shorter period of time than has ever been learned about any other viral pathogen or nonpathogen microorganism known to man.

We must not forget that host defenses actually succeed more often than they fail especially in regards to preventing infection following mucosal exposure.[42–46] Only about one in three to one in four infants born to HIV-infected women not taking PACTG 076-recommended zidovudine or currently recommended highly active antiretroviral therapy (HAART) become infected.[121] The generally low per sexual exposure transmission rate (one in 100 to one in 1,000 depending on the partner's viral load and circumcision status[122]), and strain-specific immune system recognition of "donor's" HIV virus in many of the 299 out of 300 individuals who, even without taking a post-exposure prophylaxis (PEP) regimen, do not get infected after a hollow bore needle stick exposure[123] suggest that quickly responsive innate immunity mechanisms can be quite effective at preventing and/or aborting HIV transmission, early infection, and virus dissemination events and therefore must be more intensely studied.[42,44,46]

Learning From History—Previously Successful Vaccines

Ever since Jenner's success with smallpox immunization in 1796, conventional vaccines have led to great progress in controlling other viral diseases, including smallpox, polio, rabies, measles, mumps, rubella, chickenpox, and hepatitis A and B.[23] Unfortunately, very little is actually known regarding how these successful vaccines provide their protection and, in many cases, we have benefited from serendipity. Most induce cellular immune (T-cell/CD4) responses or both antibodies and cellular responses, the possible exceptions being polio, mumps, and rubella viruses.[67] Successful vaccines have typically been generated against pathogens for which the natural immune response thwarts serious disease in a substantial fraction of those infected[14,23,67] (i.e., they recover naturally). Conventional vaccines usually protect against disease and not against infection, protect for years against viruses that do not change over time, have generally been whole killed or live-attenuated viral products, protect against infections that occur through mucosal surfaces of the respiratory or gastrointestinal tract (and not the genital tract), and are directed at free microbes (and not at cell-associated pathogens).[23]

Successful conventional vaccines have consisted of: (1) live-attenuated–virus vaccines such as the mumps and measles vaccines, which cause infection without causing disease and elicit strong and long-lasting immune responses, (2) killed whole virus vaccines, such as the original Salk killed-poliovirus–vaccine employed in widespread vaccination campaigns in the mid-20th century, and (3) recombinant viral proteins, as in the current hepatitis B vaccine.[14,23,67] Live-attenuated HIV, which has been shown to have the capacity to revert from an apathogenic virus to a pathogenic virus, is felt to be too dangerous to be tested in humans[124] although we have learned much from this vaccine technique with SIV in nonhuman primate models.[90,97,98,100]

Salk proposed and the Immune Response Corporation tested a killed HIV-derived immunogen (Remune[R]), an early therapeutic vaccine of sorts,[125] in phase I, II, and III human trials[125,126] during the 1990s. Unfortunately, there appeared to be no clear benefit with use of the agent. Although it has suffered what appeared to be fatal setbacks, the product apparently has at least four lives as it continues to be tested in patients.[127] Newer approaches to therapeutic vaccination[128] have continued, including various gene therapies,[129,130] one of which is the first HIV gene therapy to be tested in a multicenter, international, phase II clinical trial.[129] Although the completion of the trial was a milestone, none of these studies have shown benefit or had practical application to large numbers of infected patients thus far.

Recent data highlighting early transmission and infection events involving very small numbers of free virus[18,36,42] which cross mucous membranes (thus establishing small "transmitter/founder" virus focuses initially[51,67] before disseminating) reveals that there are indeed more similarities (to conventional vaccines) than initially thought and that vaccines may need to prevent both free and cell-associated virus transmission and other pathogenic events stemming from cell-associated virus [23,42] to be successful.

Vaccine Approaches and Candidates

Many male and female injection drug users, men who have sex with men (MSM), and women at heterosexual risk throughout the developed world have volunteered participation in phase I, II, and III vaccine trials since the early to mid-1990s. With the possible exception of the RV 144 phase III trial[15] of ALVAC (recombinant canarypox vector) prime, AIDSVAX B/E (rgp120 monomeric Env subunit) vaccine boost, which may have shown the earliest signal of some

TABLE 41-3	Selected HIV-1 Vaccine Efficacy Studies in Nonhuman Primates and Human Volunteers					
					Response;[a] Efficacy rate (%)[b]	
Vaccine concept	Developer	Study	Status		Rhesus macaques[c]	Humans
Monomeric gp 120 (B/B, B/E)	VaxGen	VAX 003, VAX 004 (Phase III)	Completed in 2003		100; 100	100; 0
Adenovirus vector rAd5-Gag/Pol/Nef	STEP/Merck & Co.	HVTN502/MRK023 HVTN503 Phambili (Phase IIb)	Stopped in 2007		100; 100	62; 0[d]
Canary poxvirus (ALVAC) prime, gp120 (B/E) boost	Sanofi, VaxGen (GSID)	RV 144 (Phase III)	Completed in 2009		100; 100	19/ 100;31
VEE virus vector	AVX101/ AlphaVax	HVTN040 (Phase I)	Completed		100; 100	0; ND
Multi-epitope DNA	Epimmune	HVTN048 (Phase I)	Completed		100; ND	10; ND
Multi-potpie peptides	Wyeth	HVTN056 (Phase I)	Completed		100; 84	8; ND
Canary poxvirus vector (ALVAC)	Sanofi Pasteur	HVTN039 (Phase I)	Completed		100; 100	10; ND
Canary poxvirus vector and lipopeptides	ALVAC-HIV/ANRS	HVTN041/ ANRSVAC19 (Phase I)	Completed		100; 13	4; ND
DNA plasmid	Wyeth	HVTN060 (Phase I)	Completed		100;100	40; ND
DNA plasmid and adenovirus vector	PAVE 100/VRC	HVTN204 (Phase II)	Completed		100; 100	70; 0
DNA plasmid and MVA vector	Geovax	HVTN205 (Phase II)	Ongoing		100; 100	42; 0
DNA prime, rAd5 boost Gag/Pol/EnvA/EnvB/EnvC	NIH VRC	HVTN505 (Phase Ii)	Began in 2009		100; 100	RP; RP

[a]The percentage of individuals responding to vaccination as measured by enzyme-linked immunosorbent spot assay.

[b]The percentage of individuals exhibiting some measurable level of protection against virus transmission or delay in disease progression.

[c]All results shown were in rhesus macaques except for the monomeric gp 120 (B/B, B/E), which utilized chimpanzees. MVA, modified vaccinia virus Ankara; ND, not determined;SHIV, HIV Env-expressing SIV; SIV, simian immunodefiency virus; VEE, Venezuelan equine encephalitis; VRC, Vaccine Research Center; RP, results pending.

[d]HIV transmission increased.

Source: Barouch DH, Korber B. HIV-1 vaccine development after STEP. Annu Rev Med 2010;61:153–167. Shedlock DJ, Silvestri G, Weiner DB. Monkeying around with HIV vaccines: using rhesus macaques to define "gatekeepers" for clinical trials. Nature Rev 2009;9:717–728. Modified by permission of the publishers.

protection, human HIV vaccine trials have been informative, at times unpredictable (phase I and I/II B test of concept STEP), "predictable" (original VaxGen studies, RV 144), but mostly disappointing (the three completed phase III trials) (**Table 41–3**). The lead-up to the STEP trial alone involved 12 phase I trials, which enrolled and followed more than 1,300 volunteers. Later-phase (phase IIb, III) trials required substantially greater numbers of volunteers. The time, effort, and expense involved in moving an immunogen candidate forward is quite substantial, so there is an understandable tendency to be slow to abandon a vaccine concept after years of sustained effort, especially when actual correlates of human protection are unknown. There have also been examples of successful vaccine products in which responses and mechanisms seen in the animal model were not predictive of success or failure in humans—that is, the actual result in man appeared to ignore what the animal model predicted.

The earliest work toward a vaccine targeted neutralizing antibodies with a goal of sterilizing immunity and involved efforts by scientists at the Division of Acquired Immunodeficiency Syndrome (DAIDS) of the National Institutes of Health, Institute of Allergy and Infectious Diseases (NIH/NIAID), as well as Chiron, Genentech (and later, VaxGen), MicroGeneSys, the Walter Reed Army Institute of Research, and many major U.S. academic centers involved in the HIV vaccine effort. Fueled by successes of other viral vaccines (especially the recombinant subunit surface-protein hepatitis B vaccine) and neutralizing antibody passive transfer experiments showing protection in chimpanzees,[131,132] an argument was made that without known correlates of protection, "the only way we will know a vaccine is likely to be effective is to try it in humans".[133,134] It was also reasoned that even a partially effective vaccine applied to the burgeoning pandemic, especially in developing countries unable to afford expensive ARV medications, mathematically[112,134] could prevent a great deal of death and human suffering, and slow the spread of the infection, until a more effective vaccine could be found.[133,134]

The debate regarding movement of these envelope (Env) immunogens into larger phase III trials became quite intense on a few occasions.[115,135] Protection was not seen in rhesus macaques studies. The immunogens were two monomeric Env antigens,[136] and by the time the trial started (1998), the natural turmeric envelope structure was better understood. The immunogen was also found to be type-specific—the antibodies which were produced, neutralized laboratory-adapted viral isolates but failed to neutralize primary isolates circulating in the community[94]—and it was known that the immunogen did not enter the major histocompatibility complex (MHC) class I pathway and, therefore, could not induce a cytotoxic T lymphocyte (CTL) response.

Despite this, a decision was made to proceed, so the first two phase III HIV vaccine trials went forward[115,137,138]—utilizing AIDSVAX, VaxGen's monomeric envelope recombinant glycoprotein 120 (rgp120) in alum bivalent (B/B and B/E) vaccines.[131–142] One trial took place in the U.S., Canada, and the Netherlands, and the other in Thailand. About 115 volunteers were enrolled and were followed by the Kansas City AIDS Research Consortium (principal investigator, David McKinsey), one of many communities who participated in this landmark trial (**Figure 41–2**) which evaluated 5,403 volunteers (5,095 men and 308 women) overall. The study reported that 5.7% of the vaccinated and 5.8% of the placebo recipients became infected, showing no protection. A large group of the world's most productive and respected vaccine researchers predicted this result, based on the phase II trial data.[17] When both rgp120 trials as well as an earlier MicroGeneSys/WRAIR gp160 Env trial[134] failed to how any protection,[137–140] the emphasis shifted to T-cell vaccines.

T Cell Vaccines and the STEP Trial

The precise role played by HIV-specific CTLs in HIV infection remains controversial.[65] T cell vaccines do not prevent infection; rather, it is proposed that they work by controlling viral replication. There has been shown to be a lower initial burst of virus (and, therefore, a lower peak), lower overall virus produced in the early stages of infection,[11,40] and a reduction in subsequent viral set point during chronic infection[8,10,26,39,40,41] (**Figure 41–3**). With these reduced levels of virus, there is a hope of less severe gut CD4 depletion[40] (although this occurs very rapidly in the earliest weeks of infection[45]) and a reduced risk for secondary HIV transmission in a vaccinated population.[39,47,57]

These responses do not prevent infection of latent reservoirs of viral infection.[40,41,72] Replication continues, and most individuals progress eventually to AIDS.[10,23,57] This includes those with the favorable HLA-B27 immunodominant-restricted epitope, as late escape with progression to AIDS in a patient after 9 to 12 years of epitope stability and long-term nonprogression

---

Kansas City AIDS Research Consortium
Announces the Opening of the First Phase III Trial for

AIDSVAX

a potential HIV prevention vaccine.

This trial is the first major study of a vaccine that might prevent AIDS.
5000 people at approximately 30 sites in North America will participate.
This study will test the ability of AIDSVAX, compared to placebo, to prevent HIV infection in people at risk for HIV.
It will also study the safety of AIDSVAX compared to a placebo vaccine.

To enroll, you must be: HIV-negative and a man who has sex with men or
A woman who has had one sexually-transmitted disease (STD)
and more than one sex partner in the last year
You CANNOT enroll if you are an injection drug user

Please do not enroll in this study because you believe you can then go out and have unsafe sex. YOU CAN'T!
There is no guarantee you will receive AIDSVAX rather than placebo.
There is no guarantee AIDSVAX will work.
The trial will last for up to four years.
There will be three primary shots (day 0, months 1 and 6) followed by four booster shots (months 12, 18, 24, and 30).
Each day, 16,000 people are infected with HIV worldwide.
Vaccines offer our best hope of ending the AIDS epidemic – worldwide and here in Kansas City.
This is your chance to become part of the solution.

For more information please call (816) 931-5477

Figure 41–2.

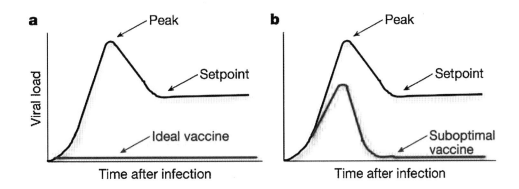

Figure 41–3. *Goals of an HIV-1 vaccine. After infection, HIV-1 replicates exponentially to a peak level and then is partially controlled to a viral set point level (black). (a) An ideal vaccine would protect against infection and afford sterilizing immunity (red). (b) A suboptimal vaccine would result in decreased peak and set point viral loads after infection (red). Source: Barouch D. Challenges in the development of an HIV-1 vaccine. Nature 2008;455:613–619. Used by permission of the publisher.*

was described by Goulder.[65] Even in the Nairobi prostitute cohort, protection eventually failed without continuous exposure to antigen.[82]

The T cell vaccine concept is based on human, in vitro, and in vivo animal model studies showing the importance of CD8 cytotoxic T cell responses in early and subsequent control of HIV infection, and SIV and chimeric SHIV infection in nonhuman primates.[39,40] The appearance of CTL responses correlates temporally with control of acute-phase viremia.[11,23,67] Highly and polyfunctional CTL responses appear to help explain long-term, nonprogressing patients, including the rare elite controllers[73,74,77,78]—individuals whose HIV RNA remains undetectable in the absence of antiretroviral treatment. Pathogenic SIV challenge in macaques vaccinated with live attenuated SIV[100] as well as DNA prime/viral vector boost strategies[98] results in controlled infection characterized by low levels of viremia, stable CD4+ cell counts, and slow (or no) disease progression up to 40 weeks (the duration of the experiment). CD8 cell depletion studies[38] indicate that cellular immune responses contribute to these effects.

A study by Wilson[98] and colleagues is particularly instructive. Eight rhesus macaques were vaccinated with three DNA primes and a single nonreplicating adenovirus type 5 (Ad5) boost, with both the DNA and Ad5 vectors expressing all the proteins in the SIV proteome except for Env (excluded as their intention was to explore the role of vaccine-induced cellular responses in control of virus replication). The animals were Mamu-A*02 (not one of the alleles associated with natural control of replication). The vaccine induced high-frequency T cell responses, as measured by interferon-gamma (INFγ) Elispot. At 61 weeks after the first DNA vaccination, the control and vaccinated animals were challenged with repeated mucosal exposures to 800 $TCID_{50}$ (1.2×10^7 viral copies/L) of heterologous swarm virus $SIV_{SM}E660$. So as to mimic the human infection situation as much as possible, the animals were given a "within-clade challenge" that was titrated so that one to three variants crossed the mucous membrane. As expected, the vaccine did not offer protection against acquisition of SIV infection. It took an average of four challenges to infect the vaccinated animals and four challenges to infect the control animals. The results however, from the challenge of the animals which received the vaccine, were quite unexpected. At 40 weeks postinfection, virus could not be detected in six of the eight vaccinated animals. Six of the eight had acute peaks of less than 1 million copies/mL, then leveled off to less than 10,000 copies/mL later in the acute phase, and an average control of virus of approximately 210 copies/mL in the chronic phase.

This is impressive control compared to that seen in control animals, in which peak viremias were over 1 million copies/mL, and chronic virus levels averaged approximately 80,000 copies/mL. The control of acute-phase viremia was postulated to have reduced damage to the all important memory CD4 compartment, allowing a robust T cell response to the infecting virus.

Letvin[53] and others, using DNA prime, adenoviral vector boost immunogens, have found a reduction in viremia restricted to the early phase of SIV infection but a prolonged survival despite loss of viral control.[53,54,55] This was determined to be associated with preserved central memory CD4+ T lymphocytes and could be predicted by the magnitude of the vaccine-induced cellular immune response.[53,55] Preservation of SIV-specific central memory CD8+ T lymphocyte response, a linked SIV-specific CD4+ T lymphocyte response as well as SIV-specific INF-γ, tumor necrosis factor-alpha (TNF-α), and interleukin (IL)-2-producing T lymphocytes were all found to be responsible for the prolonged survival.[54] Importantly, antibodies that neutralized the primary isolate of SIV used for challenge were also induced by vaccination.

Most of these T cell vaccines over the last decade have used DNA vaccination techniques,[144–150] viral vectors,[151–153] or both in a DNA prime, viral vector boost format.[154,155] There were concerns with pre-existing immunity to the viral vector, but these were primarily concerns regarding competing vector-directed immune responses lessening the HIV-specific T cell response, and the DNA prime was felt to be part of the solution.[155]

The Merck & Co. STEP trial was a ~3000 person phase IIB test of concept trial. There was no control of viremia or protection from HIV infection. However, the trial also caught us a bit off guard with the finding of a greater risk for HIV infection (than placebo) in those vaccinated who had pre-existing immunity (antibodies) to Ad5, (hazard ratio, 2.3; 95% CI, 1.2–4.3), and in those who were uncircumcised (HR 3.8; 95% CI, 1.5–9.3), but especially those with both factors.[6,7,9–14] The geometric mean plasma HIV RNA levels in placebo and vaccinated subjects who acquired HIV were comparable.

The vaccine field had embraced the more novel concept of using viral vectors with or without a DNA prime in order to induce cellular immune T cell responses, and STEP was the first test of efficacy of a T-cell–only HIV vaccine. Initiated in 2004, the trial immunogen was a trivalent, recombinant, replication-defective adenovirus serotype 5 vector expressing HIV Gag, Pol, and Nef proteins. Between 30% and 40% of individuals in the U.S. and Western Europe and 80% to 90% of persons from Sub-Saharan Africa have pre-existing neutralizing Ad5 antibodies, so the impact of the antibodies on HIV-specific immunity induction was somewhat predicted.[10]

Initial support for its use came from protection seen against the SHIV challenge model but only in monkeys with favorable (naturally protective) MHC alleles. In the more pathogenic and representative SIVmac model with differing MHC types, no protection was seen even with homologous challenge.[14] The simplest explanation for why STEP failed is that the vaccine-induced CTL responses were of insufficient magnitude and breadth as seen in phase I studies, where the vaccines induced responses to a median of only one Gag peptide epitope and a median of three epitopes (total) to any of the three expressed vaccine proteins.[7,12,13,14,179] This is far less than the median of 14 CTL epitope responses observed in natural infection in which these responses fail to prevent disease progression. Measuring the *function* of CD8+ T cell responses (e.g., cytotoxic killing, breadth of CTL, specificity of CTL, avidity, proliferation, coexpression of two or more cytokines including IL-2, INF-γ, and TNF-α), although more burdensome, may be more relevant and predictive of protection.[10–14]

When the STEP trial failed, the natural reaction was to abandon T cell approaches. David Baltimore and other experts think that this is "no time to give up" in our pursuit of a T cell vaccine or, more likely, a vaccine which elicits both T cell responses and neutralizing antibodies.[14]

Bruce Walker expressed this especially well,[14] writing: "far more selectivity than hereto in advancing immunogens to large-scale clinical trials is required. The mantra of 'the only way we will know it is likely to be effective is to try it in humans' is not appropriate, given the current state of knowledge. Trust in science, making full use of the tool kit that is provided by molecular biology, immunology, virology, structural biology, chemistry, and genomics is crucial. There is a critical need to understand how other vaccines work, with a level of detail that has never been necessary for pathogens less adapted to immune evasion. *The way forward is without question very difficult, and the possibility of failure high, but the global need is absolutely desperate, and this is an endeavor that must be pursued, now with greater passion than ever.*"

The results of STEP did have a major impact on several other trials. HVTN 503 (Phambili), a parallel phase IIb proof of concept 3000-subject trial in South Africa using the exact same vaccine, was cancelled while the NIH Vaccine Research Center (VRC) PAVE 100 trial—which was originally planned as a large phase IIb trial—was redesigned (it may only enroll *Ad5 antibody negative* subjects) and reduced significantly in size.[8]

In the wake of the STEP trial, a vaccine summit was held at which NIAID's HIV vaccine research priorities were re-examined and articulated,[11] along with a call, once again (and reminiscent of Bernard Fields' 1994 *Nature* article[156]) to get back to basic virology/immunology/pathogenesis research. The priorities discussed at the summit were as follows:

- Further define the first events leading to HIV and SIV entering the gut-associated lymphoid tissue
- Determine the rate and mechanisms by which immune cells are mobilized to the site of infection and whether innate responses can alter the course of infection
- Characterize the cellular and humoral immune responses needed to control viral replication through modulation and/or elimination of specific cell subsets in the SIV model and studies of HIV-infected populations
- Determine the three-dimensional structure of HIV envelope trimer
- Determine why broadly neutralizing antibodies are uncommon and how they can be elicited
- Define the specificities of antibodies that neutralize diverse primary isolates
- Develop more relevant animal models (and challenge viruses) to explore protection or enhancement of infection or disease, especially heterologous challenge models
- Determine why SIV is apathogenic in some nonhuman primate species
- Identify correlates of vaccine-induced immune protection, especially the mechanisms whereby nonpathogenic (e.g., attenuated) SIVs prevent infection by a pathogenic virus.

Vaccine Strategies for Dealing With Viral Diversity

Any successful HIV-1 vaccine strategy must take into account the extreme sequence diversity of the virus. It is highly unlikely that a person will encounter in the natural sexual transmission setting the exact viral strain or strains with which they were vaccinated. Since HIV made its debut in man around 70 years ago,[83,157] it has mutated and diversified rapidly now comprising a number of subtypes and circulating recombinant forms. HIV's inherently error-prone reverse transcriptase enzyme (which lacks proofreading mechanisms) leads to the creation of swarms or "quasi-species" of viruses which are antigenically heterogeneous.[47b] Circulating strains can differ from one another by up to 20% in the more conserved proteins and by as much as 35% in the envelope proteins.

This spread and the absence of an effective vaccine are to a large degree the consequence of the ability of HIV-1 to evade antibody-mediated neutralization.[83] This is highly problematic both for neutralizing antibody responses directed against the viral envelope but also for virus-specific CD8+ T cell responses. Moreover, primary isolates have no main neutralizing determinant with each isolate having distinct neutralizing targets. The predominant clade or clades causing the HIV epidemic in various regions of the world are unique and in some cases vary country to country, with viruses within clades varying by up to 20% and up to 35% between clades,[157] increasing the need for immunogens conferring cross-strain CTL responses, and neutralizing antibodies (or most likely both) that are effective against a broad diversity of HIV stains. Otherwise the very expensive approach of developing and testing (in clinical trials) several "regional HIV vaccines" will be necessary.[157,158]

Potential solutions for increasing the breadth of T cell response compared with the narrow, focused, and "type-specific" responses to natural protein immunogens used in the earlier advanced stage VaxGen and STEP vaccine trials include polyepitope vaccines (natural and

TABLE 41–4	Broadly Neutralizing Antibodies[19,21,70]	
	Broadly Neutralizing Abs	**Target Recognized**
	b12, VRC01, VRC02	CD4 binding site of gp120
	CD4i Abs	Coreceptor binding site of gp120
	447-52D, PG9, PG16	V3 loop of ggp120
	2G12	Glycans on the silent face of gp120
	2F5, 4E10	Membrane-proximal external region (MPER) of gp120

mosaic), conserved region vaccines, central vaccines[93,158–160] (using ancestral sequences, consensus sequences and center-of-tree sequences), and vaccines where immune escape has a fitness cost to the virus.

Broadly neutralizing antibody responses are known to occur (**Table 41–4**), but are rare in the infected population,[19,21,70] and designing a vaccine immunogen able to elicit them, described by some as "the holy grail of HIV vaccine development,"[10,39] will be extremely difficult and so far has eluded the best minds and teams of scientists.[25,57,113,157,159] Preclinical studies of intravenously infused broadly neutralizing monoclonal antibodies in nonhuman primates (rhesus macaques) have provided proof of principle that such antibodies are capable of conferring protection from vaginal[103,107,108] and oral[109] (model exposing newborn macaques oral cavity to SHIV shortly after birth) exposure to chimeric SIV/HIV (SHIV).

In a recent comprehensive review of the state of vaccine science which catalogs many of the most important "knowable unknowns," Drs. Herbert Virgin and Bruce Walker comment that "even if we knew what we wanted to induce in a vaccine, the science of engineering specific immune responses to exceed the capacity of natural immune response is in its infancy."[57]

HIV has evolved numerous strategies to evade host neutralizing antibody responses such as decoy mechanisms diverting immune recognition away from envelope regions critical for viral receptor binding, ineffective antibody production directed against viral debris such as monomeric gp120 rather than the intact HIV-1 Env trimer on the virion surface, glycan shielding of potential neutralization epitopes, steric occlusion, islands of variation, and conformational changes of the envelope which allows some critical structures to be available for receptor recognition of the virus but hidden from the immune system.[10,23,40,57,58,67,70]

To facilitate viral entry, the gp120 glycoprotein must bind to the cell surface,[41] alter its conformation to reveal a site for coreceptor attachment, and trigger conformational rearrangments in the gp41 glycoprotein to mediate fusion of viral and host cell membranes.[161] The conserved CD4 binding site is a target for broadly reactive neutralizing antibodies (NAbs) but is buried in a recessed pocket. The conserved chemokine receptor binding site and key epitopes in the membrane proximal external region of gp41 appear to be formed only transiently during the membrane fusion process. Additionally the virus can rapidly escape host NAbs by mutating glycans on the Env surface.[10] With established infection, the very rapid evolution of the virus will ultimately triumph by the selection of variants that are resistant to the most broadly neutralizing antibodies.[31,58-60,70] However, if the antibodies are present before infection (via vaccination) and before diversification, then they are likely to be much more effective.[70]

Two strategies are proposed to surmount all of these barriers the envelope protein poses and hopefully someday solve the "neutralizing antibody problem."[58] First is examination of known broadly neutralizing antibodies (2F5, 2G12, 4E10 and b12) and the second is analysis of functional constraints to identify potential sites of vulnerability.[161] Rational vaccine design from studies providing increased structural and functional understanding of HIV-1 Env are beginning to demonstrate that despite its tremendous complexity, solving the "HIV envelope problem" and eliciting broadly neutralizing antibodies may in fact be within our reach.[159]

Combining analysis of function with clues from the broadly neutralizing antibody (BNAb), b12, Zhou and colleagues[161] were able to structurally define a conserved neutralization epitope on gp120 which represents a site of vulnerability related to a functional requirement for efficient association of a conformationally invariant surface of the virus (overlapping a distinct subset of the CD4 binding site) with CD4, which can be targeted by antibody for neutralization. Expanded breadth of virus neutralization after immunization with a multiclade envelope vaccine candidate[162] has been demonstrated as has cross-clade binding and neutralization by a clade C Env variable (V3) region immunogen.[163] X-ray crystallographic studies allowing comparison of prefusion, unliganded SIV gp120 core to its CD4-bound structure,[164] and the comparison of two poorly binding CD4-binding site (CD4BS) antibodies complexed with gp120 with the bound conformation of the rare broadly neutralizing CD4BS antibody, b12, revealed the structural basis for immune evasion at the site of CD4 attachment on HIV-1 gp120 for the first time.[165] Another study revealed enhanced exposure of the conformationally conserved outer domain CD4-binding site to neutralizing antibodies by design of a membrane anchored HIV-1 gp120 outer domain protein[166] which the authors feel is a viable immunogen candidate.

Large-scale efforts are now focused on further dissecting these broadly neutralizing antibody binding sites on HIV and reverse engineering immunogens capable of eliciting antibodies with similar potency and breadth of neutralization.[4]

An especially large and critical segment of the neutralizing antibody mountain has been successfully scaled in the last two years. The identification of two novel potent and broadly neutralizing monoclonal antibodies, PG9 and PG16, were found from a process that involved the systematic screening of about 1800 individuals from five continents followed by high-throughput neutralization screening of antibody-containing culture supernatants from about 30,000 activated memory B-cells from a single clade A African donor.[19]

Recently a team at Merck provided reverse engineering proof of principle by showing that they could identify an HIV entry-blocking (neutralizing) immunogen (peptide mimetic of the gp41 prehairpin fusion intermediate) starting from an HIV-specific antibody.[22] A polyclonal antibody response was elicited in animals that neutralized tier 1 HIV-1 and simian HIV primary isolates in vitro, which is seen as an important starting point for the design of more potent immunogens to elicit a broadly neutralizing response against the gp42 prehairpin intermediate.[22]

In mid-2010 a team of scientists from the Vaccine Research Center at the NIAID described a process of engineering two novel exceptionally potent and broadly cross-reactive neutralizing antibodies, VCR01 and VCR02, a pair of somatic variants which target the functionally conserved and complementary CD4 binding site (CD4BS) of the HIV spike protein of gp120.[21] Using their knowledge of HIV-1 envelope (Env) structure they developed antigenically resurfaced glycoproteins specific for the structurally conserved site of CD4 binding to use as "probes" to identify sera with NAbs to the CD4BS and to isolate individual B cells from such an HIV donor. By expressing immunoglobulin genes from individual cells, they were able to identify the broadly neutralizing antibodies.

Analysis of HIV isolates susceptible to neutralization by these antibodies suggests that **the combination of the two somatic variant antibodies would be expected to neutralize more than 95% of globally diverse isolates of HIV.**

In a second equally impressive study[20] they describe how through partial receptor mimicry and extensive affinity maturation they were able to facilitate neutralization of HIV by natural human antibodies. VRC01 partially mimics CD4 interaction with gp120. A shift from the CD4-defined orientation focuses VRC01 onto the vulnerable site of initial CD4 attachment, allowing it to overcome the glycan and conformational masking that diminishes the neutralization potency of most CD4 binding site antibodies.

The Human Factor: Ethically Testing HIV Vaccines in Clinical Efficacy Trials in the Developed and the Developing World

Conducting HIV vaccine human trials in the U.S. and other industrialized nations poses some unique challenges for the research and at risk communities, government officials, and potential sponsors.[167–169] As difficult as some of these individual and community responses are to predict and prepare for, they certainly pale in comparison to the challenges and special ethical considerations involved in bringing vaccines and vaccine clinical trials to the rest of the world where the devastation of AIDS and the need for a safe and effective vaccine are so very clear.[170–172]

Ever since the world became aware of the post-ACTG 076 (the study where zidovudine reduced maternal-fetal transmission by 66%) conduct of *placebo-controlled* trials of "less intensive" and "less expensive" maternal to fetal (vertical) transmission prevention regimens[173,174] we hopefully have had our eyes opened wide to the potential for scientists, trying to design the perfect study, to treat a vulnerable person or population of persons in an unethical manner.

It also touched off a huge debate that continues to this day regarding to whose standards of care should participants, providers of care during a trial, clinical researchers, and trial sponsor's be held, and what is considered ethical and unethical care and support during a trial.[172–176]

A systematic review of HIV, TB, and malaria trials and standards of care in Sub-Saharan Africa[172] found that in the case of HIV trials only 16% provided care that met standard of care guidelines to both intervention and control patients. At the time of the review (2004, meaning articles included were likely describing studies done before 2003), only one of 34 trials in HIV-infected patients provided antiretroviral treatment. Issues of sustainability, care and research infrastructure, transparency, fairness, inclusion, and the local level of care are also important considerations. Finally, of the trials (81%) that reported on the process of ethical review, all were reviewed by a host African institution and 64% were additionally reviewed by an institution in a developed country.

The World Health Organization and the Joint United Nations Programme on HIV/AIDS (UNAIDS) indicate that if the pandemic proceeds at its current rate, there will be 45 million new infections by 2010 and nearly 70 million deaths by 2020.[157] The large majority of persons living with and dying from HIV/AIDS in the world are infected with HIV clades other than clade B (which comprises only 10% of the global HIV infection burden).

Clade C prevails in Africa and is responsible for nearly half of worldwide infections. In some areas of Sub-Saharan region the epidemiologically unlinked prevalence of subtype C infection exceeds 30% of the population.[157] Clade C is predominant in India, E/CRF01 (circulating recombinant form 01) in Southeast Asia, and a mixture of clades in other parts of the world (for example, Clades B and C in Brazil, B/CRF01/CRF07/CRF08 in China, and a "United Nations of different clades" [A, F, D, C] in the unique epidemic in the Democratic Republic of Congo).

Regarding the choice of vaccine components in developing counties, rather than using actual viruses from within the host county's population, one approach which has both economic and political advantages, is to construct either a consensus sequence or an ancestral sequence reconstructed on the basis of an evolutionary model.[157] Such sequences have the advantage of being central and most similar to currently circulating strains and may have enhanced potential to elicit cross-reactive responses. The economic advantage is that it is not feasible to duplicate vaccine design efforts using country-specific strains for every nation and region that needs a vaccine. Politically, these artificial sequences are not associated with any specific country of origin, so host nations would not need to contend with being asked to host a vaccine trial using HIV-1 antigens from distant geographic origins.[157]

In the early 1990s, the HIVNET national vaccine preparedness consortium of clinical sites did important preparatory work for eventual vaccine trials. They sought to determine how interested "at-risk" populations might be in enrolling in a preventative HIV vaccine study. What factors correlated with their interest in or intention to enroll? What were their concerns regarding vaccinations? What would likely be their risk behavior going forward in the setting of regular prevention counseling?

This last question relates to the interesting moral, ethical, and vaccine clinical trial design/power calculation assumptions dilemma. Namely, would there be enough continued risk-taking behavior, despite the site's best honest, ethical, good-faith attempts to help volunteers lower/eliminate risk through prevention counseling, for a placebo-controlled vaccine trial to have enough infection events to obtain a statistically valid answer to the question regarding a particular vaccine's preventative efficacy?

The U.S. HIVNET's study on readiness for vaccine efficacy trials[167b] found that 77% of potential volunteers would definitely (27%) or probably (50%) be willing to participate in a randomized vaccine trial, with increased willingness associated with high-risk behaviors, lower education level, being uninsured or covered by public insurance, and not having been in a previous vaccine preparedness study. Altruism and a desire for protection were major motivators, while major concerns were HIV seropositivity/reactivity due to the vaccine, safety of the vaccine, and possible problems with insurance or travel. Baseline knowledge of vaccine trial concepts was low.[167b] Other studies have found reluctance to adopt partial efficacy vaccines, and a likelihood to increase sexual risk behavior in response to vaccine availability.[168,169]

Additional considerations and issues among vaccine trial participants in the developed world include vaccine-induced seropositivity[177] (VISP), behavior disinhibition (risk compensation),[178–180] various motivators for testing outside of the trial setting,[181] and unblinding.

Interestingly, VISP occurred in 42% of those receiving vaccines overall but varied widely across different vaccine product types and testing assays: Ad5, 86.7%; poxvirus alone or as boost, 53.4%; DNA-alone products, 6.3%. For testing assays, the highest VISP was seen with HIV 1/2 (rDNA) EIA kit at 40.9% positive. Among 901 participants with VISP and a Western blot, ninety-two (10.2%) had a positive Western blot test (displaying an atypical pattern consistent with vaccine product) and 592 (65.7%) had an indeterminate Western blot result.[177]

One author wondered if behavioral disinhibition (risk compensation) might help explain the increased rate of infection among those with positive rAd5 titers in the STEP study. He also recommended administering questionnaires to detect disinhibition during vaccine trials as well as prospectively screening with biologic markers (for sexually transmitted infections) as study participants who do guess their treatment allocation might give unreliable answers to cover up any increased risk taking.[178]

The Thai RV 144 Trial—First Small Signal of Vaccine Protection?

The live replicating canarypox vector ALVAC (Aventis Pasteur)/rpg120 (the Thai RV 144 trial)[15] was the second large HIV vaccine efficacy trial for which movement out of smaller phase I, I/II trials into a larger clinical efficacy trials, (in this case, a 16,000 person phase III trial), was somewhat controversial.[17] The canarypox (ALVAC) vector was known from multiple phase I and II trials to be poorly immunogenic.[17,152–154] Patients infected during T cell vaccine clinical trials must be provided with ARV treatment where appropriate and be followed with parameters such as mean HIV RNA levels and CD4+ cell counts before ARV treatment compared by study group randomization assignment. A composite end point—for example, an HIV RNA >55,000, CD4+ count <350, or receipt of ARVs—can also be monitored for and compared. In a phase II study of ALVAC with rpg120 or rpg160 boost (HVTN 203) none of these parameters in the patients receiving vaccination were significantly different from those of the control patients.[152]

The U.S. HIV Vaccine Trials Network (HVTN), the world's largest consortium of AIDS vaccine scientists and clinicians, cancelled its plans to do a phase III trial of the vaccine just one year previous to the planned start of RV 144. In an article in *Science* in 2004, the HVTN experts/scientists wrote that they saw no rationale to believe that combining two failed or weak concepts together should somehow be more likely to elicit T cell responses adequate for viral and disease control.[17] They expressed concerns regarding a weak study hypothesis that changed for no particularly good reason at the eleventh hour, the cost (~$119 million), and the lack of independent virologist and immunologist input.[17]

They also stated:

> *Society expects the scientific community to develop a vaccine to counter the AIDS pandemic, but there are adverse consequences to conducting large-scale trials of inadequate HIV-1 vaccines. We have recently seen two large phase III trials of immunogens that, all too predictably, failed to generate protective immunity. We seriously question whether it is sensible now to conduct a third trial that, in our opinion, is no more likely to generate a meaningful level of protection against infection or disease. One price for repetitive failure could be crucial erosion of confidence by the public and politicians in our capability of developing an effective vaccine collectively. This seems to us to be another readily predictable scenario that is best prevented.[17]*

In December 2009, results of the ALVAC/rgp120 Thai trial were published in the *New England Journal of Medicine*.[15] It was interpreted as the first signal, albeit fairly small, of protection from an HIV prophylactic vaccine by some.[4,5,16] What the data showed is currently being debated by experts all over the world and the publishing of the letters to the editor is eagerly awaited. The trial[15,18] utilized ALVAC-HIV canarypox vaccine vector expressing env-gag-pol (Sanofi-Pasteur) along with AIDSVAX™ B/E, the rgp120 monomeric envelope protein of Vax-Gen as the immunogens with ALVAC given at months 0, 1 and ALVAC plus rgp120 at months 3 and 6. It was sponsored by the U.S. Military HIV Research Program, the Thai Ministry of Public Health, the NIH, and Sanofi-Pasteur. The study enrolled 16,395 heterosexual men and women ages 18–30 at "community risk" from Rayong and Chon Buri provinces with 8,197 receiving vaccine while 8,198 received a placebo. The study began in 2003 and vaccinations ended in

2006. All volunteers received HIV prevention counseling and were followed with HIV testing every 6 months. The trial ended in June 2009.

In a modified intent-to-treat analysis (excluding 7 subjects found to be HIV-positive at baseline), 51/8197 (0.62%) HIV infections occurred among those vaccinated while 74/8198 (0.90%) HIV infections occurred among the placebo group for a 31.2% vaccine efficacy (95% CI, 1.1–52.1; P=0.04) or a 3.9% possibility this could be due to random chance. In the per protocol analysis (i.e., completed all vaccinations, n=12,542) which only included a subset (86/125) of HIV-infected volunteers, 26.2% vaccine efficacy was seen (95% CI, −13.3 to 51.9; P=0.16), with a 16% possibility this could be due to random chance. There was no difference in viral set point between the groups.

Questions regarding this trial posed by Dr. Martin Hirsch at Harvard Medical School's Intensive HIV Case-Based Update Conference in January 2010[18] included: "Is this result real evidence of protection, or due to chance? What are the implications of this finding on future HIV efficacy trials and/or public policy on HIV vaccination?" Intensive study of vaccine recipients who became infected, other secondary analysis, and much discussion and debate will no doubt follow for some time in order to better understand what we are seeing in this trial result.

An HIV Vaccine—What Lies Ahead in the Future?

It is indeed frustrating to have so many extremely dedicated, bright, and talented minds working so hard for an HIV preventative vaccine and over 20 years later to still be without clear evidence of vaccine protection. In the last two years however we have continued to see important gains in knowledge which led to the groundbreaking interdisciplinary work and the discovery of the broadest, most potent neutralizing antibodies yet, ones which should respond to more than 95% of isolates worldwide. We may have finally seen a first signal of protection and we may be on the (5- to 10-year) cusp of a major breakthrough if the trends of the last 2 years continue.

Because HIV initially establishes infection in a very small number of cells appropriate pre-existing mucosal immunity has the potential to prevent infection, clear infection, or limit replication so that gut CD4 depletion is lessoned and viral set point is low enough during chronic infection to limit disease progression and prevent person to person spread of the virus.[40,42,57]

In animal models both T cell responses and broadly reactive neutralizing antibodies have provided protection. Along with natural transmission success stories previously mentioned this suggests that the "induction of even modest protective immunity at mucosal surfaces may tip the balance toward less efficient spread of HIV."[57] Detailed studies of the earliest events in transmission in animal models and humans are needed to explain the resistance to infection which is seen in the vast majority of HIV exposures.[42,57]

Three vaccine concepts have advanced through large efficacy trials yet none have controlled viral replication in those who became infected. In contrast, a small minority of infected individuals are able to control HIV to undetectable viral levels without antiretroviral therapy and some SIV vaccines control pathogenic SIV replication to low levels. To solve this paradox there is so much more we must know and so much more that needs to be done. It is daunting to acknowledge that we still do not understand the nature of the immune response needed for protection. Finding answers to Virgin and Walker's "knowable unknowns" is an obvious and excellent blueprint for basic science foundational investigation and knowledge which will help the field move forward.

Defining relationships and potential synergies between CD4 T cell, CD8 T cell, antibody, and B cell responses during vaccination and in long-term viral controllers and elite controllers will be a key step toward engineering specific immune responses found to be important to prevention or control of HIV infection.[57] Clues to potential novel immune effector mechanisms may come from analyzing cellular HIV restriction and promotion factors. A larger emphasis and understanding of the antiviral effector functions of CD4 T cells and their role in control of HIV at mucosal sites and in vaccination and a more advanced exploration of antibody responses other than neutralization (ADCC, complement fixation, interactions with Fc receptors on granulocytes, macrophages, dendritic cells, B-cells) are also recommended.[57] Even study of HIV's tremendous diversity have helped define a potential weakness whereby we may be able to achieve effective immunization via an "evolutionary trap," driving HIV into a fitness dead end by targeting epitopes in fitness-critical regions of viral proteins.[57,183]

It has been pointed out that not all answers will come efficiently from studies of HIV noting a rich history of paradigm shifts based on studies of viruses and species not normally considered "AIDS related".[57] Examples include important discoveries in the areas of T cell exhaustion, T_{reg} cells, PD1, CTLA4, and inhibitory cytokines.[57]

Better integration of novel concepts and information from other fields of study with rapid translation into the HIV field and a redefining of "HIV research" to promote the integrated study of all mechanisms that may facilitate understanding HIV pathogenesis and immunity are critically important near-term objectives.[10,16,57] Barriers between AIDS efforts and other relevant scientific areas with previously untapped human and technological resources have been articulated.[16,57] These will need to be overcome in the future. To further accelerate HIV vaccine development alternative models for the conduct of HIV vaccine clinical trials,[184] and more flexible, longer-term, large-scale grant funding of translational HIV research programmes have also been proposed.[4,16,57]

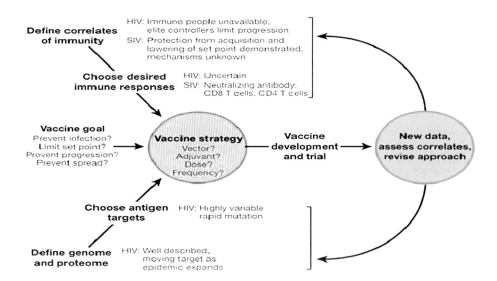

Figure 41-4. *Approach to vaccination and special challenges of HIV vaccination. Shown are the steps in development of a vaccine strategy for HIV. In **blue** are the key issues corresponding to each step that influence our capacity to immunize against HIV. Source: Virgin HW, Walker B. Immunology and the elusive AIDS vaccine. Nature 2010;464:224–231. Used by permission of the publisher.*

Barouch and Korber[10] cautioned that "it is likely that the path toward a successful HIV-1 vaccine will be a long one with multiple efficacy trial failures along the way" and that it is critical we not become paralyzed by disappointing results but rather that we continue to learn from vaccine trial failures in designing new vaccine candidates. Advances in our understanding of HIV pathogenesis and immunity should drive the movement of vaccine efficacy concepts along the clinical investigation pathway while human clinical efficacy trial results (successes and failures) must be carefully dissected and studied to inform the next generation of HIV vaccine efficacy trials (**Figure 41–4**)[57] until the goal off a safe and effective HIV vaccine is met.

It is important to remember that an HIV vaccine must be a part of a larger "prevention portfolio."[4,10,11] Bringing a partially effective HIV vaccine (one that prevents HIV transmission only partially or one that prevents or slows disease progression without preventing transmission, or does both) to regulatory approval, production, public and at-risk population acceptance, and widespread distribution will be quite challenging.[10,11] However, the future direction of the pandemic, and its tremendous toll on affected persons and society depends on our ultimate success in meeting and conquering this monumental challenge.

Acknowledgments

The authors would like to thank Ms. Amrita Burdick and Ms. Petra Bricker for their excellent assistance with literature searches, references, tables, and figures.

References

1. Gallo RC, Montagnier L. The discovery of HIV as the cause of AIDS. N Engl J Med 2003;349(24):283–285.
2. Center for Disease Control (CDC). Pneumocystis pneumonia: Los Angeles. MMWR Morb Mortal Wkly Rep 1981;30(21):250–252.
3. Center for Disease Control (CDC). Kaposi's sarcoma and Pneumocystis pneumonia among homosexual men: New York City and California. MMWR Morb Mortal Wkly Rep. 1981;30(25):305–308.
4. Koff WC, Berkley SF. The Renaissance in HIV Vaccine Development—Future Directions. N Engl J Med 2010 Jul 15. [Epub ahead of print] PubMed PMID: 20647186.
5. Folkers GK, Fauci AS. Controlling and ultimately ending the HIV/AIDS pandemic: A feasible goal. JAMA 2010;304(3):350–51.
6. Buchbinder SP, Mehrotra DV, Duerr A, et. al. Efficacy assessment of a cell-mediated immunity HIV-1 vaccine (the Step Study): a double-blind, randomized, placebo-controlled, test-of-concept trial. Lancet 2008;372(9653):1881–1893.
7. McElrath MJ, DeRosa SC, Moodie Z, et al. and the STEP Study Protocol Team. HIV-1 vaccine-induced immunity in the test of concept Step Study: A case-cohort analysis. Lancet 2008;372:1894–1905.
8. Barouch DH. Challenges in the development of an HIV-1 vaccine. Nature 2008 Oct 2;455(7213):613–619. PMID:18833271
9. Cohen J. AIDS research. Promising AIDS vaccine's failure leaves field reeling. Science 2007;318:28–29.
10. Barough HD, Korber B. HIV-1 vaccine development after STEP. Annu Rev Med 2010;61:153–167. PMID:20059334
11. Fauci AS, Johnston MI, Dieffenbach CW, et al. HIV Vaccine Research: The Way Forward. Science 2008;321(5888):530–532.
12. Panteleo G. HIV-1 T-cell vaccines: evaluating the next step. Lancet Infect Dis 2008;8:82–83.
13. Sekaly R-P. The failed HIV Merck vaccine study: a step back or a launching point for future vaccine development. J Exp Med 2008;205(1):7–12.
14. Walker BD, Burton DR. Towards an AIDS vaccine. Science 2008;320(5877):760–764.
15. Rerks-Ngarm S, Pitisuttithum P, Nitayaphan S. Vaccination with ALVAC and AIDSVAX to prevent HIV-1 infection in Thailand. N Engl J Med 2009;361:2209–2220.
16. Koff WC. Accelerating HIV vaccine development. Nature 2010;464(7286):161–162.

17. Burton DR, Desrosiers RC, Doms RW. Public health: a sound rationale needed for phase III HIV-1 vaccine trials. Science 2004;303:316.

18. Hirsch MS. Three decades of AIDS. What have we learned? Where are we going? Presented at: AIDS Medicine: An intensive case-based course 2010;Harvard Dept of Continuing Education. The Fairmont Copley Plaza, Boston, MA, January 11–12, 2010.

19. Walker LM, Phogat SK, Chan-Hui P-Y, et. al. Broad and potent neutralizing antibodies from an African donor reveal a new HIV-1 vaccine target. Science 2009;236:285–289.

20. Zhou T, Georgiev I, Wu X, et al. Structural Basis for Broad and Potent Neutralization of HIV-1 by Antibody VRC01. Science 2010 Jul 8. [Epub ahead of print] PubMed PMID:20616231.

21. Wu X, Tang ZY, Li Y, et al. Rational Design of Envelope Identifies Broadly Neutralizing Human Monoclonal Antibodies to HIV-1. Science 2010 Jul 8. [Epub ahead of print] PubMed PMID:20616233.

22. Bianchi E, Joyce JG, Miller MD, et al. Vaccination with peptide mimetics of the gp41 prehairpin fusion intermediate yields neutralizing antisera against HIV-1 isolates. Proc Natl Acad Sci 2010;107(23):10655–10660.

23. Levy JA. HIV Vaccines. In: Levy JA (Ed). HIV and the pathogenesis of AIDS (3rd Edition;2007) p. 397–428. Washington, DC: ASM Press.

24. Phillips DM. The role of cell-to-cell transmission in HIV infection. AIDS 1994;8:719–731.

25. Brander C, Frahm N, Walker BD. The challenge of host and viral diversity in HIV vaccine design. Current Opinion in Immunology. 2006;18:430–437.

26. Douek DC, Roederer M, Koup RA. Emerging concepts in the pathogenesis of AIDS. Annu Rev Med 2009;60:471–484.

27. Douek DC, Brenchley JM, Betts MR, et al. HIV preferentially infects HIV-specific CD4+ T cells. Nature 2002;95–98.

28. Yue FY, Kovacs CM, Dimayuga RC, et al. Preferential apoptosis of HIV-1-specific CD4+ T cells. J Immunol 2005;174:2196–2204.

29. Grossman Z, Meier-Schellersheim M, Sousa AE, Victorino RM, Paul WE. CD4+ T-cell depletion in HIV infection: are we closer to understanding the cause? Nature Med 2002;8:319–323.

30. Panteleo G, Soudeyns H, Demarest JF, et al. Evidence for rapid disappearance of initially expanded HIV-specific CD8+ T cell clones during primary infection. Proc Natl Acad Sci 1977;94:9848–9853.

31. Poignard P, Sabbe R, Picchio GR, et al. Neutralizing antibodies have limited effects on the control of established HIV-1 infection in vivo. Immunity 1999;10:431–438.

32. Hazenberg MD, Otto SA, Van Benthem BH, et al. Persistent immune activation in HIV-1 infection is associated with progression to AIDS. AIDS 2003;17:1881–1888.

33. Badley AD, Parato K, Cameron DW, et al. Dynamic correlation of apoptosis and immune activation during treatment of HIV infection. Cell Death Differ 1999;6:420–432.

34. Hunt PW, Martin JN, Sinclair E, et al. T cell activation is associated with lower Cd4+ T cell gains in human immunodeficiency virus-infected patients with sustained viral suppression during antiretroviral therapy. J Infect Dis 2003;187:1534–1543.

35. Ferandez S, Price P, McKinnon EJ, Nolan RC, French MA. Low CD4+ T-cell counts in HIV patients receiving effective antiretroviral therapy are associated with Cd4+ T-cell activation and senescence but not with lower effector memory T-cell function. Clin Immunol 2006;120:163–170.

36. Brenchley JM, Price DA, Schacker TW, et al. Microbial translocation is a cause of systemic immune activation in chronic HIV infection. Nat Med 2006;12:1365–1371.

37. Baum LL. Role of humoral immunity in host defense against HIV. Current HIV/AIDS Reports 2010;7(1):11–18.

38. Schmitz JE, Kuroda MJ, Santra S, et. al. Control of viremia in simian immunodeficiency virus infection by CD8+ lymphocytes. Science 1999;283:857–860.

39. Korber BT, Letvin NL, Haynes BF. T-cell vaccine strategies for human immunodeficiency virus, the virus with a thousand faces. J Virology 2009;83(17):8300–8314.

40. Johnston MI, Fauci AS. An HIV vaccine--evolving concepts. New Engl J Med 2007;356(20):2073–2081.

41. Cadogan M, Dalgleish AG. HIV immunopathogenesis and strategies for intervention. Lancet Infect Dis 2008;8(11):675–684.

42. Haase AT. Targeting early infection to prevent HIV-1 mucosal transmission. Nature 2010;464(7286):217–223.

43. Broliden K, Haase AT, Ahuja SK, Shearer GM, Andersson J. Back to basics: mucosa;immunity and novel HIV vaccine concepts. J Intern Med 2009;265(1):5–17. PMID:19093956.

44. Iqbal SM, Kaul R. Mucosal innate immunity as a determinant of HIV susceptibility. American Journal of Reproductive Immunology 2008;59(1):44–54.

45. Li Q, Duan L, Estes JD, et al. Peak SIV replications in resting memory CD4+ T cells depletes gut lamina propria CD4+ cells. Nature 2005;434:1148–1152.

151. Goepfert PA, Horton H, McElrath MJ, et al. High-dose recombinant canrypox vaccine expressing HIV-1 protein, in seronegative human subjects. J Infect Dis 2005;192:1249–1259.

152. Lee D, Graham BS, Chiu Y-L, et al. Breakthrough infections during phase 1 and 2 prime-boost HIV-1 vaccine trials with canarypox vectors (ALVAC) and booster dose of recombinant gp120 or gp160. J Infect Dis 2004;190:903–907.

153. Russell ND, Graham BS, Keefer MC. Phase 2 study of an HIV-1 canarypox vaccine (vCP1452) alone and in combination with rgp120: negative results fail to trigger a phase 3 correlates trial. J Acquir Immune Defic Syndr 2007;44:203–212.

154. Nitayaphan S, Pitisuttithum P, Karnasuta C, et al. Safety and immunogenicity of an HIV subtype B and E prime-boost vaccine in HIV-negative Thai adults. J Infect Dis 2004;190:702–706.

155. Yang ZY, Wyatt LS, Kong WP, Moodie Z, Moss B, Nabel GJ. Overcoming immunity to a viral vaccine by DNA priming before vector boosting. J Virol 203;77:799–803.

156. Fields BN. AIDS: time to turn to basic science. Nature 1994;369:94–96.

157. Gaschen B, et al. Diversity considerations in HIV-1 vaccine selection. Science 2002;296:2354.

158. Weaver EA, Lu Z, Camacho ZT, et al. Cross-subtype T-cell immune responses induced by a human immunodeficiency virus type 1 group M consensus Env immunogen. J Virol 2006;80(14):6745–6756.

159. Vaine M, Lu S, Wang S. Progress on the induction of neutralizing antibodies against HIV Type 1 (HIV-1). Biodrugs 2009;23(3):137–153.

160. Kong, W-P, Wu L, Wallstrom TC, et al. Expanded breadth of the T-cell response to mosaic human immunodeficiency virus type 1 envelope DNA vaccination. J Virol 2009;83(5):2201–2215.

161. Zhou T, Xu L, Dey B, et al. Structural definition of a conserved neutralization epitope on HIV-1 gp120. Nature 2007;445:732–737.

162. Chakrabarti BK, Ling X, Yang Z-Y, et al. Expanded breadth of neutralization after immunization with a multiclade envelope HIV vaccine candidate. Vaccine 2005;23(26): 3434–3445.

163. Wu L, Yang Z-Y, Xu L, et al. Cross-clade recognition and neutralization by the V3 region from clade C human immunodeficiency virus-1 envelope. Vaccine 2006;24(23): 4995–5002.

164. Chen B, Vogan EM, Gong H, Skehel JJ, Wiley DC, Harrison SC. Structure of an unliganded simian immunodeficiency virus gp120 core. Nature 2005;433:834–841.

165. Chen L, Kwon YD, Zhou T, et al. Structural basis of immune evasion at the site of CD4 attachment on HIV-1 gp120. Science 2009;326:1123–1127.

166. Wu L, Zhou T, Yang Z-Y, et al. Enhanced exposure of the CD4-binding site to neutralizing antibodies by structural design of a membrane anchored HIV-1 gp120 domain. J Virol 2009;83(10):5077–5086.

167. Celum CL, Buchbinder SP, Donnell D, et. al. Early human immunodeficiency virus (HIV) infection in the HIV Network for Prevention Trials Vaccine Preparedness Cohort: risk behaviors, symptoms, and early plasma and genital tract virus load. J Infect Dis 2001;183:23–35.

167b. Koblin BA, Heagery P, Sheon A, et al Readiness of high-risk populations in the HIV Network for prevention trials to participate in HIV vaccine efficacy trials in the United States. AIDS;1998;12:785–793.

168. Newman PA, Logie C. HIV vaccine acceptability: a systematic review and meta-analysis. AIDS 2010;24(11): 1749–1756.

169. Newman PA, Duan N, Rudy ET, Roberts KJ, Swendeman D. Posttrial HIV vaccine adoption: concerns, motivators, and intentions among persons at risk for HIV. J Aquir Immune Defic Syndr 2004;37(3):1393–1403.

170. Varmus H, Satcher D. Ethical complexities of conducting research in developing countries. N Engl J Med 1997;337:1003–1005.

171. Bloom BR. The highest attainable standard: ethical issues in AIDS vaccines. Science 1998;279:186–188.

172. Kent DM, Mwamburi DM, Bennish ML, Kupelnick B, Ioannidis JPA. Clinical trials in Sub-Saharan Africa and established standards of care: a systematic review of HIV, tuberculosis, and malaria trials. JAMA 2004;292:237–242.

173. Lurie P, Wolfe SM. Unethical trials of interventions to reduce perinatal transmission of the human immunodeficiency virus in developing countries. N Engl J Med 1997;337:853–856.

174. Angell M. The ethics of clinical research in the third world. N Engl J Med 1997;337:847–849.

175. Fitzgerald DW, Pape JW, Wasserheit JN, Counts GW, Corey L. Provision of treatment in HIV-1 vaccine trials in developing countries. Lancet 2003;362:993–994.

176. Douek DC, Kwong PD, Nabel GJ. The rational design of an AIDS vaccine. Cell 2006;124:677–681.

177. Cooper CJ, Metch B, Dragavon J, Coombs RW, Baden LR for the NAIAD HIV Vaccine trials Network (HVTN) vaccine-induced seropositivity (VISP) task force. Vaccine-induced seropositivity/reactivity in noninfected HIV vaccine recipients. JAMA 2010;304(3):275–283.

178. Hudson CP.HIV-1 Step study (letter to editor). Lancet 2009;373:805–806. In response to;Buchbinder SO, et al. Lancet 2008;372:1881–1893.

179. Buchbinder S, Duerr A, Robertson MN (author response to letters) Lancet 2009;373:806.

180. Eaton LA, Kalichman S. Risk compensation in HIV prevention: implications for vaccines, microbicides, and other biomedical HIV prevention technologies. Curr HIV/AIDS Rep 2007;4:165–1672.

181. Gust DA, Wiegand RE, Para M, Chen RT, Bartholow BN. HIV testing outside of the study among men who have sex with men participating in an HIV vaccine efficacy trial. J Acquir Immune Defic Syndr 2009;52(2):294–298.

182. Dolin R. HIV Vaccine Trial Results—An Opening for Further Research. N Engl J Med 2009;361: 2279-2280.

183. Fischer W, et al. Polyvalent vaccines for optimal coverage of potential T-cell epitopes in global HIV-variants. Nature Med 2007;13:100–106.

184. Excler J-L, Rida W, Priddy F, Fast P, Koff W. A strategy for accelerating development of preventative AIDS vaccines. AIDS 2007;21:2259–2263.

Chapter 42 FUTURE DIRECTIONS

PEDRO CAHN

Every man is responsible for what he didn't try to avoid

—JEAN-PAUL SARTRE

The best moment to plant a tree was twenty years ago.
The second best is today.

—ANONYMOUS AFRICAN PROVERB

The Current Situation

AIDS certainly is a different kind of disease. No other medical event in human history has generated such a variety of consequences in almost all aspects of society as the HIV/AIDS epidemic.

For instance, the only health issue that has ever become a subject for debate at the United Nations Security Council and that has also given place to a Special Session of the UN General Assembly is the AIDS pandemic. In addition, the most powerful nations have included AIDS in the G8 agenda on a regular basis. No other disease has been indicated as a "threat to the world security." In 2000, the United States National Intelligence Council (NIC) issued "The Global Infectious Disease Threat and Its Implications for the United States." Six months later, the UN Security Council passed Resolution 1308, stating that "the HIV/AIDS pandemic, if unchecked, may pose a risk to stability and security."[1]

It is not easy to look at the future in relation to this multifaceted and complex epidemic, in view of the particularly difficult time in the global response to AIDS. As stated by the International AIDS Society,[2] scaling up prevention, treatment, care, and support while fostering research are as important as ever, yet interest in AIDS is waning in some countries and complacency is growing among many political leaders and communities.

Two critical global milestones have been set by the UN General Assembly—the goal of achieving universal access to HIV prevention, treatment, care, and support by 2010, and the Millennium Development Goals (MDGs), including the goal of halting and reversing the spread of HIV by 2015. Governments and the civil society will have to redouble their efforts to reach these goals. However, there is another challenge—to think what the global response will be in case the world does not meet the 2010 and 2015 deadlines, which seems very likely. Unfortunately, AIDS continues to have a catastrophic impact on many countries and their citizens. Although global prevalence appears to be stabilizing, it is at the alarmingly high level of over 30 million people. Thousands of new cases of HIV infection continue to occur every day, and for every two people who start antiretroviral treatment, another five acquire HIV.[3]

Why is this happening? There is no single, straightforward response to this question.

Too many countries have yet to implement scientifically proven risk reduction measures (such as needle and syringe programs and opioid substitution therapy) or programs that target populations at high risk for HIV (such as men who have sex with men [MSM] and sex workers). The underlying factors that put women and girls at increased risk—including violence and unequal access to education and services—are still not tackled effectively. Human rights violations, stigmatization, and discrimination continue to fuel vulnerability and hinder effective HIV prevention, treatment, and care.

There are examples of substantial progress in the fight against AIDS, demonstrating what leadership, determination, and planning can achieve. More countries have completed national AIDS plans. More importantly, they are implementing them and gaining support to do so from political leaders. Investment in prevention has resulted in the decline in the rate of new HIV infections in some countries, including several in Sub-Saharan Africa, and the number of people receiving treatment is rising steadily.

AIDS and Poverty: The Perverse Vicious Circle

Poverty and inequality have been described as the major driving forces of our inability to curb the epidemic. There is one fundamental difference, however, between AIDS and other health problems generally linked with poverty. Unlike diseases such as tuberculosis (TB) and malaria, HIV is mostly transmitted through sex.[4]

In other words, the extent to which individuals are able to make and exercise choices about sexual behavior is, in many cases, certainly linked to economic dependence. With women, economic and social safety is largely dependent on their partners' activities and they have little choice, if any, to determine their own sexual behavior. When commercial sex work as the only chance to survive comes into the equation, the consequences can be catastrophic.

The fact that, in many regions, most of the people living with HIV are poor probably indicates the fact that the epidemic has now spread throughout the general population in a certain geographic area with a high proportion of poor people. As Piot and colleagues[4] highlight, many researchers now point not to poverty itself but to economic and gender inequalities and weakened "social cohesion" as factors influencing sexual behavior and, hence, the potential for HIV transmission. Having said that, no level of economic affluence may serve as a safe haven against HIV infection. AIDS being the so-called new epidemic among middle-class MSM in the U.S. is a good example of the absence of affluence borders that could preclude the expansion and perpetuation of the epidemic. The factors encompassing the impact of poverty on the epidemic are called the "upstream effects"; in contrast, the impact of AIDS on poverty and development has been described as the "downstream effect." AIDS increases both poverty and income inequality at the individual and family levels, but it also has a significant impact on the economy of most of the countries where the epidemic is generalized.

For instance, in Botswana, a country with a heavy burden of HIV cases, projected estimates are that the number of households living in poverty will increase at a rate that is 0.5% higher per year than if there were no AIDS.[5] Regarding the impact on GDP, a reduction of about 0.5%–

1.5% in the growth rate over a 10- to 20-year time frame is expected, compared to the same situation without AIDS.[6] In addition, Piot highlights that:

> *Some researchers have drawn attention to the longer term potential for progressive weakening of human capital, and the lost transmission of knowledge and skills between generations. This is of particular concern given the increasing recognition that AIDS is a long-term phenomenon for which long-term strategies are required.*[4]

At the individual level, people get sick and die at ages when they are supposed to work and, with their income and taxes, support the needs of people who are unable to generate their own income—for example, the elderly, children, and sick or disabled patients. Medical and funeral-related costs are to be added to the negative side of the equation.

It is worth noting that the financial implications of providing universal access to ARV therapy have not been considered in this chapter yet and will be discussed later. In any case, at least for the moment, consideration should be given to the fact that, even if drugs were provided for free, poor families may have insufficient resources to meet basic nutrition needs or the costs of travel to health clinics for care.[7]

Several issues have been mentioned as part of the hidden costs,[8] including ART interruption driven by stock shortages, binge drinking, and slimming symptoms, driving to the conclusion that "food supply programs and minimization of ARV shortage may reduce ART interruptions."

Kruk et al. studied the hidden costs for transportation and concluded that costs in health care delivery might jeopardize the success of "free services." For instance, more than 50% of the delivery costs in a TB program in rural Tanzania were for transport.[9]

The CCaSaNet cohort study (the Caribbean, Central America and South America Network, part of the International Databases to Evaluate AIDS, supported by the U.S. National Institutes of Health), addressing mortality rates in naïve patients in Latin America, showed that while the overall 1-year mortality rate was 8.3% (95% CI, 7.6%–9.1%), large variability across sites was observed: 2.6%, 3.7%, 6.0%, 13.0%, 10.8%, 3.5%, and 9.8% for clinics in Argentina, Brazil, Chile, Haiti, Honduras, Mexico, and Peru, respectively. Mortality estimates adjusting for CD4 were similar across sites (1.1%–2.8% for CD4 = 200), except for Haiti (7.5%), and Honduras (7.0%). All patients were starting HAART, so the observed differences are linked to the different health care systems and social environments in which ARV therapy is delivered.[10]

Therefore, when looking to the future and recognizing that ARV rollout is the most important component of the struggle against AIDS, it is imperative to address all the socioeconomic components that must be taken into consideration if the world really wants to drive this catastrophe to an end.

Future Directions and Challenges

ARV Treatment Scale-Up

It is encouraging that antiretroviral treatment coverage targets have been set in most countries. Four million people living with HIV in low- and middle-income countries have started ART since 2004—people who would probably have died otherwise. We need to keep in mind that we are dealing with a preventable and treatable disease, yet millions of people living with HIV still lack access to the treatment and care they need, and millions at risk are not reached by any prevention program. Many thousands of women, men, and children continue to die as a consequence of our failure as a global community.

Therefore, we need to plan ahead, aiming to honor the commitments and keep the promises made several times in different high-level meetings, conferences, and in an incredible number of declarations, papers, and documents.

Challenges for Expanding ARV Rollout: More Candidates on the Waiting List, More to Come, Patients Live Longer

More Candidates. A major issue is that, during the first decade of the new millennium, the "when to start ARV" question has seen the pendulum swinging back to earlier treatment.

Albeit when to start ARV therapy remains a matter of debate, no disagreement exists for symptomatic patients, as well as for asymptomatic individuals with CD4 T lymphocyte counts of 350 cells/mm^3 or below. In resource-poor settings, WHO recommended until late 2009 that adolescents and adults should start HAART when they have advanced HIV disease, mildly symptomatic and asymptomatic disease, or WHO Stage II or I HIV disease with CD4 cell counts <200 cells/mm^3. These recommendations were updated in November 2009 and now look closer to those released by other international bodies. Some Western countries' guidelines panels, such as the U.S. Department of Health and Human Services (DHHS),[11] recommend treatment initiation in asymptomatic patients when the CD4 count falls below 350 cells/mm^3, and opinions are divided regarding whether to consider treatment in patients with CD4 cell counts <500 cells/mm^3, particularly if the patient has a high viral load, is older than 50 years of age, and/or has comorbidities like hepatitis B (HBV) or hepatitis C (HCV coinfections), among other conditions. An increasing amount of data suggest that by starting treatment earlier, the so called "non-AIDS" diseases driving to mortality in the HAART era might be dramatically reduced. The current recommendations include starting ART before CD4 counts drop to below 350 cells/mm^3, and above 350 cells/mm^3 if there is evidence of high viral load, rapid CD4 decline, or the presence of comorbidities (including chronic HCV or HBV infection, increased cardiovascular risk, or underlying renal disease) that may be adversely affected by inflammatory events resulting from ongoing HIV replication. Data from the SMART trial[12] indicate that most morbidity and mortality is related to non-AIDS defining illnesses. Disseminated inflammation occurs while HIV is unsuppressed, irrespective of CD4 count, and it is an important driver of non-AIDS morbidities (such as malignancies) and affects the heart, liver, and kidneys. Deferring ART until patients have CD4 counts below 200 cells/mm^3 is associated with increased morbidity and mortality,[13] and an inverse correlation has been confirmed between mortality and CD4 strata—the HIV-CAUSAL collaboration studied showed corresponding hazard ratios were 0.29 (0.22–0.37) for less than 100 cells/mm^3 and 0.77 (0.58–1.01) for 500 cells/mm^3 or more for ARV initiation versus no initiation.[14]

In addition to the benefits at the individual level, ART has been shown as a prevention tool by reducing the median viral load at the community level.

The recently released WHO recommendations for ARV therapy[15] recommend earlier initiation—namely, asymptomatic patients with CD4 cell counts below 350 cells/mm^3) of antiretroviral treatment and prolonged use of antiretrovirals to prevent mother-to-child transmission.[16] According to the recommendations, *"These measures are intended to further reduce the epidemic in high-burden countries.*" The immediate implications are that the number of eligible patients has increased at least by 3 million new candidates. The financial implications are obvious, but this cannot be considered in a vacuum.

ARV therapy has been considered to be a cost-effective intervention when compared to other medical interventions,[17] even when the cost-effectiveness analysis was limited to the individual level. In his seminal paper published in 2006, Julio Montaner[18] added a new perspective regarding the benefits of ARV expansion, creating the concept of ART as prevention. Mathematical modeling done by the same group[19] and confirmed by other authors has shown that accelerating the rollout of HAART could lead to substantial reductions in the growth of the epidemic and be not only cost-saving, but cost-averting. A study published by Granich and colleagues from WHO[20] also proposed a model consisting of testing all people in a high-prevalence community (aged 15 years and older) for HIV every year and starting people on ART immediately after they are diagnosed with HIV infection. The authors conclude that the studied strategy could greatly accelerate the transition from the present endemic phase (in which most adults living with HIV are not receiving ART) to an elimination phase (in which most are on ART) within 5 years. It could reduce HIV incidence and mortality to less than one case per 1,000 people per year by 2016, or within 10 years of full implementation of the strategy, and reduce the prevalence of HIV to less than 1% within 50 years. In this model, after the year 2032, this strategy would start reducing costs, whereas the present strategy would continue to increase the amount of money spent on HIV/AIDS treatment and care. Again, this mathematical model is not a plan for action, but shows the potential benefits if the world would start to move in the right direction, reaching those patients currently eligible to be treated, as recommended by the ARV guidelines.

The idea of ART as prevention has been picked up by several stakeholders. For instance, as stated by the DHHS ARV guidelines panel, "*effective antiretroviral therapy reduces transmission of HIV.*" The most dramatic and well-established example of this effect is the use of antiretroviral therapy in pregnant women to prevent mother-to-child transmission of HIV. Effective suppression of HIV replication, as reflected in plasma HIV RNA, is a key determinant in reducing perinatal transmission. In the U.S., the use of combination antiretroviral therapy during pregnancy has reduced the HIV transmission rate from approximately 20%–30% to less than 2%. Thus, antiretroviral therapy is recommended for all HIV-infected pregnant women, both for maternal health and to prevent HIV transmission from mother to child. Emerging evidence supports the concept of "treatment as prevention" of sexual transmission of HIV. Lower plasma HIV RNA levels are associated with decreases in the concentration of the virus in genital secretions. Studies of HIV serodiscordant heterosexual couples have demonstrated a relationship between the level of plasma viremia and HIV transmission risk—when plasma HIV RNA levels are lower, transmission events are less common. Therefore, the use of effective antiretroviral therapy, regardless of CD4 count, is likely to reduce transmission to the uninfected sexual partner.

Hence, by expanding HAART coverage around the globe, we will not only benefit people living with HIV, but also billions of human beings at risk, including those yet to come. Pediatric AIDS will continue to be a shame for the international community until we reach the goal of complete eradication of perinatal transmission. Sexual transmission can be substantially reduced with HAART expansion and transmission among drug users can be halted if appropriate harm reduction programs, substitution therapies, and safe injection sites are offered where needed. These tools are to be considered in addition to, not in place of, other proven strategies including: male circumcision; timely diagnosis and treatment of sexually transmitted infections (STIs); condom promotion and distribution; behavioral interventions; sexual education for teenagers, adolescents and adults. Should a microbicide and/or a vaccine become available in the future, it will be welcome as an additional component of the strategy to get the epidemic under control. The future of HIV/AIDS is certainly linked to the progress of science, which needs further support and expansion, but it is not less dependent of the level of political will and decision by governments, donors and policy makers.

More Candidates to Come on Board for Treatment. Even taking for granted that all the resources needed are available (which is not the case in 2010, as discussed below), the challenge is to encourage more people to come earlier for HIV testing. National agencies, like the U.S. Centers for Disease Control and Prevention (CDC)[21] and international agencies like WHO[22] have endorsed new testing policies, based on the "provider-initiated" or "opt-out" approach, meaning the proactive search for HIV infections instead of the classic "client-initiated" testing.

The potential impact of the test-and-treat strategy can not be overestimated. A study performed in two hospitals in Uganda[23] showed that the acceptance rate for provider-initiated testing was 98%. Of note, 81% of those tested had not been tested previously. HIV prevalence in those accepting testing was 25%. Among 1,213 couples tested, 224 (19%) had discordant testing results, confirming the potential of timely testing as a major prevention tool, allowing for treating of the infected partner and protection of the uninfected partner.

This strategy has several logistic and ethical implications, particularly in resource-poor settings. Testing must be conducted in a manner which limits coercion and emphasizes voluntariness, while ensuring effective linkages to care and treatment for those who test HIV-positive.[24]

The WHO-UNAIDS guidance document clearly recommends an "opt-out" approach to provider-initiated HIV testing and counseling in health facilities, including simplified pretest information. With this approach, an HIV test is recommended: (1) for all patients, irrespective of epidemic setting, whose clinical presentation might result from underlying HIV infection; (2) as a standard part of medical care for all patients attending health facilities in areas with generalized HIV epidemics; and (3) more selectively in areas with concentrated and low-level epidemics. Individuals must specifically decline the HIV test if they do not want it to be performed. Additional discussion of the right to decline HIV testing, of the risks and benefits of HIV testing and disclosure, and about the social support available may be required for groups especially vulnerable to adverse consequences on disclosure of an HIV test result. An "opt-in" approach to informed consent may merit consideration for such highly vulnerable populations. Provider-initiated HIV testing and counseling should be accompanied by a recommended package of HIV-related prevention, treatment, care, and support services. How to generalize this strategy is one of the challenges for the forthcoming years.

Patients Live Longer: The Aging Population. Life expectancy for people living with HIV/AIDS has experienced a remarkable increase in the era of HAART. Also, new infections are on the rise in older adults. People 60 years of age and above are nowadays more active than those in this age group just a couple of decades ago. Obviously, this includes sexual activity, facilitated in many cases by the relatively recent introduction of medicines like sildenafil and similar compounds.

Thus, the AIDS population is aging. For instance, in the U.S. in 2005, persons aged 50 accounted for 15% of new HIV/AIDS diagnosis, 24% of persons living with HIV/AIDS, which means a net increase from 17% in 2001. Patients older than 50 years of age accounted for 19% of all AIDS diagnoses, 29% of persons living with AIDS, and 35% of all deaths of persons with AIDS in 2005.[25]

Some of the new problems linked with this population include the following:[26] (1) physicians and patients frequently don't consider this population at risk for HIV, so testing is delayed until other diseases are ruled out in patients presenting with symptoms; (2) asymptomatic patients are less likely to present spontaneously for HIV testing; and (3) older patients are more likely to have comorbid conditions requiring concomitant medications than are younger patients, with an increased potential for drug-drug interactions. In addition, toxicities from HAART— particularly dyslipidemia, insulin resistance, and pancreatitis—may also be worse in older HIV patients.[27] Furthermore, in addition to the already known higher incidence of cardiovascular disease in older patients, exposure to protease inhibitors has been pointed out as a risk factor itself.[28] In particular, drugs like indinavir and lopinavir/ritonavir, but also NRTIs like abacavir and didanosine, have been linked with an increased risk for dyslipidemia, metabolic syndrome, and myocardial infarction and other related events.[29] As some of these findings failed to be confirmed in other studies, caution is recommended when prescribing those drugs to patients with other risk factors for cardiovascular diseases. Nevertheless, our current understanding of the pathogenesis of HIV disease is that the virus induces a permanent inflammatory response which, sooner or later, affects different organs and systems, including the CNS, liver, kidneys, and bones, and also affects risk for "non-AIDS associated cancers." As shown by the SMART study and other trials, rather than increasing the risk for the above-mentioned problems, HAART plays a protective role by reducing the inflammatory status associated with unchecked viral replication.

In a nutshell, AIDS can be considered a disease that accelerates aging by inducing immune activation, which, in turn, promotes the inflammatory status that is responsible for the increased risk for severe, end organ diseases.

Thus, the immediate consequences of aging are to be considered at least in two areas: epidemiology and clinical care. A longer life span among people living with HIV means higher prevalence rates: as the incidence rates stabilize or increase, so the logistic and financial burden for society will increase over time. From a clinical point of view, the future scenario requires linking the practice of HIV medicine with the management of chronic diseases. This might be feasible in the short term in wealthy countries with reasonably organized health care systems, but it certainly adds a new challenge for low-income countries with disrupted medical care systems.

Another Challenge: The Health Care Workforce Shortage

Scaling up treatment is very difficult without working health systems. Treatment programs require affordable, effective medicines, functional supply chains, clinical care, and monitoring capacity, well-trained and motivated health workers, and support for people taking treatment. Health systems are straining to care for the growing global HIV case load. The HIV workforce is under pressure to maintain the effort year after year, often in dire circumstances, with substandard equipment and support, especially in hyperendemic countries. Everyone working in AIDS faces the challenge to keep up-to-date with new scientific findings and to translate this knowledge into practice. As a note of caution, it is necessary to consider that the possible loss of experienced staff to the better-funded and more attractive HIV treatment programs may adversely affect the health of others.[30]

But are HIV programs the main drivers of the shortage of health care workers in many developing countries? Certainly not. Rather, bad working conditions, AIDS mortality, and low salaries are fueling the brain drain of these professionals from south to north. This must be one of the major advocacy issues on the AIDS agenda.

The HIV epidemic itself is destroying the human capital at all work places, including the health systems. HIV has most heavily affected Sub-Saharan Africa, swiftly erasing decades of development gains in the world's poorest region. Although Sub-Saharan Africa accounts for more than two out of three people living with HIV/AIDS (PLWHA) worldwide, the region is home to only 3% of the world's health care providers and is responsible for only 1% of global health spending.[31] At the same time that health workers are most needed to aid their communities and countries, HIV itself is depleting health systems of critical workers due to illness and death, creating a vicious cycle that magnifies the region's human resources crisis. Modeling suggests that health systems in Africa may lose 20% of their health workers to HIV/AIDS in the coming years.[32]

As we described in an article published in the *Lancet* in 2007,[33] health care staff shortages are endemic in Sub-Saharan Africa. Overall, there is one physician for every 8,000 people in the region. In the worst affected countries, such as Malawi, the physician-to-population ratio is just 0.02:1,000 (1:50,000). Huge disparities also exist between rural and urban areas: rural parts of South Africa have 14 times fewer doctors than the national average. These figures are drastically different than in the developed world; the UK, for example, has more than 100 times more physicians per population than does Malawi,[3] but almost 1 of every 10 doctors working in the UK is from Africa. The insufficiency of health staff to provide even basic services is one of the most pressing impediments to health care delivery in resource-poor settings. The consequences are clearly shown by the inverse relationship that exists between health care worker density and mortality rates. Doctors, nurses, pharmacists, and other health workers are systematically recruited from Southern Africa, a region struggling with the greatest burden of infectious and chronic illness, and the specific challenge of HIV/AIDS. Clear, enforced regulation is required to prevent recruiting companies from enticing health workers away from their local work, and developed countries should adequately compensate less-developed countries for the human resources they have lost and continue to lose.

The Unfair Debate: AIDS versus the Strengthening of Health Care Systems

The rapid expansion of HIV care and treatment in resource-limited settings is having a positive effect in communities severely affected by this epidemic, and it enables persons living with HIV to continue to work and live productive lives that benefit themselves, their families, and their societies. Concerns have been raised, however, regarding the possible deleterious effects on other health services.

Some have expressed the opinion that the massive infusion of resources directed toward HIV programming will have a detrimental effect on other health services and responses to other health threats.[34] The major concern is that a smaller segment of the population (i.e., those with HIV infection) will gain access to much needed interventions, whereas the majority would be left with inadequate and weakened services. However, others postulate that if the resources available for the scale-up of HIV care are utilized for the design and implementation of HIV programs—with attention to benefiting the broader health services—then this effort may catalyze the transformation of health services into more effective and responsive ones capable of addressing the health needs of all individuals.[35]

For instance, in a study performed in Cote d' Ívoire, quality of antenatal and delivery care services was assessed in five urban health facilities, before and after the implementation of a prevention of mother-to-child transmission (PMTCT) program. Global scores for quality of antenatal and delivery care significantly improved in all facilities after the implementation of PMTCT.[36]

But the debate is far from being solved. Should the world phase out from the vertical programs addressing AIDS and integrate AIDS care into the global health care systems? Would this be more equitable? Or, to the contrary, would this destroy the outstanding achievements in the field, without benefiting the population at large? AIDS is an exceptional disease, but now its exceptionalism is under attack. As described by Whiteside and Smith[1]:

> *AIDS exceptionalism is under attack from two sources. The first were characterized by Stephen Lewis, speaking at the International AIDS Society Conference on Pathogenesis, Treatment and Prevention in Cape Town in July 2009, as: "he pinched bureaucrats and publicity-seeking academics who advocate exchanging the health of some for the health of others—who propose robbing Peter to pay Paul rather than arguing, in principled fashion, that money must be found for every imperative, including maternal and child health, and sexual and reproductive health, and environmental health as well as all the resources required to turn the tide of the AIDS pandemic."*

The second group is public health specialists and academics who wish to enter a serious policy debate about health priorities and resources and how they are and should be allocated. They are concerned by what appears in some contexts to be disproportionate amounts of funding targeted at AIDS, and because of the belief that AIDS activists prioritize it above other health problems. This is a valid dialogue and needs to be entered with honesty and, above all, data.

The arguments include a variety of opinions, scarcely based on evidence. The most challenging was put forward by England, when it was claimed that AIDS financing has undermined health systems in developing countries.[37] Peter Piot, former UNAIDS Executive Director, has given the opposite view about "the health system's myth," stating, "The myth that if we just, if we only strengthen health systems this will solve everything, including AIDS."[38] The Sydney Declaration called for 10% of all resources devoted to HIV programming in countries to be dedicated to research that will tell us how to make the best use of our treatment and prevention investments. We must identify which approaches are effective in the field, which are not, and why.[39]

The international AIDS Society Strategic Plan 2010–2014 addresses this issue: significant increases in life expectancy are predicted for people living with HIV who are able to access antiretroviral treatment. This raises new challenges in organizing health care services for HIV-positive people. Planning should ensure that prevention and treatment are mutually reinforced and integrated, and that these are linked with key services, including sexual and reproductive health. Psychosocial care and support for families and communities affected by HIV are also an essential component of comprehensive health care.

One of the notable impacts of investing in HIV services and programs is the flow on benefits, including the strengthening of health systems and the positive impact on related health issues such as maternal and child health, and reductions in TB and malaria deaths.

Basic science and clinical research continue to generate important new knowledge about HIV, leading to improvements in treatment, care, and prevention. Research has intensified for biomedical prevention tools that could provide an important adjunct to comprehensive prevention efforts. The effort to develop preventative and therapeutic vaccines remains strong, despite some setbacks.

Social science research is providing important insights into societal and individual impacts on persons living with HIV infection. Application of these findings can significantly improve the effectiveness of prevention, treatment, and care programs as well as inform our understanding of how scientifically validated interventions operate in "real world" settings.

Despite the tangible progress in saving lives and healing the sick in the poorest nations of the world, critics claim that HIV-targeted funding is creating more problems than it solves—that this funding could be better spent on directly funding health systems.

Health systems were weak and underresourced long before the AIDS community shifted forever the approach to global public health, before we demanded an end to the inequities that had been taken for granted for decades. Building clinics and laboratories, training health care workers, and working with ministries of health to deliver HIV programs mean stronger health systems for everyone. Ongoing efforts devoted to integrate TB, sexual and reproductive health, primary care, and perinatal health into HIV services need further support.

Health care delivery should never be a question of either/or, but of how we can work together to benefit everyone in need. It is time for collaboration, not competition.

A detailed analysis of this issue is beyond the scope of this chapter, but certainly, while sound evidence-based information becomes available from the operations research field, a couple of ideas deserve to be highlighted.

The first is the "one size does not fit all" approach, as proposed in the above-mentioned paper by Whiteside:

> *The idea that exceptionalism is somehow wrong is an oversimplification. While normalizing the response where AIDS is located largely in specific population groups can ensure equitable services and treatment by addressing stigma and discrimination. AIDS must be seen as exceptional in those places where it is having long term development impacts due to high incidences of illness and death. Critics of AIDS exceptionalism do not take into account the unique situation where international aid is literally keeping people alive. In high prevalence countries, prevention programs have yet to slow the rate of infection, and finding ways to do so will require creativity and an unprecedented political commitment. The AIDS response can not be mounted in isolation; it is part of the development agenda. It must be based on human rights principles, and it must aim to improve health and well-being of societies as a whole.*

The other approach is the so called "diagonal approach," as proposed by Ooms and coworkers.[40] These authors believe that a transformation of the Global Fund to fight AIDS, Tuberculosis and Malaria into a Global Health Fund is feasible, but only if accompanied by a substantial increase of donor commitments to the Global Fund. The transformation of the Global Fund into a "diagonal" and, ultimately, perhaps "horizontal" financing approach should happen gradually and carefully, and be accompanied by measures to safeguard its exceptional features.

Another definition for the diagonal approach would be to aim to the integration of health services without shutting down successful vertical programs. Too frequently HIV, TB, hepatitis, STIs, and sexual and reproductive health teams do not cooperate, or simply are not located in the same place, contributing to problems of duplication of material and human resources and to patient fatigue. The same individual frequently needs the services of two or more of those teams, but the inefficient organization prevents service delivery in a timely fashion.

The Financial Constraints

Last, but not least, we have to face reality. Even with the extraordinary mobilization of resources from donors, international organizations, and governments, what we are doing is not enough.

Is the investment paying off? If millions of lives saved and even more millions of infections averted would not be enough, this quote from Walensky and Kuritzkes[41] regarding the impact of the U.S. Presidential Program for AIDS Relief provides indisputable evidence:

> *PEPFAR I averted 1.2 million deaths, and HIV-related mortality decreased by 10% in PEPFAR focus countries, compared to those without such support. The perception that PEPFAR is at odds with dedicated efforts toward maternal and child health ignores the massive direct and indirect benefits PEPFAR has achieved already for mothers and children. It may be that PEPFAR—by providing health infrastructure, HIV prevention, parental survival, and the opportunity to sustain economic growth—is the most generous gift the United States can provide to future generations of those countries most in need. ...*

In 2008, the world was shocked by the worst financial crisis since 1930, this one being more global than the former. It took only a couple of days to see how governments were quickly replenishing the exhausted finances of banks and companies, frequently mismanaged by inefficient (when not corrupt) CEOs. The final figures are yet to be cleared, but the amount invested in this financial salvage was in the trillion-dollar order of magnitude. Meanwhile, in 2008, $13.7 billion U.S. dollars (USD) were allocated to the epidemic. How much money is required in 2010? Almost twice as much: $25.1 billion USD.[42] Why are we missing our targets? Because the same countries that committed to the 2010 and 2015 goals are falling short in their contributions, with few exceptions. So the answer is clear: it seems easier to rescue banks than to save lives. If we are not able to overcome this shortage of funds, then we will see people queuing and dying while they are on a waiting list to be treated. This is absolutely unacceptable. As I said in my opening speech at the XVII International AIDS Conference in Mexico in 2008:

> *We will not endorse any type of Schindler's list, by accepting that while those included save their lives, others are just left behind suffering and dying. Let's be perfectly clear: our failures have dramatic consequences: thousands of children, men and women are dying every day. They bear tragic testimony of our incapacity to transform words into action. We know what has to be done. The choice before the international community is clear: either it is time to deliver, or continue fueling the tragedy.*

As the impact of AIDS continues in all parts of the world, funding must increase, along with the political will to use it wisely. Domestic and aid funding is under added pressure because of global economic turbulence and high debt levels, with major donor countries being particularly affected. Adding to this is the reality that the AIDS epidemic has been with us for more than 25 years and no longer occupies the center stage in the media or in the political agenda. Today,

AIDS operates in a highly competitive environment with other diseases, with broader health system debates and with other pressing global issues linked to the environment and climate change.

There Is No Future Without Human Rights

The scaling up of what we know works cannot be achieved without protecting and promoting human rights. It is important to note that a number of countries have moved to change punitive laws and policies against people living with HIV, MSM, people who inject drugs, sex workers, and other marginalized populations. These changes increase the impact of prevention, improve treatment uptake, and create a supportive environment for research participation. However, discriminatory laws still exist in many countries, and widespread human rights violations continue against people with HIV and marginalized populations. Women and girls continue to be disproportionately affected by HIV, and inadequate steps have been taken to advance their needs. Services for children, including antiretroviral therapy for those living with HIV and social support for children orphaned by AIDS, are too limited. There is no chance for success without respecting and promoting human rights. More than that, there is no future for peaceful development without human rights for every human being.

The rights of sex trade workers, injecting drug users, MSM, and other vulnerable groups must be protected through legal and policy reform in every country around the world.

The epidemic has always struck harder in marginalized and vulnerable populations. Again, let's be clear: poverty is the driving force of this and other epidemics, like TB and malaria. It is hard to advocate for human rights without considering that two-thirds of the world's population lives on less than $2 a day. On this, too, it is time to deliver.

Let us redouble our efforts and make our dream come true. We shall overcome this tragedy and stop the epidemic!

Final Note: Challenges and Opportunities for the Future

Challenges

1. AIDS resource requirements will increase rapidly over the next years and will continue to rise in the future. Needs vary between $19 billion USD and $35 billion USD annually by 2031, and between $397 billion USD and $722 billion USE over the next 22-year period.[43]

2. Political will is vanishing in some donor countries, making fundraising more difficult.

3. Domestic and aid funding is under added pressure because of global economic turbulence and high debt levels, with major donor countries being particularly affected.

4. Donor fatigue is a factor. AIDS epidemic has been with us for more than 25 years and no longer occupies the center stage in the media or in the political agenda. Today, AIDS operates in a highly competitive environment with other diseases, with broader health system debates and with other pressing global issues such climate change, the energy shortage, and food security.

5. Current funding for HIV services is fragmented and, in most cases, distributed for limited periods of time.[44] Sustainability still has a question mark.

6. Resistance to first-line regimens is rising in resource-poor settings.

7. Increasing numbers of patients will require second-line ARV regimens. But in 2008, only 2% of adults and 3% of children were on second-line ART.[45]

8. Most patients lack access to viral load monitoring; access to CD4 count is limited.

9. A variety of human rights issues must be addressed. Several countries have punitive laws and policies against people living with HIV, MSM, people who inject drugs, sex workers, and other marginalized populations. Women and girls continue to be disproportionately affected by HIV and inadequate steps have been taken to advance their needs. Services for children, including antiretroviral therapy for those living with HIV and social support for children orphaned by AIDS, are too limited.

10. Specific information is needed on surveillance data, including mortality data and a direct measure of incidence, as well as better monitoring data showing the quality of interventions, including appropriate monitoring of the programmatic responses to HIV.[46]

11. Knowledge gaps persist. Several topics need evidence-based data to inform effective and efficient policies.

12. A joint meeting hosted by WHO, The Global Fund, The World Bank, and the International AIDS Society identified the following questions to be addressed, among others:[47]

   • What is the impact of HAART on HIV prevention and how can it be enhanced?
   • How can patient retention in care be improved?
   • How can adherence be improved?
   • How can first-line regimens be made more durable?
   • What are the most cost-effective first-line and second-line regimens? What and how do clinical, biological and epidemiological factors affect these cost-effective ratios?
   • What is the optimal package of prevention interventions for people living with HIV, what is the relative importance and efficiency of each component of this package and, thus, in what order should countries strive to adopt each component according to resource availability?
   • What is the most appropriate use of viral load and CD4 cell count tests in the public health approach, and how can field evaluations of existing and upcoming point of care technologies be conducted?
   • How should Quality Assurance be implemented as an integrated part of national health care systems, including laboratory services?
   • What tasks can be shifted, to whom, and what is the effect on quality and cost of care?
   • What are the optimal service delivery strategies that minimize costs, while guaranteeing quality of care?

Opportunities

The worldwide AIDS movement has generated many positive effects:

1. Commitments to halt and reverse the epidemic by 2015 have been made at the highest international level.

2. International organizations like the UN family (including all the agencies in addition to UNAIDS and WHO) and the Global Fund for AIDS, TB and Malaria are deeply involved in the struggle against AIDS

3. This is a unique global movement—a social and political movement of people living with HIV, communities vulnerable to HIV, researchers, health care workers, nongovernmental and faith-based organizations, governments, intergovernmental organizations, private foundations, the private sector, and public/private partnerships. A movement of such breadth and influence does not exist for any other health or development issue. This movement, and the economic and policy research it has generated over 3 decades, has been instrumental in shifting the paradigm from health being a consequence of development to recognizing that health is a fundamental prerequisite for development.

4. AIDS is the first disease in history to generate global mobilization in an effort to treat people, defeating the "too complex-too costly" paradigm, bridging policy with programmatic rollout—from 0% to almost 40% coverage in about 7 years.

5. Unprecedented resource mobilization, including governmental programs like PEPFAR, private donors and brokers like the Bill & Melinda Gates and the Clinton Foundations, among others.

6. Successful international initiatives have resulted in dramatic price reduction for ARV drugs.

7. A net progress in the human rights field, with stigmatization and discrimination increasingly recognized as drivers of the epidemic.

8. Most populations at risk (MSM, drug users, commercial sex workers, youngsters, women, and socially excluded populations) have become more visible, and in many countries have been able to build vocal organizations.

9. Provided that the $25.1 billion USD needed for 2010 will be gathered, the expected outcomes, as stated by UNAIDS, are:
   - An estimated 2.6 million new HIV infections will be averted, cutting HIV incidence by nearly 50%.
   - 1.3 million deaths in the next 2 years can be avoided.
   - Approximately 6.7 million individuals will be receiving antiretroviral treatment.
   - More than 70 million pregnant women will be screened and receive PMTCT services.
   - HIV prevention programs will reach 20 million MSM, 7 million sex workers, 10 million people who inject drugs, and nearly 8.1 billion male and female condoms would be distributed.
   - Seven million orphans and vulnerable children would have been supported by social support programs.

10. Outstanding progress has been made in virology, immunology, pathogenesis, and clinical care, making a life expectancy for PLWHA timely diagnosed and treated close to the one of the general population possible. This includes the ability to treat and control viral replication, even in deep salvage of patients with multidrug-resistant viruses.

11. There have been notable impacts of investments made in HIV services on related health issues such as maternal and child health and reductions in TB and malaria deaths.

12. Encouraging data have become available regarding the potential of expansion of HAART as part of a broader prevention package, allowing us to envision, for the first time, the possibility of controlling the epidemic.

Chapter 43 THE NEXT PANDEMIC: PREPAREDNESS, PREDICTION, AND PUBLICITY

PHILIP ALCABES

> *The angel of history['s] ... face is turned toward the past.*
> *Where a chain of events appears before us, he sees one single*
> *catastrophe, which keeps piling wreckage upon wreckage and hurls it*
> *at his feet.... A storm [that] is blowing from Paradise ... drives him*
> *irresistibly into the future, to which his back is turned,*
> *while the pile of debris before him grows skyward.*

—WALTER BENJAMIN, "On the Concept of History" (1940)[1]

Hindsight as Foresight

The catastrophe in view when anyone predicts a pandemic is not a future crisis at all; like Benjamin's angel, all he sees is history. The predicted pandemic is no more than a reprise of past disasters. To claim that our public health system can prepare society to fend off the next plague is to transmit the illusion that progress (or science) allows us to control the future.

A close reading of history reveals the fallacy: each of the true catastrophes, including the Black Death, Asiatic cholera in 1832, the Spanish flu of 1918, and AIDS, was beyond envisaging at the time it began. The great disasters cannot be foreseen, only seen in retrospect. Therefore, although some public health professionals never stop claiming to predict, they can never ready society for the future, only for a misreading of history.

Since the advent of AIDS, our society has asked epidemiologists for a specific kind of prediction: we have asked to be informed about risks, and expected officials to advise us as to how to avoid risks—that is, officials have become risk entrepreneurs. They use epidemiologists' information on risk to arm the population and to battle the prospect of pandemic disaster (or so they claim). They immunize against flu, spray insecticide where West Nile virus has killed an animal, or distribute condoms where AIDS is prevalent. The risk entrepreneurs show us how to defend against the catastrophe that can be foreseen.

When the foreseeable catastrophe fails to happen, risk entrepreneurs can claim that disaster was averted because of the defensive arrangements they promoted—because of the public health system, so-called biosecurity, or what is now called "preparedness." The public can enjoy the reassurance that the risk entrepreneurs' arrangements offer. That those arrangements defend against past occurrences, not future ones, and that society is no closer to impunity from the sudden appearance of new contagions, are not truths that risk entrepreneurs will divulge.

In other words, looking for the next pandemic is a paradox. With the guidance of risk entrepreneurs, society prepares itself for the eventualities that can be foreseen—flu outbreaks each winter, malaria in zones where anopheline mosquitoes thrive, dengue where *Aedes aegyptii* and *A. albopictus* live; AIDS and hepatitis C where people (forced by circumstance, habit, or police surveillance) share injecting equipment, and so forth. But it is never prepared for catastrophe—because what makes a disease outbreak catastrophic is that it cannot be foreseen. It was inconceivable that flu would kill a half of 1% of the U.S. population in 1918–1919, because—as far as policymakers of that day knew—flu had never been so deadly. It was inconceivable, in the late 1970s, that AIDS would kill 25 million people worldwide within the next 30 years—because no virus with the mutability, transmissibility, long incubation period, or delayed virulence of HIV could be imagined. The next plague will be equally unimaginable until the day it begins.

The Error of Preparedness

When officials and scientists collaborate to create massive preparedness campaigns with the aim of combating the foreseeable, they are making three errors. First, they mislead the public with the implicit claim that it's possible to forecast the future and foresee all eventualities—and to do so in such detail as to stay disaster.[2] This is the essence of risk entrepreneurship.

Second, risk entrepreneurs assert that they are uniquely capable of forecasting the fearsome future—and that this prescience entitles them to direct society's use of resources. The public is supposed to respond to reports of risk by maintaining a state of preparedness—that is, officials are supposed to make evidence-based policy by using the findings on risk to create prescriptions for risk avoidance; everyone is supposed to be ready to follow the prescriptions in order to combat the predicted disaster. Society will embrace mass flu immunization, abstinence-only sex education, condom promotion, harsh penalties for using methamphetamine or smoking in the presence of children, and other programs justified (even on thin evidence) by the risk entrepreneurs' assertions about how to reduce risk.

Third, they imply that the disaster, when it comes, will be apocalyptic.[3–8] That is, they lead people to believe that everyone, or nearly everyone, will die, and society will be changed (it's epidemiology from horror films, perhaps *I Am Legend* or *24 Days Later*). In truth, the two deadliest pandemic outbreaks of the modern West (cholera in 1832, flu in 1918–1919) each left more than 98% of the population alive and well, even in the worst-hit areas. In the U.S. and Canada, the proportion of the population dying in each of those cataclysms was below 1%. (For cholera, several sources point to a death rate just over 1% in the crowded cities, which were most severely affected, suggesting that the overall mortality rate was well under 1%.[9–12]) For Spanish flu, the death toll in the U.S. has been estimated at 550,000 to 675,000, in a population of slightly over 100 million, or about 0.5%–0.65%.[13] Data for Canada are shakier, but several sources agree that there were about 50,000 flu deaths in 1918–1919, out of a population of over 8.1 million, for a cause-specific death rate of 0.6%. (See, for instance, the article on influenza in *The Canadian Encyclopedia*. Toronto: Historica; 2009.)

AIDS was key in shaping the errors of risk entrepreneurship. With its freight of identity politics and moral judgments, AIDS was instrumental in changing how people appreciated any epidemic. Society moved from seeing any epidemic as an outbreak of disease layered with social accoutrements (typhus, typhoid, syphilis, and plague were all viewed that way), to seeing it as a nest of social problems. Shifting the language about epidemics from events to risk, eliding distinctions between cause and effect and confusing the actual untoward occurrence (illness, death) with the risk of that occurrence, AIDS cleared a path for risk entrepreneurship (for a fuller exploration of the shifts engendered by AIDS, see Alcabes[14]). After AIDS, the prediction of pandemic disaster was a matter of publicity.

Until roughly the 1970s, an epidemic was an outbreak of disease severe enough to present a policy problem: How to control contagion? By the 1980s, though, an epidemic had become a social problem. It now involved orchestrating competing claims to truth, moral authority, and civil rights. Promoting a particular reading of history was intrinsic to making authoritative claims about epidemics.

Powerful evidence that the nature of pandemic prediction was changing came in the form of the first swine flu scare, in 1976. The event occurred against a background of expanding investment in medically relevant research in the U.S., and increasing interest in the epidemiology of influenza. The possibility that viral epidemics might be limited through broad-based immunization programs had been bolstered by the effectiveness of mass polio vaccination at extinguishing the once-dreaded outbreaks of the "summer plague," paralytic poliomyelitis, and by the more recent success of measles vaccine.[15]

The 1976 Flu Fiasco

The 1976 swine flu fiasco began with a pandemic prediction. In his textbook on the epidemiology of influenza,[16] as well as a highly influential article in a 1973 issue of the *Journal of Infectious Diseases*,[17] the well-known virologist Edwin Kilbourne articulated the theory that disastrous flu pandemics occur with regular periodicity. Kilbourne noted that the pandemics of 1957 and 1968 had been relatively mild, but, on the basis of his historical theory, predicted that the U.S. was due for a flu epidemic reminiscent of the 1918 calamity.

In January 1976, amidst this new concern about a flu pandemic, a soldier at Fort Dix, an army base in New Jersey died of flu. Laboratory studies showed that the strain was partly derived from influenza viruses that infect pigs.[18] Also, it was an H1N1 strain—just like the 1918 agent. Investigation turned up 12 other cases among Fort Dix recruits, and evidence of infection among soldiers who had been in training units with the 13 sick recruits.[19] Although later investigation revealed that there was no evidence of wide spread of the new strain,[20] opinion fixed on the small Fort Dix outbreak as corroboration of the scenario Kilbourne was, however inexpertly, predicting.

Once the news from Fort Dix was out, Kilbourne rallied the disease-control warriors with a *New York Times* op-ed piece.[21] He was invited to sit in when U.S. Centers for Disease Control and Prevention (CDC) director Dr. David Sencer called the federal Advisory Committee on Immunization Practices (ACIP)[22] into session on March 10, 1976 to discuss the so-called swine flu crisis.

The deliberations at ACIP were strongly influenced by Kilbourne's thinking. They ended with Dr. Sencer backing a plan for a mass immunization program to reach all 213 million Americans. The U.S. Secretary of Health, Education, and Welfare (HEW), David Matthews, approved it. Turning ACIP's assertion that there might be an H1N1 flu outbreak into an awesome certainty, Secretary Mathews wrote that "the indication is that we will see a return of the 1918 flu virus that is the most virulent form of flu."[23]

By 1976, invoking the shade of the 1918 flu was persuasive. The anticipated epidemic, as Kilbourne's rhetoric suggested, would look like the 1918 flu. The upshot is now well known: about a quarter of the U.S. population was immunized against the so-called swine flu, but the vaccine campaign had to be halted because of a profusion of cases of Guillain-Barré syndrome, a serious neurologic disorder, among vaccine recipients. In the end, there was no outbreak of H1N1 swine flu in 1976, but there were 500 cases of Guillain-Barré syndrome, including 32 deaths.

Then came AIDS, and pandemic prediction fused with publicity.

Prediction in the AIDS Era

Infused with social and moral issues, AIDS made publicity about the epidemic inseparable from the epidemic itself.[24] The specter of epidemic disaster was part of the publicity—and so were the authorities' claims that "at-risk" groups must act to avert disaster. By depicting AIDS as a catastrophe in the making, officials, scientists, activists, religious zealots—almost anyone who had a point to make—could publicize his or her ideas. The possibility of disaster allowed AIDS to dominate the public conversation. Often, the point was not to benefit the public's health, but something more personal.

For instance, on February 11, 2005, New York City's Department of Health and Mental Hygiene convened a press conference so that the health commissioner, Dr. Thomas Frieden, could alert the public to a new epidemic threat. Frieden announced that a New York City resident, a man in his mid-40s who "reported multiple male sex partners and unprotected anal intercourse, often while using crystal methamphetamine" had been "diagnosed with [a] rare strain of multi-drug resistant HIV that rapidly progresses to AIDS."[25] The occurrence, the Commissioner declared, was a "wake-up call to...men who have sex with men." The text of the accompanying health alert named the behaviors that gay men were supposed to wake up about: anal sex, sex while high, and sex with many partners.

A few days after the alert, the commissioner conceded that he wasn't sure "whether this [occurrence] is of tremendous scientific importance,"[26] but asserted that the alert was needed because "people have not dealt with HIV as if it were an epidemic." Gay men, Frieden said, had "successfully reduced [their] risk of HIV in the 1980s" and had to "do so again to stop the devastation of HIV/AIDS and the spread of drug-resistant strains." That is, the onus would be on an imagined commonality, the bunch of victims or victims-to-be for which "gay community" was shorthand, to bring the behavior of its members into line with the standard. Adding to the sermonizing overtones, New York's mayor, Michael Bloomberg, told the *New York Times* that unprotected sex is "just a sin in our society."[27]

Ringing the epidemic alarm over a single case of AIDS in a city that, at that point, had already seen 84,000 AIDS cases, and fixing on gay sex as a new threat to 21st-century New York, would show how evoking the specter of epidemic disaster could be useful for political and moral ends. Indeed, the incident—in particular, the use of publicity to create and communicate the epidemic threat—was a piece of showmanship.

Freiden said, at the press conference, that the health department had become concerned because the HIV strain infecting the man in question was multi-drug resistant and rapidly progressed to AIDS. He asserted that this combination had never been seen before, and insisted that it warranted action. But, drug resistance to HIV was *not* new. A reading of the medical literature would have revealed that 1% to 4% of HIV infections are resistant to multiple drugs.[28-30] And rapid progression to AIDS following HIV infection had been thoroughly documented years before the 2005 alert.[31-33] Nor was the New York case the first to exhibit both drug resistance and rapid progression: in 2001, two such cases had been reported in Vancouver,[34] eliciting

predicting but merely attempting to examine scientifically the plausible upper edge of possible outcomes of the outbreak.[55] But their disavowal seemed disingenuous.

Were they really shocked that the news media seized on their scenario as a certainty and broadcast—not as conjecture but as fact—that the President's science advisors think swine flu will kill 90,000 Americans?

As of December 2009, more than 10,500 people have definitely died from swine flu worldwide,[56] and perhaps as many as 60,000, if all flu-related deaths were counted. (A CDC study estimated 3,900 flu deaths, with an upper limit of 6,000, in the U.S. between April and mid-October 2009, a period during which 1,044 U.S. deaths were confirmed to have been caused by swine flu. Assuming, at most, a 6:1—i.e., roughly 6,000/1,044—ratio of all flu deaths to confirmed deaths, there would have been no more than 63,000 flu deaths worldwide from April through December 2009, probably far fewer.)[57] Even a global mortality of 60,000 would make the 2009 swine flu outbreak about 20 times milder than typical global flu outbreaks, wherein a million or more die from a single flu strain. And it is a shadow of the terrible toll of the 1918 flu, with countless tens of millions of deaths worldwide.

The facts of comparative death tolls, important to rational planning for public health, are not quite relevant to the pandemic preparedness paradigm—just as facts had been irrelevant to bioterrorism preparedness, the HIV scare of 2005, or the Airplane Man event. The fact that, in clinical trials, the best flu vaccines protect only about 70 percent of recipients against infection with influenza virus, and are of little value in preventing shedding of virus by vaccine recipients who do experience breakthrough infection,[58] is a curiosity, not central to the preparedness case. The fact that antiviral medications like oseltamivir (sold under the trade name Tamiflu) have never been shown to reduce the extent or intensity of influenza outbreaks in a large population was not part of the discussion about distributing Tamiflu. Nor was the fact that the purchases of Tamiflu in the context of the H1N1 swine flu outbreak were often renewals of an earlier set of contracts, negotiated in 2005 and 2006 when a few hundred cases of avian (H5N1) flu had mysteriously served as sufficient evidence of the possible advent of a disastrous pandemic of avian flu. Nor was it relevant to the preparedness paradigm that that original order for Tamiflu occurred after U.S. President Bush had successfully pressed for authorization to purchase $1.7 billion worth of the drug in 2005 even while then-Secretary of State Donald Rumsfeld was reported to be in a position to earn $1 million from the country's Tamiflu purchase (through his investment in Gilead Research, the original oseltamivir patent holder).[59] Nor was it relevant that the appearance of swine flu in 2009 upped the purchase of Tamiflu worldwide to 200 million doses, representing about $1 billion in additional sales for Tamiflu's manufacturer.[60] The relevant facts were predictions of catastrophe.

Facts are a burden. The lesson of the history of pandemic forecasting is that predictions are meant to create publicity—to shape public anxieties, to support programs that consolidate power or increase profits. The facts complicate, distract, detract from the message.

The Lessons of AIDS

It seems that the main lesson taught by AIDS is that risk is everywhere. But we are continually reminded that epidemic predictions, a mainstay of government agencies and the health sector today, are written in the grammar of risk. And that the claims of the risk entrepreneurs, in the form of predictions and alerts, serve to control the public sphere and urge people to tinker with their private behavior—without offering much benefit in the way of protection from disease.

The lesson drawn from AIDS should be different. The 25 million lives[61] and uncountable years of capable living lost to AIDS in barely a quarter century should be a reminder that any reasonable public response to disease outbreaks should aim to alleviate suffering. And the enormity of the toll taken by real and present suffering, society might have learned, should count for more than any prediction.

Indeed, neither the most inflammatory nor the most optimistic forecasts about AIDS have been borne out: U.S. Secretary of Health and Human Services Margaret Heckler's 1984 assertion that a vaccine against AIDS would be ready for testing within 2 years;[62] CDC's 1987 prediction that 270,000 AIDS cases would have been diagnosed in the U.S. by 1991[63] and the U.S. General Accounting Office's 1989 prediction that there would be 300,000 to 480,000 AIDS cases in the U.S. by 1991[64] (both too high by a factor of 2 to 3); the CDC's 2001 estimate that there were only 40,000 new HIV infections each year in the U.S.;[65] the overblown forecasts about other so-called epidemics highlighted by the "risk" grammar of AIDS, like the claim that crack babies would cost New York City $2 billion by the end of the 1990s and the United States $500 million each year,[66] and the 2005 assertion by New York's health commissioner (now, perhaps significantly, director of the CDC) that a single case of AIDS was the harbinger of a new and harder-to-manage HIV outbreak.[67] "One of the things about [AIDS] is that those who make pronouncements that are proven to be untrue simply move on," the esteemed AIDS physician Joseph Sonnabend said. "They can be wrong a second, third, and fourth time and still go on."[68] Facts should be central; prediction just noise. But often it's the other way around.

Had epidemiologists been able to foresee AIDS in, say, 1975, what would have been different? Would western society have sought to block the transmission of the AIDS virus by promoting marriage and monogamy as the sexual ideal, banning heroin, controlling injection equipment, insisting on sterility in medical settings? No: forecasting AIDS would have been irrelevant, since all of those policies were in place before HIV arrived and gave them a new purpose. In fact, only the promotion of condoms might have been elected sooner than it actually was had AIDS been foreseeable. If successful, condom promotion would have made some difference to the early spread of the AIDS virus in the U.S.—but how well that would have worked is in considerable doubt, and in any case its overall impact outside of urban centers in the U.S. would have been slight. (Several studies among heterosexual populations showed that using condoms all the time is very effective, whereas substantial transmission occurs where condoms are used less than all the time. Among uninfected women who were sex partners of HIV-positive men, HIV incidence rates were 1.1% per year among consistent users of condoms and 9.7% per year among inconsistent or nonusers.[69] Transmission rates were high among people who used condoms frequently but not all the time.[70–71])

It wasn't foresight that was lacking with AIDS; it was insight. The impact of AIDS might have been less (and perhaps negligible) had society been different in a few crucial ways. Had there been adequate surveillance of the many interactions between humans and animals, it would have been easy to detect the incipient spread of HIV early on (and that would have altered the story of the severe acute respiratory syndrome [SARS], and influenza, along with those of a host of other organisms capable of doing grave damage as well[72]). Better coordination between the separate sectors of the health industry,[73] better cooperation worldwide, and better understanding of the connections between poverty, development, agriculture, commerce in food and animal feed, ecosystem change, host-species transitions on the part of viruses, and health would have made a difference. In particular, greater awareness of the potential for interactions between humans and wild animals to promote the movement of viruses might have allowed for early containment of HIV.

The insight that would have had the greatest influence on the course of the AIDS outbreak was also the most obvious one: the one afforded by experience, by history. Simply redressing the great disparities in resources between the poor and the wealthy would limit the spread of most diseases, AIDS notably. It's the oldest lesson in public health, it's the lesson of AIDS, and it remains the fundamental fact about contagion—the central fact.

Foresight is ornamentation, AIDS taught. Insight matters. Prediction is fraught, easily processed, finessed, and publicized into fact. The important facts require no prevision: we have seen them before; they are in front of us already.

Acknowledgments

Monica Serrano carried out extensive research on the 2005 HIV scare in New York City, from which some of the material in this chapter is drawn. Writing by sociologists Frank Furedi and Barry Glassner fertilized the author's thinking on pandemic prediction, as did conversations with Prof. Jack Levinson of the City College of New York and students in the Imagined Epidemic course at Hunter College.

References

1. Walter Benjamin, On the Concept of History, thesis IX. tr. Harry Zohn, in Howard Eiland and Michael W. Jennings (Eds.): Walter Benjamin: Selected Writings, vol 4: 1938–1940. Cambridge, MA: Belknap; 2003, pp. 392–393.

2. Lurie N. The need for science in the practice of public health. N Engl J Med 2009;361(26):2571–2572.

3. Osterholm MT, Schwartz J. Living Terrors: What America Nees to Know to Survive the Coming Bioterrorist Catstrophe. New York: Delacorte; 2000.

4. Hamburg MA. Addressing bioterrorist threats: where do we go from here? Emerg Infect Dis 1999;5(4):564–565.

5. Gerberding JL, Hughes JM, Koplan JP. Bioterrorism preparedness and response: clinicians and public health agencies as essential partners. JAMA 2002;287(7):898–900.

6. Henderson DA, Inglesby TV, Bartlett JG, et al. Smallpox as a biological weapon: medical and public health management. JAMA 1999;281:2127–2137.

7. Shoch-Spana M. Implications of pandemic influenza for bioterrorism response. Clin Infect Dis 2000;31:1409–1413.

8. Marwick C. Scary scenarios spark action at bioterrorism symposium. JAMA1999; 281(12):1071–1073.

9. Drasar BS, Forrest BD (Eds): Cholera and the Ecology of Vibrio cholera. London: Chapman & Hall; 1996 (p. 43).

10. Rosenberg C. The Cholera Years. U. of Chicago; 1987 (pp. 55–57).

11. Watts S. Epidemics and History: Disease, Power and Imperialism. Doubleday; 1997 (pp. 192–193).

12. McNeill W, Plagues and Peoples. New York: Anchor/Doubleday; 1977 (p. 231).

13. Barry JM. The Great Influenza. New York: Viking; 2004 (p. 397).

14. Alcabes P. The ordinariness of AIDS. Am Scholar. 2004;75(3):18–32.

15. Bloch AB, Orenstein WA, Stetler HC, et al. Health impact of measles vaccination in the United States. Pediatrics 1985;76(4):524–532.

16. Kilbourne ED. The Influenza Viruses and Influenza. New York: Academic Press; 1975.

17. Kilbourne ED. The molecular epidemiology of influenza. J Infect Dis 1973;127(4):478–487.

18. Gaydos JC, Hodder RA, Top FH Jr., Soden VJ, Allen RG, Bartley JD, Zabkar JH, Nowosiwsky T, Russell PK. Swine influenza A at Fort Dix, New Jersey (January–February 1976). I. Case finding and clinical study of cases. J Infect Dis 1976;136(suppl):S356–S362.

19. Top FH Jr., Russell PK. Swine influenza A at Fort Dix, New Jersey (January–February 1976). IV. Summary and speculation. J Infect Dis 1976;136(suppl): S376–S380.

20. Goldfield M, Bartley JD, Pizzuti W, Black HC, Altman R, Halperin WE. Influenza in New Jersey in 1976: Isolations of influenza A/New Jersey/76 virus at Fort Dix. J Infect Dis 1976;136(suppl): S347–S355.

21. Kilbourne E. Flu to Starboard! Man the harpoons! Fill 'em with vaccine! Get the captain! Hurry! New York Times 13 February 1976: 33.

22. Silverstein AM. Pure Politics and Impure Science: The Swine Flu Affair. Baltimore: Johns Hopkins; 1981 (p. 30).

23. Silverstein, ibid. p. 42.

24. Alcabes P. Dread: How Fear and Fantasy Have Fueled Epidemics from the Black Death to Avian Flu. New York: Public Affairs; 2009 (pp. 177–180).

25. New York City Department of Health and Mental Hygiene. 11 February 2005. Press release. New York City resident diagnosed with rare strain of multi-drug resistant HIV that rapidly progresses to AIDS. Accessed 4 Dec 2009 at, http://www.nyc.gov/html/doh/html/pr/pr016-05.shtml.

26. Altman LK. A public health quandary: when should the public be told? New York Times, 15 February 2005: F5.

27. Perez-Peña R, Santora M. AIDS report brings alarm, not surprise. New York Times 13 February 2005: A1.

28. Little SJ, Holte S, Routy JP, Daar ES, Markowitz M, Collier AC, et al. Antiretroviral-drug resistance among patients recently infected with HIV. N Engl J Med 2002;347:385–394.

29. Boden D, Hurley A, Zhang L, Cao Y, Guo Y, Jones E, et al. HIV-1 drug resistance in newly infected individuals. JAMA 1999; 282:1135–1141.

30. Simon V, Vanderhoeven J, Hurley A, Ramratnam B, Louie M, Dawson K, et al. Evolving patterns of HIV-1 resistance to antiretroviral agents in newly infected individuals. AIDS 2002;16:1511–1519.

31. Munoz A, Wang MC, Bass S, Taylor JM, Kingsley LA, Chmiel JS, et al. Acquired immunodeficiency syndrome (AIDS)-free time after human immunodeficiency virus type 1 (HIV-1) seroconversion in homosexual men. Am J Epidemiol 1989;130(3):530–539.

32. Keet IP, Krijnen P, Koot M, Lange JM, Miedema F, Goudsmit J, et al. Predictors of rapid progression to AIDS in HIV-1 seroconverters. AIDS 1993;7:51–57.

33. Yu XF, Wang Z, Vlahov D, Markham RB, Farzadegan H, Margolick JB. Infection with dual-tropic human immunodeficiency virus type 1 variants associated with rapid total T cell decline and disease progression in injection drug users. J Infect Dis 1998;178:388–396.

34. Skelton C. New HIV "superbug" emerges in Vancouver. Vancouver Sun, 9 August 2001: A1.

35. Brown D. Scope of unusual HIV strain is unknown, experts say. Washington Post, 13 February 2005: A16.

36. O'Brien K. New HIV strain sparks NY crisis, outreach, debate. PR Week, 21 February 2005: 3.

37. Santora M, Altman LK. H.I.V. strain adds urgency to changes in city AIDS program, New York Times, 16 February 2005: B1.

38. Stobbe M. Rare tuberculosis case prompts warning, Associated Press, 29 May 2007.

39. Neergaard L, Barrett D. U.S. probes how TB traveler crossed border, Associated Press, 30 May 2007.

40. Altman L, Schwartz J. Near misses allowed man with tuberculosis to fly to and from Europe, health officials say. New York Times, May31, 2007: A13.

41. Additional reporting in New York Times articles by J Schwartz on June 2, 2007 and L Altman on July 5, 2007.

42. Gardner A. U.S. barred 33 TB-infected people from flying over past year. HealthDay online, published in U.S. News and World Report 18 Sept 08. Accessed 20 December 09 at, http://health.usnews.com/articles/health/healthday/2008/09/18/us-barred-33-tb-infected-people-from-flying-over.html.

43. Young A. Did CDC hype TB case as a fund-raising ploy? Atlanta Journal-Constitution, 13 March 2008. Accessed 5 December 2009 at, http://www.ajc.com/search/content/health/stories/2008/03/13/tbpublicity_0113.html.

44. US Department of Health and Human Services, Project Bioshield: Progress in the War on Terror, White House website, July 2004. Accessed 16 Dec 2008 (since removed) at, http://ww.whitehouse.gov/infocus/bioshield/bioshield2.html.

45. US Department of Health and Human Services, Project Bioshield, undated document. Accessed 8 December 2009 at http://www.hhs.gov/aspr/barda/bioshield/index.html.

46. Alcabes P. The bioterrorism scare. The American Scholar 2004; 73(2):35–45.

47. Lichtblau E, Wade N. FBI details anthrax case, but doubts remain. New York Times 19 August 2008: A1. A summary and timeline of the outbreak and investigation. Accessed 8 Dec 2009 at, http://topics.nytimes.com/top/reference/timestopics/subjects/a/anthrax/index.html.

48. Associated Press (no byline), Developments in anthrax scare of 2001, 27 September 2003, reprinted. Accessed 8 Dec 2009 at, http://www.ph.ucla.edu/epi/bioter/developmentsanthrax.html.

49. US Homeland Security Council, National Strategy for Pandemic Influenza, 1 Nov 2005, introductory statement.

50. US Homeland Security Council, National Strategy for Pandemic Influenza, 1 Nov 2005, p. 2.

51. World Health Organization, Global Alert and Response. Cumulative number of confirmed human cases of avian influenza A/(H5N1) Reported to WHO, 11 December 2009. Accessed 13 December 2009 at, http://www.who.int/csr/disease/avian_influenza/country/cases_table_2009_12_11/en/index.html.

52. Harvard School of Public Health press release. In the case of an outbreak of pandemic flu, large majority of Americans willing to make major changes in their lives, 26 October 2006. Accessed 13 December 2009 at, http://www.hsph.harvard.edu/news/press-releases/2006-releases/press10262006.html.

53. World Health Organization. Influenza A (H1N1): Pandemic alert phase 6 declared, of moderate severity, 11 June 2009. Accessed 5 December 2009 at, http://www.euro.who.int/influenza/AH1N1/20090611_11.

54. President's Council of Advisors on Science and Technology, Report to the President on U.S. Preparations for 2009-H1N1 Influenza, 7 August 2009. Accessed 5 Dec 2009 at, http://www.whitehouse.gov/the_press_office/Presidents-Council-of-Advisors-on-Science-and-Technology-PCAST-releases-report-assessing-H1N1-preparations.

55. McNeil DG, Jr. Agency urges caution on estimates of swine flu, New York Times, 26 August 2009: A12.

56. European Centre for Disease Prevention and Control. ECDC daily update—pandemic (H1N1) 2009—11 December 2009. Accessed 13 December 2009 at, http://ecdc.europa.eu/en/healthtopics/Documents/091211_Influenza_AH1N1_Situation_Report_0900hrs.pdf.

57. CDC Estimates of 2009 H1N1 Influenza Cases, Hospitalizations and Deaths in the United States, April October 17, 2009, November 12, 2009. Accessed 5 December 2009 at, http://www.cdc.gov/h1n1flu/estimates_2009_h1n1.htm.

58. Jefferson T. Influenza vaccination: policy versus evidence. BMJ 2006 (28 Oct.); 333:912–915.

59. Schwartz ND. Rumsfeld's growing stake in Tamiflu. Fortune, 31 Oct 2005. Accessed 5 December 2009 at, CNN Money, http://money.cnn.com/2005/10/31/news/newsmakers/fortune_rumsfeld/.

60. Doherty D. Roche raises outlook as pandemic boosts Tamiflu sales. Bloomberg News online, 15 Oct 09. Accessed 5 December 2009 at, http://www.bloomberg.com/apps/news?pid=20601085&sid=aDSRPb5hdrP4.

61. United Programme on AIDS, Global facts and figures, December 2009. Accessed 21 December 2009 at, http://www.unaids.org/en/KnowledgeCentre/HIVData/EpiUpdate/EpiUpdArchive/2009/default.asp.

62. Heckler M, U.S. Department of Health and Human Services pres conference, 23 April 1984.

63. Coolfont Report: A PHS plan for prevention and control of AIDS and the AIDS Virus. Public Health Reports 101 (July–August 1986).

64. U.S. General Accounting Office. AIDS Forecasting: Undercount of Cases and Lack of Key Data Weaken Existing Estimates, GAO/PEMD-89-13. Washington, D.C.: GAO; June 1989 (p. 2).

65. Karon JM, Fleming PL, Steketee R, DeCock KM. HIV in the United States at the turn of the century: an epidemic in transition. Am J Public Health 2001; 91(7):1060-68. For the estimate of higher incidence see Hall HI, Song R, Rhodes P, Prejean J, et al. Estimation of HIV incidence in the United States. JAMA 2008; 300(5)520–529.

66. Will G. New York: A failed city for crack babies, $2 billion in this decade (op-ed), New York Times, 26 May1991: D7; New York Times, The Cost of not Preventing Crack Babies (editorial), 10 October1991: A26.

67. New York City Department of Health and Mental Hygiene. 11 February 2005. Press release. New York City resident diagnosed with rare strain of multi-drug resistant HIV that rapidly progresses to AIDS. Op cit.

68. Sonnabend J, reported by Fumento M, The myth of heterosexual AIDS: A nine-year retrospective of fear and (mostly) loathing, 2 November 1998. Accessed 21 December 2009 at, http://www.fumento.com/pozaids.html.

69. Saracco A, Musicco M, Nicolosi A, et al. Man-to-woman sexual transmission of HIV: Longitudinal study of 343 steady partners of infected men. J Acquir Immune Defic Syndr 1993;6:497–502.

70. De Vincenzi I. A longitudinal study of human immunodeficiency virus transmission by heterosexual partners. N Engl J Med 1994;331:341–346.

71. Guimares M et al., HIV infection among female partners of seropositive men in Brazil. Am J Epidemiol 1995;142:538–547.

72. Karesh WB, Cook RA. The human-animal link. Foreign Affairs 2005 (July–August);38–50.

73. Karesh WB. Where the wild things are: The link between the health of humans, animals, and the environment, Foreign Affairs online 8 May 2009. Accessed 21 December 2009 at, http://www.foreignaffairs.com/articles/65088/william-b-karesh/where-the-wild-things-are.

EPILOGUE

According to the World Health Organization in 2010:
- Over 7,000 young adults become infected with HIV daily.
- Over 8,500 people die from AIDS every single day.
- One child will die of AIDS every minute.

INDEX

---

*Entries with f following a page number indicate a figure; entries with t following a page number indicate a table.